Cancers of the Colon and Rectum

A Multidisciplinary Approach to Diagnosis and Management

Current Multidisciplinary Oncology Series
Charles R. Thomas, Jr., MD
Series Editor

Breast Cancer
A Multidisciplinary Approach to Diagnosis and Management
Alphonse G. Taghian, Barbara L. Smith, and John K. Erban

Lung Cancer
A Multidisciplinary Approach to Diagnosis and Management
Kemp H. Kernstine and Karen L. Reckamp

Cancers of the Colon and Rectum
A Multidisciplinary Approach to Diagnosis and Management
Al B. Benson III, A. Bapsi Chakravarthy, Stanley R. Hamilton, and Elin R. Sigurdson

Gynecologic Cancers
A Multidisciplinary Approach to Diagnosis and Management
Kunle Odunsi and Tanja Pejovic

Prostate Cancer
A Multidisciplinary Approach to Diagnosis and Management
Adam P. Dicker, Wm. Kevin Kelly, and Edouard J. Trabulsi

Current Multidisciplinary Oncology

Cancers of the Colon and Rectum

A Multidisciplinary Approach to Diagnosis and Management

Edited by

Al B. Benson III, MD

Professor of Medicine
Associate Director for Clinical Investigations
Robert H. Lurie Comprehensive Cancer Center
Northwestern University
Chicago, Illinois

A. Bapsi Chakravarthy, MD

Associate Professor
Program Director
Department of Radiation Oncology
Vanderbilt-Ingram Cancer Center
Vanderbilt University
Nashville, Tennessee

Stanley R. Hamilton, MD

Division Head
Department of Pathology
MD Anderson Cancer Center
University of Texas
Houston, Texas

Elin R. Sigurdson, MD, PhD

Chief, Division of General Surgery
Director, Department of Surgical Oncology
Fox Chase Cancer Center
Philadelphia, Pennsylvania

demosMEDICAL
New York

Acquisitions Editor: Rich Winters
Compositor: NewGen Imaging
Printer: Courier

Visit our website at www.demosmedpub.com

Library of Congress Cataloging-in-Publication Data

Cancers of the colon and rectum : a multidisciplinary approach to diagnosis and management / [edited by] Al B. Benson III, A. Bapsi Chakravarthy, Stanley R. Hamilton, Elin R. Sigurdson.
p. ; cm.—(Current multidisciplinary oncology)
Includes bibliographical references and index.
ISBN 978-1-936287-58-1 (hbk.)—ISBN 978-1-61705-105-0 (eISBN)
I. Benson, Al B., III, editor of compilation. II. Chakravarthy, A. Bapsi (Anuradha Bapsi), editor of compilation. III. Hamilton, Stanley R., editor of compilation. IV. Sigurdson, Elin R., editor of compilation. V. Series: Current multidisciplinary oncology.
[DNLM: 1. Colorectal Neoplasms—diagnosis. 2. Colorectal Neoplasms—therapy. WI 529]
RC280.C6
616.99'4347—dc23

2013020938

Printed in the United States of America
13 14 15 16 5 4 3 2 1

Contents

Series Foreword

This volume of the series Current Multidisciplinary Oncology, devoted to colorectal cancer, brings me great pleasure to introduce the practicing clinician to a valuable resource that will aid in the multidisciplinary approach of these common solid tumors.

Drs. Al B. Benson III, A. Bapsi Chakravarthy, Stanley R. Hamilton, and Elin R. Sigurdson have put together a cadre of leading-edge investigators as contributors on the multidisciplinary approach to colorectal cancer.

Over the past decade, a myriad of advances in the diagnosis and treatment of colorectal cancer have occurred. Some of the advances include, but are not limited to, diagnostic molecular tools that may aid in predicting a response to certain treatment approaches and/or in providing a guide of a prognostic outcomes for certain patients.

Colorectal neoplasms comprise some of the most common malignancies in the world and hence warrant intense efforts to find a cure. In recent years, investment of resources to help further understand the nature of this malignancy have increased.

Drs. Benson, Chakravarthy, Hamilton, and Sigurdson represent the current generation of academic, forward-thinking oncologists who have committed their careers to eradicating colorectal cancer using multidisciplinary approaches. Their collective vision and ability to assemble an outstanding group of investigators in the field have provided a very high quality product that will be a useful resource to the busy clinician as well as those along various stages of the learning spectrum. I'm sure that you will enjoy this innovative and easy-to-read volume as you look for guidance in the multidisciplinary approach of your patients with colorectal cancer.

Charles R. Thomas, Jr., MD
Series Editor
Department of Radiation Medicine
Oregon Health and Science University
Knight Cancer Institute
Portland, Oregon

Preface

Colorectal cancer (CRC) is the third most common cancer worldwide. Although largely preventable, this disease continues to engender significant morbidity and mortality. Advances in understanding the genetics of CRC (including inherited and sporadic cases), screening and prevention strategies, and treatment have resulted in improved outcomes even for patients with advanced cancer. This is the third book in the series Current Multidisciplinary Oncology, edited by Dr. Charles R. Thomas, Jr., with the intent to provide a comprehensive textbook that encompasses the entire spectrum of multidisciplinary management considerations and a significant body of evidence with references to support the decision strategies and recommendations.

The chapters in this book are arranged in a logical progression from screening and prevention to diagnosis, treatment and surveillance, which is similar to the other books in this series. Chapter 2 is composed of four in-depth sections that serve as a critical introduction to principles of screening with extensive discussion of inherited CRC, details of other risk factors including diet and inflammatory bowel disease, and review of advances in chemoprevention. Chapters that address polyps and precursor lesions and preoperative staging and endoscopic approaches such as endoscopic mucosal resection (EMR) and colonic stenting are included. Multimodality CRC imaging is reviewed in Chapter 5 revealing the utility of CT colonography, PET-CT, and MRI in rectal cancer. Principles of pathology including staging criteria and advances in molecular pathology are integrated in several chapters outlining the importance of MSI and *K-ras* mutation status as two examples.

The management of colon cancer and rectal cancer has been separated in a series of distinct chapters for each of the two disease locations since the strategies vary particularly for locally advanced disease (nonmetastatic). Neoadjuvant chemoradiation for rectal cancer and adjuvant therapy for both colon and rectal cancer are extensively reviewed. The care of patients with potentially resectable metastatic disease also is highlighted. The evolving complexity of the continuum of care for patients with advanced disease receiving systemic therapy incorporates chemotherapy regimens and the most recent evidence that guides the use of anti-VEGF and anti-EGFR agents. There are two chapters devoted to management of systemic toxicities including diarrhea, skin and neurologic toxicities, as well as a section on the use of radiation as a palliative care option for patients. In addition, Chapter 15 reviews health-related quality of life both for locally advanced and advanced disease with a discussion of the instruments to measure quality of life.

There are also unique chapters that address special topics. These include chapters with an emphasis on clinical trials encompassing phase I/II clinical trials in metastatic CRC and future directions integrating concepts of the development of targeted therapies for CRC patients, biomarker clinical trial designs, and the potential of gene profiling both as a prognostic and predictive tool. Models of care delivery, including a community practice case study and patient navigation as it supports multidisciplinary care models, are innovative chapters emphasizing some of the complexities of offering comprehensive cancer care using CRC as an example. The concluding chapters speak to the growing emphasis on health disparities, surveillance and survivorship, and patient advocacy.

This book is truly multidisciplinary in scope and is designed as a management text for the gamut of health professionals who provide care for CRC patients including medical oncologists, radiation oncologists, surgeons, gastroenterologists, radiologists, pathologists, palliative care experts, nurses and other allied health professionals, students, residents and fellows in training, as well as patients, families and advocates. The CRC thought leaders who have contributed to this volume have offered their considerable expertise to provide the most current evidence-based approach, including extensive references, to provide a valuable tool designed to enhance evaluation and management of CRC patients.

Al B. Benson III, MD

Contributors

Al B. Benson III, MD
Professor of Medicine
Associate Director for Clinical Investigations
Robert H. Lurie Comprehensive Cancer Center
Northwestern University
Chicago, IL

Adam C. Berger, MD, FACS
Department of Surgery
Kimmel Cancer Center
Thomas Jefferson University
Philadelphia, PA

Jordan Berlin, MD
Ingram Professor of Cancer Research
Division of Hematology-Oncology
Vanderbilt-Ingram Cancer Center
Nashville, TN

Kiran Bidari, MD
Fellow
Division of Gastroenterology and Hepatology
Feinberg School of Medicine
Northwestern University
Chicago, IL

Faraz Bishehasri, MD, PhD
Fellow
Division of Gastroenterology
Department of Medicine
Feinberg School of Medicine
Northwestern University
Chicago, IL

Hiliary Bownik, MD
Gastroenterology Fellow
Feinberg School of Medicine
Northwestern University
Chicago, IL

David Cella, MD
Department of Medical Social Sciences
Feinberg School of Medicine
Northwestern University
Robhert H. Lurie Comprehensive Cancer Center of Northwestern University
Chicago, IL

Emily Chan, MD, PhD
Assistant Professor
Department of Medical Oncology
Vanderbilt-Ingram Cancer Center
Nashville, TN

E. Gabriela Chiorean, MD
Associate Professor
Department of Medicine
Division of Hematology/Oncology
University of Washington
Seattle, WA

Michael V. Chiorean, MD, AGAF
Director
IBD Center of Excellence
Digestive Disease Institute
Virginia Mason Medical Center
Division of Gastroenterology and Hepatology
Seattle, WA

Yun Shin Chun, MD
Assistant Professor
Department of Surgical Oncology
Fox Chase Cancer Center
Philadelphia, PA

Jonathan Cotliar, MD
Assistant Professor
Departments of Dermatology and Medicine
Robert H. Lurie Comprehensive Cancer Center
Northwestern University Feinberg School of Medicine
Chicago, IL

Laura A. Dawson, MD
Department of Radiation Oncology
University of Toronto
Radiation Medicine Program
Princess Margaret Hospital/University Health Network
Toronto, Ontario, Canada

Kristen Drescher, PhD
Professor
Department of Microbiology and Immunology
Creighton University School of Medicine
Omaha, NE

S. Gail Eckhardt, MD
Professor and Co-Division Head Medical Oncology
University of Colorado
Aurora, CO

Jeffrey M. Farma, MD, FACS
Assistant Professor of Surgical Oncology
Fox Chase Cancer Center
Philadelphia, PA

Julio Garcia-Aguilar, MD, PhD
Colorectal Service
Department of Surgery
Memorial Sloan-Kettering Cancer Center
New York, NY

Laura Goff, MD
Assistant Professor
Department of Medical Oncology
Vanderbilt-Ingram Cancer Center
Nashville, TN

Allison Goldberg, MD
Department of Surgery
Kimmel Cancer Center
Thomas Jefferson University
Philadelphia, PA

Axel Grothey, MD
Professor of Oncology
Mayo Clinic Rochester
Rochester, MN

William A. Hall, MD
Department of Radiation Oncology
Emory University Winship Cancer Center
Atlanta, GA

Stanley R. Hamilton, MD
Division Head
Department of Pathology
MD Anderson Cancer Center
University of Texas
Houston, TX

Ernest Hawk, MD, MPH
Vice President
Division of OVP
Cancer Prevention and Population Sciences
MD Anderson Cancer Center
University of Texas
Houston, TX

Megan Hitchins, PhD
Associate Professor
Stanford Cancer Center
Department of Medicine
Division of Oncology
Stanford University
Stanford, CA

Howard S. Hochster, MD
Associate Director
Yale Cancer Center Director
GI Oncology
Professor of Medicine
Yale School of Medicine
New Haven, CT

Patrick G. Johnston
Professor, Dean of the School of Medicine
Dentistry and Biomedical Sciences
Drug Resistance Group
Centre for Cancer Research and Cell Biology
Queen's University Belfast, Belfast
Northern Ireland

Barbara H. Jung, MD
Assistant Professor
Department of Medicine
Feinberg School of Medicine
Northwestern University
Gastroenterologist
Northwestern Memorial Hospital
Chicago, IL

Lisa A. Kachnic, MD
Department of Radiation Oncology
Boston Medical Center
Boston University School of Medicine
Boston, MA

John Kauh, MD, FACP
Associate Professor of Hematology and Oncology
Department of Hematology and Oncology
Winship Cancer Institute
Emory University School of Medicine
Atlanta, GA

Fadlo R. Khuri, MD, FACP
Professor and Chair of Hematology and Medical Oncology
Winship Cancer Institute
Emory University School of Medicine
Atlanta, GA

Joseph Knezetic, PhD
Associate Professor of Pathology and Biomedical Sciences
Director of the Laboratory of Molecular Pathology
Creighton University
Omaha, NE

Srinadh Komanduri, MD, MS
Director of Interventional Endoscopy
Associate Professor
Division of Gastroenterology and Hepatology
Feinberg School of Medicine
Northwestern University
Chicago, IL

Jerome C. Landry, MD
Chief of Service
Grady Memorial Hospital
Professor
Department of Radiation Oncology
Emory University Winship Cancer Center
Atlanta, GA

Stephen J. Lanspa, MD
Senior Associate Dean of Medicine
Division of Gastroenterology
Creighton University School of Medicine
Omaha, NE

Christopher H. Lieu, MD
Assistant Professor
Division of Medical Oncology
University of Colorado
Aurora, CO

Patrick J. Loehrer, MD
Professor
Department of Medicine
Division of Hematology/Oncology
Indiana University—Purdue University of Indianapolis
Indianapolis, IN

Stephen Lutz, MD
Blanchard Valley Regional Cancer Center
Findlay, OH

Henry T. Lynch, MD
Chair of Preventive Medicine and Professor of Medicine
Hereditary Cancer Center
Creighton Univeristy School of Medicine
Omaha, NE

Jane F. Lynch, BSN
Creighton University
Department of Preventive Medicine
Omaha, NE

Sumithra J. Mandrekar, PhD
Department of Health Science Research
Mayo Clinic
Rochester, MN

Karen Colbert Maresso, MPH
Cancer Prevention and Population Sciences
University of Texas
MD Anderson Cancer Center
Houston, TX

Wells A. Messersmith, MD
Professor and Co-Division Head
Medical Oncology
University of Colorado
Aurora, CO

Julia Minocha, MD
Resident
Department of Dermatology
Feinberg School of Medicine
Northwestern University
Chicago, IL

Edith Mitchell, MD, FACP
Clinical Professor
Director
Center to Eliminate Cancer Disparities
Program Leader
Gastrointestinal Oncology
Jefferson University Hospitals
Philadelphia, PA

Rebecca A. Moss, MD
Assistant Professor
Department of Medical Oncology
The Cancer Institute of New Jersey
New Brunswick, NJ

Reid M. Ness, MD, MPH
Assistant Professor of Medicine
Vanderbilt Digestive Disease Center
Vanderbilt University Medical Center
Nashville, TN

Peter J. O'Dwyer, MD
Professor of Medicine
Abramson Cancer Center
Perelman School of Medicine
University of Pennsylvania
Philadelphia, PA

Margaret A. O'Grady, RN, MSN, OCN, FAAMA
Senior Director
Fox Chase Cancer Center Partners
Philadelphia, PA

Sherri Patterson, MD
Director
Division of Cancer Prevention and Population Science
Research Planning and Development
MD Anderson Cancer Center
Houston, TX

Rodolfo F. Perini, MD
Clinical Instructor in Radiology
University of Pennsylvania
Philadelphia, PA

Roshan S. Prabhu, MD
Department of Radiation Oncology
Emory University Winship Cancer Center
Atlanta, GA

Nancy Roach
Board Member
Fight Colorectal Cancer
Alexandria, VA

John M. Salsman, PhD
Department of Medical Social Sciences
Feinberg School of Medicine
Northwestern University
Robhert H. Lurie Comprehensive Cancer Center of Northwestern University
Chicago, IL

Julian Sanchez, MD
Assistant Professor of Surgery
Colorectal Surgery Section
Division of Surgical Oncology
Department of Surgery
City of Hope
Duarte, CA

Daniel J. Sargent, PhD
Department of Health Science Research
Mayo Clinic
Rochester, MN

Elaine Sein, RN, BSN, OCN, CBCN
Senior Project Manager
Fox Chase Cancer Center Partners
Philadelphia, PA

Prashant Shah, MD
Assistant Professor
Department of Surgical Oncology
Division of Thoracic and Esophageal Surgery
Fox Chase Cancer Center
Philadelphia, PA

Poonam Sharma, MBBS
Associate Professor
Department of Pathology
Creighton University School of Medicine
Omaha, NE

Qian Shi, PhD
Department of Health Science Research
Mayo Clinic
Rochester, MN

Elin R. Sigurdson, MD, PhD
Chief, Division of General Surgery
Director, Department of Surgical Oncology
Fox Chase Cancer Center
Philadelphia, PA

Peter Silberstein, MD
Department of Internal Medicine-Hematology
Alegent Creighton Medical Center
Omaha, NE

William Small, Jr., MD
Professor, Department of Radiation Oncology
Feinberg School of Medicine
Northwestern University
Chicago, IL

Carrie Snyder, MSN, RN, APNG, AOCNS
Cancer Genetics Nurse Specialist
Creighton University
Department of Preventive Medicine
Hereditary Cancer Prevention Clinic
Omaha, NE

Davendra P. S. Sohal, MD, MPH
Assistant Professor of Medicine
Taussig Cancer Institute
Lerner College of Medicine
Cleveland Clinic
Cleveland, OH

Charles Staley, MD
Professor of Surgery
Holland M. Ware Professor of Surgery and Chief
Division of Surgical Oncology
Department of Surgery
Emory University School of Medicine
Atlanta, GA

Jaykumar Thumar, MD, MBBS
Yale School of Medicine
Yale Cancer Center
New Haven, CT

Julia Trosman, PhD, MBA
Director
Center for Business Models in Healthcare
Assistant Adjunct Professor
Northwestern University Feinberg School of Medicine
Chicago, IL
Assistant Adjunct Professor
Department of Clinical Pharmacy
University of California
San Francisco, CA

Richard C. Turkington
Academic Clinical Lecturer (Medical Oncology)
Drug Resistance Group
Centre for Cancer Research and Cell Biology
Queen's University Belfast
Belfast, Northern Ireland

Sandra Van Schaeybroeck
Cancer Research UK Clinician Scientist
Drug Resistance Group
Centre for Cancer Research and Cell Biology
Queen's University Belfast
Belfast, Northern Ireland

Neeta K. Venepalli, MD
Assistant Professor
Division of Hematology-Oncology
Department of Medicine
University of Illinois
Chicago, IL

Maxwell T. Vergo, MD
Assistant Professor in Medicine
Geisel School of Medicine, Attending Physician
Department of Medicine
Section of Palliative Care
Dartmouth Hitchcock Medical Center
Lebanon, NH

Eduardo Vilar, MD, PhD
Assistant Professor
Department of Clinical Cancer Prevention
Division of Cancer Prevention and Population Sciences
The University of Texas MD Anderson Cancer Center
Houston, TX

Rohit Walia, MD
Assistant Professor
Department of Radiology
Fox Chase Cancer Center
Philadelphia, PA

Christine Weldon, MBA
Director
Center for Business Models in Healthcare
Adjunct Faculty
Feinberg School of Medicine
Northwestern University
Chicago, IL

Hannah Yoon, MD
Department of Radiation Oncology
The Robert H. Lurie Comprehensive Cancer Center
Northwestern University
Chicago, IL

Monique J. Youl, MBBS
Department of Radiation Oncology
Peter MacCallum Cancer Centre
Melbourne, Victoria, Australia

Susan E. Yount, PhD
Department of Medical Social Sciences
Feinberg School of Medicine
Northwestern University
Robert H. Lurie Comprehensive Cancer Center of Northwestern University
Chicago, IL

Laura Yun, MD
Assistant Professor of Medicine
Feinberg School of Medicine
Northwestern University
Chicago, IL

I Importance of the Multidisciplinary Approach to Colorectal Cancer

AL B. BENSON III

The concept of personalized or precision medicine by definition embraces the integration of a multidisciplinary approach for the care of an individual patient. Although many would emphasize the link between tumor biologic constructs and treatment selection (admittedly an important goal if not yet a realization), precision medicine should encompass the entire spectrum of not only an individual clinical situation but also the social, psychological, and physical factors that affect the individual patient. The colon and rectal cancer patient may routinely require the expertise of the surgeon, medical oncologist, pathologist, gastroenterologist, radiologist, radiation oncologist, and primary care physician to provide the most coherent, informed, comprehensive, and effective strategy for diagnosis, treatment, and in many cases, long-term surveillance. To truly personalize the individual patient's experience, the comprehensive cancer care program must also offer critical services including psychiatry/psychology, social work, physical and occupational therapy, and nutrition counseling as needed. Access to additional health care personnel in surgery, other medical disciplines, nursing and genetic counseling is also critical based on symptoms, potential complications, and long-term risks both for the patient and potentially for other family members who may also be at risk for an eventual cancer diagnosis.

Over the past 2 decades, and particularly during the last 10 years, there have emerged profound advances in the treatment of colon and rectal cancer, including public recognition of the importance of colorectal cancer (CRC), and the rise of advocacy groups, which focus on education and patient support, research, and significant advances in laboratory science and treatment opportunities. The end result has been fewer patients dying from CRC, more than doubling the survivorship for those with metastatic disease, enhanced potential for a cure for those with isolated metastatic disease, particularly in the liver and lung, and increases in the numbers of individuals screened for CRC. Since CRC is a preventable disease and one that can be cured when diagnosed at early stages, the involvement of multiple health professionals and patient organizations becomes of paramount importance to educate the population and provide access to the required services.

The unmasking of critical components of the biology of CRC, beginning with the understanding of the adenoma-to-carcinoma sequence leading to the current advances in the understanding of the molecular pathogenesis of CRC, has crystallized the importance of integrating laboratory science in the construct of the multidisciplinary team. Chapter 2 of this text, for example, highlights The identification of three major molecular pathways, which has led to refinement in genetic counseling, risk assessment, prognosis determination, and screening programs. The chromosomal instability pathway is characterized by the initial alteration of the *APC* gene, followed by genetic and epigenetic events, including the mutation of *K-ras,* the presence of global hypomethylation, and allelic deletions of other tumor suppression genes. The DNA mismatch repair pathway (mutator phenotype pathway) is characterized by the presence of microsatellite instability and contributes to approximately 15% of all CRCs. The third critical pathway includes inflammatory bowel disease resulting in increased risk for development of CRC with defined genetic and epigenetic events. In addition, there is also perhaps a fourth pathway, the serrated pathway, involving mutations including *BRAF* and hypermethylation of CpG islands generally evolving from hyperplastic polyps through serrated adenomas. These pathways further support the concept of tumor heterogeneity, reinforcing the observation that CRC does not represent a single disease entity but a growing assortment of subsets of tumors. Tumor heterogeneity also is a potentially confounding factor for individual patients, further complicated by observed biological differences comparing primary versus metastatic disease. The identification of the accumulation of molecular events within an individual patient will mandate novel clinical trial designs to incorporate molecular pathology, multiple pathway-driven drug development strategies, and sequential biopsies over time for patients with metastatic disease to determine a more optimal biologically driven treatment strategy.

Identifying individuals at risk for CRC is a responsibility across health care disciplines, particularly shared by the primary care physician and gastroenterologist. The procurement of a detailed family history and the attribution of other important risk factors linked to CRC with integration of appropriate screening methodologies and risk reduction are of paramount importance given the high incidence rate of CRC. Rising rates of obesity and diabetes linked to both poor dietary habits and lack of exercise are noteworthy because of the potential acceleration in risk for development of CRC and other comorbid conditions in the future. Rise in risk also will provide opportunities to develop chemoprevention strategies which depend on the understanding of carcinogenesis and identification of molecular derangements that can serve as targets to develop interventions that may inhibit, reverse, or delay an eventual cancer transformation.

The initial diagnosis and assessment of colon or rectal cancer is particularly dependent on the assessments of the gastroenterologist, radiologist, surgeon, pathologist, and in the case of rectal cancer, the radiation oncologist. Advances in transrectal endoscopic ultrasound (TEUS) and MRI have improved the accuracy of clinical staging for rectal cancer. Endoscopic mucosal resection has enhanced the polyp assessment and resection rate. The placement of self-expandable metal stents has evolved into the most widely used nonsurgical option for colonic decompression secondary to malignancy. Sphincter sparing rectal cancer surgeries have reduced the colostomy rate, particularly because of the emergence of neoadjuvant chemoradiation, a treatment of choice compared to the past standard of postoperative chemoradiation. Improved outcomes with total mesorectal excision (TME) have defined surgical practice for rectal cancer and the use of laparoscopically assisted colectomy for colon cancer has also emerged as a standard of care.

Collaborations between medical oncologists and surgeons, particularly since the recent era of improved response rates with combination chemotherapy, have introduced the concepts of neoadjuvant chemotherapy for patients with potentially resectable metastatic CRC and conversion chemotherapy for those who become resectable after therapy. Over the past decade, 5-year overall survival rates have improved for patients who are able to undergo R0 resections, particularly for isolated liver or lung disease. The advancements in chemotherapy have not only improved the outcomes for patients with resectable metastatic disease, but also for those with stage III colon cancer who receive adjuvant oxaliplatin with a fluoropyrimidine. CRC patients with metastatic disease that is not resectable have also experienced a survival benefit with the introduction of the concept of the continuum of care, which encourages the use of all 3 active chemotherapy agents (oxaliplatin, irinotecan, 5FU/capecitabine) over time during the course of the patient's illness, resulting in a definitive survival advantage. This last decade has introduced targeted or biological agents into treatment regimens for metastatic CRC patients, including bevacizumab and cetuximab/panitumumab for those patients with *K-ras* wild type tumors. In 2012, two additional targeted agents became available for patients, including ziv-aflibercept and regorafenib. There are significant challenges, however, to identify the patients most likely to benefit from the addition of a targeted agent, since defining predictive molecular markers has been elusive, particularly in the case of bevacizumab, ziv-aflibercept, and regorafenib.

Inclusion of experts in quality of life and symptom management has enhanced a multidisciplinary approach for CRC patients. Clinical trials comparing treatment vs best supportive care for patients with refractory CRC, for example, have demonstrated both a survival benefit as well as maintenance of quality of life for irinotecan, cetuximab, panitumumab, and regorafenib. Quality of life measures have been integrated into the design of randomized phase III clinical trials. With the introduction of new agents and the potential toxicity of such, health-related quality of life (HRQL) assessment is an important methodology to incorporate aspects of function (eg, mood, affect), as well as the patient's perspective. Treatment related symptom management strategies have incorporated algorithms to more effectively manage diarrhea as an important example. The development of oxaliplatin has resulted in the recognition of prevention and control of treatment related peripheral neuropathy. The use of anti-EGFR treatments has brought dermatologists into the multidisciplinary team to better control the treatment related rash associated with agents such as cetuximab and panitumumab.

The last decade has heralded a focus on care delivery in the United States, including patient navigation in cancer care, assessment of comprehensive CRC care, and access to care in the community with development of new models for care delivery. Patient navigation is designed to eliminate barriers to care as well as to streamline care, ensuring timely diagnosis and treatment. Since multidisciplinary CRC disease teams are essential for optimal patient care, navigation programs are increasingly integrated in cancer center programs to achieve the goal of seamless multidisciplinary delivery of care. In addition, survivorship has emerged as an integral component of comprehensive cancer care, particularly as increasing numbers of CRC patients are surviving their disease. It is estimated that there are over 11 million patients with a diagnosis of CRC living in the United States. Cancer centers must increasingly address survivorship issues including access to health care and follow-up treatment, assessment of late effects of treatment, evaluation of second cancers and quality of life. The 2006 Survivorship Report from the Institute of Medicine (IOM) states that multiple disciplines must be involved in survivorship efforts, including health care providers, patient advocates as well as other stakeholders with the intent of raising the awareness of the needs of cancer survivors and embracing the four critical components of comprehensive survivorship care, including prevention, surveillance, intervention, and coordination of care. In this text, there is also a chapter devoted to racial disparities in the care of patients with CRC, which is particularly relevant since this topic not only applies to providing access to high quality cancer care, but also reflects the importance of risk assessment. For example, the incidence and mortality rate for CRC are highest among African Americans.

The chapters in this text have been assembled to provide the current best available evidence to support the standard of care integrating multidisciplinary approaches to CRC, including prevention and screening, diagnostics, treatment, and surveillance. In addition, with an eye to the future, there is discussion of the role of phase I/II trials in metastatic CRC with an emphasis on the importance of pharmacokinetics, refinement of pharmacodynamic markers and the integration of genomics, including the identification of genetic and epigenetic changes which are potential targets for drug development. The chapter devoted to future directions discusses gene expression profiling as well as integrative genomics, clinical trials designed to validate prognostic and predictive biomarkers and surrogate endpoints, and potential biologic targets for drug development. The future continues to embrace the era of multidisciplinary CRC care and research strategies, signifying a fusion of bench to bedside strategies.

2 Prevention and Screening

■ Risk Factors, Screening, and Chemoprevention

KAREN COLBERT MARESSO
SHERRI PATTERSON
EDUARDO VILAR
ERNEST HAWK

■ EPIDEMIOLOGY

In the United States, the lifetime risk of developing colorectal cancer (CRC) in the general population is approximately 5% for both men and women (1). It is the third most commonly diagnosed cancer, the third most common cause of cancer death in each gender, and the second most common in both genders. Incidence and mortality rates are highest among African Americans (1,2) and lowest among Asian Americans (1). Overall, incidence and mortality rates have been declining among all ethnic groups for both men and women over the last 10 to 20 years.

Risk factors for CRC include a personal or family history of CRC or adenomatous polyps, a personal history of chronic inflammatory bowel disease (IBD), obesity, smoking, alcohol, and red or processed meat consumption. Support for environmental factors and dietary habits affecting the risk for CRC comes from epidemiological studies demonstrating substantial variation in incidence rates by country and world region, as well as from migration studies showing that migrant populations generally assume the risk for CRC of their adopted country within one to two generations (3). Importantly, the presence of adenomas found by screening is a strong predictor of CRC risk.

Studies have documented significantly improved survival rates for earlier-stage disease. Currently, 5-year survival rates are 90% for localized disease, 70% for regional, and just 12% for distant disease (1). Such figures provide a strong rationale for screening programs to identify early-stage CRCs and preinvasive neoplasms that can be removed to reduce cancer risk. However, current screening strategies are less than ideal and represent an area of active investigation.

In conjunction with an effective screening program, chemoprevention efforts can also impact CRC incidence and mortality. Chemoprevention is a relatively new approach to cancer prevention and relies upon our understanding of carcinogenesis in order to target drugs or nutrients that can block, reverse, or delay the process before invasive cancer develops. This section of the chapter will briefly review the biology of CRC as well as various screening modalities currently in use or in development. This background will set the stage for a more in-depth discussion of colorectal chemoprevention.

■ THE BIOLOGY OF CRC

A model for the development of CRC from adenomatous polyps (adenoma-to-adenocarcinoma sequence) was initially proposed by Hill et al in 1978 (4). Vogelstein et al built upon this work with the development of a multistep molecular tumorigenesis model requiring the mutational activation of an oncogene coupled with allelic deletions of specific chromosomal sequences harboring tumor suppressor genes (5). Subsequent research on the molecular pathogenesis of CRC has supported this model and has also resulted in the addition of alternative pathways in the adenoma-to-adenocarcinoma sequence. Currently, three major etiologic molecular pathways are recognized as leading to CRC from precursor lesions.

The first genetic pathway (the chromosomal instability pathway) is characterized by bialellic inactivation of the tumor suppressor gene *APC* and the presence of chromosomal instability. The molecular axis integrated by APC-β-catenin-Tcf-MYC is the main pathway involved in this molecular subtype of CRCs. A defective *APC* gene is found in over 80% of adenomas and colon cancers and appears as one of the earliest of all accumulated genetic defects. The initial alteration of the *APC* gene is then followed by various other genetic and epigenetic events, including the mutation of *K-ras*, the presence of global hypomethylation, and allelic deletions of other tumor suppressor genes.

The second pathway, the DNA mismatch repair pathway (also known as the mutator phenotype pathway), is characterized by the presence of microsatellite instability (MSI) and is believed to contribute to ~15%–20% of CRCs. Microsatellites are short, repetitive DNA sequences found across the genome, and several genes are devoted to correcting errors in nucleotide pairing that occurs within these sequences during DNA replication. In CRCs associated with MSI, the alteration of the multiple mismatch repair (MMR) genes *MLH1, MSH2, MSH6,* or *PMS2* through a germline mutation followed by somatic inactivation of the wild-type allele (Lynch syndrome [LS]) or by the somatic epigenetic inactivation of both alleles of *MLH1* by hypermethylation of CpG islands (sporadic cases) results in defective functioning of the MMR system. This pathway often evolves from hyperplastic polyps and sessile serrated adenomas/polyps (the so-called Serrated Pathway; 6). Subsequently, somatic secondary frame-shift mutations in the coding repeats located in tumor-suppressor and apoptosis-regulating genes generate extensive additional genetic instability (hypermutation) in this pathway (7,8). This route involves mutations occurring in *BRAF* gene.

The third distinct etiologic route to CRC development is through chronic IBD, usually ulcerative colitis (UC) or Crohn's disease. Individuals with UC have an approximate 20-fold increased risk for CRC and, although it is not a major contributor to the population burden of CRC, it provides a distinctive pathway to CRC development. Genetic and epigenetic events characteristic of this pathway include MSI, hypermethylation of CpG islands that help to control gene expression, accelerated telomere shortening, increased rates of chromosomal fusions, DNA damage and genetic instability, and the earlier appearance of *TP53* mutations compared to other pathways (9,10).

A recently identified fourth, although minor, pathway involves mutation of polymerase genes, especially POL epsilon (POLE), and MMR genes and results in hypermutated CRC with markedly high frequency of mutation ("ultramutated") but without MSI-H.

These pathways illustrate the marked heterogeneity that is characteristic of CRC and its mechanistic development. It is important to note that within each of these subsets, the development of CRC is both dependent upon the total accumulation of genetic defects and the acquisition of alterations in a preferred sequence. However, these subsets require much more study before a complete picture of CRC can fully emerge. The future of the rational design of molecularly targeted approaches to both treatment and prevention depend upon this understanding.

■ SCREENING FOR CRC

A complete discussion of colorectal screening and its related issues is beyond the scope of this section. We aim here to provide a brief background on current screening tests and issues in order to highlight these as a complementary strategy to chemoprevention in the broader context of CRC prevention and early detection.

In order for a disease to be amenable to screening, certain characteristics must be met. Ideally, a "screenable" disease must represent a significant public health burden; have a long detectable preclinical phase; safe and accurate diagnostic tests must be available; there must be evidence that earlier treatment improves outcome or survival; and appropriate and acceptable screening tests must be available. CRC exhibits all of these characteristics, thus making it suitable for screening.

CRC represents a significant public health burden in the U.S. population (1). The natural history exhibits a long, multistep process from precancerous lesions to cancer occurring over an estimated period of time of 10 to 15 years (11). Colonoscopy is considered the gold standard for diagnosis of CRC, and is the gold-standard against which all other screening tests are compared. Early detection of CRC results in significantly improved survival, with stage at diagnosis as the single most important predictor of prognosis and disease-free survival. And finally, numerous screening tests are available that are safe and cost-effective; however, these tests are less than ideal and exhibit varying levels of performance and patient compliance.

Significant barriers to CRC screening exist, and utilization of effective tests is less than desired. According to 2010 data from the Centers for Disease Control and Prevention's (CDC) Behavioral Risk Factor Surveillance System (BRFSS) on compliance with screening guidelines, more than one-third of individuals over age 50 have never had a sigmoidoscopy or colonoscopy and only 17% report having had a fecal occult blood test (FOBT) within the previous 2 years (12). Reasons for the suboptimal use of screening tests relate to poor patient acceptance due to the invasiveness of some tests and/or their required dietary restrictions; underutilization by providers; cost; and limited access, including a lack of coverage for screening tests (although this has changed under recent health care legislation), geographic proximity, and capacity constraints.

There are currently five screening tests in use: the FOBT, double-contrast barium enema, flexible sigmoidoscopy, colonoscopy, and CT colonography. It is important to keep in mind that there is no ideal screening procedure and the current modalities represent trade-offs between performance, affordability, patient acceptance, and reductions in mortality. We briefly describe each one below and provide an update on the latest findings relevant to each test.

Fecal Occult Blood Test (Stool Blood Test)

FOBT has the strongest direct evidence supporting its use as a CRC screening test. In a 2007 meta-analysis of four randomized controlled trials (RCTs), a 16% (RR, 0.84; CI, 0.78–0.90) reduction in CRC mortality was observed by intention-to-treat analysis. When adjusted for actual screening attendance in the individual studies, the reduction in mortality increased to 25% (RR, 0.75; CI, 0.66–0.84; 13). Because the FOBT is both inexpensive and noninvasive, it is the most commonly-used screening test worldwide. Nevertheless, it can have a high false-positive rate requiring additional testing, and patient compliance is often low due to the test's dietary restrictions and exposure to feces.

Double Contrast Barium Enema

This test has relatively low sensitivities for the detection of both CRC and adenomas and is also a labor-intensive procedure requiring extensive bowel preparation and radiologist expertise (14). There is also a paucity of well-designed studies assessing its effectiveness on mortality and incidence. Given these many limitations and since the introduction of CT colonography, double contrast barium enema (DCBE) is rarely employed.

Flexible Sigmoidoscopy

There is direct evidence from three randomized controlled clinical trials demonstrating significant reductions in both CRC incidence and mortality using flexible sigmoidoscopy (15–17). However, a substantial limitation of this test is that it only evaluates the distal colon (analogous to unilateral mammography), creating the possibility of significant false-negative screening exams. Furthermore, as with colonoscopy, it is operator-dependent.

Colonoscopy

Because of its high sensitivity and specificity for the identification of polyps and CRC, as well as its ability to concomitantly diagnose and reduce risks associated with biopsied precancerous lesions, diagnostic colonoscopy is considered the gold-standard against which other screening tests are compared. However, evidence for the ability of colonoscopy to reduce CRC mortality is largely indirect, coming from prospective observational and case-control studies. No RCTs to date have specifically demonstrated the effectiveness of colonoscopy in reducing CRC incidence or mortality. There is currently a large RCT underway, but results are not expected until 2026 (18; clinicaltrials.gov identifier: NCT00883792). Drawbacks of colonoscopy include its invasiveness, risk of serious complications, expense, and operator-dependence.

CT Colonography

There is currently no direct evidence establishing the effectiveness of CT colonography in reducing CRC incidence and mortality. Meta-analyses have shown it to have high sensitivity and specificity for the detection of polyps ≥ 10 mm, but reduced sensitivity and specificity for smaller polyps (19,20). While this test is relatively noninvasive, it is also operator-dependent and can result in the identification of extra-colonic findings which may or may not be clinically important. The U.S. Preventive Services Task Force (USPSTF) currently states that the evidence to assess the harms related to these extra-colonic findings is insufficient, and therefore the balance of the benefits and harms for CT colonography cannot be determined at this time (21).

There are a number of new molecular tests for feces and body fluids based upon alterations fundamental to the neoplastic process that are in development to attempt to improve upon the current tests with regard to compliance, cost, access, and performance issues (22). These tests offer significant advantages in the setting of CRC screening. They are noninvasive and generally do not require dietary restrictions, purgatives, or sedation, thus making them more acceptable to patients. These tests allow for ease in large-scale screening and, in the case of stool and urine tests, can be performed on mailed-in specimens without the need for a health care provider visit.

Some of the new tests currently being evaluated are various fecal, serum, and plasma DNA markers, as well as RNA and protein markers. Tests based on fecal DNA markers are farthest along in development and have the potential to affect the way in which current CRC screening is performed (22,23). While some opinion leaders have already asserted that stool DNA tests are now an acceptable option for CRC screening (24), the USPSTF states that there is insufficient evidence to properly assess the sensitivity and specificity of fecal DNA testing for colorectal neoplasia, and therefore, the balance of harms and benefits cannot be determined at this time (21).

■ SCREENING RECOMMENDATIONS

In 2008, the USPSTF updated their 2002 screening recommendations for individuals at average-risk of CRC (Table 2.1) based on the availability of newer screening technologies, as well as on new population models estimating the optimal ages at which to start and stop screening (21) based on their systematic review of the new evidence in the above two areas.

These recommendations differ from the prior guidelines only with respect to the age of the screened population. The 2002 recommendations applied to anyone over the age of 50, with no upper age limit on screening. New

Table 2.1 Colorectal Cancer (CRC) Screening Recommendations From the U.S. Public Health Service Task Force, 2008, for Average-Risk Individuals

A Recommendation	Screening using fecal occult blood testing, sigmoidoscopy, or colonoscopy in adults, beginning at age 50 and continuing until age 75
B Recommendation	No routine screening in adults ages 76 to 85 years
D Recommendation	No screening for CRC in adults older than 85 years
I Statement	Evidence is insufficient to assess the benefits and harms of CT colonography and fecal DNA testing as screening modalities

evidence demonstrated that while the benefits of screening outweighed the potential harms in those aged 50 to 75 years, this was not the case for those over 75. In these individuals, the likelihood of early detection yielding a mortality benefit declines due to the long average time between adenoma development and cancer diagnosis. The USPSTF continues to recommend screening with high-sensitivity FOBT annually, or sigmoidoscopy every 5 years, or high-sensitivity FOBT every 3 years, or colonoscopy every 10 years.

More aggressive screening guidelines exist for individuals at high risk for CRC due to hereditary syndromes, which are reviewed later in this chapter (25).

CHEMOPREVENTION IN CRC

The process of developing molecular preventive agents for CRC prevention is similar to those encountered in the development of agents for other cancers. The process begins with the identification of abnormalities in precancerous lesions that distinguish them from the normal epithelium from which they arise. Secondly, these abnormalities must then be assessed for their pathological relevance. Any compelling preventive target is generally both distinctive and pathologically relevant as demonstrated by various experimental manipulations confirming it is at least necessary, if not sufficient, to contribute to at least one of the characteristic abnormalities of cancer progression. Finally, such targets must be pharmacologically accessible and able to be modulated, with modulation associated with reduced risk of progression, and in some cases, regression of the premalignant lesion.

A key issue in the evaluation of any chemopreventive agent relates to the length of time required to see an effect of the agent. The ultimate long-term goal of any chemopreventive agent is a reduction in disease incidence and mortality. However, the chronic nature of carcinogenesis in general, and specifically CRC development in which the transformation of adenomas into cancer is estimated to take between 10 and 15 years (11), and current standards of care which mandate removal of polyps for histopathologic characterization, challenge efforts to demonstrate the effectiveness of molecular preventive agents on the basis of CRC incidence. Consequently, more intermediate and practical endpoints are needed that can be reliably assessed within the time constraints of typical chemopreventive trials.

The selection of endpoints in chemopreventive agent development is challenging and highly controversial. Unambiguous endpoints for agent development that are agreed upon by regulatory authorities, scientists, and patients include improvements in duration of life, quality of life, or both. While these outcomes are important, they are longer-term goals, much like reductions in incidence and mortality, and so do not truly address the issue of having more immediate and practical endpoints that can be consistently evaluated within the framework of a typical clinical trial. Given this situation, the American Association for Cancer Research (AACR) has actively engaged expert reviews on the scientific evidence in order to identify endpoints which might serve as meaningful intermediate measures of benefit or surrogates for long-term reductions in incident cancer or cancer-associated mortality. Although none of these intermediate measures are ideal, most drugs currently approved for cancer risk reduction or treatment of intra-epithelial neoplastia (dysplasia) have relied upon endpoint assessments other than cancer incidence reduction in pivotal trials.

Specifically within CRC chemoprevention, adenomas are the accepted intermediate measure generally used to assess the efficacy of potential agents. The use of adenomas as endpoints in chemopreventive trials is supported by multiple lines of evidence. First, nearly all CRC are believed to arise from adenomas, and colorectal adenomas share with CRC many molecular alterations and risk factors, suggesting a common etiology. Secondly, adenomas have been used as reasonable, if not absolute, surrogates for CRC incidence and mortality in the setting of surgical interventions. In a long-term prospective study, the National Polyp Study recently demonstrated that removal of adenomas was associated with a 53% reduction in long-term (up to 23 years) mortality from CRC (26). Preclinically, some chemopreventive agents in animal models of colorectal carcinogenesis have demonstrated sustained effects across the entire pathologic range of colorectal neoplasia (27). In humans, the chemopreventive effects on aberrant crypt foci representing the earliest identifiable morphologic lesions, adenomas, cancer, and cancer-associated mortality have been highly-correlated in data surrounding the effects of nonsteroidal anti-inflammatory drugs (NSAIDs) in reducing colorectal neoplasia across the full disease spectrum

(28–30). Finally, there is a history of adenomas being used as endpoints in chemopreventive agent efficacy trials for more than a decade, and they were the focus of the U.S. Food and Drug Administration's preliminary approval of celecoxib for familial adenomatous polyposis (FAP; 31).

The identification of potential chemopreventive agents generally occurs through one of three pathways. The first pathway is based on epidemiological data. Many agents have come to attention based on their associations in large observational studies, for example, aspirin. The efficacy of aspirin against CRC was first suggested by such studies (32–34). The analysis of secondary outcomes of RCTs represents another epidemiological source of agent identification. Conjugated equine estrogen (CEE) with medroxyprogesterone acetate (MPA) first came to attention as a potential chemopreventive agent for CRC in this manner through analysis of data from the Women's Health Initiative (WHI) where coronary heart disease was the primary outcome, but where the occurrence of various cancers was also analyzed as part of a global index summarizing the balance of risks and benefits of hormone replacement therapy (HRT; 35). Because some agents identified solely on the basis of epidemiological data have failed to show a benefit in RCTs (eg, beta-carotene and alpha-tocopherol), priority is now given to agents that have multiple lines of evidence supporting their potential chemopreventive use.

Use of animal models with various chemical carcinogens or genetic engineering for carcinogenesis is a second approach to agent identification. These animal models typically involve examining changes in the incidence, multiplicity, or volume of aberrant crypt foci, adenomas, and/or cancer. Issues for animal models center on how well these models recapitulate the various molecular and pathological mechanisms observed in human cancers, as well as their ability to predict safety and efficacy of an agent in humans. Although there is certainly no perfect animal model of human disease or chemopreventive efficacy, a retrospective comparison of the animal and human data on calcium (36–38) and COX2 inhibitors (39–48) in CRC prevention suggests there is reasonable predictiveness and consistency; and this has been additionally suggested by a systematic review and meta-analysis of colon chemoprevention studies in rodents and humans (49). Unfortunately, while there are hundreds of published chemoprevention studies in animal models of CRC, very few of the potential new agents emerging from these studies have been tested in clinical trials.

The third approach to agent identification comes from our understanding of the molecular pathogenesis of colorectal neoplasia. This mechanistic strategy suggests candidate molecular targets for chemopreventive agents. Such targets are derived from in vitro studies where the mechanisms of action, agent concentrations, essential cofactors, and downstream signaling implications can be carefully investigated. An ideal chemopreventive target meets the following criteria: (a) Differential expression in neoplasia versus normal tissue; (b) Functional significance, often demonstrated through genetic manipulation or shRNA/RNAi approaches; (c) Over-expression rather than under-expression, because down-regulation of a biologic signal is generally easier to achieve than replacement of an absent function; (d) Pharmacologic accessibility; and (e) Modulation that results in reductions in cancer incidence, burden, or mortality, at least in model systems.

■ CLINICAL EVALUATIONS TO DATE

Very few chemopreventive agents have been approved by the FDA within the last 30 years. This is due in part to a lack of validated and practical biomarkers for use in chemopreventive trials, as discussed earlier, as well as to a host of other reasons ranging from adherence and toxicity issues in healthy populations to pharmaceutical industry reluctance to engage in preventive drug development due to numerous disincentives (50). Celecoxib is currently the only agent that was historically approved for use in colorectal chemoprevention, and it was restricted to use as an adjunct to usual surgical measures in patients with the high-risk genetic condition FAP. However, the label indication was sacrificed in early 2011 when confirmatory trials to validate efficacy and toxicity estimates proved challenging.

Many RCTs have been conducted using various other agents to attempt to reduce adenoma recurrence, or much more rarely, CRC incidence or mortality. However, most of these trials have demonstrated null effects, meaning that the agents under investigation did not significantly decrease or even increased the risk of CR neoplasia during the observation period. Below we briefly review the latest findings of potential colorectal chemopreventive agents. We begin with those agents that have demonstrated positive effects on colorectal adenoma recurrence and/or CRC within RCTs, as these provide the most robust evidence for a potential agent's ability to reduce CRC risk.

Five classes of agents have demonstrated at least some degree of protective effects within RCTs. These are the anti-oxidant selenium, the mineral calcium, HRT, NSAIDs, and most recently, the omega-3 fatty acid eicosapentaenoic acid (EPA). Table 2.2 provides a summary of all RCTs for each of these five different agents.

Selenium

Ecologic studies first suggested the protective effects of selenium in cancer (51), but subsequent results from observational studies of its effects on CRC risk or adenoma formation have been mixed (52–55). A recent nested

Table 2.2 Randomized Controlled Trials With CRC or Adenoma Incidence for the 5 Agents Demonstrating Positive Effects, by Population (Average Risk vs Increased Risk)

Study	Intervention	Cohort	Primary Result
		Average Risk Populations	
Wactawski-Wende et al (69)	500 mg of elemental calcium as calcium carbonate with 200 IU of vitamin D3 bid vs placebo × 7 yr	36,282 postmenopausal women from 40 WHI centers	*CRC Incidence:* No significant difference between intervention and placebo groups. HR, 1.08 (95% CI, 0.86–1.34); *P* = .51
Lippman et al (58)	Oral selenium (200 microg/d from L-selenomethionine) and matched vitamin E placebo, vitamin E (400 IU/d of all rac-alpha-tocopheryl acetate) and matched selenium placebo, selenium + vitamin E, or placebo + placebo × 7 to 12 yr	35,533 men aged ≥ 50 (African-American) or ≥ 55 (Caucasian) with serum PSA level ≤ 4 ng/mL and a DRE not suspicious for prostate cancer	*CRC Incidence:* No significant difference between intervention and placebo groups—Vitamin E: HR, 1.09 (0.69–1.73); Selenium: HR, 1.05 (0.66–1.67); Selenium + vitamin E: HR, 1.28 (0.82–2.00). *CRC Mortality:* No significant difference between intervention and placebo groups—Vitamin E: HR, 1.30 (0.44–3.83); Selenium: HR, 1.00 (0.32–3.16); Selenium + vitamin E: HR, 1.49 (0.52–4.28)
Hulley et al (105)	0.625 mg/d conjugated estrogens + 2.5 mg/d MPA vs placebo × 4 yr	2763 postmenopausal women with coronary artery disease, average age = 67 yo	*CRC Incidence:* No significant difference between intervention and placebo groups—HR (unadjusted intention-to-treat), 0.81 (0.46–1.45). HR (adjusted, as-treated), 0.58 (0.25–1.35)
Rossouw et al (35), Chlebowski et al (103; update)	CEE 0.625 mg/d + MPA 2.5 mg/d vs placebo × 5.2 yr	16,608 healthy postmenopausal women; 50 to 79 yo	*CRC Incidence:* RR, 0.63 (0.43–0.92) Update: *CRC Stage at Diagnosis:* rate of regional or metastatic disease in hormone group (76.2%) v placebo (48.5%), *P* = .004
Anderson et al (106) Ritenbaugh et al (107; update)	CEE 0.625 mg/d vs placebo × 7.1 yr	10,738 healthy postmenopausal women with hysterectomy; 50–79 yo	*CRC Incidence:* 1.08 (0.75–1.55). Update: *Survival Following CRC Diagnosis:* 1.34 (0.58–3.19)
Gann et al (140)	325 mg aspirin or placebo every other day × 5 yr	22,071 male physicians aged 40 to 84	*CRC Incidence:* RR, 1.15 (0.80–1.65). *For In-Situ Cancers and Polyps:* RR, 0.86 (0.68–1.10)
Cook et al (139)	100 mg aspirin or placebo administered every other day × 10 yr	39,876 U.S. women aged ≥ 45 years and initially without history of cancer, CVD, or other major chronic illness	*CRC Incidence:* RR, 0.97 (0.77–1.24)
Flossman et al (141; pooled analysis of data from the UK-TIA and British Doctors' Aspirin Trials)	UK-TIA: 300 to 500 mg/d vs placebo × 1 to 7 yr British Doctors' Aspirin Trial: 300–1500 mg/d vs no aspirin × 5 to 6 yr	UK-TIA: 2449 individuals, mean age of 60.3, 73% male. British Doctors' Aspirin Trial: 5139 individuals, mean age 61.6 yo	*CRC Incidence:* HR, 0.74 (0.56–0.97), *P* = .02. Effect seen after a latency of 10 yr
		Increased Risk Populations	
Baron et al (36)	Calcium 3.0 g/d vs placebo × 4 yr	930 patients with prior adenoma	*Adenoma Incidence:* RR, 0.81 (0.67–0.99), *P* = .04. *Adenoma Number:* RR,0.76 (0.60–0.96), *P* = .02
Faivre and Bonithon-Kopp (68)	Calcium 2.0 gm/d vs 3.8 gm/d ispaghula husk vs placebo × 3 yr	655 patients with prior adenoma; 35 to 75 yo	*Adenoma Incidence:* Calcium—RR, 0.66 (0.38–1.17), *P* = .16. Fiber—RR, 1.67 (1.01–2.76), *P* = .042
Clark et al (57)	Selenium 200 µg/d vs placebo × 6.4 yr	1312 patients with prior skin cancer	*CRC Incidence:* RR, 0.42 (0.18–0.95), *P* = .03
Baron et al (39)	Aspirin 81 vs 325 mg/d vs placebo × 3 yr	1211 patients with prior adenoma	*81 mg/d, Adenoma Incidence:* RR, 0.81 (0.69–0.96). *Advanced Adenoma Incidence:* RR, 0.59 (0.38–0.92). *325 mg/d, Adenoma Incidence:* RR, 0.96 (0.81–1.13). *Advanced Adenoma Incidence:* RR, 0.83 (0.55–1.23)
Sandler et al (40)	Aspirin 325 mg/d vs placebo × 3 yr	635 patients with prior resected early-stage CRC	*Adenoma Incidence:* RR, 0.65 (0.46–0.91); prolonged time to first adenoma

(Continued)

■ **Table 2.2** *(Continued)*

Study	Intervention	Cohort	Primary Result
Benamouzig et al (137; APACC trial). Benamouzig et al (138; 4 year follow-up of APACC)	Lysine acetylsalicylate 160 to 300 mg/d vs placebo × 4 yr	291 patients with prior adenomas	*Recurrent Adenoma:* RR, 0.73 (0.52–1.04), *P* = .08. *Recurrent Adenoma ≥ 5 mm in Diameter:* RR, 0.44 (0.24–0.82), *P* = .01. Four-year follow-up: *Proportion of Patients with at Least 1 Recurrent Adenoma:* 41% in aspirin-treated group v 40% in placebo, NS. *Polyp Burden:* 3.1±5.8 mm v 3.4 ± 6.2 mm, NS. *Proportion with at Least 1 Advanced Recurrent Adenoma:* 10% v 7%, NS
Logan et al (136)	Aspirin 300 mg/d and folate supplements 0.5 mg/d vs placebo in 2 × 2 Factorial Design	939 patients with prior adenomas, mean age 57.8 yr (range, 27.6–74.6)	*Adenoma Recurrence:* RR, 0.79 (0.63–0.99). *Advanced Adenoma:* RR, 0.63 (0.43–0.91)
Burn et al (134) CAPP-1	Aspirin 600 mg/d and/or Resistant Starch (30 g/d) vs placebo × 1 to 12 yr in 2 × 2 Factorial Design	206 FAP patients, aged 10–21 yr	*Polyp count:* Aspirin—RR, 0.77 (0.54–1.10). *Size of Largest Observed Polyp:* Mean size of 3.0 mm in aspirin-treated group v 6.0 mm in placebo group, *P* = .02
Burn et al (135) CAPP-2	600 mg aspirin or aspirin placebo or 30 g resistant starch or starch placebo, for up to 4 yr	937 carriers of LS	*Time to First CRC:* HR, 0.63 (0.35–1.13), *P* = .12. For those completing 2 yr of intervention, HR, 0.41 (0.19–0.86), *P* = .02; IRR, 0.37 (0.18–00.78), *P* = .008
Steinbach et al (48)	Celecoxib, 200 mg/d or 800 mg/d vs placebo × 6 mo	77 FAP patients	*Mean Number of Polyps:* 28% reduction from baseline with 800 mg/d, *P* = .003. *Polyp Burden:* 30.7% reduction from baseline with 800 mg/d, *P* = .001
Arber et al (145)	Celecoxib, single 400-mg dose/d vs placebo	1561 patients with history of adenomas	*Adenoma Recurrence:* RR, 0.64 (0.56–0.75), *P* < .001. *Advanced adenomas:* RR, 0.49 (0.33–0.73), *P* < .001
Bertagnolli et al (146)	Celecoxib, 400 mg/d or 800 mg/d vs placebo × 3 yr	2035 patients with prior adenomas	*Recurrence of 1 or More Adenomas:* 400 mg/d—RR, 0.67 (0.59–0.77), *P* < .001. 800 mg/d—RR, 0.55 (0.48–0.64), *P* < .001. *Celecoxib significantly and dose-dependently associated with increased risk of CVD events
Labayle et al (153)	300 mg/day of sulindac vs placebo × two 4-mo periods separated by 1-mo wash-out phase	10 patients with rectal polyps previously treated by colectomy and ileorectal anastomosis	*Polyp Regression:* Sulindac induced complete (six patients) or near complete (three patients) regression of polyps compared to placebo, *P* < .01
Giardiello et al (152)	300 mg/d of sulindac vs placebo × 9 mo	22 FAP patients, including 18 with previous celectomy	*Mean Number of Polyps:* 44% reduction from baseline in sulinac group, *P* = .014. *Mean Polyp Diameter:* 35% reduction from baseline in sulindac group, *P* < .001
Nugent et al (154)	Sulindac vs placebo	24 FAP patients with previous prophylactic colectomy and advanced duodenal polyposis	*Epithelial Cell Proliferation:* Significant reduction induced by sulindac, *P* = .003. *Polyp Regression:* Trend toward regression in duodenum, *P* = .12. Significant regression in rectum, *P* = .01
Ladenheim et al (155)	150 mg of sulindac twice daily vs placebo × 4 mo	44 asymptomatic patients with sporadic colonic polyps	No significant differences noted in polyp regression or size between sulindac and placebo groups
Giardiello et al (151)	Either 150 mg/d or 300 mg/d mg of sulindac vs placebo × 4 yr	41 individuals with FAP genotype, but phenotypically unaffected, aged 8 to 25 yr	*Adenoma Incidence:* No significant difference between intervention and placebo groups, *P* = .54. *Adenoma Number and Size:* No significant differences in mean number of polyps, *P* = .69, or in their size, *P* = .17
Meyskens et al (160)	Oral DFMO 500 mg and sulindac 150 mg once daily or matched placebos × 36 mo	375 patients with history of resected adenomas	*Recurrence of 1 or More Adenomas:* RR, 0.30 (0.18–0.49) *P* < .001. *Advanced Adenomas:* RR, 0.085 (0.011–0.65) *P* < .001. *Multiple Adenomas:* RR, 0.055 (0.0075–0.41) *P* < .001
West et al (164)	Enteric-coated formulation of EPA, as the free fatty acid EPA-FFA, 2 g/d vs placebo × 6 mo	58 patients with FAP, ≥18 yo, who had previously undergone colectomy with ileorectal anastomosis	*Polyp Number:* 22.4% reduction in EPA group, *P* = .012. *Polyp Size:* 29.8% reduction in sum of polyp diameters in EPA group, *P* = .027

CEE, conjugated eguine estrogen; CRC, colorectal cancer; CVD, cardiovascular disease; DFMO, difluoromethylornithine; yo, years old.

case-control study within the WHI found no protective effect of selenium on CRC among women (56). Few RCTs have been conducted on selenium's efficacy in CRC risk or adenoma recurrence. The first trial by Clark et al tested selenium supplementation as a secondary end point in individuals with a history of skin cancer and revealed a 58% reduction in CRC incidence (57). A more recent report by Lippman et al from the Selenium and Vitamin E Cancer Prevention Trial (SELECT) did not find any significant difference in CRC incidence among men taking either oral selenium, vitamin E or both after approximately 7 years of follow-up (58). There are currently three other RCTs, including one Phase III trial, that are either planned or on-going, which will assess the effects of selenium on aberrant crypt foci, adenomatous polyps, or CRC incidence (clinicaltrials.gov identifiers: NCT00078897, NCT00706121, and NCT01211561). Final data collection is estimated to occur in 2013 for two of the studies, and in 2014 for the third.

Calcium

There is significant biological plausibility for the role of calcium in the prevention of CRC. Calcium can sequester intraluminal bile and fatty acids, which have mutagenic effects on colorectal mucosa (59,60), and can inhibit epithelial proliferation by modifying protein kinase C activity, stabilizing membranes, and/or modifying *K-ras* mutations (61).

Data from observational studies are largely consistent in suggesting an inverse association between calcium intake and recurrent polyps (62,63) or CRC risk (64–67). Two RCTs in intermediate risk populations (ie, those with a history of adenoma) demonstrated the protective effects of calcium on adenoma recurrence (36,68). The most recent trial examined calcium plus vitamin D on the risk of CRC in postmenopausal women within the WHI (69). The authors concluded that after a follow-up period of 7 years, daily supplementation of calcium with vitamin D did not have an effect on CRC incidence in this population. However, the follow-up period may not have been long enough to observe an effect. Follow-up of participants within this trial is still on-going and will assess the longer-tem effect of a calcium plus vitamin D intervention on CRC risk.

There is currently one additional ongoing RCT, the Vitamin D/Calcium Polyp Prevention Study, that is examining the effects of calcium and vitamin D on adenoma recurrence (clincaltrials.gov identifier: NCT00153816). Completion of data collection for the primary endpoint is expected in 2013. While calcium appears to reduce the risk of adenomas in intermediate risk populations, and no significant adverse events have been reported with the use of calcium/vitamin D interventions, longer-term data on their efficacy in the general population are needed.

Hormone Replacement Therapy

The biologic plausibility of HRT in the reduction of colorectal neoplasia is based on its ability to directly or indirectly reduce the production of toxic secondary bile acids and inhibit insulin-like growth factor I (IGF-1), which stimulates epithelial cell proliferation. In addition, although the role of estrogen signaling in colorectal neoplasia remains unclear at this time, recent data suggest a possible role for the estrogen receptor family in modulating CRC risk as well, with loss of the ERβ member of the estrogen receptor family being associated with advanced stages of CRC, greater tumor extent, poorer disease-free survival, and an increased risk of CRC death (70–72).

Observational data linking postmenopausal HRT use with a reduced risk for CRC and adenoma recurrence are extensive and largely consistent. The majority of prospective studies have demonstrated an inverse association with HRT use and risk of CRC and/or adenomas (73–94). Various meta-analyses have confirmed these effects, suggesting an approximate 11%–20% reduction in CRC risk for "ever" HRT users, with stronger associations seen for current use and longer duration of use (95–98). Since the publication of these meta-analyses, additional observational studies have reported similar findings (80,99,100), with the exception of the WHI observational study and the European Prospective Investigation into Cancer and Nutrition study (EPIC; 101,102). Neither of these studies documented a significant effect of either unopposed estrogen therapy or estrogen plus progestin therapy on the risk of CRC (101,102). However, the numbers of CRC cases within each formulation group of the WHI observational study, as well as in the estrogen-only group in the EPIC study, were relatively small in comparison to the numbers of cases in the formulation groups of some of the other studies documenting significant protective effects. Yet, it is noteworthy that the EPIC study included the largest number of cases to date for the estrogen plus progestin formulation and did not document an effect. The authors speculate that the relatively short duration of HRT use in that cohort may, at least in part, contribute to its null findings (102). Unlike a number of other prospective studies that have included women with longer durations of HRT use and have documented a significant protective association with CRC risk (80,99,100), both the EPIC and WHI observational cohorts included HRT use of shorter duration.

There have been three RCTs examining HRT use and risk of CRC, three testing the combined formulation of estrogen plus progestin and one testing unopposed estrogen therapy. Rossouw et al initially reported a 37% reduction in CRC incidence as a secondary outcome of the WHI randomized trial examining cardiovascular risk and the combined use of estrogen and progestin in healthy postmenopausal women (35). An update of this trial confirmed these findings; however, it also demonstrated that

CRCs were of a more advanced stage within the HRT group than in the placebo group (regional or metastatic disease, 76.2% vs 48.5%, $P = .004$), complicating the interpretation of the protective effect seen on overall risk (103). Results from the WHI observational study, as discussed previously, do not support these findings, as no significant effects were seen for combined therapy on risk or diagnosis in the observational data (101). The Heart and Estrogen/Progestin Replacement Study (HERS) was an RCT designed to test the effects of estrogen plus progestin in postmenopausal women with coronary artery disease, with disease surveillance continuing under HERS II for various outcomes, including CRC (104,105). Combining CRC cases that occurred in each of the HERS studies ($N = 21$) resulted in a nonsignificant relative hazard of 0.81 (0.46–1.45) for the effect of combined therapy on risk of CRC (105). The third RCT examined unopposed estrogen therapy in postmenopausal women with a prior hysterectomy and found that it did not reduce CRC incidence (HR, 1.08; 95% CI, 0.75–1.55; 106). This is in contrast to the findings of many of the observational studies of unopposed estrogen therapy. An update of this trial by Ritenbaugh et al confirmed these findings and also reported results on survival after diagnosis, finding no significant difference in cumulative mortality between the estrogen and placebo groups (HR, 1.34; 95% CI, 0.58–3.19; 107).

In summary, findings from randomized trials do not currently support the use of HRT in colorectal risk reduction. While numerous observational studies suggest a protective effect of HRT, it still remains unclear which formulations and dosing regimens would be optimal or the duration of treatment and observation needed to observe benefits, if they occur. Although the potential harms of HRT use currently outweigh its chemopreventive effects against CRC, its promise has stimulated much research into the mechanisms of HRT's protective effects in the hopes of improving this therapy for use in CRC risk reduction.

Nonsteroidal Antiinflammatory Drugs

NSAIDs are the most well-established chemopreventive agents for CRC and adenoma recurrence. Data supporting their chemopreventive use across the range of colorectal neoplasia is highly consistent across different agents. While NSAIDs' exact mechanisms of action against cancer are not fully understood, there has been considerable progress in understanding a particular pathway through which they exert some of their effects (108). The most well-established NSAIDs, including aspirin and the coxibs, work by inhibiting one or both of the cyclooxygenase enzymes, COX-1 and COX-2. As these enzymes serve to generate prostanoids in the inflammatory response, their inhibition results in various characteristic effects, including reduced cellular proliferation, induction of apoptosis, promotion of immunologic surveillance, and a reduction in the formation of new blood vessels. Notably, COX-2 has been shown to be overexpressed in human precancers and cancers, and this overexpression is correlated with poorer survival among patients with colorectal and other cancers (29,109–113). In addition to COX-dependent effects, various experimental data suggest NSAIDs exert some of their anti-cancer effects through COX-independent mechanisms as well (114–116).

Aspirin

The evidence for the protective effects of aspirin on CRC development and adenoma recurrence from animal and epidemiological studies is extensive (44,117–131). Data also exist suggesting that this effect is both dose-dependent and related to the duration of treatment (34,132,133). Ten RCTs focused on colorectal neoplasia have been carried out in populations with varying levels of risk; additional RCTs in the setting of cardiovascular disease prevention have evaluated CR neoplasia as a secondary endpoint.

The most recent trials have tested aspirin in high- (FAP or HNPCC) or intermediate- (history of adenomas or CRC) risk populations. The CAPP1 and CAPP2 trials examined the efficacy of aspirin in those with FAP and HNPCC, respectively. While the CAPP1 study did not find a significant effect of 600 mg/day aspirin on its primary endpoint of polyp number, it did detect a weakly significant trend toward a smaller size of the largest detected polyp in those taking aspirin compared with the nonaspirin group (134). The CAPP2 study in those with HNPCC found that 600 mg/d aspirin for a mean of 25 months significantly reduced CRC incidence after 55.7 months (135). The authors of the CAPP2 report suggest their findings provide a basis for the recommendation of aspirin chemoprevention as the standard of care in those with HNPCC. An additional study, CAPP3, aims to compare the effect of different doses of aspirin within this setting.

Four RCTs have been carried out in intermediate risk populations. Three were performed in those with a history of adenoma (39,136,137) and one in those with a history of CRC (40). The primary endpoint for all studies was adenoma recurrence, and treatment and follow-up durations ranged from 1 to 3 years. All four studies reported a significant reduction in either the risk of any recurrent adenoma, the risk of advanced adenoma, or both in those taking aspirin compared to placebo. One study recently provided an update on findings after 4 years of follow-up and found that the protective effects identified after 1 year of aspirin treatment did not remain after the 4-year follow-up period (138). It is important to note here that the intervention lasted only 1 year. The authors suggest that the discrepancy between the 1- and 4-year results may be due either to a lack of statistical power, as there were many drop-outs (32%) between years 1 and 4, or to a differential effect of aspirin on the natural history of the polyp, where an "anti-tumor" or "anti-proliferation" effect, rather than a true chemopreventive effect, was observed at year 1, suggesting that any true chemopreventive effect of aspirin requires a time frame longer than 4 years (138).

Four RCTs have tested aspirin in the setting of CRC prevention within the general population. Two of these studies are the well-known WHI (139) and the Physician's Health Study (PHS; 140). The WHI and PHS used relatively low and intermittent doses of aspirin, 100 mg every other day for 10 years or 325 mg every other day for 5 years, respectively. Neither of these studies documented a significant effect of aspirin on incidence of CRC. However, the relatively low dose of aspirin, the intermittent dosing, and the short length of follow-up time in these trials may have contributed to the null results. Results from two smaller trials using higher doses, the United Kingdom Transient Ischemic Attack Aspirin (UK-TIA) Trial and the British Doctors' Aspirin Trial, which administered 300 to 500 mg/day for 1 to 7 years and 300 to 1500 mg/day for 5 to 6 years, respectively, suggest a significant reduction in the incidence of CRC, with a greater reduction in risk if aspirin treatment lasted 5 years or more; this effect was observed only after a latency of 10 years (141). It is important to note these trials were established primarily to test aspirin in the setting of cardiovascular outcomes, not CRC. These results reflect the combined trial data recently analyzed with respect to CRC incidence (141). These findings are consistent with much of the observational data in which higher doses administered over longer time periods result in CRC protection. A recent meta-analysis of the data collected in the context of all cardiovascular prevention trials with low-dose aspirin has been communicated recently. The results of this analysis support the individual results of the above mentioned studies, confirming the effect of low-dose aspirin for CRC chemoprevention and the latency of its effect to approximately 10 years after exposure (142).

Of all the NSAIDs, aspirin may be the most promising in terms of colorectal chemoprevention because of its favorable cardiovascular profile. While the USPSTF does not currently recommend the use of aspirin for prevention of CRC due to its associated toxicities, it has recommended further investigation into optimizing the risk-benefit profile of aspirin for cancer prevention. The benefits of aspirin may outweigh the potential harms in high-risk groups; however, more research is needed. A 2009 international consensus statement calls for more studies to define aspirin's lowest effective dose, the most appropriate age at which to begin therapy, the optimum duration of therapy, and the population subsets in which benefits might outweigh potential harms (143). It is believed that some of these questions can be addressed with longer follow-up of existing RCTs, but that new RCTs will also be needed (143). As one example, a large RCT (ASPECT) of aspirin in Barrett's esophagus is on-going, focused on overall survival, but is developing additional data on the incidence of various cancers, including CRC (144).

Nonaspirin NSAIDs

Selective COX-2 inhibitors (COXIBs) and sulindac are two other NSAIDs that have demonstrated at least some efficacy in RCTs of CRC chemoprevention. Because of their ability to selectively block the COX-2 receptor and not the COX-1 receptor, blockade of which is associated with the GI toxicities seen with aspirin use, COXIBs initially generated a great deal of interest for cancer chemoprevention. Celecoxib was initially tested in a RCT of 83 FAP patients, demonstrating a 28% reduction in the number of polyps and a 31% reduction in polyp burden after 6 months of treatment at 400 mg twice daily compared to placebo (48). It was subsequently tested in two trials of individuals with a history of sporadic adenomas (145,146). After a treatment period of 2.5 years in the PreSAP Study and a treatment period of 3 years in the APC trial, significant protective effects were observed for recurrence of any adenoma and incidence of an advanced adenoma. However, the APC trial identified a dose-dependent 2- to 3-fold higher risk of cardiovascular events among those taking celecoxib which led to early termination of both the APC and PreSAP trials. This increased risk of cardiovascular events due to celecoxib was previously suggested in a study of rofecoxib, which ultimately led to rofecoxib's withdrawal from the market (147). Subsequent data have shown that the increased risk of cardiovascular events is largely confined to those with a high baseline risk of cardiovascular disease (148,149). But due to a shared set of risk factors in people at risk for CRC and cardiovascular disease, celecoxib cannot currently be recommended. However, a recent phase I dose-escalation trial of celecoxib in children (ages 10–14) with FAP demonstrated that it is safe, well-tolerated, and reasonably effective, significantly reducing the number of colorectal polyps in these patients (150).

Data from RCTs are much more limited for the other nonaspirin, nonCOXIB NSAIDs such as sulindac. Four small trials have tested sulindac in the high-risk setting of FAP. When tested in a primary prevention context, 4 years of treatment with sulindac in APC mutation carriers without adenomas did not prevent the development of adenomas, nor did it change the number or size of polyps compared to placebo (151). However, when tested in a secondary prevention context in FAP patients with adenomas, sulindac for 9 months reduced the number and size of polyps (152). Two other RCTs in Britain and France demonstrated significant effects of 4 to 6 months of treatment with sulindac on rectal polyp regression (153,154). It is important to note that results of these four trials are based on very limited sample sizes, ranging from just 10 to 41 FAP patients.

In the setting of intermediate risk, one small trial of 44 individuals with a prior history of polyps did not demonstrate significant effects of 4 months of sulindac treatment on polyp regression (155).

NSAID-based chemopreventive combinations are particularly promising in animal models where difluoromethylornithine (DFMO) given with sulindac has demonstrated synergy in preventing the growth and viability of human colon cancer cells (156–159). A subsequent RCT of sulindac with difluoromethylornithine (DFMO) versus placebo in 375 patients with prior sporadic adenomas demonstrated marked reductions in the recurrence of one of more adenomas (RR, 0.30; CI, 0.18–0.49; $P < .001$) and in the recurrence of advanced (RR, 0.085; CI, 0.011–0.65; $P < .001$) and multiple (0.055; 0.0074–0.41; $P < .001$) adenomas (160). While marked efficacy had been previously achieved in preclinical studies of chemopreventive drug combinations, this was the first trial demonstrating the ability of low doses of agent combinations to result in profound clinical efficacy.

There are currently a number of planned and ongoing RCTs for NSAIDs in colorectal chemoprevention. Two trials that will test the combination of sulindac and eflornithine in FAP patients and in those with stage 0–III colon cancer have just begun (clinicaltrials.gov identifier: NCT01483144 and NCT01349881). Two other trials are testing DFMO in combination with either aspirin (clinicaltrials.gov identifier: NCT00983580) or celecoxib (clinicaltrials.gov identifier: NCT00033371) in populations at increased risk for CRC.

Eicosapentaenoic Acid

Preclinical studies using various CRC rodent models to test EPA alone or in conjunction with DHA have consistently resulted in a 20%–50% decrease in the incidence of colorectal tumors and a 30%–70% decrease in tumor number (161,162). However, the epidemiological evidence for EPA in reducing CRC risk is inconsistent; and a recent systematic review of the literature suggests that there is no evidence to support a significant association between omega-3 fatty acids and cancer incidence (163). This review of 20 different cohorts spanning 11 different cancer types identified just one estimate of decreased risk for CRC due to omega-3 fatty acids and 17 estimates showing no association of omega-3 fatty acids with CRC (163). Nevertheless, based on the strong preclinical data, a RCT was conducted in 55 FAP patients who had previously undergone colectomy with ileorectal anastomosis (164). These patients are at high risk for the development of rectal adenomas, and hence, rectal cancer. After 6 months of treatment with an enteric-coated formulation of EPA as the free fatty acid EPA-FFA, a significant 22% reduction in polyp number and a nearly 30% significant reduction in the sum of polyp diameters was observed in the EPA-treated group when compared to placebo (164). Adverse events were similar between the treatment and placebo groups, and the authors stated that EPA-FFA was well-tolerated and achieved efficacy to a degree similar to that observed with celecoxib in FAP (164). Based on these results in the high-risk setting of FAP patients, EPA may hold promise as a chemopreventive agent in lower-risk populations as well, and warrants further investigation.

Ursodeoxycholic Acid

Ursodiol is a bile salt that reduces concentrations of the secondary bile acid deoxycholic acid (DCA) within the colon. Secondary bile acids have been implicated in colorectal carcinogenesis (165); specifically, DCA is cytoxic to the epithelial cells lining the colon and it has been shown to promote tumorigenesis, possibly through bile-acid induced DNA damage (166–168). A large RCT of 1286 patients with a history of adenomas did not identify a statistically significant reduction in total colorectal adenoma recurrence; however, it did find a significant 39% reduction in the recurrence of adenomas with high-grade dysplasia (169). In a secondary analysis of data from this trial, investigators found that gender modified the effect of Ursodiol on adenomas, with a significant reduction in the odds of advanced lesions in men, but not in women (170). The authors stated that their findings may support the use of Ursodiol in men to prevent advanced colorectal adenomas (170). However, another RCT in patients with UC and primary sclerosing cholangitis demonstrated a significantly increased risk of colorectal neoplasia in those receiving high-doses (28–30 mg/kg/day) of Ursodiol over 4 years (171). While the dosage in this study is three times higher than the dose used in the RCT of colorectal adenomas and the subjects have underlying colorectal inflammatory disease, it raises concerns regarding the use of Ursodiol as a chemopreventive agent, and therefore, further research with this agent is warranted to clarify its effects.

Dietary modifications and supplements will be addressed in the next section of this chapter including selenium, fiber, fats, and nondietary factors.

■ THE FUTURE OF CRC

There are currently only twelve drugs approved for treatment of precancerous lesions or cancer risk reduction. Of these, only one, celecoxib, was temporarily approved for CRC chemoprevention in patients with FAP. However, confirmatory trials were not completed as planned, and that preliminary approval was sacrificed. Additionally, cardiovascular safety concerns were identified. Given that CRC is the third most common cancer among both men and women, and given its associated morbidity and mortality, there is an urgent need for additional chemopreventive agents demonstrating efficacy and a favorable safety profile in phase III RCTs. However, the rate-limiting step in the identification of such agents is the pace of clinical research. The establishment of ACF or another early marker in the neoplastic process as a chemopreventive response marker can help overcome this challenge by significantly reducing the amount of time required to assess outcomes. In addition, nesting prevention endpoints as secondary goals in therapeutic trials represents a promising strategy to improve the efficiency and predictive nature of new agent identification. Combining agents that have modest efficacy or an unfavorable toxicity profile is yet another promising strategy to improve the yield of potential agents. Combinations of agents may demonstrate more potent effects than either agent alone. The trial of sulindac therapy given along with DFMO in patients with sporadic adenomas is a prime example of this concept. This trial was stopped early due to its endpoints being met sooner than anticipated, and results demonstrated a marked reduction in recurrent adenomas with low doses of each drug with no significant difference in adverse effects between the treatment and placebo groups (160). Results of RCTs testing combinations of agents, such as DFMO along with aspirin or celecoxib in high-risk CRC populations, are anticipated.

In the meantime, other promising agents remain to be tested in phase III RCTs. Curcumin has recently been tested in a phase IIa clinical trial where it was well-tolerated and decreased ACF numbers in smokers at higher concentrations over 30 days (172). Trials testing the use of curcumin in FAP (clinicaltrials.gov identifier: NCT00641147 and NCT00927485), in those with resected polyps (clinicaltrials.gov identifier: NCT00118989), and in smokers with ACF (clinicaltrials.gov identifier: NCT00365209) are currently on-going. Other promising agents, including metformin, vitamin D, and NSAIDs associated with less toxicity, such as phospho-aspirin and phospho-sulindac, are on the horizon as well. Finally, chemopreventive combinations demonstrating synthetic lethality in APC-deficient cells, as identified by Zhang et al (173) are promising as are immunovaccines under investigation for prevention by at least two groups (174,175).

Identification of High-Risk Patients: Familial and Environmental Factors

FARAZ BISHEHSARI
BARBARA H. JUNG

FAMILY HISTORY OF CRC OUTSIDE OF KNOWN GENETIC SYNDROMES

A family history of CRC increases the risk of CRC, and can be found in about one-third of all CRCs. First-degree relatives with an adenoma or CRC increase an individual's lifetime risk for CRC. A family history of CRC in any first-degree relative can slightly increase risk of rectal cancer (OR, 1.37; 95% CI, 1.02–1.85). The relative risk increases if the affected family member had cancer at age 50 or younger (OR, 2.09; 95% CI, 0.94–4.65 for rectal tumors; OR, 3.00; 95% CI, 0.98–9.20 for distal colon tumors; and OR, 7.88; 95% CI, 2.62–23.7 for proximal colon tumors; 176). A large meta-analysis of 27 case-control and cohort studies confirmed that the presence of a first-degree relative with CRC is associated with increased risk of CRC (2.25; 95% CI, 2.00–2.53). In this analysis, the risk increases further if there is more than one relative with CRC (4.25; 95% CI, 3.01–6.08) or if the relative is diagnosed with CRC before age 45 (3.87; 95% CI, 2.40–6.22; 177). These data along with several other studies show that individuals with a family history of CRC have a significantly elevated risk of developing CRC. This risk is greater for relatives of patients diagnosed young, and those with more than one affected relative.

Therefore, an earlier and more rigorous screening is recommended in these individuals. If an individual has a family history of either CRC or adenomatous polyps in a first degree relative before age 60 years or in two or more first degree relatives at any age, the screening should start at age 40 years (instead of 50) or 10 years before the youngest case in the immediate family (Table 2.3). If the first degree relative with CRC or tubular adenoma is ≥ age 60 years or two relatives with CRC are second-degree, the screening colonoscopy should start at age 40 (Table 2.3; 178,179).

Individuals (and family members of patients) with certain recognized syndromes, such as LS (formerly known as hereditary nonpolyposis CRC or HNPCC) and FAP have a much elevated risk of developing CRC. Gene positive patients have a 80% and 100% lifetime risk, respectively, of developing CRC, while untested relatives risk is at least 50% on average. These syndromes are discussed separately in the next section.

RISK CONFERRED BY PERSONAL HISTORY OF NONCOLORECTAL CANCER

A personal history of certain malignancies may confer a higher risk of CRC in the same individual. An association between breast and CRC has been suggested by a number of studies (180–182). There appears to be an increase in risk of both CRC and colorectal adenomas in breast cancer patients, however, the magnitude of the increase with the standardized incidence ratio (SIR) of less than two is not high enough to support an augmented screening program outside of average risk guidelines (183,184). The observed link between breast cancer and CRC may be due to either common environmental risk factors such as high fat intake or unknown common genetic pathways (185,186).

An increased risk of CRC in individuals with history of prostate cancer has also been reported. This risk, however, is thought to be secondary to the previous therapy received for prostate cancer. For one, androgen deprivation has been shown to be associated with an increased risk of CRC. In a study performed on a large cohort of 107,859 men from the SEER-Medicare database, the incidence rate of CRC was higher in men who either underwent surgical orchiectomies (6.3 per 1000 person-years [py]; 95% CI, 5.3–7.5), or chemical castration with GnRH agonist therapy (4.4 per 1000 py; 95% CI, 4.0–4.9; 187). Compared

Table 2.3 CRC Screening and Surveillance in Patients With Family History of CRC Outside of Known CRC Syndromes

Degree of family history of CRC	Recommendation for screening and surveillance
Single first-degree relative with CRC or advanced adenoma diagnosed at age ≥ 60	Same as average risk: the preferred CRC prevention test is colonoscopy every 10 years, beginning at age 50 in nonblack individual. In African Americans screening should begin at age 45
Single first-degree with CRC or advanced adenoma diagnosed at age < 60 or 2 first-degree relatives with CRC or advanced adenomas at any age	Colonoscopy every 5 years beginning at age 40 or 10 years younger than age at diagnosis of the youngest affected relative

Adapted from (4).

to men with prostate cancer with no androgen deprivation therapy, there was an increased risk of CRC associated with the prolonged (equal or more than 25 months) use of GnRH (hazard ratio [HR], 1.31; 95% CI, 1.12–1.53) or with orchiectomy (HR, 1.37; 95% CI, 1.14–1.66).

Patients with prostate cancer who received radiation therapy are also at higher risk of developing CRC, with the highest risk conferred to the rectum. The increased risk is usually seen in men who underwent external beam radiation therapy (EBRT) while the risk is small after brachytherapy (188,189). A recent review on secondary cancer after radiotherapy for prostate cancer confirmed an increased risk of rectal cancer after external radiation, and not after brachytherapy, but the data on new modalities such as intensity-modulated radiotherapy are limited (190).

The increased risk of CRC after abdominal radiation was also reported in other cancers such as testicular and ovarian cancers (191,192).

Patients with a history of non-Hodgkin's lymphoma (NHL) are also felt to be at elevated risk of developing CRC. However, the increased risk of CRC after diagnosis of NHL though described by some series (193–195) was not observed in other reports (196). A more recent study showed that the increased risk of CRC after chemotherapy in general is mainly due to the treatment given for NHL. Follow-up on a large cohort of 2456 patients with NHL showed that the risk of CRC was raised (RR, 2.1; 95% CI, 1.1–3.6) only if patient received chemotherapy (195). The risk of subsequent CRC was not increased in a study involving 16,540 children with history of leukemia and lymphoma (197). However, the average follow-up of patients in this study was only 6.5 years whereas CRC usually occurs later in life. There is a need for further studies determining risk by environmental as well as genetic factors to determine which individuals with previous malignancies may need intensified screening for CRC.

■ RISK RELATED TO ETHNICITY

Epidemiologic studies have shown that the risk of CRC can vary among different ethnicities. In Askenazi Jews, a specific missense mutation in the *APC* gene (I1307K) doubles the risk for adenoma development and confers an increased prevalence of CRC (198).

Among all racial groups in the United States, African Americans have the highest incidence of CRC. Although the CRC incidence rates in whites is decreasing after its peak in 1985, with 20%–25% lower incidence rate in 2000 compared to 1985, this rate has been increasing in African Americans (199). Moreover, African Americans have a younger mean age at CRC diagnosis with a higher proportion of CRCs present at younger age. The proportion of CRCs presented before the age of 50 year was almost double among African Americans compared to whites (10.6 vs 5.5%, respectively; 200).

The site distribution of CRC in African Americans is also shifted to the right relative to other ethnic groups (201). A recent large study on asymptomatic white (n = 80,061) and black (n = 5464) patients who underwent screening colonoscopy showed that compared to white, black individuals have a higher risk of polyps sized more than 9 mm. Also, black individuals older than 60 years are more likely to have proximal polyps sized more than 9 mm (202). The racial difference in the anatomic location of CRC may account for the late-stage presentation of the CRC in African Americans (201). The underlying biologic mechanism that may explain the observed racial difference in the CRC pattern is not well understood. Environmental factors such as diet, smoking, physical activity, and access to the health care as well as genetic factors all have been implicated to play a role in the distinct pattern of CRC in African Americans.

Based on the available data, the American College of Gastroenterology recommends that African Americans should undergo screening for CRC under an average-risk strategy starting at age 45 and that colonoscopy is the preferred over flexible sigmoidoscopy given the predilection for right-sided lesions (179).

■ HEREDITARY SYNDROMES OF CRC

Environmental Factors

Diet

Red Meat

The correlation between meat consumption and risk of CRC was strongly suggested by a large prospective study published over two decades ago (203). This hypothesis has been tested by several other studies. A recent meta-analysis of prospective epidemiologic studies on red meat and risk of colon cancer confirmed that the associations between red meat consumption and CRC are generally above 1.0, although most are weakly elevated (RR < 1.5) and not statistically significant (204). This is consistent with the EPIC report (205). Further, gender and tumor site may modify the relation between red meat and CRC risk. CRC in men has a stronger association with red meat consumption. Distal colon and rectal cancers are also found to have a higher correlation with use of red meat than proximal tumors (206). These differences can be possibly attributed to hormonal effects and the tendency in men to develop more distal tumors (207).

Several mechanisms could explain the association between red meat intake and CRC. Nitrite and nitrate in the processed meats under acidic environment of the stomach can form nitrosamines that are mutagenic (208). Cooking meat at higher temperature can produce carcinogens such as heterocyclic amines and polycyclic aromatic hydrocarbons (209). Heme iron in the red meat may function as a pro-oxidant at the GI tract (210). Finally, there may be genetically determined individual differences in the metabolism of meat that can partly modify the production of carcinogens and subsequently the risk of colon cancer (211,212).

Fish

While red meat is suggested to increase the risk of CRC, a protective effect of fish was shown in several studies (203,205), attributed to a potential anti-inflammatory effect of omega-3 polyunsaturated fatty acids fish oil (213). However, a systematic review of the cohort series studying the relationship between risk of CRC and omega-3 fatty acid intake showed no significant association between omega-3 fatty acid intake and CRC risk (163). Other factors such as genetic polymorphisms in genes that control the metabolism of fatty acids and the formation of inflammatory eicosanoids can alter the risk of CRC in relation to the intake of fish. It is possible that the ratio of different fatty acids and not the total fat content of the diet is most important in conferring CRC risk (214). For instance, whereas an omega-6 to omega-3 ratio of almost 1:2 may be optimal for CRC prevention, this ratio in most westernized diets is reversed and as high as 30:1 (215).

Fat

A potential association between dietary fat and risk of CRC was first described in 1974 (216), but subsequent case-control studies did not confirm this association (217). Moreover, prospective studies showed that dietary fat, after correction for other risk factors, does not increase the risk of colon cancer (203,218). This null association was recently confirmed by the large Randomized Controlled Dietary Modification Trial that included 19,541 women who modified their diet including a reduction in fat intake. However, there was no change in risk of CRC among the group that maintained a 10% reduction in fat intake (219). It is conceivable though that the total fat intake may confer a CRC risk by contributing to the total energy-intake, high body mass index (BMI) and/or low physical activity as discussed below.

Fiber

Dietary fiber was among the first factors suggested to account for the variation of the incidence of CRC among different populations (220). Lower incidence of CRC in Asia and Africa compared to Western countries has been attributed to higher consumption of nondigestible polysaccharides derived from unrefined wheat (221). Subsequent case-control studies showed an overall protective effect of fiber on CRC risk with a combined odds ratio of 0.53 (95% CI, 0.47–0.61; 222). The protective effect of fiber in CRC, however, has since remained controversial (223). Several longitudinal studies failed to confirm this effect (224–227) and a meta-analysis of prospective cohort studies showed that high dietary fiber intake was not associated with a reduced risk of CRC (228).

Further, interventional studies showed no effect of fiber supplements on colorectal adenoma recurrence (229,230). Nevertheless, most of the prospective studies may not have adequately tested the fiber hypothesis as they were carried out in populations with a relatively low and homogeneous intake of dietary fiber (218).

Moreover, the intervention trials included individuals who established vulnerability to colorectal neoplasia by developing adenoma, and therefore the effect of change in their fiber intake was only measured in the narrow window of adenoma-carcinoma development and not within a long time period. In fact, the results of the EPIC study showed a strong and significant reduction in CRC risk of approximately 9% for each uncalibrated quintile increase in fiber (*P* for linear trend was less than 0.001) after adjustment for other covariates including folate, physical activity, alcohol, smoking, and red and processed meat. This association was stronger for left-sided colon cancer. The HR for colon cancer for the highest versus lowest quintile of fiber was 0.74 (CI, 0.56–0.98; 231).

Also, the EPIC data suggest the adverse effect of red meat consumption may be offset by high intake of fiber (205). It is plausible that the fiber can have a protective effect against CRC if consumed in large quantity and for a long period of time (218).

The effect of fiber on CRC can be exerted through several suggested mechanisms. Undigested polysaccharides can function as a bulk laxative (232), which may impact CRC formation. Moreover, the fermentation of starch by the colonic microflora can lead to butyrate production, which may exert a protective effect on colonic mucosa through a variety of mechanisms (233).

Dairy Products, Calcium, and Vitamin D

Several case control and prospective studies have tested the relationship between dairy intake and CRC risk. Although the results from case-control studies were not consistent (234), prospective studies generally have suggested a protective effect for dairy products (235,236). The analysis of data from eleven cohorts showed an inverse relation between milk and risk of CRC with an RR of 0.80 (95% CI, 0.68, 0.95) for the highest compared to the lowest milk intake (237). Another meta-analysis of 10 cohorts found that consumption of more than a glass of milk (250 g) vs 70 g every day was associated with a 15% reduction of risk of developing CRC (RR, 0.85; 95% CI, 0.78, 0.94). Further, each 500 g per day increase in milk intake reduced the risk of CRC by 12% (RR, 0.88; 95% CI, 0.82, 0.95).

The data for other dairy products such as cheese, butter, and ice cream in relation to CRC risk were again not consistent and generally did not support a protective effect against CRC (234).

Dairy products also contribute to the intake of minerals such as calcium (43% of daily intake), phosphorus (24%) and magnesium (11%), as well as vitamins including riboflavin (33%), vitamin B12 (36%), and vitamin D (3%; 238).

Some data suggest that calcium intake may inversely impact CRC risk. Pooled data from cohort studies showed that the group with the highest amount of calcium consumption experienced a lower risk of CRC (RR, 0.86; 95% CI, 0.78–0.95). There seems to be a ceiling threshold for the effect of calcium intake on CRC risk as intakes greater that 1 g per day was not associated with further risk reduction (239).

The protective effect of calcium is further confirmed by interventional studies that showed a decreased risk of adenoma recurrence in individuals taking calcium supplements (240,241). Early experimental studies showed that calcium modifies crypt cell proliferation in humans and can alter the course of neoplasia (242). Calcium binds to and may neutralize tumorigenic components in the colon such secondary bile acids and phospholipids (243). Further, it may inhibit the proliferation of epithelial cells by inducing differentiation and increasing apoptosis (244).

Although calcium intake is highly associated with dairy or milk intake the protective effect of milk or dairy intake on CRC risk is not eliminated when adjusted for calcium intake, implicating other components other than calcium in the chemopreventive effects (236). For instance, adequate vitamin D levels have been suggested to confer a lower CRC risk (65,66,245). However, the source of vitamin D is not solely from dietary intake as it can be synthesized endogenously after sun exposure, and therefore the results of studies that focused on the association of solely dietary intake of vitamin D and CRC should be interpreted with caution. In fact, vitamin D and calcium can act synergistically to modify CRC risk as vitamin D has also been shown to influence cell apoptosis, proliferation, and differentiation (246). Apart from calcium and vitamin D, there are many other components such as butyric acid, conjugated linoleic acid (CLA), and probiotic bacteria in dairy products that may contribute to the protective effect of dairy against CRC (237), although the precise mechanisms and the relative contribution remain to be studied.

Fruits and Vegetables

The association between fruit and vegetable intake and risk of CRC has been investigated by many studies albeit with inconsistent results. In 1997, the first report from the World Cancer Research Fund/American Institute of Cancer Research (WCRF/AICR) concluded that there was convincing evidence that intake of vegetables, but not fruit, protects against CRC. This statement was based mainly on case-control studies (247).

Since then, several prospective studies were performed, most of which did not show a significant protective effect for fruit and vegetable against CRC (248–250). In 2007, the WCRF/AICR stated in their second report that there was limited evidence that fruit and nonstarchy vegetables protect against CRC (247).

A meta-analysis of 19 cohort studies was recently performed to investigate whether there was a nonlinear dose–response relationship between fruit and vegetable intake and CRC risk (251). This is the first study to show a significant nonlinear inverse association between both fruits and vegetables and risk of CRC. In the linear dose–response analysis, a significant inverse association was observed only for vegetables.

Several mechanisms have been proposed to explain the protective effect of fruit and vegetables. Both contain folate that is important in DNA methylation and thymine synthesis. Folate deficiency can result in chromosomal breaks (252) and has been suggested to increase the risk of CRC (253).

Other components of fruit and vegetable such as fiber, vitamins, antioxidants, and selenium may also play a role preventing cancer through a variety of different mechanisms.

Selenium

Selenium is an essential mineral important in the structure of selenoproteins. These proteins are part of antioxidant defense enzymes, which protect against oxidative damage (254). Selenium levels were found to be associated with an altered risk of several cancers including CRC (255). CRC patients have a lower serum level of selenium compared to healthy individuals (256). Similarly, plasma selenium levels were inversely correlated with the risk of colon polyps (257,258). Chemoprevention trials showed that selenium supplementation reduced the mortality from all cancers and decreased the risk of CRC (259). Several mechanisms for this anticancer effect have been proposed including inhibition of DNA methyltransferases and subsequently suppression of aberrant DNA methylation, inhibition of cyclooxygenase (COX), and induction of cell cycle arrest and apoptosis (260).

Antioxidants (Beta Carotene, Vitamins A, C, and E)

A protective effect for antioxidants in different type of cancers including CRC has been proposed and mainly attributed to the protection against oxidative stress, which is known to play a role in carcinogenesis (261,262). Several observational and randomized trials have been performed to test the antioxidants' effect on cancer.

A review of 12 randomized trials, published in 2008, found no significant effect from beta-carotene, vitamins A, C, or E on the occurrence of GI cancers (RR, 0.94; 95% CI, 0.83–1.06; 263). The effect remained nonsignificant when each antioxidant individually or in combination was tested in relation to the occurrence of GI cancers. Surprisingly, antioxidant supplements were associated with a slight increase in overall mortality in a fixed-effect model meta-analysis (RR, 1.04; 95% CI, 1.02–1.07). The authors concluded that there is no evidence of the protective effect of antioxidant on GI cancers whereas they may increase the overall mortality.

A more recent systematic review of 19 randomized trials on antioxidants and CRC showed that antioxidant use does not affect the incidence of CRC (RR, 1.00; 95% CI, 0.88–1.13; 264). Antioxidants in the general population (n = 148,922) with treatment follow-up durations between 5 and 12 years did not modify the incidence of CRC (RR, 1.00; 95% CI, 0.88–1.13).

Antioxidant use in individuals with a history of adenoma and therefore at higher risk of CRC was also not associated with protective effect against developing cancer. Analysis of the results of six studies on antioxidants in individuals with a history of adenomas (n = 1706) with treatment and follow-up durations of 2 to 5 years showed no statistically significant differences in relative risk of adenoma recurrence when either all antioxidants were analyzed together (RR, 0.78; 95% CI, 0.54–1.14) or when specific combinations were assessed separately. Therefore, despite the plausible biological protective effect of antioxidants in CRC there currently is insufficient evidence to support this hypothesis. Several explanations for the negative findings in antioxidant use and cancer prevention include inadequate duration of the follow-up in randomized trials, heterogeneity of the studied populations, and a possible complex role of a combination of many different nutrients, rather than the single nutrient or combination of a few antioxidants, which call for a more in depth analysis is the future (261,264).

In addition to the absence of strong evidence for protection against CRC, reported adverse effects of antioxidant use, and possible detrimental effects of antioxidant supplements on overall and cardiovascular mortality, as well as increased incidence in prostate cancer and lung cancer (264) will limit their clinical use in CRC chemoprevention.

Nondietary Factors

Lifestyle

Obesity, BMI, and physical activity have all been suggested to influence the risk of CRC. Attempts of delineating the relative contribution of various lifestyle attributes are discussed below.

Body Mass Index

Both case-control and prospective studies have consistently shown that obesity and high BMI are associated with an increased risk of CRC (265).

In 1992, a study was published on a cohort of men who were followed after their weight was recorded at the time of college entry. Those who developed colon cancer were compared to those that remained colon cancer free. This study showed that heaviest quintile men had an RR of 2.4 (95% CI, 1.40–4.13) compared with the lightest quintile for developing CRC (266).

Since then, several prospective studies confirmed the enhancing effect of obesity on CRC (267,268). This effect is generally most pronounced in men. The report from EPIC trial on 368,277 individuals confirmed that men with the highest versus the lowest quintile of BMI had a higher colon cancer risk (RR, 1.55; 95% CI, 1.12–2.15). This effect was not observed among women (269). It has been shown that other markers of abdominal visceral fat such as waist circumference and waist-to-hip ratio may be a better predictive for CRC risk in both genders (218).

Chronic inflammation in the colonic mucosa is suggested to account for the effect of obesity on CRC risk. In obese individuals, the adipose tissue contains macrophages that secrete proinflammatory signal molecules and cytokines (270). Several inflammatory mediators such as "adipokines," cytokines, and tumor necrosis factor alpha (TNF-β) are stored in adipose tissue (271). It is postulated that the higher percentage of body fat causes a persistent low-grade inflammatory state in obese patients. As known from inflammatory bowel syndromes, chronic inflammation may act as a precursor in colon cancer. Moreover obesity is associated with the development of insulin resistance that can affect colon cancer risk as discussed in the section on metabolism below.

Physical Activity

Physical activity (or lack thereof) has also been shown to be a risk factor for colon cancer. It has been challenging to distinguish the effect of physical activity from elevated BMI as usually individuals with higher BMI tend to have a sedentary life. Therefore, very large studies are needed to evaluate the independent effect of physical activity on colon cancer. A study on more than 400,000 individuals showed that around 2 hours of moderate physical activity per day or 1 hour of more vigorous activity was associated with a risk reduction for colon cancer of 20%–25% overall and of around 35% for right-sided colon cancer (272). The risk reduction remained significant even in overweight patients though it was stronger among individuals with a BMI of less than 25. Therefore, increased physical activity can be considered essential to any public health program for prevention of colon cancer. The risk of rectal cancer was not found to be affected by physical activity, a finding which is in agreement with previous studies (272).

Smoking

Cigarette smoking can alter the risk of colon cancer. Earlier studies consistently found that long-term smokers have an up to 3-fold higher risk of developing adenoma. Similarly, the risk of CRC was almost doubled in long-term smokers (265). A recent meta-analysis of 36 prospective studies showed that both past and current smokers have an increased risk of CRC incidence and mortality (273). This study also showed a dose-dependent effect for smoking on CRC risk. It was found that not only the duration of smoking increased the CRC risk (RR, 1.20 for an increase of 40 years of duration), but also the amount of daily consumption, pack-years and age of initiation were significantly associated with increase in CRC incidence. This suggests that for CRC, both a relatively high intensity of smoking and a long duration are required to demonstrate appreciably elevated relative risks. The mechanisms of this association are not fully understood. The colonic mucosa can be affected both by systemic effects of carcinogenic by-products from smoking in the blood or by intraluminal exposure to smoke from concomitant oral ingestion (274).

Alcohol

It has been suggested that alcohol consumption is causally associated with CRC. The first report from the WCRF and AICR concluded that alcohol drinking "probably" increases CRC risk (247). The results of the subsequent studies on alcohol consumption and CRC risk have not been consistent and therefore in 2003 the statement was downgraded by a report of a WHO/Food and Agriculture Organization (FAO) Expert Consultation that did not include CRC in the list of alcohol-related malignancies (247).

More recent studies, however, suggest a positive relation between alcohol consumption and the risk of developing CRC. A pooled analysis of 8 cohort studies recorded a dose-response relation between risk of CRC and amount of alcohol consumption (275). Another recently published meta-analysis of cohort studies found a dose-response between alcohol intake and CRC risk. This study also suggested that although the risk of distal colon and rectum malignancies is increased by alcohol intake this effect may not be seen for proximal tumors (276). In fact, it has been shown that alcohol consumption of more than 30 g every day is associated with an increased risk of CRC (277,278). It is suggested that the effect of alcohol on the risk of colon cancer is modified by sex. One-fourth of CRCs in men were attributable to alcohol use of more than 23 g every day (279). The main mechanism of alcohol influence on CRC is thought to be via anti-folate effects, as alcohol adversely affects folate metabolism leading to folate deficiency, which in turn may induce DNA hypomethylation (280).

Metabolic

Type II Diabetes Mellitus (DM)

Type II diabetes and colon cancer are both very common in industrial or westernized countries and share common risk factors such as high BMI, increased central obesity, physical inactivity, and dietary patterns that stimulate secretion of insulin (281). The results from studies that analyzed the association of type II DM and colon cancer are not entirely consistent. One of the first case-control studies reporting this association was published in 1991 and showed an RR of 1.7 for colon cancer among type 2 diabetics (282). In another case-control study this association was only significant in women (RR, 5 1.8; 95% CI, 5 1.2–2.8) and was stronger for colon than rectal cancer (283). A prospective study of 15,487 subjects with diabetes showed that the risk of developing CRC increased significantly only in men (RR, 1.30; 95% CI, 5 1.03–1.65; 284).

Several other prospective studies confirmed an association of type II diabetes and colon cancer after controlling for other covariates such as BMI and physical activity (285,286). These associations in general differ by colonic subsite, and also gender. Recently, elevated HbA1c, a marker for long-term glycemia, was found to be an independent predictor of aggressive clinical behavior in patients with CRC (287).

Several mechanisms have been proposed for the observed relationship between DM and CRC. Hyperinsulinemia and high IGF-1 are present in type 2 diabetes and play important roles in metabolism, cell growth, proliferation, and apoptosis favoring tumorigenesis (288).

Pharmacologic

See previous section "Chemoprevention in CRC" in this chapter discussing chemoprevention.

Peroxisome Proliferator-Activated Receptor Gamma (PPARγ)

The peroxisome proliferator-activated receptor γ (PPARγ) is a member of the nuclear receptor superfamily that is expressed in the intestinal epithelium (289).

PPARγ expression is also found in several malignancies and has been shown to play a role in colon cancer carcinogenesis (290–292). Studies using human colon cancer cells suggested a tumor suppressive role for PPARγ in CRC (293–295), whereas some experiments using animal models showed that PPARγ ligands can enhance colon cancer progression under certain circumstances (296).

The antineoplastic effect of PPARγ may be exerted through inhibition of cell proliferation partly via inhibition of β-catenin translocation into the nucleus and inhibition of subsequent transcriptional neoplastic effects affecting cell turnover, apoptosis, and angiogenesis. Further, PPARγ can inhibit NF-κB–mediated inflammation (297–299). The clear understanding of how PPARγ plays a role in colon cancer pathogenesis warrants further investigation and is of considerable importance since PPARγ agonists are commonly used in management of individuals with type II diabetes (298).

Statins

Some case control studies suggested that use of statins is associated with a risk reduction in CRC (300–302). Statins are suggested to reduce the risk of CRC through several putative mechanisms: in vivo carcinogenesis may be inhibited via reduction of chronic inflammation and associated inflammatory markers (303,304).

Statins also inhibit GTPases (Ras and Rho) to affect cell proliferation and to induce apoptosis (303, 305–307). However, a pooled analysis of prospective studies including 6 RCTs and 3 cohorts in a meta-analysis reported no significant association between statins and CRC (308). This is similar to findings reported by another more recently published meta- and pool analysis of 11 published RCTs that showed no significant correlation of statin use and the risk of CRC (309). Only the subanalysis of the eight cohort studies showed a small but nonsignificant reduction in risk of CRC among statin users (HR, 0.89; 95% CI, 0.75–1.05; 309). Further, a recent prospective study on 159,219 postmenopausal women with an average follow up of 10.7 years showed no significant association between the use of any type of statin and risk of CRC (310). However, when different types of statins (simvastatin, fluvastatin, and lovastatin) were tested separately in relation to the CRC risk, lovastatin was associated with a lower risk of CRC with HR of 0.62 (95% CI, 0.39–0.99; 310). In conclusion, based on the existing literature currently there are no sufficient data to support the role of statins as CRC chemopreventive agents.

Lynch Syndrome as a Model for Identification of Hereditary High-Risk Patients

HENRY T. LYNCH
KRISTEN DRESCHER
POONAM SHARMA
CARRIE SNYDER
JANE F. LYNCH
JOSEPH KNEZETIC
MEGAN HITCHINS
PETER SILBERSTEIN
STEPHEN LANSPA

INTRODUCTION

CRC is relatively common as reflected by its worldwide incidence of 1,200,000, with approximately 50% mortality (311). CRC in the United States is estimated to have an incidence of 142,570 cases with a mortality of 51,370 (~36%; 312). Lynch syndrome (LS) is the most common hereditary form of CRC and is estimated to account for approximately 3%–5% of all CRCs (36,000–60,000 incident cases worldwide; approximately 4277 to 7129 cases in the United States; 313,314). In contrast, FAP accounts for less than 1% of the total CRC burden. Familial CRC, meaning one or more (and, by some definitions, two or more) first-degree and/or second-degree relatives of the index case manifesting CRC, indicates that the index case has an approximate 2-fold increased CRC risk; familial CRC by this definition constitutes about 20% of the total CRC incident burden (248,000 cases worldwide; 28,514 in the United States; 315).

LS is a multifaceted hereditary disorder where these patients have a strong predilection for developing CRC, endometrial carcinoma, and a number of additional extracolonic cancers, which include cancers of the ovary, upper urinary tract, small bowel, hepatobiliary tract, stomach, brain (as in the Turcot's syndrome variant of LS), as well as cutaneous lesions (sebaceous adenomas, sebaceous carcinomas, multiple keratoacanthomas) in the Muir-Torre syndrome (MTS) variant of LS, and more recently breast and prostate cancer. Molecular genetic evidence demonstrates that these extracolonic cancers may have similar underlying pathologies and clinical presentations comparable to the LS CRCs, thus demonstrating that these carcinomas are not spontaneously developing cancers, but rather are part of the LS spectrum (see Table 2.4).

FAMILY CONSIDERATIONS

Importance of Family History

Each hereditary cancer case emanates from a family that could benefit from genetic counseling, molecular genetic testing, surveillance, and targeted management (316–318). Guttmacher et al (9) note that when a patient's family risk of disease development is overlooked "... so too are opportunities for early screening" (319). Furthermore, the United States Surgeon General was concerned enough to launch a campaign promoting awareness of the medical value of family history and encouraging collection and analysis of data (319,320).

The Amsterdam Criteria (AC; 321,322) were developed two decades ago with the goal of developing a consistent criteria for describing and defining LS families. However, current guidelines for LS diagnosis harbor major limitations. Most critically, Boland and Shike (323) determined that screening of all CRC patients meeting the AC would fail to detect half of the cases of LS; screening those age 50 years or younger would also detect only half of all cases, while screening of all patients meeting Bethesda Guidelines for MSI testing would fail to detect about one-third of these cases. The inability of the AC to identify such a large number of affected individuals clearly outlines the need to further refine tools in assisting clinicians in their identification of patients at risk for developing CRC and other LS tumors.

Approximately 60% of families fulfilling the AC have identified MMR germline mutations consistent with a diagnosis of LS (313). A subset of the remaining 40% families include patients with a hereditary cancer syndrome of unknown origin in the absence of a MMR mutation, known as familial CRC type X (324).

Family History in Concert With Molecular Genetics

While the Hampel et al model (testing every single CRC for LS; 313) demonstrates the importance of the role

Table 2.4 Cardinal Features of Lynch Syndrome (LS)

- Autosomal dominant inheritance pattern seen for syndrome cancers in the family pedigree
- Earlier average age of CRC onset than in the general population:
  Average age of 45 years in LS vs 63 years in the general population
- Proximal (right-sided) colonic cancer predilection:
  70%–85% of LS CRCs are proximal to the splenic flexure
- Accelerated carcinogenesis: (tiny adenomas can develop into carcinomas more quickly):
  Within 2 to 3 years in LS versus 8 to 10 years in the general population
- High risk of additional CRCs: 25%–30% of patients having surgery for an LS-associated CRC will have a second primary CRC within 10 years of surgical resection if the surgery was less than a subtotal colectomy
- Increased risk for malignancy at certain extracolonic sites:
  - Endometrium (40%–60% lifetime risk for female mutation carriers)
  - Ovary (12%–15% lifetime risk for female mutation carriers)
  - Stomach (higher risk in families indigenous to the Orient, reason unknown at this time)
  - Small bowel
  - Hepatobiliary tract
  - Pancreas
  - Upper uroepithelial tract (transitional cell carcinoma of the ureter and renal pelvis)
  - Prostate cancer
  - Breast cancer
  - Adrenal cortical carcinomas
  - Brain (glioblastomas in the Turcot's syndrome variant of the LS)
  - Sebaceous adenomas, sebaceous carcinomas, and multiple keratoacanthomas in the Muir-Torre syndrome variant of LS
- Pathology of CRCs is more often poorly differentiated, with an excess of mucoid and signet cell features, a Crohn's-like reaction, and a significant excess of infiltrating lymphocytes within the tumor.
- Increased survival from CRC
- The sine qua non for diagnosis of LS is the identification of a germline mutation in a MMR gene (most commonly *MLH1*, *MSH2*, or *MSH6*) that segregates in the family; that is, members who carry the mutation show a much higher rate of syndrome-related cancers than those who do not carry the mutation

of molecular genetics in identifying LS cases, we must remain fully cognizant of the importance of the family history. Delgado-Plasencia et al (325) assessed the usefulness of a detailed genealogical tree as a screening method for identifying families showing a high probability of LS. The genealogical pedigrees of the families were classified as high or low probability of LS in context with their fulfillment of the AC II. In addition, they analyzed the level of tumor MSI and identified a likely founder mutation in exon 13 of the *MSH2* gene. Ten families with high probability of LS and 30 families with low probability of LS were identified. Those families that were identified as likely to have LS all had high levels of microsatellite instability (MSI-H), while those that were unlikely to have LS had microsatellite stable (MSS) tumors. These investigators concluded that the genealogical tree is an extremely valuable mechanism for determining the possibility that a diagnosis of LS will be made before molecular genetic testing occurs. MSI testing, while showing high sensitivity, nevertheless, has low specificity, due to the fact that MSI-H occurs in approximately 15%–17% of sporadic CRCs (315,326). Those patients with MSI-H findings are referred for additional genetic evaluation, including genetic counseling.

There have been indications that informed consent should be recommended for MSI testing (327) although in clinical practice these recommendations remain inconsistent. However, in the end analysis patient knowledge is rather limited about the MSI test and they remain inadequately informed relevant to its purpose and implications (328).

In virtually all hereditary cancer syndromes, attention is given to ascertaining the proband and completing an extensive medical and family history workup and, when indicated, germline mutation testing. However, physicians, medical geneticists, and genetic counselors often do not extend the same vigor toward other at-risk members of the extended family. In part, this is because insurance coverage is extremely limited for the clinically ideal completion of the genetic counseling process; in short, while the insurance carrier may fund the process for the proband, extension of this funding to the patient's high-risk relatives is often unavailable. As a consequence, the intrinsic value of the crucial and potentially lifesaving message inherent in the genetic information derived from the proband and applicable for diagnosis among family members may not be communicated to the patient's high-risk relatives. This is a pity and it is clearly exemplified in the following example of a family which poses an extremely informative case: A married-in spouse and her two daughters visited our office simply to establish a social relationship, at the suggestion of a hometown acquaintance with LS. The family of the visitor's husband also has LS and she wanted to meet Dr. Lynch to say "Hello." After appropriate introductions, she was asked about her husband's family history but readily admitted that she had limited information on the topic. She knew that her father-in-law, who had nine children, had been diagnosed with LS and had had four metachronous colon cancers, prostate cancer, kidney cancer, and gastric lymphoma. Additionally, the father-in-law had been tested and was negative for *MLH1* and *MSH2* mutations, but *MSH6* testing revealed a variant of unknown significance. Immunohistochemistry (IHC) testing had been performed on one of his colon tumors, wherein the *PMS2* protein was absent, *MLH1* protein was weakly present, and *MSH2* and *MSH6* proteins were present.

Should the *PMS2* mutation be confirmed in his father, her husband (the proband) would automatically be at approximately 50% LS risk, given the autosomal dominant mode of inheritance of *PMS2*. However, he has been exceedingly reluctant to seek genetic counseling or enter into any genetic testing. His main concern is insurance discrimination which he believes could affect his three children as well as other members of his family, if an LS status were confirmed. The presence of the deleterious gene, coupled with its profound cancer risk to his father's nine offspring and their children, created interest and concern by our hereditary cancer clinical and research team. According to his wife, few of the family members at risk had any detailed medical-genetic knowledge of LS and the significance of testing for a pathogenic germline mutation. Importantly, they had virtually no knowledge about the available cancer control measures, in particular colonoscopy which could prove of lifesaving benefit to those relatives who are harbingers of the deleterious mutation.

If this case were an isolated event, it would still be worth reporting. However, the fact of the matter is that this clinical genetic challenge is frequently encountered by us and poses a highly prevalent problem in hereditary cancer settings; soberingly, this issue remains the responsibility of the proband and, unless action is taken by him, may give rise to severe neglect of all of his accompanying high-risk relatives.

Direct Contact and Cancer Control for High-Risk Family Members

Aktan-Collan et al (329) in their review of the literature pertinent to the role of communication in hereditary cancer-prone families note that informing relatives may be challenging for the patient, "... especially when distant relatives are concerned (330) discussing this type of information is discomforting (331–333), and probands tend to inform the nuclear family rather than more distant relatives (334). Therefore, some relatives may remain unaware of the serious genetic condition segregating in the family." As a consequence, they fail to be tested and effectively screened and managed.

The active recruitment of potential high-risk patients who could benefit from education, testing, screening, and management, is a novel approach which Aktan-Collan et al note raises the ethical dilemma of respect for autonomy and privacy versus beneficence which relates to the duty to warn. Theirs may be the first prospective large-scale study of hereditary cancer investigation with concern about attitudes toward a direct contact recruitment method with comparison of psychosocial responses.

Aktan-Collan et al (329) note that in their early experience involving their predictive genetic testing program (335) those who had not applied for genetic counseling and developed colon cancer, without exception, expressed disappointment "... that their relatives had not warned them of their at-risk status...." In addition, their large-scale genetic-testing program "... had been encouraging, confirming high levels of satisfaction and no serious psychological side-effects related to testing [335–337]. These results have since been confirmed by other studies showing similar trends [338–340]. Several groups have proposed that the duty to warn patients may help waive the requirement for confidentiality in cases of life-threatening disease where prevention exists [341–345]...." Of the literature surveyed by Aktan-Collan et al, they found studies that acknowledged that in the interest of preventing harm when serious imminent or treating conditions are present (346), confidentiality can be breached. "... Thus, the resolution of the conflict between confidentiality and the duty to warn is not unambiguous..." (349).

■ LS CHARACTERISTICS

LS Colorectal Cancers

LS CRCs manifest MSI-H, and typically have the following distinctive clinical and pathologic features: (a) predominance of CRC in proximal colon; (b) lymphocyte infiltration within tumor; (c) poorly differentiated mucinous or signet cell appearance; (d) medullary and mucoid features; (e) accelerated rate of progression from adenoma to carcinoma;

(f) better prognosis as evidenced by increased survival; (g) differing response to chemotherapeutics, particularly reduced response to 5-fluorouracil (5-FU); 326,347,348). and favorable preventive response to aspirin (349).

Thanks to the prodigious advances in molecular genetics, the diagnosis of LS can be aided significantly by demonstrating the presence of MSI within the tumor and/or by IHC that identifies a loss of MMR proteins. Diagnosis of LS can be verified by the identification of a germline mutation in one of the MMR genes, the sine qua non for LS's confirmation. Ideally, this molecular testing is performed on high-risk individuals from families that show the clinical-pathology features of LS (see Table 2.4). The goal of targeted, intensive testing for LS in at-risk individuals is of extreme clinical importance to maximize cancer control potential in a person once hereditary cancer risk status has been confirmed (340).

LS is caused by a germline mutation that results in loss of function of one of the DNA MMR genes (315). The MMR proteins are key participants in assuring DNA fidelity during DNA replication. The disorder is inherited in a classic autosomal dominant manner, but at the tissue level the defect in MMR genes functions in a recessive fashion. With the risk of transmission of the mutant allele being 50%, half of the offspring of affected individuals inherit the cancer predisposing mutation. All cells in the body of an LS patient have normal DNA MMR activity, since one functioning MMR allele is sufficient to make adequate amounts of the DNA MMR protein. In an LS tumor, however, there is a "second hit" that inactivates the other (unmutated or "wild type") MMR gene allele inherited from the unaffected parent. Because of the biallelic inactivation of one of the MMR genes that occurs in LS CRCs, the tumor cells have reduced/absent ability to repair DNA mismatches that occur during DNA replication. In addition, these cells have defective repair of DNA damage acquired by other mechanisms (reviewed by Boland and Goel [16]). The lack of an intact DNA MMR system results in a substantial increase in the rate of mutations within the tumor. The short repetitive sequences (microsatellites) are particularly sensitive to the loss of DNA MMR activity resulting in high levels of mutations in these microsatellites, and can be utilized as a bellwether for defects in the MMR proteins. MSI-H is a key feature of LS.

Microsatellite Instability, Immunohistochemistry, and Mismatch Repair Mutations

Most CRCs in LS have MSI; these tumors represent a fundamentally different disease than most sporadic CRCs. The stepwise accumulation of genetic mutations, worked out elegantly by Vogelstein and others two decades ago (351), demonstrated the contributions of these mutations to cancer development through a pathway distinct from that which occurs in most sporadic CRC. Regions of the genome containing repetitive sequences (microsatellites) are extremely vulnerable to extensions and deletions of bases during DNA replication. The MMR proteins maintain genetic fidelity by repairing these errors. MMR mutations do not permit adequate repair processes to occur. In LS, mutations accumulate in genes that contain repetitive elements (microsatellites) within their coding regions, resulting in mutated reading frames and/or premature stop codons, both of which can result in the synthesis of novel proteins referred to as "neopeptides." MSI-H in tumor tissue is routinely detected using PCR.

The DNA MMR system requires a complex interaction among a variety of proteins; some are specialized in recognizing the DNA mismatches as they occur during DNA replication in S phase, others are involved in excision of the erroneously synthesized DNA, and still others are involved in matchmaking between the DNA chain, DNA polymerase, DNA docking proteins, and DNA synthetic enzymes. Initially, only four of the DNA MMR genes have been found to be associated with LS: *MSH2, MLH1, MSH6* and *PMS2* (352,353; Please refer to discussion of epithelial cell adhesion molecule (EPCAM) and epimutation phenomena on pages 31–32). About 90% of LS cases with identified MMR mutations have germline mutations in *MSH2* or *MLH1* and, consequently, these are considered to be the critical DNA MMR genes involved in LS development.

Most of the mutations identified are loss-of-function point mutations disseminated throughout the genes, identified by exonic sequencing. However, *MLH1* and *MSH2* are also frequently subject to structural alterations, accounting for 10%–20% of LS cases (354–357). In the case of *MSH2*, large deletions encompassing at least one exon are typically caused by homologous unequal recombination between Alu elements located within the introns kbs apart, with loss of the intervening sequence (355). The high density of Alu repeat elements scattered throughout the *MSH2* gene increases its susceptibility to genomic deletion and most of these are heterogeneous and occur independently (357). Structural alterations are detected using multiple ligation-dependent probe assay (MLPA; 358–359).

Patients with mutations in *MSH6* develop LS tumors later in life than individuals with mutations in the other MMR genes. Mutations in *PMS2* are associated with an attenuated phenotype (weaker family history and a later age of disease onset compared with individuals with mutations in *MSH2* or *MLH1*; 360, 361) for reasons that are not entirely clear. Therefore, an increased proportion of *MSH6* and *PMS2* mutation carriers may not develop cancer but can nevertheless pass the mutation on to their children, who may develop CRC, often before the age of 50, even with a minimal cancer family history. While these molecular factors provide sound explanations for CRC's etiology and pathogenesis, they ultimately require attention to the complex role of environmental perturbation in this molecular-based carcinogenic process.

While gene sequencing is expensive and limited in availability, and patients may view DNA sequencing as threatening and/or intrusive, IHC testing for the presence or absence of MMR protein expression in the tumor may provide clinicians with guidance regarding need for more intensive monitoring of family members at risk for the development of LS cancers.

Molecular Genetic Screening of All CRC Patients

Given that cancer treatment is most effective when the cancer is in its earliest stages and that there are straightforward means to identify patients at risk for LS cancers, should we test all cases of CRC? Hampel et al (313) answered this question when they investigated 500 consecutive CRC patients and found that 18 (3.6% or 1 in 35 cases) had met the AC. All of these patients had CRCs with MSI. LS was correctly diagnosed in 17 (94%) of these 18 cases by IHC. Of interest was the finding that only eight cases (44%) were diagnosed at less than 50 years and 13 cases (72%) met the revised Bethesda Guidelines. The Evaluation of Genomic Applications in Practice and Prevention (EGAPP) Working Group (314) supports the Hampel et al findings (313) and concluded that using genetic testing strategies to reduce morbidity and mortality in CRC probands and their relatives at high risk for and/or affected by LS is a sound and prudent measure. The EGAPP Working Group (314), using published data from Mvundura et al (362), conducted a cost-effectiveness analysis and found that such screening for LS is cost effective. Using IHC as the preliminary diagnostic test was shown to be the most efficient screening method, since it reduces the need for sequencing all four of the genes normally tested for the diagnosis of LS, to sequencing of only one or two of these genes.

Ladabaum et al (363) investigated cost effectiveness of a Markov model to identify LS considering attention to sex, age at screening, and differential effects for probands and relatives. The target population comprised all those with newly diagnosed CRC and their relatives. The time horizon was lifetime, and the perspective was third-party payer. The outcome measures were life-years, cancer cases and deaths, and costs coupled with incremental cost-effectiveness ratios. The results considered current rates of germline testing, screening, and prophylactic surgery, which "... reduced deaths from CRC by 7%–42% and deaths from endometrial and ovarian cancer by 1%–6%. Among tumor-testing strategies, immunohistochemistry followed by *BRAF* mutation testing for all persons with CRC was preferred, with an incremental cost-effectiveness ratio of $36,200 per life-year gained."

The authors concluded that widespread CRC testing led to LS diagnosis yielding substantial benefits at acceptable cost. This was particularly noteworthy for women with an LS mutation, enabling them to begin regular screening and consider the option of risk-reducing gynecologic surgery with the result of cost effectiveness of this testing, which was dependent on the participation of relatives at risk for LS. In an accompanying editorial (364), Burt notes that the cost effectiveness of these approaches "... was very sensitive to the number of relatives who would undergo mutation-specific testing after a disease-causing mutation was found in an index case. It is interesting that success of tumor testing first has already led some institutions and health policy organizations to recommend MSI or IHC testing in all patients with colon cancer and perhaps in all women with endometrial cancer to find those who should then have genetic testing for Lynch syndrome" (362,365,366).

The findings of Hampel et al (313) and the EGAPP Working Group (314) were based upon meticulous clinical and molecular methodologies, but such an approach to cancer prevention and control may not be practical in most clinical practice settings where a broad gap exists between cancer genetics knowledge and its clinical translation in the medical practice setting at the community level. Nevertheless, the rapid development of centers with molecular genetic expertise, heightened by the ongoing veritably explosive advances in molecular genetics, harbors the potential to provide even more personalized genetic screening services to high-risk families. Undoubtedly, public awareness is increasing about the intrinsic importance of understanding one's genetic information in cancer development as well as common hereditary predispositions to a multitude of noncancer disorders including but not limited to coronary artery disease, hypertension, multiple sclerosis, type 1 diabetes, and the more rare muscular dystrophies. The long list of additional disorders with a hereditary basis is increasingly raising the level for greater attention to one's genetic endowment; thereby, advances can be made in the prevention or, at least, amelioration of genetically based diseases, whenever possible.

■ CANCER SPECTRUM IN LS

Integral Cancers

The known cancer spectrum in LS has become more extensive since early reports by us in the 1960s showed a predominance of only CRC and endometrial cancer in LS patients (367–369). The list of LS-associated cancers has now expanded significantly (see Table 2.4). Carcinomas of the breast and prostate, both of which are extremely common in the general population, have posed a challenge in their inclusion as integral tumors of LS. These cancers are discussed in further detail below.

Breast Cancer and LS

Early anecdotal support for breast cancer's integral association with LS was based upon molecular genetic findings by Risinger et al (370) and Boyd et al (371). Risinger et al described MSI-H in breast cancers in LS kindreds, while Boyd et al (371) reported a case of male breast cancer in an individual with a germline mutation in *MLH1* who was a member of a large LS family. Since these initial reports, many studies have examined the hypothesis that breast cancer is part of the LS cancer spectrum. For example, Walsh et al (372) examined 107 cases of breast cancer from 90 families in the CRC Family Registry (Colon CFR) wherein both breast and colon cancer occurred in families with either modified AC or there was at least one early-onset (less than 50 years) CRC which included available breast tissue as part of the biospecimen registry for MMR. Sections of breast tumors were stained for the MMR proteins (*MLH1, PMS2, MSH2, MSH6*) and then tested for MSI. Breast cancer had arisen in 35 mutation carriers, of which 18 (51%) were negative for an MMR protein as determined by IHC. The missing MMR protein corresponded to the specific MMR germline mutation segregating in the family. Other features of these MMR-deficient breast cancers are that these cancers are more likely to be poorly differentiated, have a high mitotic index, are negative for the estrogen and progesterone receptors, have peritumoral lymphocytes present, and grow in solid sheets. Interestingly, some of these histological features are also those observed in LS CRCs, supporting the inclusion of breast cancer as an integral LS cancer.

Prostate Cancer and LS

Soravia et al (373) described prostate cancer with MSI and an absence of positive staining for *MSH2* and *MSH6* by IHC, suggesting that prostate cancer should be included in LS's tumor spectrum. Grindedal et al (374) further investigated whether germline mutations in MMR genes were associated with prostate cancer in 106 male carriers or obligate carriers of MMR mutations. Prostate cancer developed in nine (8.5%) individuals. IHC was performed on tumor tissue from eight of the nine tumors and in seven of the eight cases, the gene product from the mutated MMR gene was absent. The incidence of prostate cancer was significantly elevated in this population compared to the predicted incidence of the disease (1.52 cases). Furthermore, the age of disease onset was approximately 6 years earlier than in patients without mutated MMR genes, and the risk of developing prostate cancer was almost four times greater in patients with mutated MMR genes compared to the general population.

Other GI Cancers Integral to LS

Extracolonic GI cancers associated with LS include gastric, hepatobiliary, small bowel, and pancreatic adenocarcinomas. In Brazilian families with LS, the most frequent extracolonic cancers are breast, endometrial, uterine cervix, and prostate. Gastric cancer was a more common tumor in men by 3-fold (12 of 77 extracolonic cancers) over hepatobiliary or pancreatic cancer. Only one small bowel cancer was reported among the extracolonic cancers in these men (375). In the women from these families, gastric cancer was the most common extracolonic cancer after breast and gynecologic malignancy. No pancreas or small bowel cancers were reported in the women.

In the Netherlands, Capelle et al also report a significant risk of gastric cancer in LS (8.0% lifetime risk in males; 5.3% in females) and suggest screening by gastroscopy (376).

The median age of onset of gastric cancer was 52 years (range, 24–81 years) in a report from the French Cancer Genetics Network (377).

In the Orient, particularly Korea and Japan, gastric cancer, rather than endometrial cancer, is the most common extracolonic cancer in LS (378).

The risk of pancreatic cancer was reported as 3.7% up to age 70 (379). The National Comprehensive Cancer Network states there are no current recommendations for screening LS patients for pancreatic cancer (380).

In 2005, the German HNPCC Consortium reported on 32 small bowel cancers in LS patients. Median age at diagnosis was 39 years (range, 15–73 years). Fifty percent were in the duodenum (381). Onset of small bowel cancers in LS patients in the French Cancer Genetics Network ranged from age 29 to 71 years (377).

Muir-Torre Syndrome and Its LS Connection

In the late 1960s, Muir and associates (382) and Torre (383) described isolated patients who had MTS, a syndrome characterized by sebaceous adenomas, sebaceous carcinomas, and multiple keratoacanthomas, associated with visceral system cancers, particularly CRC. These early reports did not mention any significant family histories of cancer (382,383) to suggest that a hereditary cancer associated genodermatosis was involved. In the early 1980s, Fusaro et al (384) and Lynch et al (385) reported the cutaneous features of MTS as integral components in five classic LS families (384,385). A review of MTS patients' pedigrees in our Creighton University hereditary cancer resource showed that MTS patients share certain common systemic visceral cancers. At that time, this was called the Cancer Family Syndrome (384–386). The MTS patients were subsequently designated as a variant of LS (386). These classic examples of LS had differing patterns of cutaneous expressions of sebaceous proliferations and keratoacanthomas of the MTS occurring in certain high-risk cancer-affected family members in association with differing phenotypic patterns of expression of colonic and extracolonic visceral cancers (315,317,387). These clinical findings led us to postulate that MTS was a manifestation of an apparently unrelated cancer syndrome, namely LS (384,387).

Since that time, more has been understood about MTS's genotypic and phenotypic heterogeneity, which includes mutations in the MMR genes *MSH2, MSH6, MLH1,* and *PMS2* (388). Biallelic MYH mutations have also been described as causing the MTS phenotype in some cases (389,390).

South et al (391) determined the frequency of MTS among 50 LS families from a population-based series of cancer patients who were newly diagnosed with CRC or endometrial cancer. MTS was identified in families with mutations in *MLH1* (4 of 9 families with *MLH1* mutations), and mutations in *MSH2* (10 of 24 families with *MSH2* mutations). Interestingly, MTS did not develop in families with mutations in *MSH6* or *PMS2*. Furthermore, a specific *MSH2* mutation (c.942+3A>T) had a higher frequency of MTS than families who carried other mutations in the *MSH2* gene (75% vs 25%; $P = .026$). It was concluded that MTS is a variant of LS and therein screening for MTS-associated cutaneous lesions among LS patients is recommended. Clearly, the MTS cutaneous phenotypes are of particular concern when evaluating families with cancers as well as certain noncancer phenotypic features (386,387,392–396). Cutaneous signs are of particular clinical and pathologic significance in the comprehension of the diagnosis, management, and ultimately the etiologic-pathologic-physiologic elements of MTS.

Unusual LS Tumors

Broaddus et al (397) described two young patients, each with a known *MSH2* mutation in the family, who developed rare tumors (adrenal cortical carcinoma and anaplastic carcinoma of the thyroid) that are not usually associated with LS. Both tumors showed complete loss of *MSH2* protein expression as determined by IHC. Additionally, both patients were members of families that fulfilled Amsterdam-II criteria for LS.

Over the years, sarcomas have been described in LS patients, although this is not typically a part of LS. Nilbert et al (398) examined the occurrence of sarcomas in a cohort of patients in the Danish LS registry, which encompassed 164 families and a total of 1570 malignancies. Sarcomas occurred in 14 patients. The sarcomas included, but were not limited to, liposarcomas, gliosarcomas, leiomyosarcomas, and osteosarcomas. *MSH2* mutations were identified in seven of the 14 cases, *MLH1* mutations in four cases, and *MLH6* in three cases. Similar to MTS, no cases developed in patients with mutations in *PMS2*. Undoubtedly, other cancer types will likely be identified as integral lesions in LS.

Germline Biallelic MMR Mutations and GI Phenotype: Constitutional Mismatch Repair Deficiency Syndrome

Jasperson et al (399) described what is referred to as constitutional mismatch repair-deficiency (CMMR-D) syndrome, inherited as an autosomal recessive disorder, in two sisters with biallelic *MSH6* mutations. Hematologic malignancies, brain tumors, and the spectrum of LS-associated cancers may be found in these patients. Patients with CMMR-D syndrome also experience skin manifestations that mimic neurofibromatosis type 1 (NF1). CMMR-D is extremely rare and disease manifestations frequently occur during early childhood. This condition may also involve colonic polyps that are often sparser than is observed in its classical FAP counterpart, but tends to mimic attenuated familial adenomatous polyposis (AFAP) or MUTYH-associated polyposis (MAP). In the report by Jasperson et al (399) it was determined that the two sisters, both with biallelic *MSH6* MMR mutations, were older than patients typically identified with CMMR-D. Their parents were heterozygous for the *MSH6* mutation while their half-sister (sharing the same mother) was heterozygous for *MSH6* mutation. No consanguinity was present in this family.

As the biallelic sisters wanted children, potential concerns were also addressed. They were informed that all children of the biallelic sisters would have a pathogenic *MSH6* germline mutation, and that this would constitute a 100% risk in each pregnancy. An alternative would be fertilization of a donor egg with the husband's sperm, followed by implantation in the sister's uterus. We emphasized that this must be a purely personal decision by these sisters in concert with wishes of the respective husbands.

Jasperson et al (399) in their literature review of cases of CMMR-D syndrome, found 78 patients from 46 families wherein only five of the 78 cases lacked any evidence of cancer, but all of these were 10 years of age or younger (400). The mean age of onset for hematologic malignancies and brain tumors in these studies was 5.5 and 8 years, respectively, while a mean age of onset for LS-associated cancers in CMMR-D syndrome is 16 years. This is striking as it is approximately 30 years earlier than the average age of onset of LS-associated CRCs.

Multiple colonic polyps were identified in one of the mentioned sisters with biallelic mutations at age 23, who subsequently underwent further colonoscopies and sigmoidoscopies over a 4-month period. More than 20 cumulative tubular and tubulovillous adenomas were removed. The patient eventually underwent a total colectomy with ileorectal anastomosis. The proband's 21-year-old sister underwent screening colonoscopy and was found to have a 4-cm or larger cecal polyp and a 7-mm polyp of the sigmoid colon, and these were removed by partial snare polypectomy. Esophagogastroduodenoscopy in this patient identified a tubulovillous adenoma in the duodenum and at the ampulla.

IHC results revealed a possible germline defective *MSH6* sequence. Molecular studies demonstrated 2 mutations in both the proband's and her sister's *MSH6* genes. Both of the mutations are considered deleterious—one mutation is predicted to result in a frameshift mutation (c.1421_1422dupTG) while the other mutation (c.3226C>T [R1076C]) is predicted to result in an amino acid substitution (cysteine to arginine) in a conserved domain in the gene. The sisters' mother carried the c.3226C>T mutation, as did their maternal half-sister; their father had the c.1421_1422dupTG mutation.

The authors note that this is the first reported adult CMMR-D syndrome case presenting as colonic polyposis without a significant personal or family history of cancer. The authors also noted that the more than 20 colonic adenomas identified in the proband could easily be misdiagnosed as AFAP or MAP.

Childhood-onset GI tract cancers presenting as a novel cancer syndrome are often associated with a biallelic MMR mutation. Durno et al (401) studied 237 patients from a Canadian GI cancer registry who had intestinal cancer diagnosed prior to age 35; 5 (2.1%) of these were found to have a biallelic MMR mutation. Using both the registry and a literature review, 32 individuals from 29 families were identified with biallelic MMR germline mutations and GI cancers, 29 of these cancers being CRCs. The mean age of first cancer diagnosis in this cohort was 16.4 years (range, 5–28) among the 29 patients with CRCs. Of these patients, more than a third had multiple colorectal adenomas (greater than 10 polyps). In addition, six patients with biallelic MMR gene mutations had small bowel adenocarcinomas (mean age, 20 years [range, 11–41]). Café au lait macules were reported in 72%; consanguinity was suspected in 52% of kindreds. Interestingly, *PMS2* mutations were highly overrepresented (19 of 29 kindreds or 66%), followed by *MSH6* mutations (6% or 21%), *MLH1* mutations (3% or 10%), and *MSH2* mutation (1% or 3%). It was concluded that biallelic MMR mutations portend an underrecognized etiology for small bowel cancer and CRCs in children and young adults.

Krüger et al (402) also described a distinctive childhood cancer syndrome (CCS) manifesting hematologic malignancies, brain tumors, and bowel cancer in childhood that is frequently associated with NF1. CCS was described in six children from two consanguineous families harboring homozygous *PMS2* germline mutations. In 1 family, all four children harbored the homozygous p.I590Xfs mutation. Two children were diagnosed with glioblastomas at 6 years of age and one of them had three additional LS-associated tumors at age 15. A third sibling was diagnosed with a glioblastoma at age 9, while a fourth sibling was diagnosed with infantile myofibromatosis at age one. In the second family, two of four siblings were homozygous for the p.G271V mutation. One child had two CRCs diagnosed at ages 13 and 14, while the second child had NHL at age 10 and a CRC at age 11. All of the children with cancer showed multiple café au lait spots.

Epithelial Cell Adhesion Molecule and LS

The underlying molecular defect responsible for a portion of AC families without an identified MMR mutation, is a mutation in the *EPCAM* gene, located immediately 5′ of *MSH2* (403–405). A germline deletion removing the 3′ end of *EPCAM* results in tissue-specific methylation and silencing of the otherwise intact *MSH2* gene.

Ligtenberg et al (405) were the first to describe a subset of families with cancer-prone phenotypes consonant with LS, including MSI and IHC, wherein a deletion at the 3′ end of the gene encoding *EPCAM* was identified. These individuals with *EPCAM* mutations harbored *MSI-H* and therein IHC tests showed a loss of *MSH2* protein in the absence of an identifiable mutation of the *MSH2* gene (403,405). Importantly, the *EPCAM* mutations cosegregated with the LS phenotype in approximately 19% of LS families that lacked *MLH1*/*MSH2* mutations (403). *EPCAM* deletions accounted for about 2.3% of explained *MSH2*-deficient families (406).

EPCAM deletions encompass its transcription termination (polyadenylation) signal, permitting transcription to proceed from *EPCAM* downstream across the intervening sequence into *MSH2*, essentially overriding the *MSH2* promoter. This results in promoter methylation and *MSH2* gene silencing. However, since expression of the *EPCAM* gene is restricted primarily to epithelial tissues, it therefore appears to be due to the inactivation of *MSH2* in deletion carriers. Thus, the functional impact that germline *EPCAM* deletions have on *MSH2* activity is confined to epithelial tissues, such as colonic mucosa. This in turn appears to influence the phenotypic expression associated with this type of mutation.

EPCAM deletion carriers may have phenotypic features that differ from carriers of *MSH2* mutations, namely, an almost exclusive expression of cancers in the colon and rectum, with a paucity of endometrial cancers. CRC occurs in *EPCAM* deletion-positive individuals with a frequency comparable to that of carriers of an *MSH2* mutation. Of great interest, however, is the minimal risk of endometrial cancer in individuals with some *EPCAM* deletions when compared with *MSH2* mutation carriers. Importantly, though, when the *EPCAM* gene extends into, or is in close proximity to, the *MSH2* gene, the risk for endometrial cancer becomes equivalent to those with *MSH2* mutations, a higher risk than in those whose deletion is farther from *MSH2*. Determination of the precise boundaries of deletions involving *EPCAM* is likely to be of importance for personalized clinical management of these families.

We have studied an extremely large family (Figure 2.1) containing more than 700 individuals wherein 50 individuals manifested CRC (407). A deletion confined to *EPCAM* was identified in this highly-extended kindred, which has been studied by us for more than 35 years (407). The breadth and size of this *EPCAM*-prone family is testament to the potential impact of a single mutation event (407).

Epigenetics and LS

Epigenetics is defined as "heritable changes in gene expression that are not due to any alteration in the DNA sequence" (408,409). Epigenetic modifications of the DNA sequence (or chromatin) serve as a secondary code, providing functional instructions on whether a gene should be active or suppressed. The best-described epigenetic modification is DNA methylation, which occurs almost exclusively at cytosines within CpG dinucleotides. Hypermethylation of a gene promoter, of which many are embedded within CpG-dense sequences termed CpG islands, results in silencing of gene expression. Acquired epigenetic silencing of tumor suppressor and DNA repair genes, via somatic promoter methylation, is a frequent event in sporadically arising CRC and other cancers. Acquired hypermethylation of the MLH1 promoter accounts for the vast majority of sporadic CRCs demonstrating MSI, which comprise 10%–15% of all incident CRCs (410). Van Engeland et al (411) reviewed recent evidence that indicates that epigenetic alterations add to the complexity of the pathogenesis of CRC, wherein they characterize a subgroup of CRCs that harbor distinct etiology and prognosis. A number of epigenetic changes were highlighted including histone modifications, chromatic looping, microRNAs expression, DNA methylation, and nucleosomal positioning.

In recent years, epigenetic silencing of cancer-associated genes has been found in the normal somatic tissues of individuals who developed a young-onset cancer phenotype synonymous with a familial cancer syndrome, as has been observed in LS. These so-called "constitutional epimutations" manifest as promoter methylation and transcriptional silencing of a single allele within normal somatic tissues, thereby predisposing to cancer (412,413). Hitchins et al demonstrated that hypermethylation of one allele of *MLH1* in somatic cells throughout the body results in transcriptional silencing, thereby predisposing an individual to the development of *MLH1*-deficient, MSI cancers in a pattern typical of LS (414). Tumors associated with constitutional *MLH1* epimutations typically arise following somatic loss of the unmethylated allele through an acquired genetic alteration, further demonstrating that epimutations serve as the "first hit" in cancer susceptibility (415).

Recent evidence has emerged that shows constitutional *MLH1* epimutations exist in two distinct forms: those that arise in the context of a normal gene sequence and are reversible between generations, and those that are linked to an underlying genetic defect and demonstrate classic autosomal dominant inheritance. In the former cases, carriers tend to have a personal history of LS-associated cancer and the *MLH1* epimutations were shown to have arisen de novo in the absence of an identifiable sequence mutation within or in the vicinity of the *MLH1* gene. This type of epimutation is reversible between successive generations, since the offspring of epimutation carriers can inherit the very same genetic allele (that bore the epimutation in the parent), but in an unmethylated and transcriptionally active state (413). In these offspring, the allele has reverted from an inactive epimutant state back to the normal functional state during transmission through the germ line. However, this type of epimutation can also be transmitted from one generation to the next but in an unpredictable non-Mendelian fashion, as observed in one family. Hitchins et al showed that a mother who had presented with multiple LS-associated cancers transmitted her *MLH1* epimutation to just one of her three sons who had each inherited the genetically-identical maternal *MLH1* allele. The epimutation was thus transmitted with this allele to one son, but reverted back to the normal functional state in his two brothers (413). How this stochastic pattern of inheritance occurred remains unknown; however, it seems unlikely that the epimutation was transmitted intact through the maternal germline. It has been shown that *MLH1* epimutations are erased in the spermatozoa of male epimutation carriers, including in the son with the maternally inherited epimutation. This is observed as a complete absence of methylation and reactivation of the allele in spermatozoa, despite the methylation and allelic silencing throughout the somatic tissues of these individuals (413,416). Thus, it seems this type of epimutation is erased in the germ line, then reestablished in a proportion of the members of the next generation but not in others. The risk and mode of inheritance and onset in these cases remain unknown at present, which is a confounding factor in genetic counseling of these families.

On the other hand, soma-wide *MLH1* methylation and transcriptional loss has also been described in conjunction with a genetic alteration of the *MLH1* gene in a small number of LS cases. These genetic alterations presumably act in cis to induce the epimutation, although the precise mechanism by which this occurs has not been defined. A deletion encompassing the first exon of *MLH1*, with constitutional methylation of the intact promoter sequence upstream (consistent with an *MLH1* epimutation), has been described in one individual (417). Another

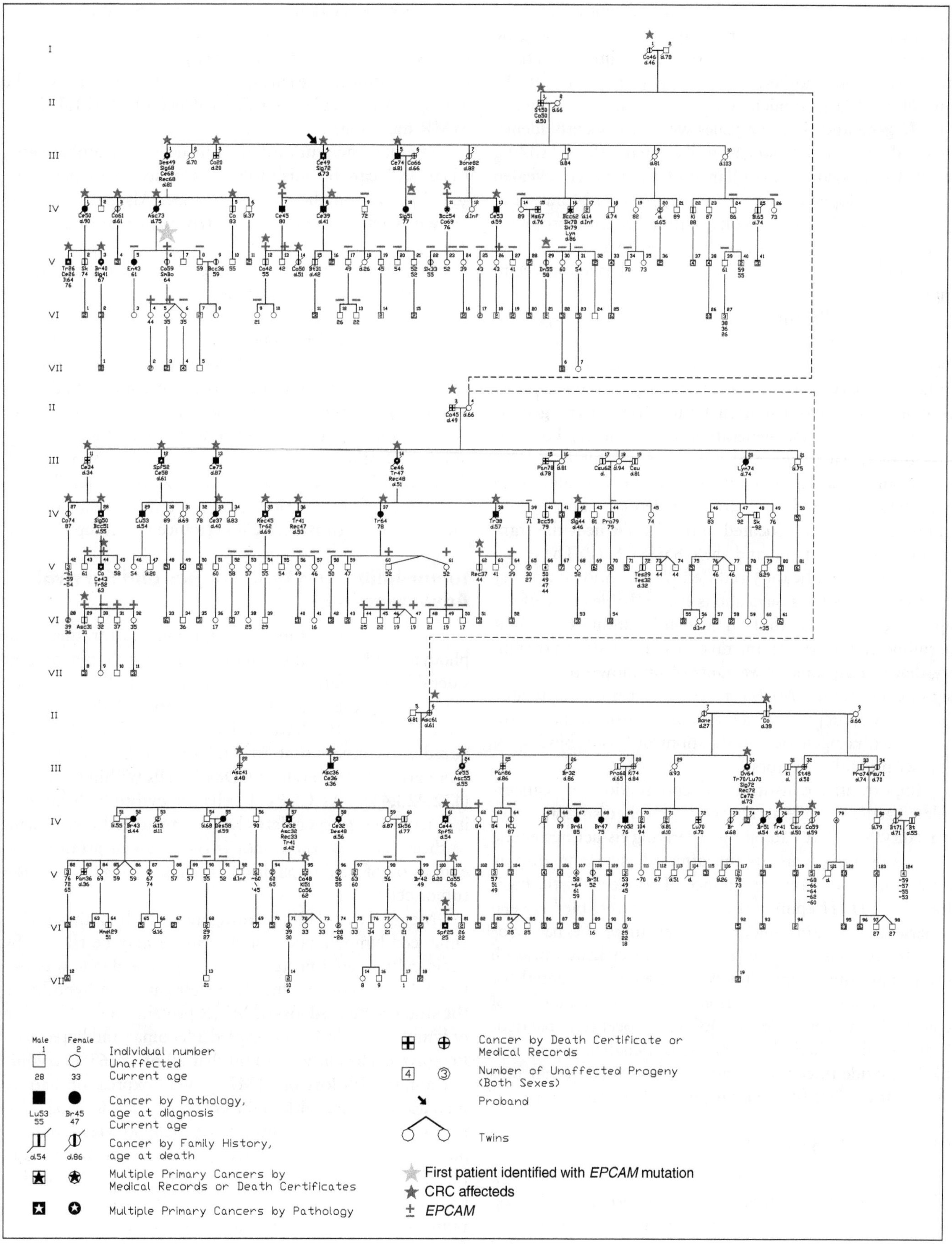

FIGURE 2.1 Pedigree of large family with *EPCAM* mutation. Numbers below the symbols refer to the age in years of last clinical follow up. Published with permission from Lynch et al, *American Journal of Gastroenterology,* 2011;106:1829–1836.

seemingly sporadic proband identified with low-level soma-wide *MLH1* promoter methylation and partial gene silencing was found to have inherited the epimutation from his 64-year-old mother, who was asymptomatic at the time (418). A large tandem duplication spanning the entire *MLH1* gene and flanking genes was subsequently identified in the mother and son, as well as an unaffected sibling (419). Colonoscopic surveillance of the mother revealed she had developed a CRC at 65 years of age. Morak et al (418) cautioned that "... constitutional *MLH1* promoter methylation may therefore in rare cases be a heritable disease mechanism and should not be overlooked in seemingly sporadic patients."

Recently, Hitchins et al described a three-generation LS pedigree meeting the AC with soma-wide highly mosaic *MLH1* methylation and transcriptional repression linked to a particular variant genetic haplotype (420). The epimutation was transmitted faithfully with the genetic haplotype from one generation to the next, but was erased in spermatozoa and reinstated on this haplotype in the somatic cells of the next generation. The affected haplotype harbored two single nucleotide substitutions in tandem; c.-27C>A located in the 5′UTR near the transcription initiation site and the c.85G>T SNP. The c.-27-C>A variant significantly reduced transcriptional activity in in vitro reporter assays and is the probable cause of the epimutation in this family. The identification of a 5′UTR germline c.-27C>A variant raises the interesting possibility that other promoter variants of unknown pathogenic significance within *MLH1* as well as other cancer-related genes may confer cancer susceptibility through their association with epigenetic modifications or loss of binding of transcriptional activators.

Importantly, constitutional epimutations of cancer-related genes provide an alternative mechanism for cancer causality. Some are caused by underlying cis-acting genetic alterations proximate to the affected gene and display autosomal dominant inheritance. The mechanistic basis for other *MLH1* epimutations that are reversible between generations remains undefined. Certainly, the basis for *MLH1* epimutations will need to be investigated in each individual family, since this will dictate the potential for transmission to new generations. A full understanding of epigenetics and its role in CRC carcinogenesis, particularly its role in heritable cancers, is a challenge that will likely provide researchers and clinicians with insight into how best to identify and manage familial CRC cases.

Familial CRC Type X

As many as 30%–40% of families who fulfill AC lack MSI-H and MMR mutations and are referred to as having familial CRC type X (424). This phenotype varies from LS as the familial CRC type X CRCs are more often left-sided in the colon, and extracolonic cancers are less frequent in these patients than is observed in LS patients. There is also a later age of onset in patients with familial CRC type X than those CRCs that are positive for MMR germline mutations. The sine qua non for this diagnosis is the absence of molecular genetic evidence of LS (MSI, IHC, MMR mutation).

The nomenclature for this phenotype is problematic. "Type X" can be misleading, as it seems to place the genetic cause on the X chromosome. Also, it is not yet known whether these families represent one or multiple disorders (423).

The phenomenon of clinical presentation of a well-defined hereditary disease in the absence of the known genetic markers of the disease is not peculiar to familial CRC type X. For example, Fernández-Ramires et al (421) note that while *BRCA1* and *BRCA2* account for approximately 25% of the hereditary breast-ovarian cancer syndrome, the etiology of the remaining familial breast cancer cases (so-called *BRCAX* cases) remains elusive. Mutations in a number of other genes including *TP53, PTEN, CHEK2, ATM, BRIP1/FANCJ,* and *PALB2/FANCN* contribute to some cases of familial breast cancer, but our knowledge of the mechanism of *BRCAX* inheritance is incomplete.

Tumor-Infiltrating Lymphocytes and Survival Advantage in LS

The presence and function of tumor infiltrating lymphocytes (TILs) in any tumor has been a matter of considerable speculation and debate (422–437). Numerous studies over the years have demonstrated that patients with MSI-H CRCs have an increased level of TILs compared with tumors that are MSS or MSI-L; in particular, there are elevated levels of CD8+ T cells within the tumor (422,423,435). As CD8+ T cells are cytotoxic in nature, it is tempting to speculate that the enhanced recruitment of these cells into the tumor is the result of priming and expansion of a subpopulation of lymphocytes that lyse the tumor cells.

Meijer et al (438) investigated the hypothesis that enhanced lymphocytic response in LS may be elicited by genetically altered proteins that may arise due to a defective DNA MMR system. To investigate this hypothesis, the study correlated loss of MMR proteins and infiltration of lymphocytes in LS-associated adenomas and hyperplastic polyps. The authors found that 20 of 32 (63%) colonic adenomas with loss of MMR protein expression had an increase in TILs, with eight adenomas (25% of 32) displaying many tumor-infiltrating lymphocytes, and 12 adenomas (38% of 32) showing a minor increase. In adenomas that did not lose MMR protein expression, neither sporadic nor LS-associated tumors showed an increased number of TILs. In LS patients, hyperplastic polyps manifested neither loss of MMR expression nor an increase in TILs. These authors concluded that there was a correlation between loss of MMR proteins and infiltration of TILs in LS-associated adenomas.

One mechanism to account for the increase in TILs within MSI-H tumors is that the defect in MMR genes has reduced the level of fidelity in the DNA replication process. Because of insertions, deletions, and premature stop codons, novel proteins are generated by the tumor when MSI-H is present. These novel proteins are presented as neopeptides to infiltrating T cells by antigen specific cells. Because the neopeptides were not expressed in the thymus during development, central tolerance has not developed to the peptides, thereby resulting in the likelihood that neopeptide-reactive T cells exist in the periphery. This is in contrast to the situation that occurs in MSS tumors. The tumors are weakly immunogenic, as the antigens expressed by the tumor are closely related to the host; therefore, the immune system ignores these proteins. The presence of the neopeptides in the tumor enhances the immunogenicity of the tumor, making it appear less like self and permitting a robust immune response to develop. While the immune response does not clear the tumor, it does appear to be sufficient to control the spread of the tumor, as LS patients experienced fewer metastases than individuals with non-LS CRCs.

In addition to the increased number of CD8+ T cells in LS CRCs, there are other features of the immune response that may contribute to the survival advantage in LS patients. There have been studies characterizing the levels of T regulatory cells (CD4+CD25+) within the tumors (439). In general, this subset of T cells is considered antiinflammatory via their production of cytokines such as transforming growth factor-β (TGF-β) and IL-17, which dampen the cellular immune response and increase the potential for metastatic events by enhancing angiogenesis (440,441). Some studies have shown that tumors from LS patients have fewer T regulatory cells infiltrating the tissue than do MSS tumors (443). Together with the increased levels of CD8+ T cells which lyse tumor cells, the resultant immune response in LS patients assists in the control of tumor growth and metastasis, ultimately resulting in increased survival time. Table 2.5 outlines the immunological factors that are ultimately postulated to impact survival in LS patients.

Figure 2.2 shows a graphic representation of this process. Tumors with intact MMR genes express peptides that are very similar to those found throughout the body. The body recognizes these peptides within the tumor as self. A strong immune response is not generated and the tumor grows and metastasizes. When there is a defect in the MMR genes, frameshift peptides are generated due to the lack of proofreading that occurs during DNA replication. Because these altered peptides are expressed only in the tumor, the immune system has not developed central tolerance to them. The host can generate a strong immune response to the tumor that may control the growth of the tumor.

Pathology of LS CRC

LS cancers reveal a variety of specific pathologic associations that are an important first step in identifying individuals with LS. These patients usually present with adenocarcinoma of the proximal colon, with or without synchronous or metachronous colorectal or other primary malignancy typical of the syndrome (eg, stomach, urinary tract, skin, and in women ovarian and endometrial carcinomas). LS CRCs are more likely to be multiple, have a polypoid or exophytoic growth pattern, and are less likely to present as diffuse growth or tight stricture. They show sharply circumscribed pushing margins. Although the majority of colorectal carcinomas arising in LS patients are generally similar to sporadic nonMSI H CRC, a variety of tumor types and histologic features are identified with increased frequency in LS and MSI-H CRCs: mucinous, signet ring cell, and medullary carcinoma, tumor infiltrating, and peritumoral lymphocytes, a "Crohn-like" inflammatory response, poor differentiation and tumor heterogeneity (442,443). These histologic features can thus further aid in the identification of patients with LS-associated CRC.

An increased incidence of mucinous carcinomas (see Figure 2.3a) in cancer family syndrome was first noted in 1986, predating the recognition of MSI and the genetic basis of Lynch syndrome by 7 years (444,445). Mucinous carcinoma, defined as tumors with greater than 50% extracellular mucin, is identified in approximately 20% of MSI-H tumors (446). Of note, the association between mucinous histology and DNA MMR deficiency is high even when less than 50% of the tumor reveals this feature (443,446).

Signet ring cell carcinomas (see Figure 2.3b) are defined as tumors containing more than 50% of signet

Table 2.5 Potential Immunological Factors Involved in Enhancing Survival in Lynch Syndrome (LS) Patients

Factor	Function
Increased level of CD8+T cell infiltration	Enhanced killing of tumor cells
Generation of neopeptides	Increased immunogenicity of tumor
Decreased T regulatory cells	Enhanced cellular immunity
Decreased TGF-β levels	Enhanced cellular immunity/ decreased metastases
Decreased IL-17 levels	Decreased angiogenesis/ metastases
Increased granzyme B levels	Increased CD8+ killing
Decreased IL-6 levels	Enhanced cellular immunity

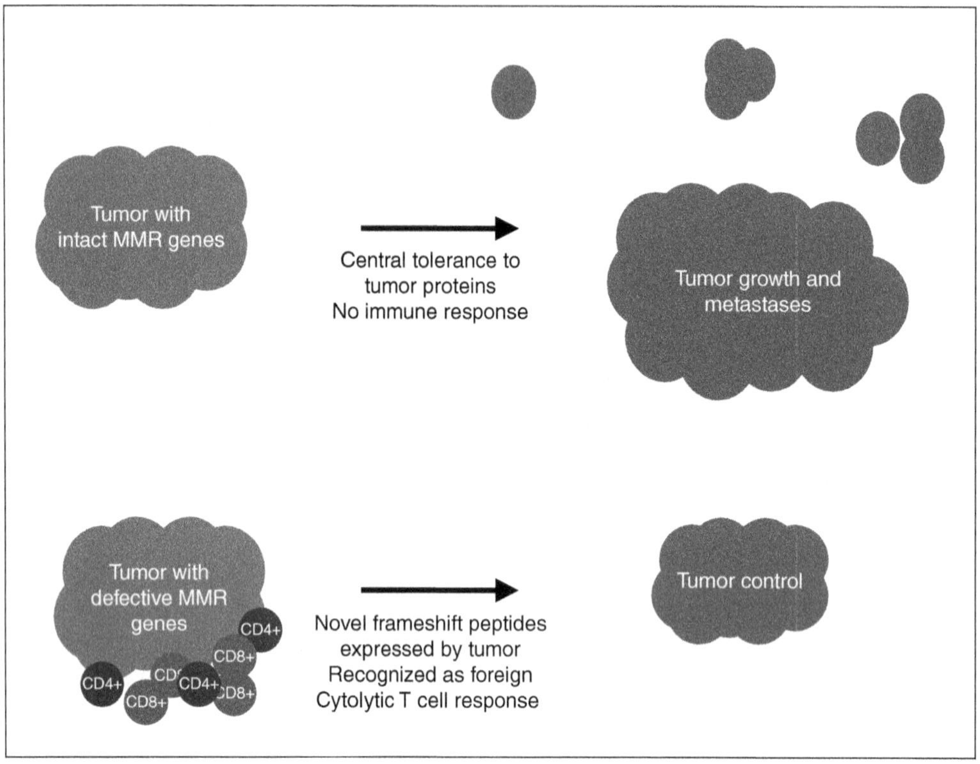

FIGURE 2.2 Defects in DNA mismatch repair genes leads to the generation of immunogenic peptides expressed by the tumor.

ring cells. Signet ring cells contain prominent intracytoplasmic mucin, typically displacing nucleus to one side of the cell. The American Joint Committee on Cancer and the College of American Pathologists accept signet ring cell morphology to be an independent adverse prognostic factor. Approximately, one-third of signet ring cell carcinomas of the colorectum are MSI-H. The MSI-H status is a predictor of favorable outcome in colorectal carcinomas. However, the correlation of MSI status with signet ring cell morphology indicates that the MSI-H status does not confer survival advantage in signet ring cell carcinomas of the colorectum (447).

Medullary carcinoma, a subtype of colorectal carcinoma, is composed of sheets of polygonal cells with vesicular nuclei, prominent nucleoli, and abundant cytoplasm, and is associated with a marked intratumoral and peritumoral lymphocytic response. Tumor cells may have an organoid or trabecular architecture, and a well-circumscribed margin. Medullary-type carcinoma shows high specificity (99%) for MSI-H status but the low frequency of this tumor type (prevalence of only 4%) results in low sensitivity of only 14% (448).

Pathology Perspective of Tumor Infiltrating Lymphocytes

As discussed earlier in this chapter, a wide variety of host lymphocytic responses have been noted in LS cancers. These include TILs, peritumoral lymphocytic and "Crohn-like" reaction. TILs refer to the lymphoid component intimately admixed with the tumor. They have been shown to consist largely of CD3/CD8 coexpressing cytotoxic T cells and their prominence is speculated to represent a possible basis for the improved prognosis in MSI-H tumors. The presence of TILs, which can be evaluated with ordinary light microscopy, is highly predictive of MSI-H cancer type (434,445). Various methods and thresholds for counting TILs have been reported, including evaluation of hematoxylin and eosin or CD3-immunostained slides (443,449,450). Peritumoral lymphocytic reaction is defined as a conspicuous band of lymphocytes found at the leading edge of the tumor. The "Crohn-like" reaction is composed of at least four nodular lymphoid aggregates counted in low power field (4× magnification; Figure 2.3c) beyond the advancing edge of the tumor, typically identified at the junction of the muscularis propria and pericolonic adipose tissue. Thresholds for a positive "Crohn-like" reaction range from two or more large lymphoid Aggregates in a section to four nodular aggregates in a low-power field (4× magnification; Figure 2.3d; 442,449).

Histologic evaluation is an efficient and cost-effective method compared with collecting and confirming a detailed family history, and is more sensitive and specific at identifying MSI-H tumors. Pathologic evaluation is also more useful in situations where an informative family history is not available. Histology-based models, such as PREDICT and MsPath, for prediction of MSI in CRC have been proposed where the pathologists score parameters such as patient age, anatomic site, and pathologic features while conducting routine histologic valuations of CRCs

(442,446,449). These models can be valuable in identifying cases that have high probability of MSI-H status and thus require further testing of microsatellite status.

The pathology of LS cancer is similar to that of sporadic MSI-H colorectal carcinoma. Some studies highlight subtle differences between the two. Compared with sporadic MSI-H CRCs, LS cancers are more likely to occur in men, present at a younger age (generally less than 60 years), and be associated with prior CRCs or LS extracolonic cancers. LS CRCs are also typically associated with a residual precursor adenoma, compared with a high association with serrated polyps (see Figures 2.4 a and b) in the sporadic counterpart. When microscopic features are considered, lymphocytic infiltration is more common in LS cancers, whereas poor differentiation, tumor heterogeneity, and glandular serration are more common in sporadic MSI-H CRCs.

Histopathological features alone cannot reliably discriminate between MSI-H tumors of LS and MSS tumors. In one study, histopathologic evaluation alone could not reliably detect approximately 40% of MSI-H cancers and 6% were never detected by histopathology (448). Therefore, specific MSI testing is recommended if clinical criteria alone indicated the presence of LS.

IHC is available as part of the routine service in the general pathology laboratories and constitutes a convenient screening tool for identification of LS. Around 1996, monoclonal antibodies against MMR proteins started to become available (451,452). IHC testing that assesses all four MMR proteins (*MLH1, MSH2, MSH6*, and *PMS2*)

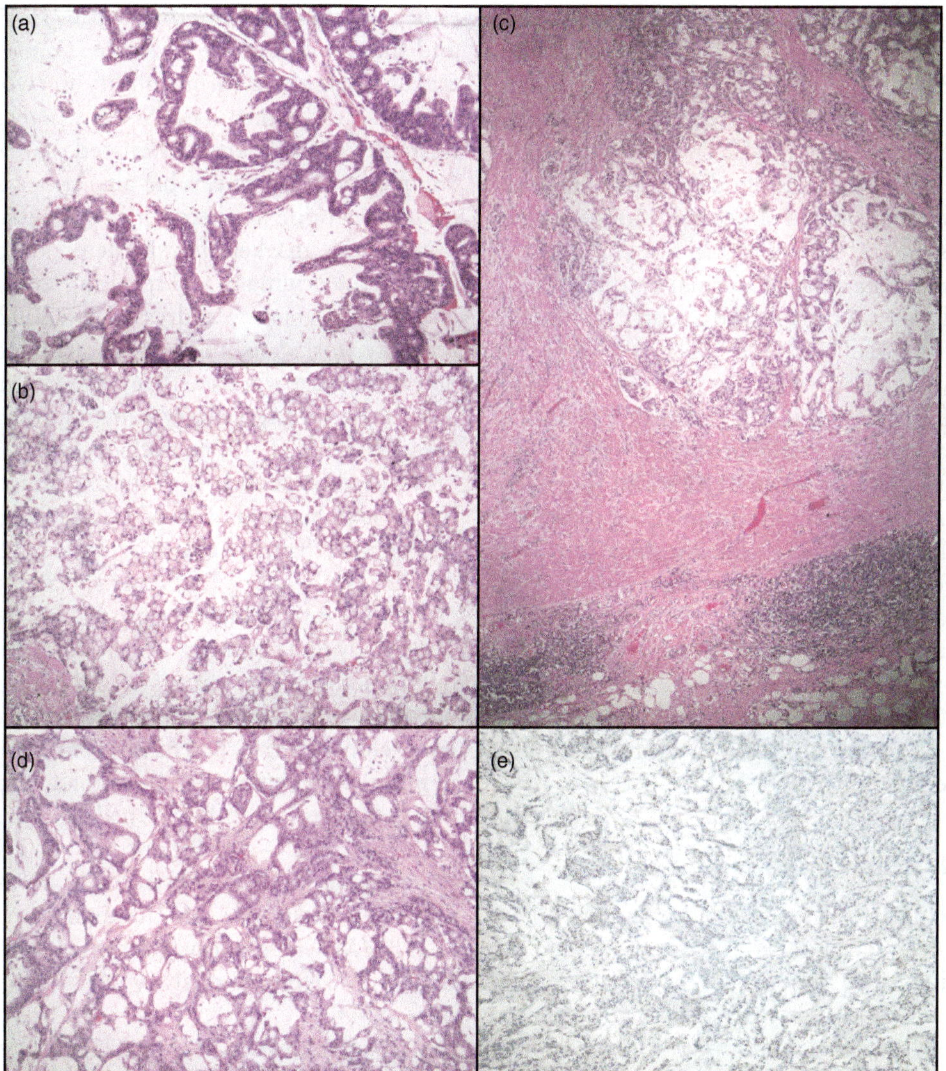

FIGURE 2.3 (a) Mucinous adenocarcinoma (20× magnification). (b) Signet ring cell carcinoma (20× magnification). (c) Mucinous adenocarcinoma with "Crohn-like" inflammatory response below the advancing edge of tumor (4× magnification). (d) Mucinous adenocarcinoma with "Crohn-like inflammatory response (4× magnification). (e) *MLH1* immunohistochemical stain. No staining is observed in the tumor cells indicating loss of *MLH1* MMR protein.

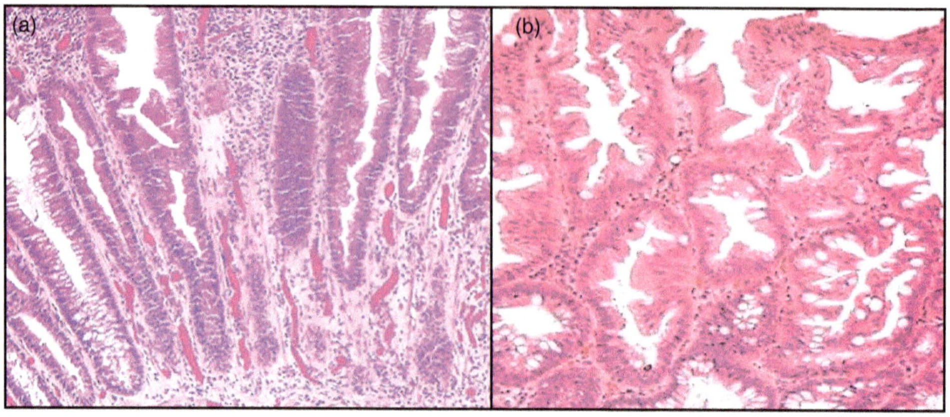

FIGURE 2.4 (a) Serrated adenoma (4× magnification). (b) Serrated adenoma (10× magnification).

has a sensitivity of 92% in predicting germline mutation in these genes, which is equivalent to that of MSI. The specificity is believed to be high; one study reports 95% specificity for IHC testing of both *MLH1* and *MSH2* (453). Thus, loss of expression of MMR proteins serves as a reasonably reliable test of MMR deficiency. In evaluating the expression of these antibodies, any tumor cell nuclear expression is considered positive due to the heterogeneity of expression and difficulties in test standardization. Nuclear immunostaining of normal epithelial cells, lymphocytes, and stromal cells served as internal positive controls (see Figure 2.3e).

IHC is readily available, rather inexpensive, and helps identify the mutated gene. IHC may also detect MMR-deficient cases that can potentially be missed by MSI testing. Limitations to IHC do exist. IHC staining pattern may vary, resulting in uncertainty in interpretation, and it may not be reliable in a small biopsy specimen. IHC is reliable in screening for mutations that result in truncation or degradation of the protein. However, in some cases missense mutations will result in loss of function of MMR enzymes but the protein will still be expressed and detectable by IHC (454). IHC results may be interpreted as genetic information, which can complicate the use of IHC as a first-line screening tool.

Microsatellite Instability Testing

MSI testing is being used as a surrogate marker of LS and has been widely accepted as a primary method for identifying individuals at risk for LS. Frameshift mutations in microsatellites can be identified by extraction of DNA from both normal and tumor tissue (usually paraffin-embedded tissue), amplification of selected microsatellites by PCR, and analysis of fragment size by gel electrophoresis or an automated sequencer. The original Bethesda Guidelines (1997) proposed a panel of five microsatellite markers for the uniform analysis of MSI in LS (454,455). This panel, which is referred to as the Bethesda panel, includes two mononucleotide (BAT-25 and BAT-26) and three dinucleotide (D5S346, D2S123, and D17S250) repeats. Samples with instability in two or more of these markers are defined as MSI-H, whereas, those with one unstable marker are designated as MSI-low (MSI-L). Samples with no detectable alterations are MSS. Because mononucleotide markers appear to be more sensitive than dinucleotide markers for the detection of MSI-H, limitations in the original panel resulting from inclusion of dinucleotide repeats were addressed at a 2002 National Cancer Institute workshop, and revised recommendations for MSI detection were proposed (456). The revision mainly recommends testing a secondary panel of mononucleotide markers, such as BAT-40, to exclude MSI-L in cases in which only the dinucleotide repeats are mutated. According to the revised Bethesda Guidelines, strategies based on MSI testing are effective in identifying *MLH1/MSH2* mutation carriers (sensitivity 81.8% and specificity 98.0%).

MSI testing is highly reproducible. MSI analysis could potentially identify a tumor that has defective DNA MMR but intact IHC staining possibly due to nontruncating missense alterations or mutations in other MMR proteins not included in the current IHC panel. Unlike IHC, which requires well experienced pathologists, molecular laboratory directors can be trained to read MSI test results. Although MSI is a hallmark for LS, it is not specific for LS. MSI has been demonstrated in 10%–15% of sporadic CRCs. Although the *MSH6* gene is a component of the DNA MMR machinery, LS tumors with germline mutations in *MSH6* tend to show MSI-L and therefore may be missed (457).

To some extent, MSI and IHC are complementary to each other in identifying LS. MSI can provide a fallback position in situations where IHC is normal and yet clinical suspicion exists, or IHC is inconclusive. MSI testing will also remain a significant research tool for discovering new MMR gene abnormalities (454).

BRAF Testing

MSI has been demonstrated in 10%–15% of sporadic CRCs. MSI-H status in sporadic CRC is largely attributed to hypermethylation of the 5′ CpG island in the *MLH1* promoter. The methylation is typically associated with loss of *MLH1* protein expression on IHC. This so-called epigenetic silencing affects gene function by aberrant methylation of DNA without genetic changes at the DNA sequence level. *BRAF* (V600E) mutation is frequently present in sporadic CRCs with *MLH1* hypermethylation, but not present in LS (458,459). Therefore, the incorporation of *BRAF* V600E mutation testing into the laboratory algorithm is recommended for patients with suspected LS, whose CRCs show loss of expression of *MLH1* (460,461). This approach can avoid costly and labor consuming germline sequencing and rearrangement analysis of *MLH1* in such cases.

Hyperplastic Polyps and Serrated Adenomas

The etiology of hyperplastic polyposis syndrome (HPS) remains elusive. Buchanan et al (462) identified a significant increase in these polyp numbers in association with direct exposure to cigarette smoking. Therein, they suggested that cigarette smoke exposure may play a modulation role in the phenotype and cause increased polyp numbers. Specifically, these authors showed, as in previous studies, that the cigarette smoking effect and CRC was "... largely due to the strong effect of smoking on the subset of CRC which arose through the serrated hyperplasia pathway...(463) with the most significant association between smokers and serrated neoplasia in the population having both hyperplastic and adenomatous polyps (464), a phenotype shared with individuals with HPS.... "

Roberts et al (465) discussed the examination of linkage in nonsyndromic CRC families and in their review they found reports of statistically significant associations at 3q22, 7q31, and 9q22. Their recent study found linkage to 7q31 in CRC families, which confirmed the region at 3q22 as a susceptibility locus for CRC (466). They discussed families with multiple cases of neoplasia wherein serrated polyps were prominent and therein facilitated the exploration "... of a proportion of the remaining unexplained familial aggregation. Such families were initially reported from New Zealand by the late Professor Jass and colleagues in the mid-1990s (467,468), and a further publication demonstrated the familial involvement of hyperplastic polyposis (463), associated with loss of heterogeneity (LOH) at chromosome 1p. Families fulfilling the Amsterdam I criteria with mixed epithelial polyps and variable levels of microsatellite instability (MSI) in which LS could be excluded, and which showed some overlap with hyperplastic polyposis, were reported in 2005 (469). Such families are characterized by a mixture of serrated and adenomatous polyps, and, in contrast to LS, somatic *BRAF* mutation is commonly observed in CRC. Only a minority of cancers demonstrate MMR deficiency, attributable to methylation of the *MLH1* gene promoter. We refer to this condition of serrated neoplasia and adenomas clustered in families as Jass syndrome, after the pathologist who first described it" (467,468).

Roberts et al (465) also studied genomic regions associated with Jass syndrome through genome-wide linkage screen in one large family, and finemapping in an additional 10 families, and therein they presented evidence "... for linkage to chromosome 2q32.2-q33.3. Through further finemapping analysis, we also provide evidence that previously reported CRC susceptibility loci at 3q22, 7q31, and 9q22 are unlikely to contribute to Jass syndrome."

Young and Jass (470) studied an alternative pathway of CRC that showed serrated polyps replacing the traditional adenoma as the precursor lesion. Therein, they noted that serrated polyps in a subset of CRC harbor "... largely nonoverlapping mutation profiles to those found in adenomas and the majority of CRC. These genetic alterations include activating mutation of the *BRAF* proto-oncogene and widespread gene promoter hypermethylation (CpG island methylator phenotype or CIMP)...." They note that FAP and LS both develop via the adenoma-carcinoma pathway and the 2 syndromes together account for approximately one-third of familial CRC.

Young and Jass (470) had described 11 CRC-prone families with evidence of an autosomal dominant CRC phenomenon that is linked to the serrated pathway, which has been referred to as serrated pathway syndrome (Jass syndrome), in concert with the related disorder hyperplastic polyposis with suggestion of a recessive mode of hereditary transmission. Therein, the *BRAF* mutation and methylation co-occur within serrated precursor lesions. Furthermore, "... CIMP is observed in the normal colonic mucosa of individuals with hyperplastic polyposis consistent with a field defect in epigenetic regulation. The spectrum of serrated neoplasia may also implicate the apparently sporadic and later onset subset of CRC with high levels of microsatellite instability. The tendency for these lesions to be multiple, associated with smoking, and to show frequent *BRAF* mutation and CIMP points to a defect that may result from interactions between the environment and a weakly penetrant genetic alteration."

Boparai et al (471) found that hyperplastic polyps (HPs) and sessile serrated adenomas (SSAs) are a common finding in MYH-associated polyposis (MAP), which is due to a biallelic germline MYH mutation and is characterized by multiple colorectal adenomas. From the molecular genetic standpoint, they note that "... The detection of almost exclusively G:C>T:A transversions in the *K-ras* gene of HPs/SSAs strongly suggests that these polyps are related causally to MYH deficiency. This implies that distinct pathways, that is, *APC*-gene related in adenomas and non-related in HPs/SSAs, appear to be operational in MAP."

The majority of sporadic CRCs that have deficient MMR (dMMR) are believed to arise in SSA/P (472,473) in the proximal colon of older patients (474). The morphology of SSA/P differs from traditional colonic adenomatous polyps, which are the precursors for sporadic CRCs with proficient MMR (pMMR) and LS dMMR CRCs (472, 473).

Jass (472) and Snover (473) have shown that SSA/P with dysplasia is the precursor for sporadic dMMR CRC. Its molecular features include BRAFc1799T>A mutation, a generalized increase in CpG island methylation (the CpG island methylator phenotype, CIMP), *MLH1* promotor hypermethylation, and MSI-H.

Snover (473) recognizes fully that adenocarcinoma of the colorectum is not a single disease entity but rather constitutes a family of diseases with differing precursor lesions, differing molecular pathways, as well as different end-stage carcinomas associated with varying prognoses. While approximately 60% of CRCs are attributable to precursor conventional adenomas via the suppressor pathway and going on to MSS carcinomas, nevertheless the carcinogenic pathway has been targeted for cancer control.

In addition, about 35% of these CRCs are attributable to the serrated pathway "... developing from the precursor lesion known as the sessile serrated adenoma (also referred to as the sessile serrated polyp). Sessile serrated adenomas/polyps lead to carcinomas with extensive CpG island promoter methylation (CpG island methylated phenotype positive carcinomas), which can be either microsatellite instable high or microsatellite stable. The remaining 5% of carcinomas arise from conventional adenomas in patients with germ line mutations of mismatch repair genes (Lynch syndrome), leading to CpG island methylated phenotype negative microsatellite instable carcinomas...." Furthermore, CRCs attributable to sessile serrated adenomas/polyps are not prevented when conventional adenomas are removed and thereby may be missed through routine screening programs wherein "... a subset of these lesions may potentially progress rapidly to carcinoma; hence, it is likely that these lesions will require a different screening strategy from that used for conventional adenomas...." Clearly, more research will be necessary to fully understand the etiology and pathogenesis of the serrated pathway to CRC.

■ MANAGEMENT

Screening Colonoscopy in LS

The ability to reduce cancer mortality through colonoscopic surveillance in LS has been fully demonstrated (475, 476). Colonoscopy for mutation carriers in LS families is mandated, given CRC's proximal occurrence (70%–80% proximal to the splenic flexure) and needs to start by age 25 due to LS's early age of onset (average 45 years of age). Should CRC occur in an individual with a defect in a MMR gene, subtotal colectomy may be necessary, given the marked frequency of synchronous and metachronous CRC (477).

Because of accelerated carcinogenesis, observed in LS patients, colonoscopy should be repeated every 1 to 2 years through age 40 and then annually thereafter. Järvinen et al (478), studying a highly compliant LS population over a 10-year period, demonstrated that while not all deaths could be prevented (due to noncompliance or missed lesions), colonoscopy at intervals of 2 to 3 years can reduce mortality in LS patients. The advantage of more frequent colonoscopy was studied by Vasen et al (479) who showed a lower risk for CRC in LS using 1 to 2 year screening intervals compared to 2 to 3 year intervals. Edelstein et al (480) evaluated serial colonoscopy findings from 54 individuals representing 29 pedigrees with pathogenic mutations in *MSH2* or *MLH1* to determine the development of colorectal neoplasia relevant to age, sex, tumor location, and number. The mean follow-up time in this study was 9.3 years, and the mean colonoscopy interval was 1.7 ± 1.2 years. In the cohort, 112 adenomas and 31 cancers were identified. "Dwell time" was calculated from individual instances where one colonoscopy was clear, and the next showed neoplasia. The dwell time for advanced adenomas (containing a villous component) was 33.0 ± 16.2 months. Dwell time for CRC was 35.2 ± 22.3 months. The authors conclude that the dwell time is short for colon neoplasia in LS and annual colonoscopy is warranted. The study reported an excellent CRC 5-year survival rate that supported data that colonoscopy screening-surveillance is a life-saving tool.

Efficacy of colonoscopic surveillance can be improved. Recommendations for screening intervals in U.S. patients are often not followed; patients who had genetic testing/counseling and genetic testing were more compliant with surveillance (481). Also, adenoma miss rate may be high (55% in one report by Stoffel et al [482]). Improved detection rates may be achieved with chromoendoscopy (483–485).

Natarajan et al (486) investigated advantages and disadvantages of subtotal colectomy for CRC in patients with LS. Cases were patients who underwent subtotal colectomy in one of two settings, namely, no CRC diagnosis (prophylactic) or at diagnosis of initial CRC; controls for these 2 types of cases were, respectively, patients who either underwent no colon surgery or those who had a limited resection at the time of diagnosis of their first CRC. Results showed that event-free survival did not reach 50%, so event-free survival at 5 years was used as the parameter for comparing the two groups. Therein, "... The event-free survival for subsequent CRC, subsequent abdominal surgery, and death was 94%, 84%, and 93%, respectively, for cases and 74%, 63%, and 88% respectively, for controls. Times to subsequent CRC and subsequent abdominal surgery were significantly shorter in the control group ($P < .006$ and $P < .04$, respectively). No significant difference was identified with respect to survival between the cases and controls." The authors concluded that even in the *absence* of survival benefit between cases and controls, the increased incidence of metachronous CRC and therein increased abdominal surgeries among controls clearly fostered the use of subtotal colectomy in patients with LS.

Testing Women With Endometrial Cancer to Detect LS

Kwon et al (486) noted that endometrial cancer as part of LS may not be identified through Amsterdam II criteria, so they developed a Markov Monte Carlo simulation model in order to compare the following criteria for LS testing among women diagnosed with endometrial cancer: (a) Amsterdam II Criteria; (b) diagnosed earlier than 50 years of age with at least 1 first-degree relative having an LS-associated cancer at any age; (c) IHC triage if age at diagnosis is less than 50 years; (d) IHC triage if age at diagnosis is less than 60 years; (e) IHC triage with diagnosis at any age if at least 1 first-degree relative has had an LS-associated cancer; (f) IHC triage of all endometrial cancers. Results showed that IHC triage of women with endometrial cancer having at least 1 first-degree relative with an LS-associated cancer was cost effective for identifying LS; this method gave a favorable incremental cost-effectiveness ratio (ICCR) of $9126 per year of life gained. IHC triage of all endometrial carcinomas identified the most mutation carriers, but at a cost of $648,494 per year of life gained. Using age thresholds of 50 or 60 years would submit more women to testing while identifying fewer mutation carriers.

Prophylactic Surgery and Risk Reduction for Endometrial and Ovarian Cancer in LS

Schmeler et al (487) have shown significant risk reduction for carcinoma of the endometrium and ovary through prophylactic surgery in women at inordinately high risk for LS who have completed their families, have had genetic counseling relevant to the pros and cons of this surgery, and have signed informed consent. We found it extremely important that these patients fully understood the reduced penetrance of carcinoma of the endometrium and ovary, as well as the limitations of screening, particularly in ovarian carcinoma. Schmeler's findings were based on 61 women who had undergone prophylactic hysterectomy with 210 mutation-positive women who had not undergone the surgery acting as controls, and 47 women who had undergone prophylactic bilateral salpingo-oophorectomy with 223 mutation-positive women who had not undergone the surgery as controls. Those who had undergone prophylactic surgery had no manifestations of endometrial, ovarian, or primary peritoneal cancer. On the other hand, among the control group for endometrial cancer, 69 women (33%) had been diagnosed with this cancer before the end of the study; among the control group for ovarian cancer, 12 women (5%) were diagnosed with ovarian cancer during that time. These findings suggest that prophylactic hysterectomy with bilateral salpingo-oophorectomy is effective in preventing endometrial and ovarian cancer in women carrying a mutation for LS.

Satisfaction With Ovarian Cancer Risk-Reduction Strategies

Westin et al (488) examined patients' overall satisfaction rate with ovarian periodic screening (PS) versus risk-reducing salpingo-oophorectomy (RRSO), and therein they identified factors that may influence patient satisfaction with ovarian cancer management options for reducing the risk of ovarian cancer.

The median satisfaction with decision (SWD) scale "... was significantly higher in the RRSO group compared with the PS group ($P < .001$). *BRCA* mutation carriers had higher median SWD scores regardless of management type ($P = .01$). Low satisfaction scores were associated with high levels of uncertainty and the perception that the decision between PS and RRSO was difficult to make ($P = .001$). Satisfaction was unrelated to demographics, clinical factors, or concerns of cancer risk."

They concluded that those women who showed the highest risk for breast and ovarian cancer were satisfied with their choice of risk reduction strategy. When decision making was difficult, the satisfaction levels were lower. It was further concluded that the decision-making process may enhance overall levels of satisfaction.

■ FUTURE RESEARCH DEVELOPMENTS

miRNAs

Balaguer et al (489) investigated microRNAs (miRNAs), namely small noncoding transcripts that appear to harbor an important pathogenic role in carcinogenesis and that discriminate between different types of cancer. This study involved an analysis of "... genome-wide miRNA expression profiles in 54 CRC tissues [22 with Lynch syndrome, 13 with sporadic MSI due to *MLH1* methylation, 19 without MSI (or microsatellite stable, MSS)] and 20 normal colonic tissues by miRNA microarrays...." A miRNA-based predictor was developed in order to differentiate both types of MSI by quantitative reverse transcriptase PCR. Importantly, results showed that a subset of nine miRNAs "... significantly discriminated between tumor and normal colonic mucosa tissues (overall error rate = 0.04). More importantly, LS tumors displayed a unique miRNA profile compared with sporadic MSI tumors;...[and the investigators] developed a miRNA predictor capable of differentiating between types of MSI and an independent sample set." It was concluded that these CRC tissues manifested distinct miRNA profiles when compared with normal colonic mucosa. This is an exceedingly important molecular genetic finding, given their discovery of a unique miRNA expression profile "... that can successfully discriminate between LS, sporadic MSI, and sporadic MSS CRCs ..." These findings are scientifically provocative and therein will play an important role for advancements in diagnosis, prognosis, and therapy that will likely evolve from these discoveries (489).

Exomes: Novel Molecular Genetic Developments

Newly developed "next-generation" DNA sequencing (NGS) technologies provide remarkable power for genomic studies (490,491). This new molecular genetic development is of keen interest and power, and harbors the following attributes: low sequencing cost; simple sample preparation; high speed; mass production; and ability to sequence individual and population genomes.

This exome sequencing involves only the exome part of the genome through NGS sequencing. Mutations in the protein-coding region contribute approximately 85% of the genetic disease-causing mutations. Cost is substantially lower (currently under $2000 per sample, compared with approximately $5000 to $50,000 per sample for whole genome sequencing). Further advantages are its focus on analyzing exon sequences, which is simpler than that for whole genome sequencing and, finally, information identified in affected genes can be biologically translated.

Genetically Based Therapeutic Differences in CRC

Microsatellite Instability, LS, and Therapeutic Implications

In vitro responses of LS CRCs suggest that chemoresistance is observed to many chemotherapeutic agents (492). Virtually all studies on MSI-H tumors and LS-associated CRC demonstrate either no benefit or adverse effects in response to 5-FU-based adjuvant chemotherapy (326). However, current treatment guidelines do not recommend using MSI status to determine whether or not a patient should receive 5-FU chemotherapy; this recommendation merits a second look, given the wealth of emerging data showing the inadequacy of 5-FU for CRC with MSI. Ideally, the effectiveness of 5-FU should be tested in the context of a randomized clinical trial (326).

Ribic et al (493) investigated MSI-H status as a predictor of benefit of adjuvant chemotherapy with 5-FU among stage II and III CRCs. Their findings showed that the benefit of treatment differed in accord with MSI status (P = .01). Patients with MSS tumors or those exhibiting MSI-L had an overall improved survival with adjuvant chemotherapy in accord with multivariate analysis, which was adjusted for stage and grade (HR for death, 0.72; 95% CI, 0.53–0.99; P = .04). However, the group with MSI-H showed no benefit from adjuvant chemotherapy.

Lanza et al (494) provide further verification of the prognostic significance of MMR status in a series of 393 stage II and 325 III CRC patients who underwent curative surgical resection. CRCs were tested for the presence of *MLH1* and *MSH2* proteins. Results showed that patients whose carcinomas had abnormal MMR protein expression (MMRP) showed marked reduction in the risk of cancer-related deaths when compared with patients with tumors having normal MMRP (HR, 0.2579; 95% CI, 0.1289–0.5159). A better clinical outcome for patients with abnormal MMRP was observed in both stage II (P = .0006) and stage III (P = .0052) disease. In stage III disease, the survival advantage associated with abnormal MMRP was more evident among patients treated with surgery alone than among patients who received adjuvant chemotherapy. A nonsignificant trend for survival benefit from adjuvant chemotherapy was observed among patients with normal MMRP carcinomas but not among those with abnormal MMRP carcinomas. It was concluded that testing for *MLH1/MSH2* expression yields important prognostic information for both stage II and III CRC patients.

Sinicrope et al (495) studied CRCs with defective DNA MMR that, while having a favorable prognosis when compared with those with proficient MMR, may lack benefit from 5-FU-based adjuvant chemotherapy. They, therefore, developed models to predict MMR deficiency in sporadic CRC and therein studied "... TNM stage II and III colon carcinomas (n = 982) from 6 5-fluorouracil-based adjuvant therapy trials... for microsatellite instability and/or MMR protein expression...." Mathematical modeling was performed to identify predictive factors for MMR status. Fifteen percent of the cancers had dMMR. The authors concluded that because dMMR is rare in distal, sporadic colon cancers, MMR testing of these cancers is not advised. Females with tumors that are located proximally and are poorly differentiated account for 51% of the sporadic tumors that are dMMR. When levels of TILs are included in the analysis instead of the tumor stage, the positive predictive value increases to 81%. These findings can increase the adequacy of MMR testing to assist in clinical treatment decisions.

Sinicrope et al (496) studied 2141 patients with stage II and III CRC who were treated in randomized trials of 5-FU-based adjuvant therapy. MSI and IHC were performed to determine dMMR or pMMR status. dMMR was detected in 344 of 2141 (16.1%) tumors. When compared with pMMR tumors, "... dMMR was associated with reduced 5-year recurrence rates (33% vs 22%; $P < .001$), delayed TTR ($P < .001$) and fewer distant recurrences (22% vs 12%; $P < .001$). In multivariable models, dMMR was independently associated with delayed TTR (time to recurrence 0.72, 95% HR, 0.56 to 0.91, $P = .005$) and improved DFS (disease-free survival; $P = .035$) and OS (overall survival; $P = .031$)...."

In stage III cancers, findings disclosed that "... 5-FU-based treatment vs surgery alone or no 5-FU was associated with reduced distant recurrence for dMMR tumors (11% vs 29%; $P = .011$) and reduced recurrence to all sites for pMMR tumors ($P < .001$). The dMMR tumors with suspected germline mutations were associated with improved DFS after 5-FU-based treatment compared with sporadic tumors where no benefit was observed ($P = .006$)."

Carethers et al (348) showed improved survival in patients with non-MSI-H CRCs following 5-FU that failed to extend to patients with MSI-H CRCs, thereby providing further confirmation that MSI status of CRC affected patients may indicate differences in 5-FU-based chemosensitivity which they had found to be consistent with in vitro investigations.

Sargent et al (347) demonstrated that adjuvant therapy provided improved DFS (HR, 0.67; 95% CI, 0.48–0.93; $P = .02$) among patients with pMMR tumors. In contrast, those patients with dMMR tumors who received 5-FU failed to show improvement in DFS (HR, 1.10; 95% CI, 0.42–2.91; $P = .85$) when compared with those randomly assigned to surgery only. Furthermore, "... In the pooled data set of 1027 patients ($n = 165$ with dMMR) these findings were maintained; in patients with stage II disease and with dMMR tumors, treatment was associated with reduced overall survival (HR, 2.95; 95% CI, 1.02–8.54; $P = .04$)." These authors concluded that a more tailored approach to CRC adjuvant therapy should involve MMR status. Therein, their data support "... MMR status assessment for patients being considered for FU therapy alone and consideration of MMR status in treatment decision making."

But what about stage II and stage III CRCs in MMR mutation-confirmed LS patients? Unfortunately, to the best of our knowledge, 5-FU-based adjuvant therapy studies have not yet been investigated in a sufficiently large number of MMR mutation confirmed LS patients manifesting stage II and stage III CRC to provide an answer to this question.

Aspirin and Polyp Regression

Burn et al (497) conducted the largest ever clinical trial in the setting of FAP and identified a trend of reduced polyp mode, both number and size, with administration of 600 mg of aspirin daily. Resistant starch did not have an effect on adenomas. Chan (498), in a perspective account of the Burn et al (497) study, notes that the role of aspirin in the clinical management of FAP patients fosters its role as a chemopreventive agent for CRC among broader populations.

A similar study conducted on a large cohort of LS patients failed to reveal significant polyp regression (499). However, a recent study by Burn et al (349) has, through an extension of time in the interest of greater maturity of the study, shown evidence for polyp regression.

Burn et al (349) in the CAPP2 randomized trial, assigned carriers of LS germline mutations to be randomly assigned by a 2 × 2 factorial design for receipt of 600 mg aspirin or aspirin placebo or 30 g resistant starch or starch placebo, for up to 4 years, with the primary endpoint being CRC occurrence. This study involved 861 participants who were assigned to aspirin or aspirin placebo with a mean follow-up of 55.7 months. Findings showed 48 participants to have developed 53 CRCs (18 of 427 randomly assigned to aspirin; 30 of 434 to aspirin placebo). Results showed that "... Poisson regression taking account of multiple primary events gave an incidence rate ratio (IRR) of 0.56 (95% CI, 0.32–0.99; $P = .05$). For participants completing 2 years of intervention (258 aspirin, 250 aspirin placebo), per-protocol analysis yielded an HR of 0.41 (0.19–0.86, $P = .02$) and an IRR of 0.37 ([91%CI] 0.18–0.78, $P = .008$)." It was concluded that "600 mg aspirin per day for a mean of 25 months substantially reduced cancer incidence after 55.7 months in carriers of hereditary CRC. Further studies are needed to establish the optimum dose and duration of aspirin treatment."

Other LS cancers showed an aspirin effect. Specifically, 18 participants manifested endometrial cancer, of whom five were randomly assigned to aspirin and 13 to aspirin placebo. Furthermore, "... in total, 38 participants developed cancer at a site other than the colorectum... of whom 16 were randomly assigned to aspirin and 22 to aspirin placebo... The HR for those randomly assigned to aspirin was 0.63 (95% CI, 0.34–1.19; $P = .16$ ...) and the IRR was 0.63 (95% CI, 0.34–1.16; $P = .14$) compared with the aspirin placebo group. ..."

The findings in this study support the hypothesis "... of a delayed effect of aspirin on CRC by showing that aspirin reduced incidence of CRC with the effect becoming apparent after 3–4 years from the start of aspirin intervention, a difference consistent with faster cancer development in those with Lynch syndrome." A second hypothesis pertains to whether LS cancers are more responsive to aspirin, a concern that remains elusive. However, in CAPP2, "... non-Lynch syndrome extracolonic cancers seemed unaffected by aspirin intervention ..."

This study raised several important questions, as follows: "(1) whether aspirin targets the minority of adenomas with the greatest malignant potential; (2) whether some Lynch syndrome CRCs arise from lesions other than adenomas (500); and (3) why do some tumors seem to be resistant to the effects of aspirin? The mechanism by which aspirin suppresses cancer development long after cessation of exposure to the drug is unclear...."

■ SUMMARY

LS has emerged as an important clinical model for the study of all varieties of hereditary cancer during the past several decades, comparable in many ways to the intense interest given to its FAP counterpart beginning in the 1950s and 1960s. The breadth and scope of cancer of multiple anatomic sites, a cardinal feature of LS, has intrigued clinicians and basic scientists with respect to molecular genetic pathways that might help explain its etiology and pathogenesis. Clearly, such discovery could ultimately lead to a better understanding of cancer control measures for LS, inclusive of chemoprevention, the role of chemotherapy, radiation therapy, and surgery, once a site-specific cancer has emerged. Such discovery should impact upon the overwhelming larger burden of cancer in the general population.

■ Colorectal Cancer in Inflammatory Bowel Disease

HILIARY BOWNIK
MICHAEL V. CHIOREAN
LAURA YUN

Inflammatory bowel diseases, namely UC and Crohn's disease (CD) are chronic, immune-mediated inflammatory disorders that affect only the colon in the case of UC, or the colon and the small bowel in patients with Crohn's disease. In 1925, Dr. Crohn first described IBD associated CRC (501). The risk of CRC is increased in patients with long-standing chronic colitis regardless of the specific diagnosis, although risk of CRC in IBD reported in studies varies widely, likely due to variations in study methodology and patient populations, that is, tertiary referral centers vs population based studies. Most of the initial studies evaluated patients with UC. In a population-based Swedish cohort, Ekbom et al reported that the risk of colon cancer in patients with UC was increased almost 6-fold compared to the general population (502). The same group reported that patients with Crohn's colitis also have an increased risk of colon cancer with a relative risk of 2.5 (503). A subsequent meta-analysis of 116 studies estimated the incidence of colon cancer in patients with UC at 3/1000. The cumulative probability of colon cancer 10 years after diagnosis was 2% but increased to 8% by 20 years and 18% by 30 years (504). More recent studies, however, seem to indicate that the risk of colon cancer may be lower than initially estimated. A population-based study from Manitoba, Canada, found the relative risk of colon cancer in both UC and Crohn's to be 2.7 (505). Two population-based studies, one from Denmark and one from Olmsted county, MN found no increased risk of colon cancer in patients with IBD compared to the general population (506,507). A nationwide Danish cohort study of 47,374 IBD patients followed over a 30-year period found that the risk of CRC among patients with UC was comparable to the general population (RR, 1.07). However, the relative risk of CRC decreased from the first to the last decade of the study by more than 2-fold (1.34 in 1979–1988 vs 0.57 from 1999–2008). The reason for this recent time trend is unclear but it is speculated that the increased use of 5-aminosalicylate (5-ASA) compounds, and possibly immunosuppressives such as azathioprine or anti-TNF biologics and surgery may be important contributors (508).

A recent study by Herrinton et al published in 2012 looking at the Kaiser Permanente patient population found the incidence of CRC in patients with IBD was 60% higher than in the general population (509).

Overall, the risk of CRC development in Crohn's colitis is similar to that of UC when comparable disease duration, extent, and age exists (510–513). A meta-analysis of population based studies looking at intestinal cancer in CD found the SIR for CRC was 1.9 (95% CI 1.4–2.5; 514). Another meta-analysis, found an overall CRC relative risk in CD to be 2.5 (1.3–4.7) and 4.5 (1.3–14.9) for patients with colonic disease. The cumulative risk of CRC overall, regardless of disease location was 2.9%, 5.6%, 8.3% after 10, 20, and 30 years of disease, respectively (515).

Overall, IBD patients are younger compared to the general population when diagnosed with CRC. The mean age for sporadic CRC is 60 years old whereas the mean age at diagnosis in UC is 43 and CD 55 years old. Several studies show that the most common location of CRC development in UC is in the rectosigmoid colon (516,517). In contrast, CRC in CD is evenly distributed throughout the colon.

■ RISK FACTORS FOR CRC IN CHRONIC COLITIS

The most important risk factor for colon cancer in patients with colitis are the anatomical or histological disease extent, time since diagnosis or symptom onset (disease duration), family history of colon cancer, coexistent diagnosis of primary sclerosing cholangitis (PSC), previous history of dysplasia, medication noncompliance and nonuse of 5-ASA drugs. Determination of disease extent has traditionally been based on endoscopic rather than histological inflammation. On the other hand, histological inflammation may be a more accurate marker of disease extent as mucosal healing with normal macroscopic appearance can occur, thus falsely decreasing the amount of bowel estimated at risk for neoplasia (518–520). Regardless how the disease extent is appreciated, studies have consistently showed that the more extensive the colon involvement, the higher the cancer risk. This has been demonstrated in both earlier and recent publications regardless of the overall reported cancer risk. For instance, in the meta-analysis by Eaden et al, the overall prevalence of CRC among patients with UC in all 116 studies was 3.7%, but this rose to 5.4% in patients with extensive colitis (504). Furthermore, in the Olmsted county study, where the overall cancer risk was not significantly elevated compared to the general population, a subgroup analysis showed that the relative risk increased from 0 in patients with proctitis, to 0.8 in patients with left-sided colitis and 2.4 in patients with extensive or pancolonic disease (507).

Longer disease duration since diagnosis or symptom onset has been associated with an increased colon cancer risk in several studies in patients with UC. In the meta-analysis by Eaden et al, the annual incidence of CRC in the first decade was 0.2% and increased to 0.7% and 1.2% annually in the second and third decade of disease, respectively (504). Other recently published studies show no clear-cut association between disease duration and cancer risk; for instance, in the large cohort study from St. Mark's Hospital, the slope of the actuarial cumulative CRC incidence curve remained constant over the 30 years of the study surveillance (519).

Patients with coexistent primary sclerosing cholangitis (PSC) are at especially high risk for colorectal dysplasia or cancer based on several case-control and population-based studies (521–524). A meta-analysis found PSC patients with UC had a 4.8-fold increased CRC risk compared to the baseline risk in UC (525). The cumulative CRC risk in patients with UC and PSC has been reported as high as 10% at 10 years, 33% at 20 years, and 40% at 30 years after UC diagnosis (526). Whether this association represents a true biological phenomenon or rather a marker of more extensive colitis or longer disease duration is unclear (527). The challenging aspect in patients with PSC-IBD is the fact that the risk of cancer seems to be substantially increased even if most patients have milder IBD activity compared with patients without PSC (528,529).

A family history of CRC appears to be an independent risk factor for colon cancer in patients with IBD with a relative risk of 2 to 3 (530–533). Patients with a first degree relative diagnosed with CRC before age 50 have a 9-fold increased risk (532). Therefore, a careful family history should be elicited in all patients with IBD regardless of disease duration or activity.

Severity of inflammation may be an important risk factor for neoplasia in patients with colitis (520). Both macroscopic and microscopic inflammation was found to be associated with an increased risk of neoplasia in a case-control study from the St. Mark's group (534). Several studies have suggested that most dysplastic lesions are visible at standard colonoscopy (535,536). Endoscopic features that are predictive of neoplasia include the presence of multiple inflammatory pseudopolyps (which by themselves are not premalignant) or colonic strictures (517, 533, 537, 538). In addition, others found that the acquisition of mucosal healing actually decreases the risk of CRC (533). However, other studies have found that patients with mucosal healing and those with no evidence of active disease have similar risk to developing CRC compared to those with active disease (539). Because children diagnosed with IBD at a young age often have more extensive, severe disease with longer disease duration, the data are mixed as to whether young age at diagnosis itself is an independent risk factor for CRC. Together, these findings suggest that more severe and perhaps protracted inflammation may increase the risk of cancer. In contrast, patients with an endoscopically normal-appearing colon seem to have a lower risk of neoplasia, which is similar to the general population (540).

■ DYSPLASIA AS A PRECURSOR FOR CANCER IN IBD

In the chronically inflamed bowel, the mucosa undergoes morphological changes with eventual development of precancerous cytological and histological abnormalities called dysplasia. In this regard, the neoplastic transformation in IBD seems to follow a similar pattern to the adenoma-carcinoma sequence in sporadic colon cancer. For this reason, dysplasia has been used as the main target for endoscopic surveillance in patients with colitis. The current definition of dysplasia was proposed in the landmark paper by Riddell et al in 1983 and it entails an unequivocal neoplastic transformation of the epithelium confined to the basement membrane without invasion into the lamina propria (541). Dysplasia was divided into high-grade (HGD), low-grade (LGD), and indefinite (IND) based on the histological appearance of the epithelial cells and their nuclei. Although this system continues to be in use today, it has several important limitations. The inter-observer agreement for dysplasia is often poor, particularly for LGD and IND (542–544). Although HGD seems to fare a little better, one study showed that the agreement for HGD among expert GI pathologists was only average ($\kappa = 0.5$; 545).

The pathogenesis of dysplasia in colitis is complex and it is likely to share some common pathways with the traditional adenoma-carcinoma sequence in patients with sporadic CRC. As in other chronic inflammatory conditions, IBD could theoretically predispose to cancer by inducing cellular injury with associated DNA damage as well as by the local production of carcinogens, tumor promoters or growth factors at the site of inflammation. Repeated cycles of mucosal damage, ulceration, and regeneration in IBD create a particularly fertile ground for expansion of cell clones that have acquired a growth advantage through mutations or epigenetic transformation. Therefore, colonic carcinogenesis in IBD is thought to arise through sequential episodes of somatic genetic mutations and clonal expansion (546). This theory has been supported by flow cytometry and tissue histochemistry studies using surgical specimens from patients with colitis (547–549). Genetic alterations such as mutations or epigenetic silencing (through methylation) have been demonstrated in a variety of proto-oncogenes such as *K-ras,* tumor suppressor genes such as *p53, APC, DCC,* and *Rb,* and DNA repair genes such as *MLH1, MSH2, MSH6,* and *PMS2* in patients with colitis-associated colon cancer and dysplasia (549–558).

From the clinico-pathological standpoint, dysplasia is classified as flat (no raised lesion visible endoscopically) or elevated (obvious endoscopic lesion). An elevated dysplastic lesion surrounded by flat dysplasia is also called a DALM (dysplasia-associated lesion or mass) whereas polypoid dysplasia (without concomitant surrounding dysplasia) is also known as ALM (adenoma-like mass) if situated within an area of colitis or a sporadic adenoma if the surrounding mucosa was not inflamed (559). The grade and appearance of dysplasia in an individual with colitis helps stratify the cancer risk. A retrospective cohort analysis from Mount Sinai Hospital found that among 46 patients with UC who had flat LGD but did not undergo immediate surgery, seven were found to have CRC by the time of their subsequent colectomy; in addition, four out of 17 patients undergoing colectomy for flat LGD were found to have unexpected advanced neoplasia (560). The experience reported from the group at St. Mark's Hospital in their surveillance database study seems to mirror these findings. In this case, 20% of patients with LGD who underwent direct colectomy had concurrent adenocarcinoma while 39.1% of those followed up for several years developed HGD or CRC (519). In a recent meta-analysis, the finding of either flat or elevated LGD at colonoscopy carried a 9-fold, long-term risk of developing CRC and a 12-fold risk of developing HGD or cancer over a mean of 5.2 years (561). The highest risk of synchronous or metachronous cancer is associated with the presence of HGD or DALM. In the original study by Blackstone et al, 7 of 12 patients with DALM were found to harbor adenocarcinoma at the time of colectomy (559). In a more recent review of 10 prospective studies, 43% of patients with DALMs and 42% of those with HGD at colonoscopy who had immediate colectomy were found to have cancer. In contrast, 19% of those with LGD at colonoscopy had concurrent CRC. Patients with LGD who continue surveillance colonoscopy had a risk of progression to a more advanced lesion—HGD, DALM or cancer—of 16%–29% (562; Figure 2.5).

■ MANAGEMENT OF DYSPLASIA IN FLAT MUCOSA

When a biopsy confirms the presence of HGD, colectomy is recommended. Colectomy is recommended because of the high rate of concurrent CRC, 42%–67%, as well as the subsequent development of CRC, 32%, as reported by Bernstein et al (540,562).

The management of LGD management is controversial. Thus, if a single focus of low-grade dysplasia is found, the patient should be educated about the risks and benefits of colectomy vs continued surveillance (563). If colectomy is not performed, the patient should undergo surveillance within 3 months (no longer than 6 months) from the initial acquisition of the biopsy (563). Subsequent surveillance colonoscopies should be performed every 6 months, even if all repeat surveillance exams show no further evidence of dysplasia (560). Most experts agree that multifocal low-grade dysplasia (2 or more biopsies showing low grade dysplasia obtained from 1 colonoscopy) should be managed with a total colectomy (564,565).

A specimen read as indefinite for dysplasia should be confirmed by an expert GI pathologist (563). If confirmed, a surveillance colonoscopy should be performed within 3 to 6 months (563). Underlying inflammation should be treated prior to the subsequent examination (see Figure 2.6 for flat dysplasia management algorithm).

■ MANAGEMENT OF RAISED DYSPLASTIC LESIONS

One of the most important features of a raised dysplastic lesion is its resectability. If a dysplastic lesion is not able to be completely resected endoscopically, colectomy is recommended (510,563,566). If a dysplastic lesion is able to be completely removed and the surrounding mucosa does not show dysplasia, the patient should undergo surveillance colonoscopy in 6 months (563,566). If no further evidence of dysplasia is seen on subsequent colonoscopy, the patient can return to annual surveillance colonoscopy (563,566). An adenoma removed in an area of colon that has not been involved in colitis can be managed according to standard recommendations for the general population (567; see Figure 2.7 for raised dysplastic lesion algorithm).

Surveillance for Colorectal Neoplasia in IBD

The rationale for surveillance colonoscopy in IBD is based on the premise that detection of neoplasia in its early stages (ie, dysplasia) is possible and an intervention at this juncture can prevent progression to cancer and death. Despite this logical argument, no prospective comparative studies have been performed to validate this approach.

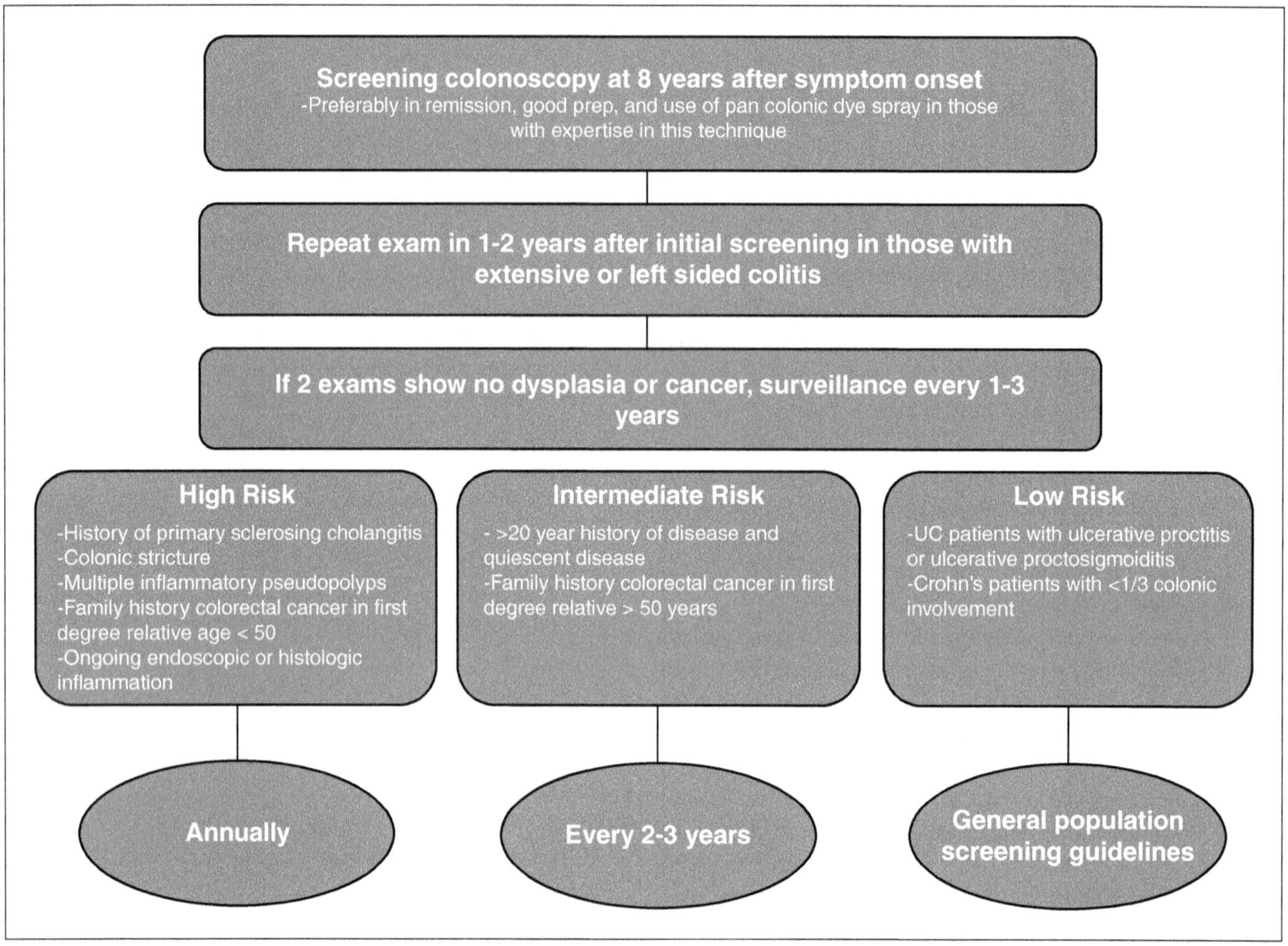

FIGURE 2.5 Guidelines for surveillance colonoscopy in IBD.

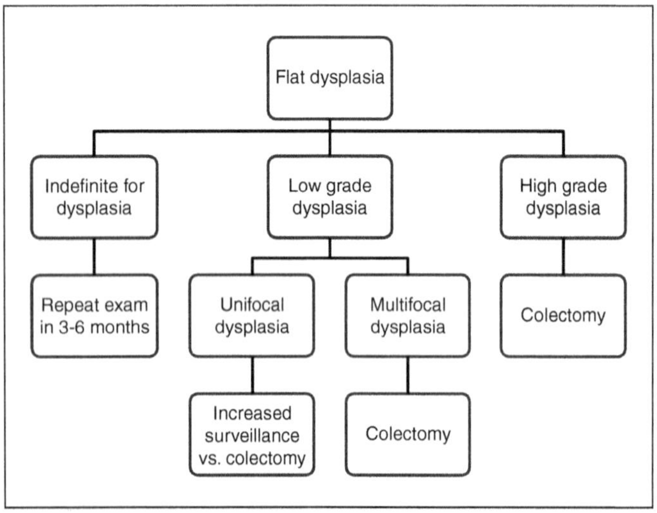

FIGURE 2.6 Flat dysplasia management algorithm.

A number of earlier observational studies suggested a benefit by diagnosing neoplasia through periodic surveillance colonoscopy (568–571). In contrast, three case-control studies have attempted to assess the impact of surveillance colonoscopy compared to usual care in patients with UC, all with limited results (572–574). A subsequent Cochrane review concluded that there was a nonsignificant trend toward improved survival through earlier cancer detection in patients with UC undergoing surveillance colonoscopy but lead-time bias may contribute substantially to this benefit (575). There is much less evidence for the benefit, or lack thereof, of surveillance colonoscopy in patients with Crohn's colitis. Friedman et al, in their updated study of 259 patients with CD undergoing surveillance and of which the majority had extensive disease, found dysplasia or cancer in 7% of patients at the first screening colonoscopy and 14% at follow up. In addition, the cumulative risk of dysplasia or cancer after an initial negative colonoscopy was 25% after the 10th surveillance examination, suggesting that the risk of neoplasia in patients with extensive Crohn's colitis is similar to that of patients with UC (576).

Surveillance Techniques in Patients With IBD

Colonoscopy with random biopsies is the current standard for surveillance in patients with chronic colitis in

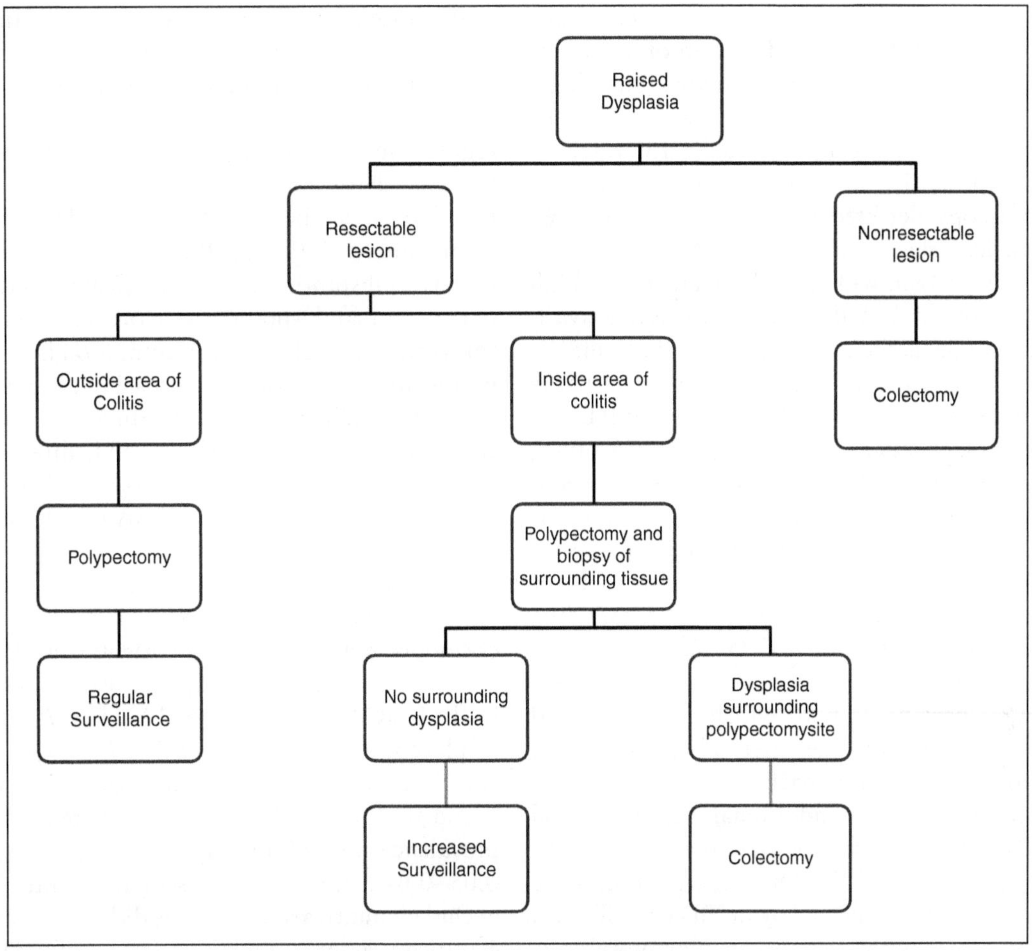

FIGURE 2.7 Raised dysplasia management algorithm.

many countries including the United States. Traditionally, random biopsies were deemed necessary in the era of standard definition endoscopes, based on the assumption that some of the dysplasia is flat and therefore invisible with standard white light colonoscopy. However, a typical biopsy covers less than 0.05% of the colon surface, thus raising concerns for sampling errors even with a large number of such biopsies (577). Based on a mathematical model, Rubin et al determined that 33 and 64 random biopsies, respectively, are necessary to detect dysplasia in UC with 90% and 95% probability (578). It is unclear if this approach has either clinical or economical merit as the incremental cost-effectiveness ratio of yearly surveillance colonoscopy is probably in excess of $300,000 per year of life saved (579,580). The large number of biopsies required under this strategy is undoubtedly a primary cost driver as the prevalence of dysplasia in random samples of flat colonic mucosa is extremely low (540).

In an effort to increase the yield of colonoscopy, several image enhancing or "red flag" technologies have been developed. The common assumption shared by these techniques is that all neoplasia is, in fact, uneven from the surrounding mucosa (either elevated or depressed) and therefore should be detectable using a variety of image enhancements. The main purpose of these methods is to decrease the need for random biopsies or eliminate it altogether. A widely available method named chromoendoscopy involves the use of dye spraying in the colon (581). Several randomized and case-control studies consistently showed a superiority of chromoendoscopy over white light colonoscopy with a per-patient and per-lesion incremental yield for dysplasia of 3-and 5-fold, respectively (535, 581–583). Narrow-band imaging (NBI) is another technique readily available in some modern endoscopes in which blue-green spectrum light (narrow-band) is projected on the bowel mucosa instead of the traditional white light. Because the peak absorption of hemoglobin occurs at these wavelengths, blood vessels appear very dark in contrast with the surrounding epithelium. However, mucosal unevenness and pit pattern, which make the basis for diagnosing neoplasia in IBD, are not as accurately visualized as with chromoendoscopy. In fact, several studies showed no advantage of NBI over high-definition white light endoscopy (584–586). Furthermore, a small study showed that NBI was inferior to chromoendoscopy although the study lacked the power to detect a significant difference (587).

Confocal endomicroscopy uses a miniaturized confocal microscope integrated into the distal tip of a specialized colonoscope. This enables a true "in vivo" histologic evaluation of the colonic mucosa after the intravenous administration of a contrast agent (usually fluorescein). In a randomized study, chromoendoscopy combined with endomicroscopy detected five times more neoplastic lesions with half the number of biopsies (582). This method is not currently in widespread use due to the high cost of the technology and the limited expertise available. Autofluorescence is the property of certain tissues to reflect light at a different wavelength than the one that is originally projected on them (excitation wavelength) based on the different biochemical composition. For instance, green light will be reflected by normal tissue as green and neoplastic tissue as magenta. Although the technology is not available for clinical use, a small pilot trial showed that autofluorescence imaging can increase the yield of surveillance endoscopy by 2-fold over standard white light endoscopy in patients with UC (588). Among currently available methods, chromoendoscopy appears to be the technology to beat being both widely accessible and more accurate compared to other methods for detecting neoplasia in IBD. Its major drawback is that it is relatively time consuming and requires additional periprocedural implements. The British Society of Gastroenterology and the European Crohn's and Colitis Organization both have endorsed the use of chromoendoscopy in IBD surveillance, somewhat in contrast with societies in North America (Table 2.6).

Chemoprevention for Colorectal Neoplasia

The role of chemoprevention for colorectal neoplasia in patients with IBD is unclear. Although frequently used in practice, the benefit of 5-ASA drugs such as sulfasalazine and mesalamine is controversial. A review of nine observational studies suggested a substantial benefit with regard to colon cancer reduction (OR= 0.51) in patients with UC (508). A large case-control study from the UK also indicated a modest reduction in cancer risk among regular versus intermittent users (589). In contrast, 2 large database studies from Canada and the United States failed to show a benefit of 5-ASA in decreasing the risk of colon cancer (590,591). Both positive and negative studies have substantial limitations related to their retrospective design and should therefore be interpreted within this context. As chronic inflammation is believed to be an important risk factor for neoplasia, it is plausible that any agent that induces mucosal healing can reduce the risk of cancer thus extenuating the possible direct antineoplastic effect of specific drugs such as 5-ASA. The suggested dose for chemoprevention with 5-ASA is at least 1.2 g per day (592).

Ursodeoxycholic (UDCA) is the only medication for which we have random controlled studies to support a chemopreventative effect in patients with PSC and colitis. The relative risk for developing CRC or dysplasia was .26 in the UDCA treated group (13–15 mg/kg/day) compared to placebo (95% CI, 0.06–0.92; P = .034; 593). A retrospective, cross sectional study from Tung and colleagues found that ursodiol use was associated with a decreased prevalence of colonic dysplasia (OR, 0.18; 95% CI, 0.05–0.61), but when cases of indefinite dysplasia were excluded, multivariate analysis did not reveal a statistically significant association with UDCA (594). Data from Wolf et al did not show a statistically significant decreased risk of developing dysplasia or cancer with UDCA use in UC/PSC patients but did show a decrease in mortality (595). In addition, a study looking at high dose ursodiol 28 to 30 mg/kg/day actually showed a 4-fold increased risk (HR, 4.44; 95% CI, 1.30–20.1; P = .02) of CRC and dysplasia compared to placebo (596). Since the drug is overall ineffective for patients with PSC, its use for colon cancer

Table 2.6 Societal Guidelines for Surveillance in Patients With IBD-Related Chronic Colitis

	ECCO '08	BSG '10	AGA '10	ACG '10
Disease duration at first screening	• Pancolitis: 8–10 yr • L-sided: 15 yr	• Pan: 10 yr • L-sided: 15 yr	• Pan: 8 yr • L-sided: 15 yr	• Pan: 8–10 yr • L-sided: 15 yr
Surveillance interval	• Extensive: 2 yearly up to 20 yr then yearly • Left-sided: 2 yearly after 15 years • PSC: yearly	• Low risk: 5 yr • Intermediate: 3 yr • High risk: 1 yr	• Average risk: 1 to 3 yr • High-risk, PSC: yearly	• 1–2 yr
Chromoendoscopy	Superior to white light endoscopy	Recommended	Special cases	No recommendation
Biopsies	Min 32 if no chromo	Min 32 if no chromo	Min 32	Min 32

ECCO, European Crohn's and Colitis Organization; BSG, British Society of Gastroenterology; AGA, American Gastroenterological Association; ACG, American College of Gastroenterology.

prevention in IBD cannot be justified. Further studies are needed to look at the role statins, folic acid, corticosteroids, thiopurines, and anti-TNF in decreasing CRC risk in IBD.

■ REFERENCES

1. ACS ACS. *Colorectal Cancer Facts & Figures, 2011–2013*. Atlanta, GA: American Cancer Society; 2011.
2. Sylvester BE, Huo D, Khramtsov A, et al. Molecular analysis of colorectal tumors within a diverse patient cohort at a single institution. *Clin Cancer Res*. 2012;18(2):350–359.
3. Parkin DM. International variation. *Oncogene*. 2004;23(38):6329–6340.
4. Hill MJ, Morson BC, Bussey HJ. Aetiology of adenoma–carcinoma sequence in large bowel. *Lancet*. 1978;1(8058):245–247.
5. Vogelstein B, Fearon ER, Hamilton SR, et al. Genetic alterations during colorectal-tumor development. *N Engl J Med*. 1988;319(9):525–532.
6. Rampino N, Yamamoto H, Ionov Y, et al. Somatic frameshift mutations in the BAX gene in colon cancers of the microsatellite mutator phenotype. *Science*. 1997;275(5302):967–969.
7. Markowitz S, Wang J, Myeroff L, et al. Inactivation of the type II TGF-beta receptor in colon cancer cells with microsatellite instability. *Science*. 1995;268(5215):1336–1338.
8. O'Sullivan JN, Bronner MP, Brentnall TA, et al. Chromosomal instability in ulcerative colitis is related to telomere shortening. *Nat Genet*. 2002;32(2):280–284.
9. Burmer GC, Rabinovitch PS, Haggitt RC, et al. Neoplastic progression in ulcerative colitis: histology, DNA content, and loss of a p53 allele. *Gastroenterology*. 1992;103(5):1602–1610.
10. Mäkinen MJ. Colorectal serrated adenocarcinoma. *Histopathology*. 2007;50(1):131–150.
11. Winawer SJ. Natural history of colorectal cancer. *Am J Med*. 1999;106(1A):3S–6S; discussion 50S.
12. CDC CfDCaP. Behavioral risk factor surveillance system survey data. In: Atlanta, GA: Department of Health and Human Services, Centers for Disease Control and Prevention; 2010.
13. Hewitson P, Glasziou P, Irwig L, Towler B, Watson E. Screening for colorectal cancer using the faecal occult blood test, Hemoccult. *Cochrane Database Syst Rev*. 2007:CD001216.
14. Nelson RS, Thorson AG. Colorectal cancer screening. *Curr Oncol Rep*. 2009;11(6):482–489.
15. Schoen RE, Pinsky PF, Weissfeld JL, et al.; PLCO Project Team. Colorectal-cancer incidence and mortality with screening flexible sigmoidoscopy. *N Engl J Med*. 2012;366(25):2345–2357.
16. Atkin WS, Edwards R, Kralj-Hans I, et al.; UK Flexible Sigmoidoscopy Trial Investigators. Once-only flexible sigmoidoscopy screening in prevention of colorectal cancer: a multicentre randomised controlled trial. *Lancet*. 2010;375(9726):1624–1633.
17. Segnan N, Armaroli P, Bonelli L, et al.; SCORE Working Group. Once-only sigmoidoscopy in colorectal cancer screening: follow-up findings of the Italian Randomized Controlled Trial–SCORE. *J Natl Cancer Inst*. 2011;103(17):1310–1322.
18. Kaminski MF, Bretthauer M, Zauber AG, et al. The NordICC Study: rationale and design of a randomized trial on colonoscopy screening for colorectal cancer. *Endoscopy*. 2012;44(7):695–702.
19. Sosna J, Morrin MM, Kruskal JB, Lavin PT, Rosen MP, Raptopoulos V. CT colonography of colorectal polyps: a metaanalysis. *AJR Am J Roentgenol*. 2003;181(6):1593–1598.
20. Rosman AS, Korsten MA. Meta-analysis comparing CT colonography, air contrast barium enema, and colonoscopy. *Am J Med*. 2007;120(3):203–210.e4.
21. Screening for colorectal cancer: U.S. Preventive Services Task Force recommendation statement. *Ann Intern Med*. 2008;149:627–37.
22. Ahlquist DA. Molecular detection of colorectal neoplasia. *Gastroenterology*. 2010;138(6):2127–2139.
23. Berger BM, Ahlquist DA. Stool DNA screening for colorectal neoplasia: biological and technical basis for high detection rates. *Pathology*. 2012;44(2):80–88.
24. Levin B, Lieberman DA, McFarland B, et al.; American Cancer Society Colorectal Cancer Advisory Group; US Multi-Society Task Force; American College of Radiology Colon Cancer Committee. Screening and surveillance for the early detection of colorectal cancer and adenomatous polyps, 2008: a joint guideline from the American Cancer Society, the US Multi-Society Task Force on Colorectal Cancer, and the American College of Radiology. *CA Cancer J Clin*. 2008;58(3):130–160.
25. ACS ACS. Colorectal Cancer Early Detection. Atlanta, GA: American Cancer Society; 2012.
26. Zauber AG, Winawer SJ, O'Brien MJ, et al. Colonoscopic polypectomy and long-term prevention of colorectal-cancer deaths. *N Engl J Med*. 2012;366(8):687–696.
27. Corpet DE, Taché S. Most effective colon cancer chemopreventive agents in rats: a systematic review of aberrant crypt foci and tumor data, ranked by potency. *Nutr Cancer*. 2002;43(1):1–21.
28. Takayama T, Katsuki S, Takahashi Y, et al. Aberrant crypt foci of the colon as precursors of adenoma and cancer. *N Engl J Med*. 1998;339(18):1277–1284.
29. Hawk ET, Viner JL, Umar A, et al. Cancer and the cyclo-oxygenase enzyme: implications for treatment and prevention. *Am J Cancer*. 2003;2:27–55.
30. Shpitz B, Klein E, Buklan G, et al. Suppressive effect of aspirin on aberrant crypt foci in patients with colorectal cancer. *Gut*. 2003;52(11):1598–1601.
31. http://www.fda.gov/Drugs/DevelopmentApprovalProcess/HowDrugsareDevelopedandApproved/DrugandBiologicApprovalReports/ucm121597.htm. Accessed August 30, 2012.
32. Kune GA, Kune S, Watson LF. Colorectal cancer risk, chronic illnesses, operations, and medications: case control results from the Melbourne Colorectal Cancer Study. *Cancer Res*. 1988;48(15):4399–4404.
33. Cancer Prevention Study II. The American cancer society prospective study. *Stat Bull Metrop Insur Co*. 1992;73:21–9.
34. Giovannucci E, Egan KM, Hunter DJ, et al. Aspirin and the risk of colorectal cancer in women. *N Engl J Med*. 1995;333(10):609–614.
35. Rossouw JE, Anderson GL, Prentice RL, et al.; Writing Group for the Women's Health Initiative Investigators. Risks and benefits of estrogen plus progestin in healthy postmenopausal women: principal results From the Women's Health Initiative randomized controlled trial. *JAMA*. 2002;288(3):321–333.
36. Baron JA, Beach M, Mandel JS, et al. Calcium supplements for the prevention of colorectal adenomas. Calcium Polyp Prevention Study Group. *N Engl J Med*. 1999;340(2):101–107.
37. Li H, Kramer PM, Lubet RA, Steele VE, Kelloff GJ, Pereira MA. Effect of calcium on azoxymethane-induced aberrant crypt foci and cell proliferation in the colon of rats. *Cancer Lett*. 1998;124(1):39–46.
38. Wargovich MJ, Allnutt D, Palmer C, Anaya P, Stephens LC. Inhibition of the promotional phase of azoxymethane-induced colon carcinogenesis in the F344 rat by calcium lactate: effect of simulating two human nutrient density levels. *Cancer Lett*. 1990;53(1):17–25.
39. Baron JA, Cole BF, Sandler RS, et al. A randomized trial of aspirin to prevent colorectal adenomas. *N Engl J Med*. 2003;348(10):891–899.
40. Sandler RS, Halabi S, Baron JA, et al. A randomized trial of aspirin to prevent colorectal adenomas in patients with previous colorectal cancer. *N Engl J Med*. 2003;348(10):883–890.
41. Craven PA, DeRubertis FR. Effects of aspirin on 1,2-dimethylhydrazine-induced colonic carcinogenesis. *Carcinogenesis*. 1992;13(4):541–546.

42. Barnes CJ, Lee M. Chemoprevention of spontaneous intestinal adenomas in the adenomatous polyposis coli Min mouse model with aspirin. *Gastroenterology.* 1998;114(5):873–877.
43. Davis AE, Patterson F. Aspirin reduces the incidence of colonic carcinoma in the dimethylhydrazine rat animal model. *Aust N Z J Med.* 1994;24(3):301–303.
44. Reddy BS, Rao CV, Rivenson A, Kelloff G. Inhibitory effect of aspirin on azoxymethane-induced colon carcinogenesis in F344 rats. *Carcinogenesis.* 1993;14(8):1493–1497.
45. Shpitz B, Bomstein Y, Kariv N, Shalev M, Buklan G, Bernheim J. Chemopreventive effect of aspirin on growth of aberrant crypt foci in rats. *Int J Colorectal Dis.* 1998;13(4):169–172.
46. Jacoby RF, Seibert K, Cole CE, Kelloff G, Lubet RA. The cyclooxygenase-2 inhibitor celecoxib is a potent preventive and therapeutic agent in the min mouse model of adenomatous polyposis. *Cancer Res.* 2000;60(18):5040–5044.
47. Reddy BS, Hirose Y, Lubet R, et al. Chemoprevention of colon cancer by specific cyclooxygenase-2 inhibitor, celecoxib, administered during different stages of carcinogenesis. *Cancer Res.* 2000;60(2):293–297.
48. Steinbach G, Lynch PM, Phillips RK, et al. The effect of celecoxib, a cyclooxygenase-2 inhibitor, in familial adenomatous polyposis. *N Engl J Med.* 2000;342(26):1946–1952.
49. Corpet DE, Pierre F. How good are rodent models of carcinogenesis in predicting efficacy in humans? A systematic review and meta-analysis of colon chemoprevention in rats, mice and men. *Eur J Cancer.* 2005;41(13):1911–1922.
50. Meyskens FL Jr, Curt GA, Brenner DE, et al.; C-Change Chemoprevention Clinical Trials and Biomarkers Subcommittee. Regulatory approval of cancer risk-reducing (chemopreventive) drugs: moving what we have learned into the clinic. *Cancer Prev Res (Phila).* 2011;4(3):311–323.
51. Shamberger RJ, Tytko SA, Willis CE. Antioxidants and cancer. Part VI. Selenium and age-adjusted human cancer mortality. *Arch Environ Health.* 1976;31(5):231–235.
52. Knekt P, Aromaa A, Maatela J, et al. Serum vitamin E, serum selenium and the risk of gastrointestinal cancer. *Int J Cancer.* 1988;42(6):846–850.
53. Knekt P, Aromaa A, Maatela J, et al. Serum selenium and subsequent risk of cancer among Finnish men and women. *J Natl Cancer Inst.* 1990;82(10):864–868.
54. Clark LC, Hixson LJ, Combs GF Jr, Reid ME, Turnbull BW, Sampliner RE. Plasma selenium concentration predicts the prevalence of colorectal adenomatous polyps. *Cancer Epidemiol Biomarkers Prev.* 1993;2(1):41–46.
55. Nelson RL, Davis FG, Sutter E, et al. Serum selenium and colonic neoplastic risk. *Dis Colon Rectum.* 1995;38(12):1306–1310.
56. Takata Y, Kristal AR, King IB, et al. Serum selenium, genetic variation in selenoenzymes, and risk of colorectal cancer: primary analysis from the Women's Health Initiative Observational Study and meta-analysis. *Cancer Epidemiol Biomarkers Prev.* 2011; 20(9):1822–1830.
57. Clark LC, Combs GF Jr, Turnbull BW, et al. Effects of selenium supplementation for cancer prevention in patients with carcinoma of the skin. A randomized controlled trial. Nutritional Prevention of Cancer Study Group. *JAMA.* 1996;276(24):1957–1963.
58. Lippman SM, Klein EA, Goodman PJ, et al. Effect of selenium and vitamin E on risk of prostate cancer and other cancers: the Selenium and Vitamin E Cancer Prevention Trial (SELECT). *JAMA.* 2009;301(1):39–51.
59. Giovannucci E, Goldin B. The role of fat, fatty acids, and total energy intake in the etiology of human colon cancer. *Am J Clin Nutr.* 1997;66(6 Suppl):1564S–1571S.
60. Narisawa T, Magadia NE, Weisburger JH, Wynder EL. Promoting effect of bile acids on colon carcinogenesis after intrarectal instillation of N-methyl-N'-nitro-N-nitrosoguanidine in rats. *J Natl Cancer Inst.* 1974;53(4):1093–1097.
61. Bautista D, Obrador A, Moreno V, et al. Ki-ras mutation modifies the protective effect of dietary monounsaturated fat and calcium on sporadic colorectal cancer. *Cancer Epidemiol Biomarkers Prev.* 1997;6(1):57–61.
62. Peters U, Chatterjee N, McGlynn KA, et al. Calcium intake and colorectal adenoma in a US colorectal cancer early detection program. *Am J Clin Nutr.* 2004;80(5):1358–1365.
63. Kesse E, Boutron-Ruault MC, Norat T, Riboli E, Clavel-Chapelon F; E3N Group. Dietary calcium, phosphorus, vitamin D, dairy products and the risk of colorectal adenoma and cancer among French women of the E3N-EPIC prospective study. *Int J Cancer.* 2005;117(1):137–144.
64. Martínez ME, Willett WC. Calcium, vitamin D, and colorectal cancer: a review of the epidemiologic evidence. *Cancer Epidemiol Biomarkers Prev.* 1998;7(2):163–168.
65. Flood A, Peters U, Chatterjee N, Lacey JV Jr, Schairer C, Schatzkin A. Calcium from diet and supplements is associated with reduced risk of colorectal cancer in a prospective cohort of women. *Cancer Epidemiol Biomarkers Prev.* 2005;14(1):126–132.
66. McCullough ML, Robertson AS, Rodriguez C, et al. Calcium, vitamin D, dairy products, and risk of colorectal cancer in the Cancer Prevention Study II Nutrition Cohort (United States). *Cancer Causes Control.* 2003;14(1):1–12.
67. Terry P, Baron JA, Bergkvist L, Holmberg L, Wolk A. Dietary calcium and vitamin D intake and risk of colorectal cancer: a prospective cohort study in women. *Nutr Cancer.* 2002; 43(1):39–46.
68. Bonithon-Kopp C, Kronborg O, Giacosa A, Räth U, Faivre J. Calcium and fibre supplementation in prevention of colorectal adenoma recurrence: a randomised intervention trial. European Cancer Prevention Organisation Study Group. *Lancet.* 2000; 356(9238):1300–1306.
69. Wactawski-Wende J, Kotchen JM, Anderson GL, et al.; Women's Health Initiative Investigators. Calcium plus vitamin D supplementation and the risk of colorectal cancer. *N Engl J Med.* 2006;354(7):684–696.
70. Rudolph A, Toth C, Hoffmeister M, et al. Expression of oestrogen receptor ß and prognosis of colorectal cancer. *Br J Cancer.* 2012;107(5):831–839.
71. Fang YJ, Lu ZH, Wang F, et al. Prognostic impact of ERß and MMP7 expression on overall survival in colon cancer. *Tumour Biol.* 2010;31(6):651–658.
72. Jassam N, Bell SM, Speirs V, Quirke P. Loss of expression of oestrogen receptor beta in colon cancer and its association with Dukes' staging. *Oncol Rep.* 2005;14(1):17–21.
73. Calle EE, Miracle-McMahill HL, Thun MJ, Heath CW Jr. Estrogen replacement therapy and risk of fatal colon cancer in a prospective cohort of postmenopausal women. *J Natl Cancer Inst.* 1995;87(7):517–523.
74. Corrao G, Zambon A, Conti V, et al. Menopause hormone replacement therapy and cancer risk: an Italian record linkage investigation. *Ann Oncol.* 2008;19(1):150–155.
75. Fernandez E, La Vecchia C, Braga C, et al. Hormone replacement therapy and risk of colon and rectal cancer. *Cancer Epidemiol Biomarkers Prev.* 1998;7(4):329–333.
76. Folsom AR, Mink PJ, Sellers TA, Hong CP, Zheng W, Potter JD. Hormonal replacement therapy and morbidity and mortality in a prospective study of postmenopausal women. *Am J Public Health.* 1995;85(8 Pt 1):1128–1132.
77. Furner SE, Davis FG, Nelson RL, Haenszel W. A case-control study of large bowel cancer and hormone exposure in women. *Cancer Res.* 1989;49(17):4936–4940.
78. Hammond CB, Jelovsek FR, Lee KL, Creasman WT, Parker RT. Effects of long-term estrogen replacement therapy. II. Neoplasia. *Am J Obstet Gynecol.* 1979;133(5):537–547.
79. Jacobs EJ, White E, Weiss NS. Exogenous hormones, reproductive history, and colon cancer (Seattle, Washington, USA). *Cancer Causes Control.* 1994;5(4):359–366.
80. Johnson JR, Lacey JV Jr, Lazovich D, et al. Menopausal hormone therapy and risk of colorectal cancer. *Cancer Epidemiol Biomarkers Prev.* 2009;18(1):196–203.

81. Kampman E, Potter JD, Slattery ML, Caan BJ, Edwards S. Hormone replacement therapy, reproductive history, and colon cancer: a multicenter, case-control study in the United States. *Cancer Causes Control.* 1997;8(2):146–158.
82. Nachtigall LE, Nachtigall RH, Nachtigall RD, Beckman EM. Estrogen replacement therapy II: a prospective study in the relationship to carcinoma and cardiovascular and metabolic problems. *Obstet Gynecol.* 1979;54(1):74–79.
83. Paganini-Hill A. Estrogen replacement therapy and colorectal cancer risk in elderly women. *Dis Colon Rectum.* 1999;42(10):1300–1305.
84. Persson I, Yuen J, Bergkvist L, Schairer C. Cancer incidence and mortality in women receiving estrogen and estrogen-progestin replacement therapy–long-term follow-up of a Swedish cohort. *Int J Cancer.* 1996;67(3):327–332.
85. Peters RK, Pike MC, Chang WW, Mack TM. Reproductive factors and colon cancers. *Br J Cancer.* 1990;61(5):741–748.
86. Potter JD, McMichael AJ. Large bowel cancer in women in relation to reproductive and hormonal factors: a case-control study. *J Natl Cancer Inst.* 1983;71(4):703–709.
87. Prihartono N, Palmer JR, Louik C, Shapiro S, Rosenberg L. A case-control study of use of postmenopausal female hormone supplements in relation to the risk of large bowel cancer. *Cancer Epidemiol Biomarkers Prev.* 2000;9(4):443–447.
88. Rennert G, Rennert HS, Pinchev M, Lavie O, Gruber SB. Use of hormone replacement therapy and the risk of colorectal cancer. *J Clin Oncol.* 2009;27(27):4542–4547.
89. Slattery ML, Potter JD, Curtin K, et al. Estrogens reduce and withdrawal of estrogens increase risk of microsatellite instability-positive colon cancer. *Cancer Res.* 2001;61(1):126–130.
90. Jacobson JS, Neugut AI, Garbowski GC, et al. Reproductive risk factors for colorectal adenomatous polyps (New York City, NY, United States). *Cancer Causes Control.* 1995;6(6):513–518.
91. Peipins LA, Newman B, Sandler RS. Reproductive history, use of exogenous hormones, and risk of colorectal adenomas. *Cancer Epidemiol Biomarkers Prev.* 1997;6(9):671–675.
92. Potter JD, Bostick RM, Grandits GA, et al. Hormone replacement therapy is associated with lower risk of adenomatous polyps of the large bowel: the Minnesota Cancer Prevention Research Unit Case-Control Study. *Cancer Epidemiol Biomarkers Prev.* 1996;5(10):779–784.
93. Wolf LA, Terry PD, Potter JD, Bostick RM. Do factors related to endogenous and exogenous estrogens modify the relationship between obesity and risk of colorectal adenomas in women? *Cancer Epidemiol Biomarkers Prev.* 2007;16(4):676–683.
94. Woodson K, Lanza E, Tangrea JA, et al. Hormone replacement therapy and colorectal adenoma recurrence among women in the Polyp Prevention Trial. *J Natl Cancer Inst.* 2001;93(23):1799–1805.
95. MacLennan SC, MacLennan AH, Ryan P. Colorectal cancer and oestrogen replacement therapy. A meta-analysis of epidemiological studies. *Med J Aust.* 1995;162(9):491–493.
96. Hébert-Croteau N. A meta-analysis of hormone replacement therapy and colon cancer in women. *Cancer Epidemiol Biomarkers Prev.* 1998;7(8):653–659.
97. Grodstein F, Newcomb PA, Stampfer MJ. Postmenopausal hormone therapy and the risk of colorectal cancer: a review and meta-analysis. *Am J Med.* 1999;106(5):574–582.
98. Nanda K, Bastian LA, Hasselblad V, Simel DL. Hormone replacement therapy and the risk of colorectal cancer: a meta-analysis. *Obstet Gynecol.* 1999;93(5 Pt 2):880–888.
99. Hildebrand JS, Jacobs EJ, Campbell PT, et al. Colorectal cancer incidence and postmenopausal hormone use by type, recency, and duration in cancer prevention study II. *Cancer Epidemiol Biomarkers Prev.* 2009;18(11):2835–2841.
100. Delellis Henderson K, Duan L, Sullivan-Halley J, et al. Menopausal hormone therapy use and risk of invasive colon cancer: the California Teachers Study. *Am J Epidemiol.* 2010;171(4):415–425.
101. Prentice RL, Pettinger M, Beresford SA, et al. Colorectal cancer in relation to postmenopausal estrogen and estrogen plus progestin in the Women's Health Initiative clinical trial and observational study. *Cancer Epidemiol Biomarkers Prev.* 2009;18(5):1531–1537.
102. Tsilidis KK, Allen NE, Key TJ, et al. Menopausal hormone therapy and risk of colorectal cancer in the European Prospective Investigation into Cancer and Nutrition. *Int J Cancer.* 2011;128(8):1881–1889.
103. Chlebowski RT, Wactawski-Wende J, Ritenbaugh C, et al.; Women's Health Initiative Investigators. Estrogen plus progestin and colorectal cancer in postmenopausal women. *N Engl J Med.* 2004;350(10):991–1004.
104. Grady D, Herrington D, Bittner V, et al.; HERS Research Group. Cardiovascular disease outcomes during 6.8 years of hormone therapy: Heart and Estrogen/progestin Replacement Study follow-up (HERS II). *JAMA.* 2002;288(1):49–57.
105. Hulley S, Furberg C, Barrett-Connor E, et al.; HERS Research Group. Noncardiovascular disease outcomes during 6.8 years of hormone therapy: Heart and Estrogen/progestin Replacement Study follow-up (HERS II). *JAMA.* 2002;288(1):58–66.
106. Anderson GL, Limacher M, Assaf AR, et al.; Women's Health Initiative Steering Committee. Effects of conjugated equine estrogen in postmenopausal women with hysterectomy: the Women's Health Initiative randomized controlled trial. *JAMA.* 2004;291(14):1701–1712.
107. Ritenbaugh C, Stanford JL, Wu L, et al.; Women's Health Initiative Investigators. Conjugated equine estrogens and colorectal cancer incidence and survival: the Women's Health Initiative randomized clinical trial. *Cancer Epidemiol Biomarkers Prev.* 2008;17(10):2609–2618.
108. Maxwell PH. Tumor strengths and frailties: Aspiring to prevent colon cancer. *Nat Med.* 2012;18(1):32–33.
109. Sheehan KM, Sheahan K, O'Donoghue DP, et al. The relationship between cyclooxygenase-2 expression and colorectal cancer. *JAMA.* 1999;282(13):1254–1257.
110. Ristimäki A, Sivula A, Lundin J, et al. Prognostic significance of elevated cyclooxygenase-2 expression in breast cancer. *Cancer Res.* 2002;62(3):632–635.
111. Gaffney DK, Holden J, Davis M, Zempolich K, Murphy KJ, Dodson M. Elevated cyclooxygenase-2 expression correlates with diminished survival in carcinoma of the cervix treated with radiotherapy. *Int J Radiat Oncol Biol Phys.* 2001;49(5):1213–1217.
112. Buskens CJ, Van Rees BP, Sivula A, et al. Prognostic significance of elevated cyclooxygenase 2 expression in patients with adenocarcinoma of the esophagus. *Gastroenterology.* 2002;122(7):1800–1807.
113. Khuri FR, Wu H, Lee JJ, et al. Cyclooxygenase-2 overexpression is a marker of poor prognosis in stage I non-small cell lung cancer. *Clin Cancer Res.* 2001;7(4):861–867.
114. Lehmann JM, Lenhard JM, Oliver BB, Ringold GM, Kliewer SA. Peroxisome proliferator-activated receptors alpha and gamma are activated by indomethacin and other non-steroidal anti-inflammatory drugs. *J Biol Chem.* 1997;272(6):3406–3410.
115. Hsu AL, Ching TT, Wang DS, Song X, Rangnekar VM, Chen CS. The cyclooxygenase-2 inhibitor celecoxib induces apoptosis by blocking Akt activation in human prostate cancer cells independently of Bcl-2. *J Biol Chem.* 2000;275(15):11397–11403.
116. Waskewich C, Blumenthal RD, Li H, Stein R, Goldenberg DM, Burton J. Celecoxib exhibits the greatest potency amongst cyclooxygenase (COX) inhibitors for growth inhibition of COX-2-negative hematopoietic and epithelial cell lines. *Cancer Res.* 2002;62(7):2029–2033.
117. Breuer-Katschinski B, Nemes K, Rump B, et al. Long-term use of nonsteroidal antiinflammatory drugs and the risk of colorectal adenomas. The Colorectal Adenoma Study Group. *Digestion.* 2000;61(2):129–134.

118. Coogan PF, Rosenberg L, Louik C, et al. NSAIDs and risk of colorectal cancer according to presence or absence of family history of the disease. *Cancer Causes Control.* 2000;11(3):249–255.
119. Friedman GD, Coates AO, Potter JD, Slattery ML. Drugs and colon cancer. *Pharmacoepidemiol Drug Saf.* 1998;7(2):99–106.
120. Friis S, Poulsen AH, Sørensen HT, et al. Aspirin and other non-steroidal anti-inflammatory drugs and risk of colorectal cancer: a Danish cohort study. *Cancer Causes Control.* 2009;20(5):731–740.
121. Friis S, Sørensen HT, McLaughlin JK, Johnsen SP, Blot WJ, Olsen JH. A population-based cohort study of the risk of colorectal and other cancers among users of low-dose aspirin. *Br J Cancer.* 2003;88(5):684–688.
122. García Rodríguez LA, Huerta-Alvarez C. Reduced incidence of colorectal adenoma among long-term users of nonsteroidal antiinflammatory drugs: a pooled analysis of published studies and a new population-based study. *Epidemiology.* 2000;11(4):376–381.
123. Grau MV, Sandler RS, McKeown-Eyssen G, et al. Nonsteroidal anti-inflammatory drug use after 3 years of aspirin use and colorectal adenoma risk: observational follow-up of a randomized study. *J Natl Cancer Inst.* 2009;101(4):267–276.
124. Jacobs EJ, Thun MJ, Bain EB, Rodriguez C, Henley SJ, Calle EE. A large cohort study of long-term daily use of adult-strength aspirin and cancer incidence. *J Natl Cancer Inst.* 2007;99(8):608–615.
125. Juarranz M, Calle-Purón ME, González-Navarro A, et al. Physical exercise, use of Plantago ovata and aspirin, and reduced risk of colon cancer. *Eur J Cancer Prev.* 2002;11(5):465–472.
126. Kahn HS, Tatham LM, Thun MJ, Heath CW Jr. Risk factors for self-reported colon polyps. *J Gen Intern Med.* 1998;13(5):303–310.
127. La Vecchia C, Negri E, Franceschi S, et al. Aspirin and colorectal cancer. *Br J Cancer.* 1997;76(5):675–677.
128. Morimoto LM, Newcomb PA, Ulrich CM, Bostick RM, Lais CJ, Potter JD. Risk factors for hyperplastic and adenomatous polyps: evidence for malignant potential? *Cancer Epidemiol Biomarkers Prev.* 2002;11(10 Pt 1):1012–1018.
129. Sandler RS, Galanko JC, Murray SC, Helm JF, Woosley JT. Aspirin and nonsteroidal anti-inflammatory agents and risk for colorectal adenomas. *Gastroenterology.* 1998;114(3):441–447.
130. Sørensen HT, Friis S, Nørgård B, et al. Risk of cancer in a large cohort of nonaspirin NSAID users: a population-based study. *Br J Cancer.* 2003;88(11):1687–1692.
131. Tangrea JA, Albert PS, Lanza E, et al.; Polyp Prevention Study Group. Non-steroidal anti-inflammatory drug use is associated with reduction in recurrence of advanced and non-advanced colorectal adenomas (United States). *Cancer Causes Control.* 2003;14(5):403–411.
132. Chan AT, Giovannucci EL, Meyerhardt JA, Schernhammer ES, Curhan GC, Fuchs CS. Long-term use of aspirin and nonsteroidal anti-inflammatory drugs and risk of colorectal cancer. *JAMA.* 2005;294(8):914–923.
133. Chan AT, Giovannucci EL, Meyerhardt JA, Schernhammer ES, Wu K, Fuchs CS. Aspirin dose and duration of use and risk of colorectal cancer in men. *Gastroenterology.* 2008;134(1):21–28.
134. Burn J, Bishop DT, Chapman PD, et al.; International CAPP consortium. A randomized placebo-controlled prevention trial of aspirin and/or resistant starch in young people with familial adenomatous polyposis. *Cancer Prev Res (Phila).* 2011;4(5):655–665.
135. Burn J, Gerdes AM, Macrae F, et al.; CAPP2 Investigators. Long-term effect of aspirin on cancer risk in carriers of hereditary colorectal cancer: an analysis from the CAPP2 randomised controlled trial. *Lancet.* 2011;378(9809):2081–2087.
136. Logan RF, Grainge MJ, Shepherd VC, Armitage NC, Muir KR; ukCAP Trial Group. Aspirin and folic acid for the prevention of recurrent colorectal adenomas. *Gastroenterology.* 2008;134(1):29–38.
137. Benamouzig R, Deyra J, Martin A, et al. Daily soluble aspirin and prevention of colorectal adenoma recurrence: one-year results of the APACC trial. *Gastroenterology.* 2003;125(2):328–336.
138. Benamouzig R, Uzzan B, Deyra J, et al.; Association pour la Prévention par l'Aspirine du Cancer Colorectal Study Group (APACC). Prevention by daily soluble aspirin of colorectal adenoma recurrence: 4-year results of the APACC randomised trial. *Gut.* 2012;61(2):255–261.
139. Cook NR, Lee IM, Gaziano JM, et al. Low-dose aspirin in the primary prevention of cancer: the Women's Health Study: a randomized controlled trial. *JAMA.* 2005;294(1):47–55.
140. Gann PH, Manson JE, Glynn RJ, Buring JE, Hennekens CH. Low-dose aspirin and incidence of colorectal tumors in a randomized trial. *J Natl Cancer Inst.* 1993;85(15):1220–1224.
141. Flossmann E, Rothwell PM; British Doctors Aspirin Trial and the UK-TIA Aspirin Trial. Effect of aspirin on long-term risk of colorectal cancer: consistent evidence from randomised and observational studies. *Lancet.* 2007;369(9573):1603–1613.
142. Rothwell PM, Fowkes FG, Belch JF, Ogawa H, Warlow CP, Meade TW. Effect of daily aspirin on long-term risk of death due to cancer: analysis of individual patient data from randomised trials. *Lancet.* 2011;377(9759):31–41.
143. Cuzick J, Otto F, Baron JA, et al. Aspirin and non-steroidal anti-inflammatory drugs for cancer prevention: an international consensus statement. *Lancet Oncol.* 2009;10(5):501–507.
144. Das D, Chilton AP, Jankowski JA. Chemoprevention of oesophageal cancer and the AspECT trial. *Recent Results Cancer Res.* 2009;181:161–169.
145. Arber N, Eagle CJ, Spicak J, et al.; PreSAP Trial Investigators. Celecoxib for the prevention of colorectal adenomatous polyps. *N Engl J Med.* 2006;355(9):885–895.
146. Bertagnolli MM, Eagle CJ, Zauber AG, et al.; APC Study Investigators. Celecoxib for the prevention of sporadic colorectal adenomas. *N Engl J Med.* 2006;355(9):873–884.
147. Bresalier RS, Sandler RS, Quan H, et al.; Adenomatous Polyp Prevention on Vioxx (APPROVe) Trial Investigators. Cardiovascular events associated with rofecoxib in a colorectal adenoma chemoprevention trial. *N Engl J Med.* 2005;352(11):1092–1102.
148. Solomon SD, Wittes J, Finn PV, et al.; Cross Trial Safety Assessment Group. Cardiovascular risk of celecoxib in 6 randomized placebo-controlled trials: the cross trial safety analysis. *Circulation.* 2008;117(16):2104–2113.
149. Bertagnolli MM, Eagle CJ, Zauber AG, et al.; Adenoma Prevention with Celecoxib Study Investigators. Five-year efficacy and safety analysis of the Adenoma Prevention with Celecoxib Trial. *Cancer Prev Res (Phila).* 2009;2(4):310–321.
150. Lynch PM, Ayers GD, Hawk E, et al. The safety and efficacy of celecoxib in children with familial adenomatous polyposis. *Am J Gastroenterol.* 2010;105(6):1437–1443.
151. Giardiello FM, Yang VW, Hylind LM, et al. Primary chemoprevention of familial adenomatous polyposis with sulindac. *N Engl J Med.* 2002;346(14):1054–1059.
152. Giardiello FM, Hamilton SR, Krush AJ, et al. Treatment of colonic and rectal adenomas with sulindac in familial adenomatous polyposis. *N Engl J Med.* 1993;328(18):1313–1316.
153. Labayle D, Fischer D, Vielh P, et al. Sulindac causes regression of rectal polyps in familial adenomatous polyposis. *Gastroenterology.* 1991;101(3):635–639.
154. Nugent KP, Farmer KC, Spigelman AD, Williams CB, Phillips RK. Randomized controlled trial of the effect of sulindac on duodenal and rectal polyposis and cell proliferation in patients with familial adenomatous polyposis. *Br J Surg.* 1993;80(12):1618–1619.
155. Ladenheim J, Garcia G, Titzer D, et al. Effect of sulindac on sporadic colonic polyps. *Gastroenterology.* 1995;108(4):1083–1087.
156. Nigro ND, Bull AW, Boyd ME. Inhibition of intestinal carcinogenesis in rats: effect of difluoromethylornithine with piroxicam or fish oil. *J Natl Cancer Inst.* 1986;77(6):1309–1313.

157. Meyskens FL Jr, Gerner EW. Development of difluoromethylornithine (DFMO) as a chemoprevention agent. *Clin Cancer Res.* 1999;5(5):945–951.
158. Gerner EW, Meyskens FL Jr, Goldschmid S, Lance P, Pelot D. Rationale for, and design of, a clinical trial targeting polyamine metabolism for colon cancer chemoprevention. *Amino Acids.* 2007;33(2):189–195.
159. Lawson KR, Ignatenko NA, Piazza GA, Cui H, Gerner EW. Influence of K-ras activation on the survival responses of Caco-2 cells to the chemopreventive agents sulindac and difluoromethylornithine. *Cancer Epidemiol Biomarkers Prev.* 2000;9(11):1155–1162.
160. Meyskens FL Jr, McLaren CE, Pelot D, et al. Difluoromethylornithine plus sulindac for the prevention of sporadic colorectal adenomas: a randomized placebo-controlled, double-blind trial. *Cancer Prev Res (Phila).* 2008;1(1):32–38.
161. Hull MA. Omega-3 polyunsaturated fatty acids. *Best Pract Res Clin Gastroenterol.* 2011;25(4–5):547–554.
162. Cockbain AJ, Toogood GJ, Hull MA. Omega-3 polyunsaturated fatty acids for the treatment and prevention of colorectal cancer. *Gut.* 2012;61(1):135–149.
163. MacLean CH, Newberry SJ, Mojica WA, et al. Effects of omega-3 fatty acids on cancer risk: a systematic review. *JAMA.* 2006;295(4):403–415.
164. West NJ, Clark SK, Phillips RK, et al. Eicosapentaenoic acid reduces rectal polyp number and size in familial adenomatous polyposis. *Gut.* 2010;59(7):918–925.
165. McMichael AJ, Potter JD. Host factors in carcinogenesis: certain bile-acid metabolic profiles that selectively increase the risk of proximal colon cancer. *J Natl Cancer Inst.* 1985;75(2):185–191.
166. Perez MJ, Briz O. Bile-acid-induced cell injury and protection. *World J Gastroenterol.* 2009;15(14):1677–1689.
167. Amaral JD, Castro RE, Solá S, Steer CJ, Rodrigues CM. p53 is a key molecular target of ursodeoxycholic acid in regulating apoptosis. *J Biol Chem.* 2007;282(47):34250–34259.
168. Amaral JD, Viana RJ, Ramalho RM, Steer CJ, Rodrigues CM. Bile acids: regulation of apoptosis by ursodeoxycholic acid. *J Lipid Res.* 2009;50(9):1721–1734.
169. Alberts DS, Martínez ME, Hess LM, et al.; Phoenix and Tucson Gastroenterologist Networks. Phase III trial of ursodeoxycholic acid to prevent colorectal adenoma recurrence. *J Natl Cancer Inst.* 2005;97(11):846–853.
170. Thompson PA, Wertheim BC, Roe DJ, et al. Gender modifies the effect of ursodeoxycholic acid in a randomized controlled trial in colorectal adenoma patients. *Cancer Prev Res (Phila).* 2009;2(12):1023–1030.
171. Eaton JE, Silveira MG, Pardi DS, et al. High-dose ursodeoxycholic acid is associated with the development of colorectal neoplasia in patients with ulcerative colitis and primary sclerosing cholangitis. *Am J Gastroenterol.* 2011;106(9):1638–1645.
172. Carroll RE, Benya RV, Turgeon DK, et al. Phase IIa clinical trial of curcumin for the prevention of colorectal neoplasia. *Cancer Prev Res (Phila).* 2011;4(3):354–364.
173. Zhang L, Ren X, Alt E, et al. Chemoprevention of colorectal cancer by targeting APC-deficient cells for apoptosis. *Nature.* 2010;464(7291):1058–1061.
174. Silk AW, Schoen RE, Potter DM, Finn OJ. Humoral immune response to abnormal MUC1 in subjects with colorectal adenoma and cancer. *Mol Immunol.* 2009;47(1):52–56.
175. Schlom J. Therapeutic cancer vaccines: current status and moving forward. *J Natl Cancer Inst.* 2012;104(8):599–613.
176. Slattery ML, Levin TR, Ma K, Goldgar D, Holubkov R, Edwards S. Family history and colorectal cancer: predictors of risk. *Cancer Causes Control.* 2003;14(9):879–887.
177. Johns LE, Houlston RS. A systematic review and meta-analysis of familial colorectal cancer risk. *Am J Gastroenterol.* 2001;96(10):2992–3003.
178. Levin B, Lieberman DA, McFarland B, et al.; American Cancer Society Colorectal Cancer Advisory Group; US Multi-Society Task Force; American College of Radiology Colon Cancer Committee. Screening and surveillance for the early detection of colorectal cancer and adenomatous polyps, 2008: a joint guideline from the American Cancer Society, the US Multi-Society Task Force on Colorectal Cancer, and the American College of Radiology. *Gastroenterology.* 2008;134(5):1570–1595.
179. Rex DK, Johnson DA, Anderson JC, Schoenfeld PS, Burke CA, Inadomi JM; American College of Gastroenterology. American College of Gastroenterology guidelines for colorectal cancer screening 2009 [corrected]. *Am J Gastroenterol.* 2009;104(3):739–750.
180. Buiatti E, Crocetti E, Acciai S, et al. Incidence of second primary cancers in three Italian population-based cancer registries. *Eur J Cancer.* 1997;33(11):1829–1834.
181. Agarwal N, Ulahannan MJ, Mandile MA, Cayten CG, Pitchumoni CS. Increased risk of colorectal cancer following breast cancer. *Ann Surg.* 1986;203(3):307–310.
182. Eisen GM, Sandler RS. Are women with breast cancer more likely to develop colorectal cancer? Critical review and meta-analysis. *J Clin Gastroenterol.* 1994;19(1):57–63.
183. Khalil S, Ceccarelli F. Colorectal cancer after breast cancer: magnitude of risk in clinical practice and in the literature. *Tumori.* 2009;95(1):28–31.
184. Bremond A, Collet P, Lambert R, Martin JL. Breast cancer and polyps of the colon. A case-control study. *Cancer.* 1984;54(11):2568–2570.
185. Willett WC. Diet and cancer. *Oncologist.* 2000;5(5):393–404.
186. Bartsch H, Nair J, Owen RW. Dietary polyunsaturated fatty acids and cancers of the breast and colorectum: emerging evidence for their role as risk modifiers. *Carcinogenesis.* 1999;20(12):2209–2218.
187. Gillessen S, Templeton A, Marra G, Kuo YF, Valtorta E, Shahinian VB. Risk of colorectal cancer in men on long-term androgen deprivation therapy for prostate cancer. *J Natl Cancer Inst.* 2010;102(23):1760–1770.
188. Brenner DJ, Curtis RE, Hall EJ, Ron E. Second malignancies in prostate carcinoma patients after radiotherapy compared with surgery. *Cancer.* 2000;88(2):398–406.
189. Brown AP, Neeley ES, Werner T, Soisson AP, Burt RW, Gaffney DK. A population-based study of subsequent primary malignancies after endometrial cancer: genetic, environmental, and treatment-related associations. *Int J Radiat Oncol Biol Phys.* 2010;78(1):127–135.
190. Bostrom PJ, Soloway MS. Secondary cancer after radiotherapy for prostate cancer: should we be more aware of the risk? *Eur Urol.* 2007;52(4):973–982.
191. Tarin TV, Sonn G, Shinghal R. Estimating the risk of cancer associated with imaging related radiation during surveillance for stage I testicular cancer using computerized tomography. *J Urol.* 2009;181(2):627–32; discussion 632.
192. Kaldor J. Second cancer following chemotherapy and radiotherapy. An epidemiological perspective. *Acta Oncol.* 1990;29(5):647–655.
193. Travis LB, Curtis RE, Glimelius B, et al. Second cancers among long-term survivors of non-Hodgkin's lymphoma. *J Natl Cancer Inst.* 1993;85(23):1932–1937.
194. Brennan P, Coates M, Armstrong B, Colin D, Boffetta P. Second primary neoplasms following non-Hodgkin's lymphoma in New South Wales, Australia. *Br J Cancer.* 2000;82(7):1344–1347.
195. Mudie NY, Swerdlow AJ, Higgins CD, et al. Risk of second malignancy after non-Hodgkin's lymphoma: a British Cohort Study. *J Clin Oncol.* 2006;24(10):1568–1574.
196. Dong C, Hemminki K. Second primary neoplasms among 53 159 haematolymphoproliferative malignancy patients in Sweden, 1958–1996: a search for common mechanisms. *Br J Cancer.* 2001;85(7):997–1005.
197. Maule M, Scélo G, Pastore G, et al. Risk of second malignant neoplasms after childhood leukemia and lymphoma: an international study. *J Natl Cancer Inst.* 2007;99(10):790–800.

198. Woodage T, King SM, Wacholder S, et al. The APCI1307K allele and cancer risk in a community-based study of Ashkenazi Jews. *Nat Genet.* 1998;20(1):62–65.
199. Ries LA, Eisner M, Kosary CL, et al. SEER cancer statistics review, 1975–2000. National Cancer Institute; 2000.
200. Theuer CP, Wagner JL, Taylor TH, et al. Racial and ethnic colorectal cancer patterns affect the cost-effectiveness of colorectal cancer screening in the United States. *Gastroenterology.* 2001;120(4):848–856.
201. Agrawal S, Bhupinderjit A, Bhutani MS, et al.; Committee of Minority Affairs and Cultural Diversity, American College of Gastroenterology. Colorectal cancer in African Americans. *Am J Gastroenterol.* 2005;100(3):515–23; discussion 514.
202. Lieberman DA, Holub JL, Moravec MD, Eisen GM, Peters D, Morris CD. Prevalence of colon polyps detected by colonoscopy screening in asymptomatic black and white patients. *JAMA.* 2008;300(12):1417–1422.
203. Willett WC, Stampfer MJ, Colditz GA, Rosner BA, Speizer FE. Relation of meat, fat, and fiber intake to the risk of colon cancer in a prospective study among women. *N Engl J Med.* 1990;323(24):1664–1672.
204. Alexander DD, Miller AJ, Cushing CA, Lowe KA. Processed meat and colorectal cancer: a quantitative review of prospective epidemiologic studies. *Eur J Cancer Prev.* 2010;19(5):328–341.
205. Norat T, Bingham S, Ferrari P, et al. Meat, fish, and colorectal cancer risk: the European Prospective Investigation into cancer and nutrition. *J Natl Cancer Inst.* 2005;97(12):906–916.
206. Larsson SC, Wolk A. Meat consumption and risk of colorectal cancer: a meta-analysis of prospective studies. *Int J Cancer.* 2006;119(11):2657–2664.
207. Jacobs ET, Thompson PA, Martínez ME. Diet, gender, and colorectal neoplasia. *J Clin Gastroenterol.* 2007;41(8):731–746.
208. Bingham SA, Pignatelli B, Pollock JR, et al. Does increased endogenous formation of N-nitroso compounds in the human colon explain the association between red meat and colon cancer? *Carcinogenesis.* 1996;17(3):515–523.
209. Cross AJ, Ferrucci LM, Risch A, et al. A large prospective study of meat consumption and colorectal cancer risk: an investigation of potential mechanisms underlying this association. *Cancer Res.* 2010;70(6):2406–2414.
210. Sesink AL, Termont DS, Kleibeuker JH, Van der Meer R. Red meat and colon cancer: the cytotoxic and hyperproliferative effects of dietary heme. *Cancer Res.* 1999;59(22):5704–5709.
211. Le Marchand L, Hankin JH, Wilkens LR, et al. Combined effects of well-done red meat, smoking, and rapid N-acetyltransferase 2 and CYP1A2 phenotypes in increasing colorectal cancer risk. *Cancer Epidemiol Biomarkers Prev.* 2001;10(12):1259–1266.
212. Nöthlings U, Yamamoto JF, Wilkens LR, et al. Meat and heterocyclic amine intake, smoking, NAT1 and NAT2 polymorphisms, and colorectal cancer risk in the multiethnic cohort study. *Cancer Epidemiol Biomarkers Prev.* 2009;18(7):2098–2106.
213. Hall MN, Campos H, Li H, et al. Blood levels of long-chain polyunsaturated fatty acids, aspirin, and the risk of colorectal cancer. *Cancer Epidemiol Biomarkers Prev.* 2007;16(2):314–321.
214. Nkondjock A, Shatenstein B, Maisonneuve P, Ghadirian P. Assessment of risk associated with specific fatty acids and colorectal cancer among French-Canadians in Montreal: a case-control study. *Int J Epidemiol.* 2003;32(2):200–209.
215. Simopoulos AP. Evolutionary aspects of diet, the omega-6/omega-3 ratio and genetic variation: nutritional implications for chronic diseases. *Biomed Pharmacother.* 2006;60(9):502–507.
216. Wynder EL, Reddy BS. Metabolic epidemiology of colorectal cancer. *Cancer.* 1974;34(3):suppl:801–suppl:806.
217. Howe GR, Aronson KJ, Benito E, et al. The relationship between dietary fat intake and risk of colorectal cancer: evidence from the combined analysis of 13 case-control studies. *Cancer Causes Control.* 1997;8(2):215–228.
218. Johnson IT, Lund EK. Review article: nutrition, obesity and colorectal cancer. *Aliment Pharmacol Ther.* 2007;26(2):161–181.
219. Beresford SA, Johnson KC, Ritenbaugh C, et al. Low-fat dietary pattern and risk of colorectal cancer: the Women's Health Initiative Randomized Controlled Dietary Modification Trial. *JAMA.* 2006;295(6):643–654.
220. Burkitt DP. Possible relationships between bowel cancer and dietary habits. *Proc R Soc Med.* 1971;64(9):964–965.
221. Trowell H, Burkitt D. Physiological role of dietary fiber: a ten-year review. *ASDC J Dent Child.* 1986;53(6):444–447.
222. Howe GR, Benito E, Castelleto R, et al. Dietary intake of fiber and decreased risk of cancers of the colon and rectum: evidence from the combined analysis of 13 case-control studies. *J Natl Cancer Inst.* 1992;84(24):1887–1896.
223. Tan KY, Seow-Choen F. Fiber and colorectal diseases: separating fact from fiction. *World J Gastroenterol.* 2007;13(31):4161–4167.
224. Fuchs CS, Giovannucci EL, Colditz GA, et al. Dietary fiber and the risk of colorectal cancer and adenoma in women. *N Engl J Med.* 1999;340(3):169–176.
225. Terry P, Giovannucci E, Michels KB, et al. Fruit, vegetables, dietary fiber, and risk of colorectal cancer. *J Natl Cancer Inst.* 2001;93(7):525–533.
226. Otani T, Iwasaki M, Ishihara J, Sasazuki S, Inoue M, Tsugane S; Japan Public Health Center-Based Prospective Study Group. Dietary fiber intake and subsequent risk of colorectal cancer: the Japan Public Health Center-based prospective study. *Int J Cancer.* 2006;119(6):1475–1480.
227. Shin A, Li H, Shu XO, Yang G, Gao YT, Zheng W. Dietary intake of calcium, fiber and other micronutrients in relation to colorectal cancer risk: Results from the Shanghai Women's Health Study. *Int J Cancer.* 2006;119(12):2938–2942.
228. Park Y, Hunter DJ, Spiegelman D, et al. Dietary fiber intake and risk of colorectal cancer: a pooled analysis of prospective cohort studies. *JAMA.* 2005;294(22):2849–2857.
229. Alberts DS, Martínez ME, Roe DJ, et al. Lack of effect of a high-fiber cereal supplement on the recurrence of colorectal adenomas. Phoenix Colon Cancer Prevention Physicians' Network. *N Engl J Med.* 2000;342(16):1156–1162.
230. Schatzkin A, Lanza E, Corle D, et al. Lack of effect of a low-fat, high-fiber diet on the recurrence of colorectal adenomas. Polyp Prevention Trial Study Group. *N Engl J Med.* 2000;342(16):1149–1155.
231. Bingham SA, Norat T, Moskal A, et al. Is the association with fiber from foods in colorectal cancer confounded by folate intake? *Cancer Epidemiol Biomarkers Prev.* 2005;14(6):1552–1556.
232. Eastwood MA, Morris ER. Physical properties of dietary fiber that influence physiological function: a model for polymers along the gastrointestinal tract. *Am J Clin Nutr.* 1992;55(2):436–442.
233. Gibson GR, Willems A, Reading S, Collins MD. Fermentation of non-digestible oligosaccharides by human colonic bacteria. *Proc Nutr Soc.* 1996;55(3):899–912.
234. Pufulete M. Intake of dairy products and risk of colorectal neoplasia. *Nutr Res Rev.* 2008;21(1):56–67.
235. Park SY, Murphy SP, Wilkens LR, Nomura AM, Henderson BE, Kolonel LN. Calcium and vitamin D intake and risk of colorectal cancer: the Multiethnic Cohort Study. *Am J Epidemiol.* 2007;165(7):784–793.
236. Larsson SC, Bergkvist L, Rutegård J, Giovannucci E, Wolk A. Calcium and dairy food intakes are inversely associated with colorectal cancer risk in the Cohort of Swedish Men. *Am J Clin Nutr.* 2006;83(3):667–73; quiz 728.
237. Norat T, Riboli E. Dairy products and colorectal cancer. A review of possible mechanisms and epidemiological evidence. *Eur J Clin Nutr.* 2003;57(1):1–17.
238. Henderson N, Gregory J, Irving K, et al. The National Diet and Nutrition Survey: Adults Aged 19 to 64 years. Vitamin and Mineral Intake and Urinary Analytes. Vol. 3. http://www.food.gov.uk/multimedia/pdfs/ndnsv3.pdf

239. Cho E, Smith-Warner SA, Spiegelman D, et al. Dairy foods, calcium, and colorectal cancer: a pooled analysis of 10 cohort studies. *J Natl Cancer Inst.* 2004;96(13):1015–1022.
240. Martínez ME, Marshall JR, Sampliner R, Wilkinson J, Alberts DS. Calcium, vitamin D, and risk of adenoma recurrence (United States). *Cancer Causes Control.* 2002;13(3):213–220.
241. Hartman TJ, Albert PS, Snyder K, et al.; Polyp Prevention Study Group. The association of calcium and vitamin D with risk of colorectal adenomas. *J Nutr.* 2005;135(2):252–259.
242. Lipkin M, Friedman E, Winawer SJ, Newmark H. Colonic epithelial cell proliferation in responders and nonresponders to supplemental dietary calcium. *Cancer Res.* 1989;49(1):248–254.
243. Govers MJ, Termont DS, Lapré JA, Kleibeuker JH, Vonk RJ, Van der Meer R. Calcium in milk products precipitates intestinal fatty acids and secondary bile acids and thus inhibits colonic cytotoxicity in humans. *Cancer Res.* 1996;56(14):3270–3275.
244. Lipkin M, Newmark H. Calcium and the prevention of colon cancer. *J Cell Biochem Suppl.* 1995;22:65–73.
245. Garland CF, Garland FC. Do sunlight and vitamin D reduce the likelihood of colon cancer? *Int J Epidemiol.* 2006;35(2):217–220.
246. Harris DM, Go VL. Vitamin D and colon carcinogenesis. *J Nutr.* 2004;134(12 Suppl):3463S–3471S.
247. Food nutrition and the prevention of cancer: a global prespective. Washington, DC: World Cancer Research Fund/American Institute for Cancer Research; 1997.
248. Voorrips LE, Goldbohm RA, Verhoeven DT, et al. Vegetable and fruit consumption and lung cancer risk in the Netherlands Cohort Study on diet and cancer. *Cancer Causes Control.* 2000; 11(2):101–115.
249. Michels KB, Edward Giovannucci, Joshipura KJ, et al. Prospective study of fruit and vegetable consumption and incidence of colon and rectal cancers. *J Natl Cancer Inst.* 2000;92(21): 1740–1752.
250. Lin J, Zhang SM, Cook NR, et al. Dietary intakes of fruit, vegetables, and fiber, and risk of colorectal cancer in a prospective cohort of women (United States). *Cancer Causes Control.* 2005;16(3):225–233.
251. Aune D, Lau R, Chan DS, et al. Nonlinear reduction in risk for colorectal cancer by fruit and vegetable intake based on meta-analysis of prospective studies. *Gastroenterology.* 2011;141(1):106–118.
252. Blount BC, Mack MM, Wehr CM, et al. Folate deficiency causes uracil misincorporation into human DNA and chromosome breakage: implications for cancer and neuronal damage. *Proc Natl Acad Sci USA.* 1997;94(7):3290–3295.
253. Kim DH, Smith-Warner SA, Spiegelman D, et al. Pooled analyses of 13 prospective cohort studies on folate intake and colon cancer. *Cancer Causes Control.* 2010;21(11):1919–1930.
254. el-Bayoumy K, Chae YH, Upadhyaya P, Meschter C, Cohen LA, Reddy BS. Inhibition of 7,12-dimethylbenz(a)anthracene-induced tumors and DNA adduct formation in the mammary glands of female Sprague-Dawley rats by the synthetic organoselenium compound, 1,4-phenylenebis(methylene)selenocyanate. *Cancer Res.* 1992;52(9):2402–2407.
255. Whanger PD. Selenium and its relationship to cancer: an update. *Br J Nutr.* 2004;91(1):11–28.
256. Russo MW, Murray SC, Wurzelmann JI, Woosley JT, Sandler RS. Plasma selenium levels and the risk of colorectal adenomas. *Nutr Cancer.* 1997;28(2):125–129.
257. Jacobs ET, Jiang R, Alberts DS, et al. Selenium and colorectal adenoma: results of a pooled analysis. *J Natl Cancer Inst.* 2004;96(22):1669–1675.
258. Peters U, Chatterjee N, Church TR, et al. High serum selenium and reduced risk of advanced colorectal adenoma in a colorectal cancer early detection program. *Cancer Epidemiol Biomarkers Prev.* 2006;15(2):315–320.
259. Reid ME, Duffield-Lillico AJ, Sunga A, Fakih M, Alberts DS, Marshall JR. Selenium supplementation and colorectal adenomas: an analysis of the nutritional prevention of cancer trial. *Int J Cancer.* 2006;118(7):1777–1781.
260. Nelson MA, Goulet AC, Jacobs ET, Lance P. Studies into the anticancer effects of selenomethionine against human colon cancer. *Ann N Y Acad Sci.* 2005;1059:26–32.
261. Lee IM. Antioxidant vitamins in the prevention of cancer. *Proc Assoc Am Physicians.* 1999;111(1):10–15.
262. Seifried HE. Oxidative stress and antioxidants: a link to disease and prevention? *J Nutr Biochem.* 2007;18(3):168–171.
263. Bjelakovic G, Nikolova D, Simonetti RG, Gluud C. Systematic review: primary and secondary prevention of gastrointestinal cancers with antioxidant supplements. *Aliment Pharmacol Ther.* 2008;28(6):689–703.
264. Cooper K, Squires H, Carroll C, et al. Chemoprevention of colorectal cancer: systematic review and economic evaluation. *Health Technol Assess.* 2010;14(32):1–206.
265. Giovannucci E, Liu Y, Willett WC. Cancer incidence and mortality and vitamin D in black and white male health professionals. *Cancer Epidemiol Biomarkers Prev.* 2006;15(12): 2467–2472.
266. Lee IM, Paffenbarger RS Jr. Quetelet's index and risk of colon cancer in college alumni. *J Natl Cancer Inst.* 1992; 84(17):1326–1331.
267. MacInnis RJ, English DR, Hopper JL, Gertig DM, Haydon AM, Giles GG. Body size and composition and colon cancer risk in women. *Int J Cancer.* 2006;118(6):1496–1500.
268. Samanic C, Chow WH, Gridley G, Jarvholm B, Fraumeni JF Jr. Relation of body mass index to cancer risk in 362,552 Swedish men. *Cancer Causes Control.* 2006;17(7):901–909.
269. Pischon T, Lahmann PH, Boeing H, et al. Body size and risk of colon and rectal cancer in the European Prospective Investigation Into Cancer and Nutrition (EPIC). *J Natl Cancer Inst.* 2006; 98(13):920–931.
270. Fantuzzi G. Adipose tissue, adipokines, and inflammation. *J Allergy Clin Immunol.* 2005;115(5):911–9; quiz 920.
271. Rondinone CM. Adipocyte-derived hormones, cytokines, and mediators. *Endocrine.* 2006;29(1):81–90.
272. Friedenreich C, Norat T, Steindorf K, et al. Physical activity and risk of colon and rectal cancers: the European prospective investigation into cancer and nutrition. *Cancer Epidemiol Biomarkers Prev.* 2006;15(12):2398–2407.
273. Liang PS, Chen TY, Giovannucci E. Cigarette smoking and colorectal cancer incidence and mortality: systematic review and meta-analysis. *Int J Cancer.* 2009;124(10):2406–2415.
274. Marshall JR. Prevention of colorectal cancer: diet, chemoprevention, and lifestyle. *Gastroenterol Clin North Am.* 2008;37(1):73–82, vi.
275. Cho E, Smith-Warner SA, Ritz J, et al. Alcohol intake and colorectal cancer: a pooled analysis of 8 cohort studies. *Ann Intern Med.* 2004;140(8):603–613.
276. Moskal A, Norat T, Ferrari P, Riboli E. Alcohol intake and colorectal cancer risk: a dose-response meta-analysis of published cohort studies. *Int J Cancer.* 2007;120(3):664–671.
277. Mizoue T, Inoue M, Wakai K, et al.; Research Group for Development and Evaluation of Cancer Prevention Strategies in Japan. Alcohol drinking and colorectal cancer in Japanese: a pooled analysis of results from five cohort studies. *Am J Epidemiol.* 2008;167(12):1397–1406.
278. Tsong WH, Koh WP, Yuan JM, Wang R, Sun CL, Yu MC. Cigarettes and alcohol in relation to colorectal cancer: the Singapore Chinese Health Study. *Br J Cancer.* 2007;96(5):821–827.
279. Ferrari P, Jenab M, Norat T, et al. Lifetime and baseline alcohol intake and risk of colon and rectal cancers in the European prospective investigation into cancer and nutrition (EPIC). *Int J Cancer.* 2007;121(9):2065–2072.
280. Giovannucci E. Alcohol, one-carbon metabolism, and colorectal cancer: recent insights from molecular studies. *J Nutr.* 2004;134(9):2475S–2481S.

281. Giovannucci E. Insulin, insulin-like growth factors and colon cancer: a review of the evidence. *J Nutr.* 2001;131(11 Suppl):3109S–3120S.
282. La Vecchia C, D'Avanzo B, Negri E, Franceschi S. History of selected diseases and the risk of colorectal cancer. *Eur J Cancer.* 1991;27(5):582–586.
283. Le Marchand L, Wilkens LR, Kolonel LN, Hankin JH, Lyu LC. Associations of sedentary lifestyle, obesity, smoking, alcohol use, and diabetes with the risk of colorectal cancer. *Cancer Res.* 1997;57(21):4787–4794.
284. Will JC, Galuska DA, Vinicor F, Calle EE. Colorectal cancer: another complication of diabetes mellitus? *Am J Epidemiol.* 1998;147(9):816–825.
285. Hu FB, Manson JE, Liu S, et al. Prospective study of adult onset diabetes mellitus (type 2) and risk of colorectal cancer in women. *J Natl Cancer Inst.* 1999;91(6):542–547.
286. Limburg PJ, Vierkant RA, Fredericksen ZS, et al. Clinically confirmed type 2 diabetes mellitus and colorectal cancer risk: a population-based, retrospective cohort study. *Am J Gastroenterol.* 2006;101(8):1872–1879.
287. Siddiqui AA, Spechler SJ, Huerta S, Dredar S, Little BB, Cryer B. Elevated HbA1c is an independent predictor of aggressive clinical behavior in patients with colorectal cancer: a case-control study. *Dig Dis Sci.* 2008;53(9):2486–2494.
288. Giouleme O, Diamantidis MD, Katsaros MG. Is diabetes a causal agent for colorectal cancer? Pathophysiological and molecular mechanisms. *World J Gastroenterol.* 2011;17(4):444–448.
289. Fajas L, Auboeuf D, Raspé E, et al. The organization, promoter analysis, and expression of the human PPARgamma gene. *J Biol Chem.* 1997;272(30):18779–18789.
290. DuBois RN, Gupta R, Brockman J, Reddy BS, Krakow SL, Lazar MA. The nuclear eicosanoid receptor, PPARgamma, is aberrantly expressed in colonic cancers. *Carcinogenesis.* 1998;19(1):49–53.
291. Sarraf P, Mueller E, Smith WM, et al. Loss-of-function mutations in PPAR gamma associated with human colon cancer. *Mol Cell.* 1999;3(6):799–804.
292. Ikezoe T, Miller CW, Kawano S, et al. Mutational analysis of the peroxisome proliferator-activated receptor gamma gene in human malignancies. *Cancer Res.* 2001;61(13):5307–5310.
293. Sarraf P, Mueller E, Jones D, et al. Differentiation and reversal of malignant changes in colon cancer through PPARgamma. *Nat Med.* 1998;4(9):1046–1052.
294. Brockman JA, Gupta RA, Dubois RN. Activation of PPARgamma leads to inhibition of anchorage-independent growth of human colorectal cancer cells. *Gastroenterology.* 1998;115(5):1049–1055.
295. Shimada T, Kojima K, Yoshiura K, Hiraishi H, Terano A. Characteristics of the peroxisome proliferator activated receptor gamma (PPARgamma) ligand induced apoptosis in colon cancer cells. *Gut.* 2002;50(5):658–664.
296. Lefebvre AM, Chen I, Desreumaux P, et al. Activation of the peroxisome proliferator-activated receptor gamma promotes the development of colon tumors in C57BL/6J-APCMin/+ mice. *Nat Med.* 1998;4(9):1053–1057.
297. Suzawa M, Takada I, Yanagisawa J, et al. Cytokines suppress adipogenesis and PPAR-gamma function through the TAK1/TAB1/NIK cascade. *Nat Cell Biol.* 2003;5(3):224–230.
298. Thompson EA. PPARgamma physiology and pathology in gastrointestinal epithelial cells. *Mol Cells.* 2007;24(2):167–176.
299. Fujisawa T, Nakajima A, Fujisawa N, et al. Peroxisome proliferator-activated receptor gamma (PPARgamma) suppresses colonic epithelial cell turnover and colon carcinogenesis through inhibition of the beta-catenin/T cell factor (TCF) pathway. *J Pharmacol Sci.* 2008;106(4):627–638.
300. Poynter JN, Gruber SB, Higgins PD, et al. Statins and the risk of colorectal cancer. *N Engl J Med.* 2005;352(21):2184–2192.
301. Farwell WR, Scranton RE, Lawler EV, et al. The association between statins and cancer incidence in a veterans population. *J Natl Cancer Inst.* 2008;100(2):134–139.
302. Karp I, Behlouli H, Lelorier J, Pilote L. Statins and cancer risk. *Am J Med.* 2008;121(4):302–309.
303. Yasuda Y, Shimizu M, Shirakami Y, et al. Pitavastatin inhibits azoxymethane-induced colonic preneoplastic lesions in C57BL/KsJ-db/db obese mice. *Cancer Sci.* 2010;101(7):1701–1707.
304. Yasui Y, Suzuki R, Miyamoto S, et al. A lipophilic statin, pitavastatin, suppresses inflammation-associated mouse colon carcinogenesis. *Int J Cancer.* 2007;121(10):2331–2339.
305. Riganti C, Aldieri E, Doublier S, Bosia A, Ghigo D. Statins-mediated inhibition of rho GTPases as a potential tool in anti-tumor therapy. *Mini Rev Med Chem.* 2008;8(6):609–618.
306. Cho SJ, Kim JS, Kim JM, Lee JY, Jung HC, Song IS. Simvastatin induces apoptosis in human colon cancer cells and in tumor xenografts, and attenuates colitis-associated colon cancer in mice. *Int J Cancer.* 2008;123(4):951–957.
307. Shibata MA, Ito Y, Morimoto J, Otsuki Y. Lovastatin inhibits tumor growth and lung metastasis in mouse mammary carcinoma model: a p53-independent mitochondrial-mediated apoptotic mechanism. *Carcinogenesis.* 2004;25(10):1887–1898.
308. Bonovas S, Filioussi K, Flordellis CS, Sitaras NM. Statins and the risk of colorectal cancer: a meta-analysis of 18 studies involving more than 1.5 million patients. *J Clin Oncol.* 2007;25(23):3462–3468.
309. Bardou M, Barkun A, Martel M. Effect of statin therapy on colorectal cancer. *Gut.* 2010;59(11):1572–1585.
310. Simon MS, Rosenberg CA, Rodabough RJ, et al. Prospective analysis of association between use of statins or other lipid-lowering agents and colorectal cancer risk. *Ann Epidemiol.* 2012;22(1):17–27.
311. International Agency for Research on Cancer. Globocan 2008. URL. http://www-dep.iarc.fr/. Accessed July 28, 2010.
312. Jemal A, Siegel R, Xu J, Ward E. Cancer statistics, 2010. *CA Cancer J Clin.* 2010;60(5):277–300.
313. Hampel H, Frankel WL, Martin E, et al. Feasibility of screening for Lynch syndrome among patients with colorectal cancer. *J Clin Oncol.* 2008;26(35):5783–5788.
314. Evaluation of Genomic Applications in Practice and Prevention (EGAPP) Working Group. Recommendations from the EGAPP Working Group: genetic testing strategies in newly diagnosed individuals with colorectal cancer aimed at reducing morbidity and mortality from Lynch syndrome in relatives. *Genet Med.* 2009;11:35–41.
315. Lynch HT, Lynch PM, Lanspa SJ, Snyder CL, Lynch JF, Boland CR. Review of the Lynch syndrome: history, molecular genetics, screening, differential diagnosis, and medicolegal ramifications. *Clin Genet.* 2009;76(1):1–18.
316. Lynch HT, de la Chapelle A. Genetic susceptibility to non-polyposis colorectal cancer. *J Med Genet.* 1999;36(11):801–818.
317. Lynch HT, de la Chapelle A. Hereditary colorectal cancer. *N Engl J Med.* 2003;348(10):919–932.
318. Lynch HT, Boland CR, Gong G, et al. Phenotypic and genotypic heterogeneity in the Lynch syndrome: diagnostic, surveillance and management implications. *Eur J Hum Genet.* 2006;14(4):390–402.
319. Guttmacher AE, Collins FS, Carmona RH. The family history–more important than ever. *N Engl J Med.* 2004;351(22):2333–2336.
320. United States Department of Health & Human Services. U.S. surgeon general's family history initiative. 2004. URL. http://www.hhs.gov/familyhistory/. Accessed October 10, 2011.
321. Vasen HF, Mecklin JP, Khan PM, Lynch HT. The International Collaborative Group on Hereditary Non-Polyposis Colorectal Cancer (ICG-HNPCC). *Dis Colon Rectum.* 1991;34(5):424–425.
322. Vasen HF, Watson P, Mecklin JP, Lynch HT. New clinical criteria for hereditary nonpolyposis colorectal cancer (HNPCC, Lynch syndrome) proposed by the International Collaborative group on HNPCC. *Gastroenterology.* 1999;116(6):1453–1456.
323. Boland CR, Shike M. Report from the Jerusalem Workshop on Lynch Syndrome-Hereditary Nonpolyposis Colorectal Cancer. *Gastroenterology.* 2010;138:2197.e1–2197.e7.

324. Lindor NM, Rabe K, Petersen GM, et al. Lower cancer incidence in Amsterdam-I criteria families without mismatch repair deficiency: familial colorectal cancer type X. *JAMA*. 2005;293(16):1979–1985.
325. Delgado-Plasencia L, Medina-Arana V, Barrios Del Pino Y, Fernández-Peralta A, González-Aguilera JJ. Genealogical tree study as screening method in the Lynch syndrome prior to genetic test. *Am J Clin Oncol*. 2010;33(4):376–380.
326. Boland CR, Goel A. Microsatellite instability in colorectal cancer. *Gastroenterology*. 2010;138(6):2073–2087.e3.
327. Palomaki GE, McClain MR, Melillo S, Hampel HL, Thibodeau SN. EGAPP supplementary evidence review: DNA testing strategies aimed at reducing morbidity and mortality from Lynch syndrome. *Genet Med*. 2009;11(1):42–65.
328. Manne SL, Chung DC, Weinberg DS, et al. Knowledge and attitudes about microsatellite instability testing among high-risk individuals diagnosed with colorectal cancer. *Cancer Epidemiol Biomarkers Prev*. 2007;16(10):2110–2117.
329. Aktan-Collan K, Haukkala A, Pylvänäinen K, et al. Direct contact in inviting high-risk members of hereditary colon cancer families to genetic counselling and DNA testing. *J Med Genet*. 2007;44(11):732–738.
330. Claes E, Evers-Kiebooms G, Boogaerts A, Decruyenaere M, Denayer L, Legius E. Communication with close and distant relatives in the context of genetic testing for hereditary breast and ovarian cancer in cancer patients. *Am J Med Genet A*. 2003;116A(1):11–19.
331. Hallowell N, Ardern-Jones A, Eeles R, et al. Communication about genetic testing in families of male BRCA1/2 carriers and non-carriers: patterns, priorities and problems. *Clin Genet*. 2005;67(6):492–502.
332. Hughes C, Lerman C, Schwartz M, et al. All in the family: evaluation of the process and content of sisters' communication about BRCA1 and BRCA2 genetic test results. *Am J Med Genet*. 2002;107(2):143–150.
333. Kenen R, Arden-Jones A, Eeles R. We are talking, but are they listening? Communication patterns in families with a history of breast/ovarian cancer (HBOC). *Psychooncology*. 2004;13(5):335–345.
334. Mesters I, Ausems M, Eichhorn S, Vasen H. Informing one's family about genetic testing for hereditary non-polyposis colorectal cancer (HNPCC): a retrospective exploratory study. *Fam Cancer*. 2005;4(2):163–167.
335. Aktan-Collan K, Mecklin JP, Järvinen H, et al. Predictive genetic testing for hereditary non-polyposis colorectal cancer: uptake and long-term satisfaction. *Int J Cancer*. 2000;89(1): 44–50.
336. Aktan-Collan K, Haukkala A, Mecklin JP, Uutela A, Kääriäinen H. Psychological consequences of predictive genetic testing for hereditary non-polyposis colorectal cancer (HNPCC): a prospective follow-up study. *Int J Cancer*. 2001;93(4): 608–611.
337. Aktan-Collan K, Haukkala A, Mecklin JP, Uutela A, Kääriäinen H. Comprehension of cancer risk one and 12 months after predictive genetic testing for hereditary non-polyposis colorectal cancer. *J Med Genet*. 2001;38(11):787–792.
338. Meiser B, Collins V, Warren R, et al. Psychological impact of genetic testing for hereditary non-polyposis colorectal cancer. *Clin Genet*. 2004;66(6):502–511.
339. Claes E, Denayer L, Evers-Kiebooms G, et al. Predictive testing for hereditary nonpolyposis colorectal cancer: subjective perception regarding colorectal and endometrial cancer, distress, and health-related behavior at one year post-test. *Genet Test*. 2005;9(1):54–65.
340. Gritz ER, Peterson SK, Vernon SW, et al. Psychological impact of genetic testing for hereditary nonpolyposis colorectal cancer. *J Clin Oncol*. 2005;23(9):1902–1910.
341. de Wert G. Cascade screening: whose information is it anyway? *Eur J Hum Genet*. 2005;13(4):397–398.
342. Newson AJ, Humphries SE. Cascade testing in familial hypercholesterolaemia: how should family members be contacted? *Eur J Hum Genet*. 2005;13(4):401–408.
343. Godard B, Hurlimann T, Letendre M, Egalité N; INHERIT BRCAs. Guidelines for disclosing genetic information to family members: from development to use. *Fam Cancer*. 2006;5(1):103–116.
344. Svendsen MN, Koch L. Genetics and prevention: a policy in the making. *New Genet Soc*. 2006;25(1):51–68.
345. Tupasela A. When legal worlds collide: from research to treatment in hereditary cancer prevention. *Eur J Cancer Care (Engl)*. 2006;15(3):257–266.
346. Kääriäinen H, Rantanen E, Hietala M. Summary of the guidelines for genetic counselling, 2006. *Eurogentest* 2006; URL. http://eurogentest.org/web/files/public/unit3/summaryofguidelinesMay06.pdf. Accessed October 12, 2011.
347. Sargent DJ, Marsoni S, Monges G, et al. Defective mismatch repair as a predictive marker for lack of efficacy of fluorouracil-based adjuvant therapy in colon cancer. *J Clin Oncol*. 2010;28(20):3219–3226.
348. Carethers JM, Smith EJ, Behling CA, et al. Use of 5-fluorouracil and survival in patients with microsatellite-unstable colorectal cancer. *Gastroenterology*. 2004;126(2):394–401.
349. Burn J, Gerdes AM, Macrae F, et al. Aspirin reduces cancer risk in carriers of hereditary colorectal cancer: the CAPP2 Randomised Controlled Trial. *Lancet*. 2011;378(9809):2081–2087.
350. Lynch HT, Boland CR, Rodriguez-Bigas MA, Amos C, Lynch JF, Lynch PM. Who should be sent for genetic testing in hereditary colorectal cancer syndromes? *J Clin Oncol*. 2007;25(23):3534–3542.
351. Fearon ER, Vogelstein B. A genetic model for colorectal tumorigenesis. *Cell*. 1990;61(5):759–767.
352. Peltomäki P. Lynch syndrome genes. *Fam Cancer*. 2005;4(3):227–232.
353. Nyström-Lahti M, Parsons R, Sistonen P, et al. Mismatch repair genes on chromosomes 2p and 3p account for a major share of hereditary nonpolyposis colorectal cancer families evaluable by linkage. *Am J Hum Genet*. 1994;55(4):659–665.
354. Nyström-Lahti M, Kristo P, Nicolaides NC, et al. Founding mutations and Alu-mediated recombination in hereditary colon cancer. *Nat Med*. 1995;1(11):1203–1206.
355. Wijnen J, van der Klift H, Vasen H, et al. MSH2 genomic deletions are a frequent cause of HNPCC. *Nat Genet*. 1998;20(4):326–328.
356. Charbonnier F, Olschwang S, Wang Q, et al. MSH2 in contrast to MLH1 and MSH6 is frequently inactivated by exonic and promoter rearrangements in hereditary nonpolyposis colorectal cancer. *Cancer Res*. 2002;62(3):848–853.
357. van der Klift H, Wijnen J, Wagner A, et al. Molecular characterization of the spectrum of genomic deletions in the mismatch repair genes MSH2, MLH1, MSH6, and PMS2 responsible for hereditary nonpolyposis colorectal cancer (HNPCC). *Genes Chromosomes Cancer*. 2005;44(2):123–138.
358. Wang Y, Friedl W, Sengteller M, et al. A modified multiplex PCR assay for detection of large deletions in MSH2 and MLH1. *Hum Mutat*. 2002;19(3):279–286.
359. Taylor CF, Charlton RS, Burn J, Sheridan E, Taylor GR. Genomic deletions in MSH2 or MLH1 are a frequent cause of hereditary non-polyposis colorectal cancer: identification of novel and recurrent deletions by MLPA. *Hum Mutat*. 2003;22(6):428–433.
360. Goel A, Nagasaka T, Spiegel J, Meyer R, Lichliter WE, Boland CR. Low frequency of Lynch syndrome among young patients with non-familial colorectal cancer. *Clin Gastroenterol Hepatol*. 2010;8(11):966–971.
361. Giráldez MD, Balaguer F, Bujanda L, et al. MSH6 and MUTYH deficiency is a frequent event in early-onset colorectal cancer. *Clin Cancer Res*. 2010;16(22):5402–5413.
362. Mvundura M, Grosse SD, Hampel H, Palomaki GE. The cost-effectiveness of genetic testing strategies for Lynch syndrome

among newly diagnosed patients with colorectal cancer. *Genet Med.* 2010;12(2):93–104.
363. Ladabaum U, Wang G, Terdiman J, et al. Strategies to identify the Lynch syndrome among patients with colorectal cancer: a cost-effectiveness analysis. *Ann Intern Med.* 2011;155(2): 69–79.
364. Burt RW. Who should have genetic testing for the Lynch syndrome? *Ann Intern Med.* 2011;155(2):127–128.
365. Teutsch SM, Bradley LA, Palomaki GE, et al.; EGAPP Working Group. The Evaluation of Genomic Applications in Practice and Prevention (EGAPP) Initiative: methods of the EGAPP Working Group. *Genet Med.* 2009;11(1):3–14.
366. Vasen HF, Möslein G, Alonso A, et al. Recommendations to improve identification of hereditary and familial colorectal cancer in Europe. *Fam Cancer.* 2010;9(2):109–115.
367. Lynch HT, Shaw MW, Magnuson CW, Larsen AL, Krush AJ. Hereditary factors in cancer. Study of two large midwestern kindreds. *Arch Intern Med.* 1966;117(2):206–212.
368. Lynch HT, Krush AJ. Heredity and adenocarcinoma of the colon. *Gastroenterology.* 1967;53(4):517–527.
369. Lynch HT, Krush AJ, Larsen AL. Heredity and endometrial carcinoma. *South Med J.* 1967;60(3):231–235.
370. Risinger JI, Barrett JC, Watson P, Lynch HT, Boyd J. Molecular genetic evidence of the occurrence of breast cancer as an integral tumor in patients with the hereditary nonpolyposis colorectal carcinoma syndrome. *Cancer.* 1996;77(9):1836–1843.
371. Boyd J, Rhei E, Federici MG, et al. Male breast cancer in the hereditary nonpolyposis colorectal cancer syndrome. *Breast Cancer Res Treat.* 1999;53(1):87–91.
372. Walsh MD, Buchanan DD, Cummings MC, et al. Lynch syndrome-associated breast cancers: clinicopathologic characteristics of a case series from the colon cancer family registry. *Clin Cancer Res.* 2010;16(7):2214–2224.
373. Soravia C, van der Klift H, Bründler MA, et al. Prostate cancer is part of the hereditary non-polyposis colorectal cancer (HNPCC) tumor spectrum. *Am J Med Genet A.* 2003;121A(2): 159–162.
374. Grindedal EM, Møller P, Eeles R, et al. Germ-line mutations in mismatch repair genes associated with prostate cancer. *Cancer Epidemiol Biomarkers Prev.* 2009;18(9):2460–2467.
375. da Silva FC, de Oliveira LP, Santos EM, et al. Frequency of extracolonic tumors in Brazilian families with Lynch syndrome: analysis of a hereditary colorectal cancer institutional registry. *Fam Cancer.* 2010;9(4):563–570.
376. Capelle LG, Van Grieken NC, Lingsma HF, et al. Risk and epidemiological time trends of gastric cancer in Lynch syndrome carriers in the Netherlands. *Gastroenterology.* 2010;138(2):487–492.
377. Bonadona V, Bonaïti B, Olschwang S, et al.; French Cancer Genetics Network. Cancer risks associated with germline mutations in MLH1, MSH2, and MSH6 genes in Lynch syndrome. *JAMA.* 2011;305(22):2304–2310.
378. Park YJ, Shin KH, Park JG. Risk of gastric cancer in hereditary nonpolyposis colorectal cancer in Korea. *Clin Cancer Res.* 2000;6(8):2994–2998.
379. Kastrinos F, Mukherjee B, Tayob N, et al. Risk of pancreatic cancer in families with Lynch syndrome. *JAMA.* 2009;302(16): 1790–1795.
380. National Comprehensive Cancer Network. *National Comprehensive Cancer Network* 2011. URL. nccn.org. Accessed June 30, 2009.
381. Schulmann K, Brasch FE, Kunstmann E, et al.; German HNPCC Consortium. HNPCC-associated small bowel cancer: clinical and molecular characteristics. *Gastroenterology.* 2005;128(3): 590–599.
382. Muir EG, Bell AJ, Barlow KA. Multiple primary carcinomata of the colon, duodenum, and larynx associated with kerato-acanthomata of the face. *Br J Surg.* 1967;54(3):191–195.
383. Torre D. Multiple sebaceous tumors. *Arch Dermatol.* 1968;98(5):549–551.
384. Fusaro RM, Lynch HT, Pester J, Lynch PM. Torre's syndrome as phenotypic expression of cancer family syndrome. *Arch Dermatol.* 1980;116(9):986–987.
385. Lynch HT, Lynch PM, Pester J, Fusaro RM. The cancer family syndrome. Rare cutaneous phenotypic linkage of Torre's syndrome. *Arch Intern Med.* 1981;141(5):607–611.
386. Lynch HT, Fusaro RM, Roberts L, Voorhees GJ, Lynch JF. Muir-Torre syndrome in several members of a family with a variant of the Cancer Family Syndrome. *Br J Dermatol.* 1985;113(3):295–301.
387. Abdel-Rahman WM, Peltomäki P. Lynch syndrome and related familial colorectal cancers. *Crit Rev Oncog.* 2008;14(1):1–22; discussion 23.
388. Ponti G, Losi L, Pedroni M, et al. Value of MLH1 and MSH2 mutations in the appearance of Muir-Torre syndrome phenotype in HNPCC patients presenting sebaceous gland tumors or keratoacanthomas. *J Invest Dermatol.* 2006;126(10):2302–2307.
389. Guillén-Ponce C, Castillejo A, Barberá VM, et al. Biallelic MYH germline mutations as cause of Muir-Torre syndrome. *Fam Cancer.* 2010;9(2):151–154.
390. Ponti G, Ponz de Leon M, Maffei S, et al. Attenuated familial adenomatous polyposis and Muir-Torre syndrome linked to compound biallelic constitutional MYH gene mutations. *Clin Genet.* 2005;68(5):442–447.
391. South CD, Hampel H, Comeras I, Westman JA, Frankel WL, de la Chapelle A. The frequency of Muir-Torre syndrome among Lynch syndrome families. *J Natl Cancer Inst.* 2008;100(4):277–281.
392. Fusaro RM, Lemon SJ, Lynch HT. The Muir-Torre syndrome: a variant of hereditary nonpolyposis colorectal cancer syndrome. *J Tumor Marker Oncol.* 1996;11:19–31.
393. Watson P, Lynch HT. The tumor spectrum in HNPCC. *Anticancer Res.* 1994;14(4B):1635–1639.
394. Lynch HT, Lynch PM, Pester JA, Fusaro RM. Sebaceous neoplasia and visceral cancer (Torre's syndrome) and its relationship to the cancer family syndrome. In: Lynch HT, Fusaro RM, eds. *Cancer-associated Genodermatoses.* New York, NY: Van Nostrand Reinhold; 1982:366–393.
395. Lynch HT, Fusaro RM. Muir-Torre syndrome: heterogeneity, natural history, diagnosis, and management. *Prob Gen Surg.* 1993;10:1–14.
396. Lynch HT, Leibowitz R, Smyrk T, et al. Colorectal cancer and the Muir-Torre syndrome in a Gypsy family: a review. *Am J Gastroenterol.* 1999;94(3):575–580.
397. Broaddus RR, Lynch PM, Lu KH, Luthra R, Michelson SJ. Unusual tumors associated with the hereditary nonpolyposis colorectal cancer syndrome. *Mod Pathol.* 2004;17(8):981–989.
398. Nilbert M, Therkildsen C, Nissen A, Akerman M, Bernstein I. Sarcomas associated with hereditary nonpolyposis colorectal cancer: broad anatomical and morphological spectrum. *Fam Cancer.* 2009;8(3):209–213.
399. Jasperson KW, Samowitz WS, Burt RW. Constitutional mismatch repair-deficiency syndrome presenting as colonic adenomatous polyposis: clues from the skin. *Clin Genet.* 2011;80(4): 394–397.
400. Wimmer K, Etzler J. Constitutional mismatch repair-deficiency syndrome: have we so far seen only the tip of an iceberg? *Hum Genet.* 2008;124(2):105–122.
401. Durno CA, Holter S, Sherman PM, Gallinger S. The gastrointestinal phenotype of germline biallelic mismatch repair gene mutations. *Am J Gastroenterol.* 2010;105(11):2449–2456.
402. Krüger S, Kinzel M, Walldorf C, et al. Homozygous PMS2 germline mutations in two families with early-onset haematological malignancy, brain tumours, HNPCC-associated tumours, and signs of neurofibromatosis type 1. *Eur J Hum Genet.* 2008;16(1):62–72.
403. Kovacs ME, Papp J, Szentirmay Z, Otto S, Olah E. Deletions removing the last exon of TACSTD1 constitute a distinct class of mutations predisposing to Lynch syndrome. *Hum Mutat.* 2009;30(2):197–203.

404. Kobelka CE. Silencing is not-so golden: a new model for inheritance of Lynch syndrome. *Clin Genet.* 2009;75:522–523.
405. Ligtenberg MJ, Kuiper RP, Chan TL, et al. Heritable somatic methylation and inactivation of MSH2 in families with Lynch syndrome due to deletion of the 3' exons of TACSTD1. *Nat Genet.* 2009;41(1):112–117.
406. Kuiper RP, Vissers LE, Venkatachalam R, et al. Recurrence and variability of germline EPCAM deletions in Lynch syndrome. *Hum Mutat.* 2011;32(4):407–414.
407. Lynch HT, Riegert-Johnson DL, Snyder C, et al. Lynch syndrome-associated extracolonic tumors are rare in two extended families with the same EPCAM deletion. *Am J Gastroenterol.* 2011;106(10):1829–1836.
408. Esteller M. Epigenetics in cancer. *N Engl J Med.* 2008;358(11): 1148–1159.
409. Holliday R. The inheritance of epigenetic defects. *Nature.* 1983;301:89–92.
410. Cunningham JM, Christensen ER, Tester DJ, et al. Hypermethylation of the hMLH1 promoter in colon cancer with microsatellite instability. *Cancer Res.* 1998;58(15): 3455–3460.
411. van Engeland M, Derks S, Smits KM, Meijer GA, Herman JG. Colorectal cancer epigenetics: complex simplicity. *J Clin Oncol.* 2011;29(10):1382–1391.
412. Hitchins MP, Ward RL. Constitutional (germline) MLH1 epimutation as an aetiological mechanism for hereditary non-polyposis colorectal cancer. *J Med Genet.* 2009;46(12):793–802.
413. Hitchins MP, Wong JJ, Suthers G, et al. Inheritance of a cancer-associated MLH1 germ-line epimutation. *N Engl J Med.* 2007;356(7):697–705.
414. Hitchins M, Williams R, Cheong K, et al. MLH1 germline epimutations as a factor in hereditary nonpolyposis colorectal cancer. *Gastroenterology.* 2005;129(5):1392–1399.
415. Goel A, Nguyen TP, Leung HC, et al. De novo constitutional MLH1 epimutations confer early-onset colorectal cancer in two new sporadic Lynch syndrome cases, with derivation of the epimutation on the paternal allele in one. *Int J Cancer.* 2011;128(4):869–878.
416. Hitchins MP, Lin VA, Buckle A, et al. Epigenetic inactivation of a cluster of genes flanking MLH1 in microsatellite-unstable colorectal cancer. *Cancer Res.* 2007;67(19):9107–9116.
417. Gylling A, Ridanpää M, Vierimaa O, et al. Large genomic rearrangements and germline epimutations in Lynch syndrome. *Int J Cancer.* 2009;124(10):2333–2340.
418. Morak M, Schackert HK, Rahner N, et al. Further evidence for heritability of an epimutation in one of 12 cases with MLH1 promoter methylation in blood cells clinically displaying HNPCC. *Eur J Hum Genet.* 2008;16(7):804–811.
419. Morak M, Koehler U, Schackert HK, et al.; German HNPCC consortium. Biallelic MLH1 SNP cDNA expression or constitutional promoter methylation can hide genomic rearrangements causing Lynch syndrome. *J Med Genet.* 2011;48(8):513–519.
420. Hitchins MP, Rapkins RW, Kwok CT, et al. Dominantly inherited constitutional epigenetic silencing of MLH1 in a cancer-affected family is linked to a single nucleotide variant within the 5'UTR. *Cancer Cell.* 2011;20(2):200–213.
421. Fernández-Ramires R, Gómez G, Muñoz-Repeto I, et al. Transcriptional characteristics of familial non-BRCA1/BRCA2 breast tumors. *Int J Cancer.* 2011;128(11):2635–2644.
422. Dolcetti R, Viel A, Doglioni C, et al. High prevalence of activated intraepithelial cytotoxic T lymphocytes and increased neoplastic cell apoptosis in colorectal carcinomas with microsatellite instability. *Am J Pathol.* 1999;154(6):1805–1813.
423. Drescher KM, Sharma P, Watson P, Gatalica Z, Thibodeau SN, Lynch HT. Lymphocyte recruitment into the tumor site is altered in patients with MSI-H colon cancer. *Fam Cancer.* 2009;8(3):231–239.
424. Bennett MW, O'Connell J, O'Sullivan GC, et al. The Fas counterattack in vivo: apoptotic depletion of tumor-infiltrating lymphocytes associated with Fas ligand expression by human esophageal carcinoma. *J Immunol.* 1998;160(11):5669–5675.
425. Fisk B, Anderson BW, Gravitt KR, et al. Identification of naturally processed human ovarian peptides recognized by tumor-associated CD8+ cytotoxic T lymphocytes. *Cancer Res.* 1997;57(1):87–93.
426. Murray D, Hreno A, Dutton J, Hampson LG. Prognosis in colon cancer: a pathologic reassessment. *Arch Surg.* 1975;110(8):908–913.
427. Mann B, Gratchev A, Böhm C, et al. FasL is more frequently expressed in liver metastases of colorectal cancer than in matched primary carcinomas. *Br J Cancer.* 1999;79(7–8): 1262–1269.
428. Buckowitz A, Knaebel HP, Benner A, et al. Microsatellite instability in colorectal cancer is associated with local lymphocyte infiltration and low frequency of distant metastases. *Br J Cancer.* 2005;92(9):1746–1753.
429. Le Gouvello S, Bastuji-Garin S, Aloulou N, et al. High prevalence of Foxp3 and IL17 in MMR-proficient colorectal carcinomas. *Gut.* 2008;57(6):772–779.
430. Morris M, Platell C, Iacopetta B. Tumor-infiltrating lymphocytes and perforation in colon cancer predict positive response to 5-fluorouracil chemotherapy. *Clin Cancer Res.* 2008;14(5):1413–1417.
431. Bennett MW, O'connell J, O'sullivan GC, et al. Expression of Fas ligand by human gastric adenocarcinomas: a potential mechanism of immune escape in stomach cancer. *Gut.* 1999;44(2): 156–162.
432. Okada K, Komuta K, Hashimoto S, Matsuzaki S, Kanematsu T, Koji T. Frequency of apoptosis of tumor-infiltrating lymphocytes induced by fas counterattack in human colorectal carcinoma and its correlation with prognosis. *Clin Cancer Res.* 2000;6(9):3560–3564.
433. Okano K, Maeba T, Moroguchi A, et al. Lymphocytic infiltration surrounding liver metastases from colorectal cancer. *J Surg Oncol.* 2003;82(1):28–33.
434. Smyrk TC, Watson P, Kaul K, Lynch HT. Tumor-infiltrating lymphocytes are a marker for microsatellite instability in colorectal carcinoma. *Cancer.* 2001;91(12):2417–2422.
435. Prall F, Dührkop T, Weirich V, et al. Prognostic role of CD8+ tumor-infiltrating lymphocytes in stage III colorectal cancer with and without microsatellite instability. *Hum Pathol.* 2004;35(7):808–816.
436. Menon AG, Janssen-van Rhijn CM, Morreau H, et al. Immune system and prognosis in colorectal cancer: a detailed immunohistochemical analysis. *Lab Invest.* 2004;84(4):493–501.
437. Pagès F, Kirilovsky A, Mlecnik B, et al. In situ cytotoxic and memory T cells predict outcome in patients with early-stage colorectal cancer. *J Clin Oncol.* 2009;27(35):5944–5951.
438. Meijer TW, Hoogerbrugge N, Nagengast FM, Ligtenberg MJ, van Krieken JH. In Lynch syndrome adenomas, loss of mismatch repair proteins is related to an enhanced lymphocytic response. *Histopathology.* 2009;55(4):414–422.
439. Le Gouvello S, Bastuji-Garin S, Aloulou N, et al. High prevalence of Foxp3 and IL17 in MMR-proficient colorectal carcinomas. *Gut.* 2008;57(6):772–779.
440. Numasaki M, Fukushi J, Ono M, et al. Interleukin-17 promotes angiogenesis and tumor growth. *Blood.* 2003;101(7):2620–2627.
441. Tartour E, Fossiez F, Joyeux I, et al. Interleukin 17, a T-cell-derived cytokine, promotes tumorigenicity of human cervical tumors in nude mice. *Cancer Res.* 1999;59(15):3698–3704.
442. Jenkins MA, Hayashi S, O'Shea AM, et al.; Colon Cancer Family Registry. Pathology features in Bethesda guidelines predict colorectal cancer microsatellite instability: a population-based study. *Gastroenterology.* 2007;133(1):48–56.
443. Greenson JK, Huang SC, Herron C, et al. Pathologic predictors of microsatellite instability in colorectal cancer. *Am J Surg Pathol.* 2009;33(1):126–133.

444. Mecklin JP, Sipponen P, Järvinen HJ. Histopathology of colorectal carcinomas and adenomas in cancer family syndrome. *Dis Colon Rectum.* 1986;29(12):849–853.
445. Michael-Robinson JM, Biemer-Hüttmann A, Purdie DM, et al. Tumour infiltrating lymphocytes and apoptosis are independent features in colorectal cancer stratified according to microsatellite instability status. *Gut.* 2001;48(3):360–366.
446. Hyde A, Fontaine D, Stuckless S, et al. A histology-based model for predicting microsatellite instability in colorectal cancers. *Am J Surg Pathol.* 2010;34(12):1820–1829.
447. Kakar S, Smyrk TC. Signet ring cell carcinoma of the colorectum: correlations between microsatellite instability, clinicopathologic features and survival. *Mod Pathol.* 2005;18(2):244–249.
448. Alexander J, Watanabe T, Wu TT, Rashid A, Li S, Hamilton SR. Histopathological identification of colon cancer with microsatellite instability. *Am J Pathol.* 2001;158(2):527–535.
449. Román R, Verdú M, Calvo M, et al. Microsatellite instability of the colorectal carcinoma can be predicted in the conventional pathologic examination. A prospective multicentric study and the statistical analysis of 615 cases consolidate our previously proposed logistic regression model. *Virchows Arch.* 2010;456(5):533–541.
450. Greenson JK, Bonner JD, Ben-Yzhak O, et al. Phenotype of microsatellite unstable colorectal carcinomas: Well-differentiated and focally mucinous tumors and the absence of dirty necrosis correlate with microsatellite instability. *Am J Surg Pathol.* 2003;27(5):563–570.
451. Wilson TM, Ewel A, Duguid JR, et al. Differential cellular expression of the human MSH2 repair enzyme in small and large intestine. *Cancer Res.* 1995;55(22):5146–5150.
452. Leach FS, Polyak K, Burrell M, et al. Expression of the human mismatch repair gene hMSH2 in normal and neoplastic tissues. *Cancer Res.* 1996;56(2):235–240.
453. Shia J, Klimstra DS, Nafa K, et al. Value of immunohistochemical detection of DNA mismatch repair proteins in predicting germline mutation in hereditary colorectal neoplasms. *Am J Surg Pathol.* 2005;29(1):96–104.
454. Shia J. Immunohistochemistry versus microsatellite instability testing for screening colorectal cancer patients at risk for hereditary nonpolyposis colorectal cancer syndrome. Part I. The utility of immunohistochemistry. *J Mol Diagn.* 2008;10(4): 293–300.
455. Boland CR, Thibodeau SN, Hamilton SR, et al. A National Cancer Institute Workshop on Microsatellite Instability for cancer detection and familial predisposition: development of international criteria for the determination of microsatellite instability in colorectal cancer. *Cancer Res.* 1998;58(22):5248–5257.
456. Umar A, Boland CR, Terdiman JP, et al. Revised Bethesda Guidelines for hereditary nonpolyposis colorectal cancer (Lynch syndrome) and microsatellite instability. *J Natl Cancer Inst.* 2004;96(4):261–268.
457. Zhang L. Immunohistochemistry versus microsatellite instability testing for screening colorectal cancer patients at risk for hereditary nonpolyposis colorectal cancer syndrome. Part II. The utility of microsatellite instability testing. *J Mol Diagn.* 2008;10(4):301–307.
458. Domingo E, Niessen RC, Oliveira C, et al. BRAF-V600E is not involved in the colorectal tumorigenesis of HNPCC in patients with functional MLH1 and MSH2 genes. *Oncogene.* 2005;24(24):3995–3998.
459. Morán A, Ortega P, de Juan C, et al. Differential colorectal carcinogenesis: Molecular basis and clinical relevance. *World J Gastrointest Oncol.* 2010;2(3):151–158.
460. Loughrey MB, Waring PM, Tan A, et al. Incorporation of somatic BRAF mutation testing into an algorithm for the investigation of hereditary non-polyposis colorectal cancer. *Fam Cancer.* 2007;6(3):301–310.
461. Gatalica Z, Torlakovic E. Pathology of the hereditary colorectal carcinoma. *Fam Cancer.* 2008;7(1):15–26.
462. Buchanan DD, Sweet K, Drini M, et al. Phenotypic diversity in patients with multiple serrated polyps: a genetics clinic study. *Int J Colorectal Dis.* 2010;25(6):703–712.
463. Rashid A, Houlihan PS, Booker S, Petersen GM, Giardiello FM, Hamilton SR. Phenotypic and molecular characteristics of hyperplastic polyposis. *Gastroenterology.* 2000;119(2):323–332.
464. Ji BT, Weissfeld JL, Chow WH, Huang WY, Schoen RE, Hayes RB. Tobacco smoking and colorectal hyperplastic and adenomatous polyps. *Cancer Epidemiol Biomarkers Prev.* 2006;15(5):897–901.
465. Roberts A, Nancarrow D, Clendenning M, et al. Linkage to chromosome 2q32.2-q33.3 in familial serrated neoplasia (Jass syndrome). *Fam Cancer.* 2011;10(2):245–254.
466. Neklason DW, Kerber RA, Nilson DB, et al. Common familial colorectal cancer linked to chromosome 7q31: a genome-wide analysis. *Cancer Res.* 2008;68(21):8993–8997.
467. Jass JR, Cottier DS, Pokos V, Parry S, Winship IM. Mixed epithelial polyps in association with hereditary non-polyposis colorectal cancer providing an alternative pathway of cancer histogenesis. *Pathology.* 1997;29(1):28–33.
468. Jeevaratnam P, Cottier DS, Browett PJ, Van De Water NS, Pokos V, Jass JR. Familial giant hyperplastic polyposis predisposing to colorectal cancer: a new hereditary bowel cancer syndrome. *J Pathol.* 1996;179(1):20–25.
469. Young J, Barker MA, Simms LA, et al. Evidence for BRAF mutation and variable levels of microsatellite instability in a syndrome of familial colorectal cancer. *Clin Gastroenterol Hepatol.* 2005;3(3):254–263.
470. Young J, Jass JR. The case for a genetic predisposition to serrated neoplasia in the colorectum: hypothesis and review of the literature. *Cancer Epidemiol Biomarkers Prev.* 2006;15(10):1778–1784.
471. Boparai KS, Dekker E, Van Eeden S, et al. Hyperplastic polyps and sessile serrated adenomas as a phenotypic expression of MYH-associated polyposis. *Gastroenterology.* 2008;135(6):2014–2018.
472. Jass JR. Classification of colorectal cancer based on correlation of clinical, morphological and molecular features. *Histopathology.* 2007;50(1):113–130.
473. Snover DC. Update on the serrated pathway to colorectal carcinoma. *Hum Pathol.* 2011;42(1):1–10.
474. Samowitz WS, Albertsen H, Herrick J, et al. Evaluation of a large, population-based sample supports a CpG island methylator phenotype in colon cancer. *Gastroenterology.* 2005;129(3):837–845.
475. de Jong AE, Hendriks YM, Kleibeuker JH, et al. Decrease in mortality in Lynch syndrome families because of surveillance. *Gastroenterology.* 2006;130(3):665–671.
476. Mecklin JP, Aarnio M, Läärä E, et al. Development of colorectal tumors in colonoscopic surveillance in Lynch syndrome. *Gastroenterology.* 2007;133(4):1093–1098.
477. Natarajan N, Watson P, Silva-Lopez E, Lynch HT. Comparison of extended colectomy and limited resection in patients with Lynch syndrome. *Dis Colon Rectum.* 2010;53(1):77–82.
478. Järvinen HJ, Renkonen-Sinisalo L, Aktán-Collán K, Peltomäki P, Aaltonen LA, Mecklin JP. Ten years after mutation testing for Lynch syndrome: cancer incidence and outcome in mutation-positive and mutation-negative family members. *J Clin Oncol.* 2009;27(28):4793–4797.
479. Vasen HF, Abdirahman M, Brohet R, et al. One to 2-year surveillance intervals reduce risk of colorectal cancer in families with Lynch syndrome. *Gastroenterology.* 2010;138(7): 2300–2306.
480. Edelstein DL, Axilbund J, Baxter M, et al. Rapid development of colorectal neoplasia in patients with Lynch syndrome. *Clin Gastroenterol Hepatol.* 2011;9(4):340–343.
481. Stoffel EM, Mercado RC, Kohlmann W, et al. Prevalence and predictors of appropriate colorectal cancer surveillance in Lynch syndrome. *Am J Gastroenterol.* 2010;105(8):1851–1860.

482. Stoffel EM, Turgeon DK, Stockwell DH, et al.; Great Lakes-New England Clinical Epidemiology and Validation Center of the Early Detection Research Network. Missed adenomas during colonoscopic surveillance in individuals with Lynch Syndrome (hereditary nonpolyposis colorectal cancer). *Cancer Prev Res (Phila).* 2008;1(6):470–475.
483. Lecomte T, Cellier C, Meatchi T, et al. Chromoendoscopic colonoscopy for detecting preneoplastic lesions in hereditary nonpolyposis colorectal cancer syndrome. *Clin Gastroenterol Hepatol.* 2005;3(9):897–902.
484. Hurlstone DP, Karajeh M, Cross SS, et al. The role of high-magnification-chromoscopic colonoscopy in hereditary nonpolyposis colorectal cancer screening: a prospective "back-to-back" endoscopic study. *Am J Gastroenterol.* 2005;100(10):2167–2173.
485. Hüneburg R, Lammert F, Rabe C, et al. Chromocolonoscopy detects more adenomas than white light colonoscopy or narrow band imaging colonoscopy in hereditary nonpolyposis colorectal cancer screening. *Endoscopy.* 2009;41(4):316–322.
486. Kwon JS, Scott JL, Gilks CB, Daniels MS, Sun CC, Lu KH. Testing women with endometrial cancer to detect Lynch syndrome. *J Clin Oncol.* 2011;29(16):2247–2252.
487. Schmeler KM, Lynch HT, Chen LM, et al. Prophylactic surgery to reduce the risk of gynecologic cancers in the Lynch syndrome. *N Engl J Med.* 2006;354(3):261–269.
488. Westin SN, Sun CC, Lu KH, et al. Satisfaction with ovarian carcinoma risk-reduction strategies among women at high risk for breast and ovarian carcinoma. *Cancer.* 2011;117(12):2659–2667.
489. Balaguer F, Moreira L, Lozano JJ, et al. Colorectal cancers with microsatellite instability display unique miRNA profiles. *Clin Cancer Res.* 2011;17(19):6239–6249.
490. Ng SB, Turner EH, Robertson PD, et al. Targeted capture and massively parallel sequencing of 12 human exomes. *Nature.* 2009;461(7261):272–276.
491. Cooper DN, Krawczak M, Antonorakis SE. The nature and mechanisms of human gene mutation. In: Scriver C, Beaudet AL, Sly WS, Valle D, eds. *The Metabolic and Molecular Bases of Inherited Disease.* 7th ed. New York, NY: McGraw-Hill; 1995:259–291.
492. Aebi S, Kurdi-Haidar B, Gordon R, et al. Loss of DNA mismatch repair in acquired resistance to cisplatin. *Cancer Res.* 1996;56(13):3087–3090.
493. Ribic CM, Sargent DJ, Moore MJ, et al. Tumor microsatellite-instability status as a predictor of benefit from fluorouracil-based adjuvant chemotherapy for colon cancer. *N Engl J Med.* 2003;349(3):247–257.
494. Lanza G, Gafà R, Santini A, Maestri I, Guerzoni L, Cavazzini L. Immunohistochemical test for MLH1 and MSH2 expression predicts clinical outcome in stage II and III colorectal cancer patients. *J Clin Oncol.* 2006;24(15):2359–2367.
495. Sinicrope F, Foster NR, Sargent DJ, Thibodeau SN, Smyrk TC, O'Connell MJ; North Central Cancer Treatment Group. Model-based prediction of defective DNA mismatch repair using clinicopathological variables in sporadic colon cancer patients. *Cancer.* 2010;116(7):1691–1698.
496. Sinicrope FA, Foster NR, Thibodeau SN, et al. DNA mismatch repair status and colon cancer recurrence and survival in clinical trials of 5-fluorouracil-based adjuvant therapy. *J Natl Cancer Inst.* 2011;103(11):863–875.
497. Burn J, Bishop DT, Chapman PD, et al.; International CAPP consortium. A randomized placebo-controlled prevention trial of aspirin and/or resistant starch in young people with familial adenomatous polyposis. *Cancer Prev Res (Phila).* 2011;4(5):655–665.
498. Chan AT. Aspirin and familial adenomatous polyposis: coming full circle. *Cancer Prev Res (Phila).* 2011;4(5):623–627.
499. Burn J, Bishop DT, Mecklin JP, et al.; CAPP2 Investigators. Effect of aspirin or resistant starch on colorectal neoplasia in the Lynch syndrome. *N Engl J Med.* 2008;359(24):2567–2578.
500. Jass JR, Walsh MD, Barker M, Simms LA, Young J, Leggett BA. Distinction between familial and sporadic forms of colorectal cancer showing DNA microsatellite instability. *Eur J Cancer.* 2002;38(7):858–866.
501. Crohn B, Rosenberg H. The sigmoidoscopic picture of chronic ulcerative colitis (non-specific). *Am J Med Sci.* 1925;170:220–228.
502. Ekbom A, Helmick C, Zack M, Adami HO. Increased risk of large-bowel cancer in Crohn's disease with colonic involvement. *Lancet.* 1990;336(8711):357–359.
503. Ekbom A, Helmick C, Zack M, Adami HO. Ulcerative colitis and colorectal cancer. A population-based study. *N Engl J Med.* 1990;323(18):1228–1233.
504. Eaden JA, Abrams KR, Mayberry JF. The risk of colorectal cancer in ulcerative colitis: a meta-analysis. *Gut.* 2001;48(4):526–535.
505. Bernstein CN, Blanchard JF, Kliewer E, Wajda A. Cancer risk in patients with inflammatory bowel disease: a population-based study. *Cancer.* 2001;91(4):854–862.
506. Winther KV, Jess T, Langholz E, Munkholm P, Binder V. Long-term risk of cancer in ulcerative colitis: a population-based cohort study from Copenhagen County. *Clin Gastroenterol Hepatol.* 2004;2(12):1088–1095.
507. Jess T, Loftus EV Jr, Velayos FS, et al. Risk of intestinal cancer in inflammatory bowel disease: a population-based study from olmsted county, Minnesota. *Gastroenterology.* 2006;130(4):1039–1046.
508. Velayos FS, Terdiman JP, Walsh JM. Effect of 5-aminosalicylate use on colorectal cancer and dysplasia risk: a systematic review and metaanalysis of observational studies. *Am J Gastroenterol.* 2005;100(6):1345–1353.
509. Herrinton LJ, Liu L, Levin TR, Allison JE, Lewis JD, Velayos F. Incidence and mortality of colorectal adenocarcinoma in persons with inflammatory bowel disease from 1998 to 2010. *Gastroenterology.* 2012;143(2):382–389.
510. Cairns SR, Scholefield JH, Steele RJ, et al.; British Society of Gastroenterology; Association of Coloproctology for Great Britain and Ireland. Guidelines for colorectal cancer screening and surveillance in moderate and high risk groups (update from 2002). *Gut.* 2010;59(5):666–689.
511. Choi PM, Zelig MP. Similarity of colorectal cancer in Crohn's disease and ulcerative colitis: implications for carcinogenesis and prevention. *Gut.* 1994;35(7):950–954.
512. Levin B. Inflammatory bowel disease and colon cancer. *Cancer.* 1992;70(5 Suppl):1313–1316.
513. Gillen CD, Andrews HA, Prior P, Allan RN. Crohn's disease and colorectal cancer. *Gut.* 1994;35(5):651–655.
514. Jess T, Gamborg M, Matzen P, Munkholm P, Sørensen TI. Increased risk of intestinal cancer in Crohn's disease: a meta-analysis of population-based cohort studies. *Am J Gastroenterol.* 2005;100(12):2724–2729.
515. Canavan C, Abrams KR, Mayberry J. Meta-analysis: colorectal and small bowel cancer risk in patients with Crohn's disease. *Aliment Pharmacol Ther.* 2006;23(8):1097–1104.
516. Choi PM. Predominance of rectosigmoid neoplasia in ulcerative colitis and its implication on cancer surveillance. *Gastroenterology.* 1993;104(2):666–667.
517. Rutter MD, Saunders BP, Wilkinson KH, Kamm MA, Williams CB, Forbes A. Most dysplasia in ulcerative colitis is visible at colonoscopy. *Gastrointest Endosc.* 2004;60(3):334–339.
518. Mathy C, Schneider K, Chen YY, Varma M, Terdiman JP, Mahadevan U. Gross versus microscopic pancolitis and the occurrence of neoplasia in ulcerative colitis. *Inflamm Bowel Dis.* 2003;9(6):351–355.
519. Rutter MD, Saunders BP, Wilkinson KH, et al. Thirty-year analysis of a colonoscopic surveillance program for neoplasia in ulcerative colitis. *Gastroenterology.* 2006;130(4):1030–1038.
520. Gupta RB, Harpaz N, Itzkowitz S, et al. Histologic inflammation is a risk factor for progression to colorectal neoplasia in ulcerative

colitis: a cohort study. *Gastroenterology.* 2007;133(4):1099–105; quiz 1340.
521. Broomé U, Löfberg R, Veress B, Eriksson LS. Primary sclerosing cholangitis and ulcerative colitis: evidence for increased neoplastic potential. *Hepatology.* 1995;22(5):1404–1408.
522. Loftus EV Jr, Sandborn WJ, Tremaine WJ, et al. Risk of colorectal neoplasia in patients with primary sclerosing cholangitis. *Gastroenterology.* 1996;110(2):432–440.
523. Nuako KW, Ahlquist DA, Sandborn WJ, Mahoney DW, Siems DM, Zinsmeister AR. Primary sclerosing cholangitis and colorectal carcinoma in patients with chronic ulcerative colitis: a case-control study. *Cancer.* 1998;82(5):822–826.
524. Shetty K, Rybicki L, Brzezinski A, Carey WD, Lashner BA. The risk for cancer or dysplasia in ulcerative colitis patients with primary sclerosing cholangitis. *Am J Gastroenterol.* 1999;94(6):1643–1649.
525. Soetikno RM, Lin OS, Heidenreich PA, Young HS, Blackstone MO. Increased risk of colorectal neoplasia in patients with primary sclerosing cholangitis and ulcerative colitis: a meta-analysis. *Gastrointest Endosc.* 2002;56(1):48–54.
526. Kornfeld D, Ekbom A, Ihre T. Is there an excess risk for colorectal cancer in patients with ulcerative colitis and concomitant primary sclerosing cholangitis? A population based study. *Gut.* 1997;41(4):522–525.
527. Broomé U, Löfberg R, Lundqvist K, Veress B. Subclinical time span of inflammatory bowel disease in patients with primary sclerosing cholangitis. *Dis Colon Rectum.* 1995;38(12):1301–1305.
528. Lundqvist K, Broomé U. Differences in colonic disease activity in patients with ulcerative colitis with and without primary sclerosing cholangitis: a case control study. *Dis Colon Rectum.* 1997;40(4):451–456.
529. Loftus EV Jr, Harewood GC, Loftus CG, et al. PSC-IBD: a unique form of inflammatory bowel disease associated with primary sclerosing cholangitis. *Gut.* 2005;54(1):91–96.
530. Nuako KW, Ahlquist DA, Mahoney DW, Schaid DJ, Siems DM, Lindor NM. Familial predisposition for colorectal cancer in chronic ulcerative colitis: a case-control study. *Gastroenterology.* 1998;115(5):1079–1083.
531. Eaden J, Abrams K, Ekbom A, Jackson E, Mayberry J. Colorectal cancer prevention in ulcerative colitis: a case-control study. *Aliment Pharmacol Ther.* 2000;14(2):145–153.
532. Askling J, Dickman PW, Karlén P, et al. Family history as a risk factor for colorectal cancer in inflammatory bowel disease. *Gastroenterology.* 2001;120(6):1356–1362.
533. Velayos FS, Loftus EV Jr, Jess T, et al. Predictive and protective factors associated with colorectal cancer in ulcerative colitis: A case-control study. *Gastroenterology.* 2006;130(7):1941–1949.
534. Rutter M, Saunders B, Wilkinson K, et al. Severity of inflammation is a risk factor for colorectal neoplasia in ulcerative colitis. *Gastroenterology.* 2004;126(2):451–459.
535. Rutter MD, Saunders BP, Schofield G, Forbes A, Price AB, Talbot IC. Pancolonic indigo carmine dye spraying for the detection of dysplasia in ulcerative colitis. *Gut.* 2004;53(2):256–260.
536. Rubin DT, Rothe JA, Hetzel JT, Cohen RD, Hanauer SB. Are dysplasia and colorectal cancer endoscopically visible in patients with ulcerative colitis? *Gastrointest Endosc.* 2007;65(7):998–1004.
537. Gumaste V, Sachar DB, Greenstein AJ. Benign and malignant colorectal strictures in ulcerative colitis. *Gut.* 1992;33(7):938–941.
538. Reiser JR, Waye JD, Janowitz HD, Harpaz N. Adenocarcinoma in strictures of ulcerative colitis without antecedent dysplasia by colonoscopy. *Am J Gastroenterol.* 1994;89(1):119–122.
539. Lakatos L, Mester G, Erdelyi Z, et al. Risk factors for ulcerative colitis-associated colorectal cancer in a Hungarian cohort of patients with ulcerative colitis: results of a population-based study. *Inflamm Bowel Dis.* 2006;12(3):205–211.
540. Rutter MD, Saunders BP, Wilkinson KH, et al. Cancer surveillance in longstanding ulcerative colitis: endoscopic appearances help predict cancer risk. *Gut.* 2004;53(12):1813–1816.
541. Riddell RH, Goldman H, Ransohoff DF, et al. Dysplasia in inflammatory bowel disease: standardized classification with provisional clinical applications. *Hum Pathol.* 1983;14(11):931–968.
542. Riddell RH. Grading of dysplasia. *Eur J Cancer.* 1995; 31A(7–8):1169–1170.
543. McKenna BJ, Appelman HD. Dysplasia can be a pain in the gut. *Pathology.* 2002;34(6):518–528.
544. Lim CH, Dixon MF, Vail A, Forman D, Lynch DA, Axon AT. Ten year follow up of ulcerative colitis patients with and without low grade dysplasia. *Gut.* 2003;52(8):1127–1132.
545. Eaden J, Abrams K, McKay H, Denley H, Mayberry J. Inter-observer variation between general and specialist gastrointestinal pathologists when grading dysplasia in ulcerative colitis. *J Pathol.* 2001;194(2):152–157.
546. Rosman-Urbach M, Niv Y, Birk Y, et al. A high degree of aneuploidy, loss of p53 gene, and low soluble p53 protein serum levels are detected in ulcerative colitis patients. *Dis Colon Rectum.* 2004;47(3):304–313.
547. Levine DS, Rabinovitch PS, Haggitt RC, et al. Distribution of aneuploid cell populations in ulcerative colitis with dysplasia or cancer. *Gastroenterology.* 1991;101(5):1198–1210.
548. Ahnen DJ. Abnormal DNA content as a biomarker of large bowel cancer risk and prognosis. *J Cell Biochem Suppl.* 1992;16G:143–150.
549. Burmer GC, Rabinovitch PS, Haggitt RC, et al. Neoplastic progression in ulcerative colitis: histology, DNA content, and loss of a p53 allele. *Gastroenterology.* 1992;103(5):1602–1610.
550. Burmer GC, Levine DS, Kulander BG, Haggitt RC, Rubin CE, Rabinovitch PS. c-Ki-ras mutations in chronic ulcerative colitis and sporadic colon carcinoma. *Gastroenterology.* 1990;99(2):416–420.
551. Chen J, Compton C, Cheng E, Fromowitz F, Viola MV. c-Ki-ras mutations in dysplastic fields and cancers in ulcerative colitis. *Gastroenterology.* 1992;102(6):1983–1987.
552. Yin J, Harpaz N, Tong Y, et al. p53 point mutations in dysplastic and cancerous ulcerative colitis lesions. *Gastroenterology.* 1993;104(6):1633–1639.
553. Brentnall TA, Crispin DA, Rabinovitch PS, et al. Mutations in the p53 gene: an early marker of neoplastic progression in ulcerative colitis. *Gastroenterology.* 1994;107(2):369–378.
554. Kern SE, Redston M, Seymour AB, et al. Molecular genetic profiles of colitis-associated neoplasms. *Gastroenterology.* 1994;107(2):420–428.
555. Suzuki H, Harpaz N, Tarmin L, et al. Microsatellite instability in ulcerative colitis-associated colorectal dysplasias and cancers. *Cancer Res.* 1994;54(18):4841–4844.
556. Redston MS, Papadopoulos N, Caldas C, Kinzler KW, Kern SE. Common occurrence of APC and K-ras gene mutations in the spectrum of colitis-associated neoplasias. *Gastroenterology.* 1995;108(2):383–392.
557. Sato F, Shibata D, Harpaz N, et al. Aberrant methylation of the HPP1 gene in ulcerative colitis-associated colorectal carcinoma. *Cancer Res.* 2002;62(23):6820–6822.
558. Olaru AV, Cheng Y, Agarwal R, et al. Unique patterns of CpG island methylation in inflammatory bowel disease-associated colorectal cancers. *Inflamm Bowel Dis.* 2012;18(4):641–648.
559. Blackstone MO, Riddell RH, Rogers BH, Levin B. Dysplasia-associated lesion or mass (DALM) detected by colonoscopy in long-standing ulcerative colitis: an indication for colectomy. *Gastroenterology.* 1981;80(2):366–374.
560. Ullman T, Croog V, Harpaz N, Sachar D, Itzkowitz S. Progression of flat low-grade dysplasia to advanced neoplasia in patients with ulcerative colitis. *Gastroenterology.* 2003;125(5):1311–1319.
561. Thomas T, Abrams KA, Robinson RJ, Mayberry JF. Meta-analysis: cancer risk of low-grade dysplasia in chronic ulcerative colitis. *Aliment Pharmacol Ther.* 2007;25(6):657–668.
562. Bernstein CN, Shanahan F, Weinstein WM. Are we telling patients the truth about surveillance colonoscopy in ulcerative colitis? *Lancet.* 1994;343(8889):71–74.

563. Itzkowitz SH, Present DH; Crohn's and Colitis Foundation of America Colon Cancer in IBD Study Group. Consensus conference: Colorectal cancer screening and surveillance in inflammatory bowel disease. *Inflamm Bowel Dis.* 2005;11(3):314–321.
564. Bernstein CN, Blanchard JF, Kliewer E, Wajda A. Cancer risk in patients with inflammatory bowel disease: a population-based study. *Cancer.* 2001;91(4):854–862.
565. Neumann H, Vieth M, Langner C, Neurath MF, Mudter J. Cancer risk in IBD: how to diagnose and how to manage DALM and ALM. *World J Gastroenterol.* 2011;17(27):3184–3191.
566. Farraye FA, Odze RD, Eaden J, et al.; AGA Institute Medical Position Panel on Diagnosis and Management of Colorectal Neoplasia in Inflammatory Bowel Disease. AGA medical position statement on the diagnosis and management of colorectal neoplasia in inflammatory bowel disease. *Gastroenterology.* 2010;138(2):738–745.
567. Winawer S, Fletcher R, Rex D, et al.; Gastrointestinal Consortium Panel. Colorectal cancer screening and surveillance: clinical guidelines and rationale-Update based on new evidence. *Gastroenterology.* 2003;124(2):544–560.
568. Leidenius M, Kellokumpu I, Husa A, Riihelä M, Sipponen P. Dysplasia and carcinoma in longstanding ulcerative colitis: an endoscopic and histological surveillance programme. *Gut.* 1991;32(12):1521–1525.
569. Connell WR, Lennard-Jones JE, Williams CB, Talbot IC, Price AB, Wilkinson KH. Factors affecting the outcome of endoscopic surveillance for cancer in ulcerative colitis. *Gastroenterology.* 1994;107(4):934–944.
570. Rozen P, Baratz M, Fefer F, Gilat T. Low incidence of significant dysplasia in a successful endoscopic surveillance program of patients with ulcerative colitis. *Gastroenterology.* 1995;108(5):1361–1370.
571. Lindberg B, Persson B, Veress B, Ingelman-Sundberg H, Granqvist S. Twenty years' colonoscopic surveillance of patients with ulcerative colitis. Detection of dysplastic and malignant transformation. *Scand J Gastroenterol.* 1996;31(12):1195–1204.
572. Lashner BA, Kane SV, Hanauer SB. Colon cancer surveillance in chronic ulcerative colitis: historical cohort study. *Am J Gastroenterol.* 1990;85(9):1083–1087.
573. Choi PM, Nugent FW, Schoetz DJ Jr, Silverman ML, Haggitt RC. Colonoscopic surveillance reduces mortality from colorectal cancer in ulcerative colitis. *Gastroenterology.* 1993;105(2):418–424.
574. Karlén P, Kornfeld D, Broström O, Löfberg R, Persson PG, Ekbom A. Is colonoscopic surveillance reducing colorectal cancer mortality in ulcerative colitis? A population based case control study. *Gut.* 1998;42(5):711–714.
575. Mpofu, C., A. J. Watson, et al. Strategies for detecting colon cancer and/or dysplasia in patients with inflammatory bowel disease. *Cochrane Database Syst Rev.* 2004;(2):CD000279.
576. Friedman S, Rubin PH, Bodian C, Harpaz N, Present DH. Screening and surveillance colonoscopy in chronic Crohn's colitis: results of a surveillance program spanning 25 years. *Clin Gastroenterol Hepatol.* 2008;6(9):993–8; quiz 953.
577. Itzkowitz SH, Harpaz N. Diagnosis and management of dysplasia in patients with inflammatory bowel diseases. *Gastroenterology.* 2004;126(6):1634–1648.
578. Rubin CE, Haggitt RC, Burmer GC, et al. DNA aneuploidy in colonic biopsies predicts future development of dysplasia in ulcerative colitis. *Gastroenterology.* 1992;103(5):1611–1620.
579. Provenzale D, Wong JB, Onken JE, Lipscomb J. Performing a cost-effectiveness analysis: surveillance of patients with ulcerative colitis. *Am J Gastroenterol.* 1998;93(6):872–880.
580. Rubenstein JH, Waljee AK, Jeter JM, Velayos FS, Ladabaum U, Higgins PD. Cost effectiveness of ulcerative colitis surveillance in the setting of 5-aminosalicylates. *Am J Gastroenterol.* 2009;104(9):2222–2232.
581. Hurlstone DP, Sanders DS, Lobo AJ, McAlindon ME, Cross SS. Indigo carmine-assisted high-magnification chromoscopic colonoscopy for the detection and characterisation of intraepithelial neoplasia in ulcerative colitis: a prospective evaluation. *Endoscopy.* 2005;37(12):1186–1192.
582. Kiesslich R, Goetz M, Lammersdorf K, et al. Chromoscopy-guided endomicroscopy increases the diagnostic yield of intraepithelial neoplasia in ulcerative colitis. *Gastroenterology.* 2007;132(3):874–882.
583. Marion JF, Waye JD, Present DH, et al.; Chromoendoscopy Study Group at Mount Sinai School of Medicine. Chromoendoscopy-targeted biopsies are superior to standard colonoscopic surveillance for detecting dysplasia in inflammatory bowel disease patients: a prospective endoscopic trial. *Am J Gastroenterol.* 2008;103(9):2342–2349.
584. Dekker E, van den Broek FJ, Reitsma JB, et al. Narrow-band imaging compared with conventional colonoscopy for the detection of dysplasia in patients with longstanding ulcerative colitis. *Endoscopy.* 2007;39(3):216–221.
585. van den Broek FJ, Fockens P, van Eeden S, et al. Narrow-band imaging versus high-definition endoscopy for the diagnosis of neoplasia in ulcerative colitis. *Endoscopy.* 2011;43(2): 108–115.
586. Ignjatovic A, East JE, Subramanian V, et al. Narrow band imaging for detection of dysplasia in colitis: a randomized controlled trial. *Am J Gastroenterol.* 2012;107(6):885–890.
587. Pellisé M, Lópcz-Cerón M, Rodríguez de Miguel C, et al. Narrow-band imaging as an alternative to chromoendoscopy for the detection of dysplasia in long-standing inflammatory bowel disease: a prospective, randomized, crossover study. *Gastrointest Endosc.* 2011;74(4):840–848.
588. van den Broek FJ, Fockens P, van Eeden S, et al. Endoscopic tri-modal imaging for surveillance in ulcerative colitis: randomised comparison of high-resolution endoscopy and autofluorescence imaging for neoplasia detection; and evaluation of narrow-band imaging for classification of lesions. *Gut.* 2008;57(8):1083–1089.
589. van Staa TP, Card T, Logan RF, Leufkens HG. 5-Aminosalicylate use and colorectal cancer risk in inflammatory bowel disease: a large epidemiological study. *Gut.* 2005;54(11):1573–1578.
590. Terdiman JP, Steinbuch M, Blumentals WA, Ullman TA, Rubin DT. 5-Aminosalicylic acid therapy and the risk of colorectal cancer among patients with inflammatory bowel disease. *Inflamm Bowel Dis.* 2007;13(4):367–371.
591. Bernstein CN, Nugent Z, Blanchard JF. 5-aminosalicylate is not chemoprophylactic for colorectal cancer in IBD: a population based study. *Am J Gastroenterol.* 2011;106(4):731–736.
592. Eaden JA. The data supporting a role for aminosalicylates for the chemoprevention of colorectal cancer in patients with inflammatory bowel disease. Aliment Pharmacol Ther, 2003;18 Suppl 2:15–21. Review
593. Pardi DS, Loftus EV Jr, Kremers WK, Keach J, Lindor KD. Ursodeoxycholic acid as a chemopreventive agent in patients with ulcerative colitis and primary sclerosing cholangitis. *Gastroenterology.* 2003;124(4):889–893.
594. Tung BY, Emond MJ, Haggitt RC, et al. Ursodiol use is associated with lower prevalence of colonic neoplasia in patients with ulcerative colitis and primary sclerosing cholangitis. *Ann Intern Med.* 2001;134(2):89–95.
595. Wolf JM, Rybicki LA, Lashner BA. The impact of ursodeoxycholic acid on cancer, dysplasia and mortality in ulcerative colitis patients with primary sclerosing cholangitis. *Aliment Pharmacol Ther.* 2005;22(9):783–788.
596. Eaton JE, Silveira MG, Pardi DS, et al. High-dose ursodeoxycholic acid is associated with the development of colorectal neoplasia in patients with ulcerative colitis and primary sclerosing cholangitis. *Am J Gastroenterol.* 2011;106(9):1638–1645.

3 Navigation Programs in Colorectal Cancer Care

MARGARET A. O'GRADY
ELAINE SEIN

■ RATIONALE FOR COLORECTAL NAVIGATION SERVICES

Patient navigation in cancer care is defined by the National Cancer Institute (2005) as the assistance offered to health care consumers to help them access and chart a course through the health care system and overcome barriers to care (1,2). Patient navigation eliminates barriers, streamlines care, ensures timely diagnosis and treatment, and provides resource support (3).

With the development of multidisciplinary colorectal cancer (CRC) disease teams or CRC-specific service lines within health care settings, the growth in patient navigation programs for CRC has increased exponentially. The driving forces are multiple—overcoming barriers to care, such as colonoscopy screening practices, assistance/education on cost of care, evidence of better clinical outcomes from multimodality treatments and the overarching goal of seamless delivery of care for better customer satisfaction. A preassessment tool has been developed by the Association of Community Cancer Centers to identify areas of need as well as readiness to execute a navigation program (Table 3.1; 4). Carroll discusses barriers to care and estimates of navigation intensity leading to time-to-care issues. With increasing barriers, more navigation time is needed per patient and potential delay of care is increased unless these issues are addressed. This helps identify staffing trends (5). Lebwohl discusses the effect of patient navigation on the volume and quality of colonoscopy. Of the 749 patients assessed by the patient navigators, 678 (91%) underwent colonoscopy. Volume increased 56% for Medicaid outpatients. Preparation quality was superior to nonnavigated patients (40% vs 34%; 6). Ma discusses community based CRC screening and use of navigators for underserved Korean populations. One hundred sixty-seven Koreans were enrolled from six churches in the Philadelphia area. A tailored education program in their native language by a Korean-speaking navigator was used vs control group who received general health education that included cancer-related issues for screening. At 12- month postintervention follow up, 74% of the intervention group had received colorectal screening compared to 10.8% of the control group (7).

There exists a number of treatment options for patients with CRCs. An example is the treatment of liver metastasis. Potential treatment options include: surgical c-resection, cryoablation, radiofrequency ablation, intraarterial chemotherapy, intraarterial radioembolization, and hyperthermia treatment (8). Newer techniques have made the treatment discussion more complex and, therefore, clinical navigation becomes a critical element to help sort out the plethora of technology, processes, options, and cost for patients and their family.

Also of critical importance to comprehensive cancer centers is the role of clinical trials and patient education. Navigation is paramount for this discussion. The National Cancer Institute has developed a Patient Navigation Research Program (1) whereby trained, culturally competent health care workers work with patients/families, clinicians, and health care systems to ensure patients needs are appropriately and effectively addressed. Developed by the Center to Reduce Cancer Health Disparities (CRCHD) this program has been operational since October 2005 with support from the National Cancer Institute and American Cancer Society. Nine sites have been funded to date to develop innovative strategies to reduce or eliminate cancer health disparities and test efficacy and cost effectiveness.

With many treatment options available and the need for patients to see multiple specialists, it becomes a barrier to the patient and family to coordinate services and decide best care options. There rests an opportunity for clinicians and health systems to coordinate these services and provide seamless care. If the multidisciplinary experience is well coordinated, patients will be retained. Thus clinically navigating the patient/family through the continuum is an imperative.

Table 3.1 Patient Navigation Program Pre-Assessment Tool

This pre-assessment tool can help you assess your organization and consider all aspects of a patient navigation program. This tool can also help you assess your readiness for implementation or identify areas that need to be addressed before rolling out a patient navigation program.

GOALS AND CHALLENGES

1. **Goals** for my navigator program:

2. **Barriers/Challenges** to my navigator program:

OPERATIONS

1. Tumor types to be covered by navigator program:

2. Will each tumor type have its own navigation program or will one navigator cover more than one tumor type?

3. Do you have team(s) to set up program(s) by disease state(s)?

4. Timeline for implementation:

5. How many patients per year will participate in the navigator program?

6. What is your anticipated patient to navigator ratio?

7. How will you identify patients eligible for the program?
   - ☐ Pathology reports
   - ☐ Inpatients
   - ☐ MD referrals
   - ☐ Surgical reports
   - ☐ Other ______________

(Continued)

■ **Table 3.1** *(Continued)*

8. What are the biggest challenges facing the patient that need to be addressed by the navigator?
____
____
____
____

9. Where will the navigator(s) be housed?

10. What other space is allocated for the program:
    ☐ Patient library/education space ☐ Counseling rooms
    ☐ Other offices ☐ Other ____________________

11. How will the program be funded?
    ☐ Grants ☐ Patient pays ☐ Insurance
    ☐ Other ______________________________

12. Will patients be charged for any part of the service?

13. Which salaries will be supported solely by program budget (navigator, administrative assistant, etc.)?

14. Which salaries will be partially supported by program budget (social work, PT/OT, etc.)?

15. What else will the budget be used for (patient education materials, journals, etc.)?
____
____
____
____

16. Do you have an electronic charting system?

17. How will you communicate between practitioners?
____
____
____
____

ROLE OF NAVIGATOR

18. Who do you see as the navigator in your program?
    ☐ RN ☐ Social worker ☐ Lay person/survivor
    ☐ Other ______________________________

19. When would you like the navigator to become involved with the patient?
    ☐ Prior to entering the health care system ☐ At time of screening
    ☐ At time of suspicious finding ☐ At time of diagnosis
    ☐ Other (please specify) ____________________

20. What are the primary functions you would like the navigator to fulfill? Please rank them with 1 being the most important.
    ☐ Community education ☐ Patient education ☐ Care coordinator
    ☐ Psychosocial counselor ☐ Financial counselor ☐ Other (please specify)

(Continued)

Table 3.1 *(Continued)*

21. What other activities would you like the navigator to be involved in? Please rank them with 1 being the most important.
    - ☐ QI/PI activities
    - ☐ Community educational programs
    - ☐ Screenings
    - ☐ Staff educational programs
    - ☐ Survivorship program
    - ☐ Help set up program(s) by disease state(s)
    - ☐ Other (specify)

RESOURCES

22. What resources do you currently have in place?
    - ☐ Case managers
    - ☐ Social workers
    - ☐ Registered dietitians
    - ☐ Financial counselors
    - ☐ Genetic counselors
    - ☐ Health psychologists
    - ☐ Chaplain
    - ☐ PT/OT
    - ☐ Speech therapy
    - ☐ Home care services
    - ☐ Hospice services
    - ☐ Palliative care services
    - ☐ Patient advisory committee
    - ☐ Support groups

    (specify)____
    - ☐ Other (specify)

    ____

23. Do you currently have a relationship with community patient support agencies such as the American Cancer Society (ACS) or local support groups other than hospital-based groups?

    ____
    ____
    ____
    ____
    ____

OTHER CONSIDERATIONS

24. Do you have an MD champion for patient navigation program?

25. Do MDs support the program? If not, will MDs need convincing of need of program?

26. Administration level support/commitment or lack of support/commitment?

27. What percentage of your population has?
    - ☐ Private health insurance
    - ☐ Medicare
    - ☐ Medicaid
    - ☐ No insurance

28. What percentage of your population is?
    - ☐ Caucasian
    - ☐ Hispanic
    - ☐ Asian
    - ☐ African American
    - ☐ Native American
    - ☐ Other (please specify) ______________________________

Reprinted with permission of The Association of Community Cancer Centers (4).

OVERVIEW OF THE ROLE OF NAVIGATION AS IT SUPPORTS MULTIDISCIPLINARY CARE MODELS

Engineering Care Management

There are two key communication factors in developing a colorectal multidisciplinary program. The first is coordination of entry into the health care system as an outpatient or inpatient. The second is a point in time for specialists to review jointly their recommendations to develop a coordinated plan of care for the patient. Programs may or may not be housed together for these care aspects. Offering a patient "one-stop-shopping" is attractive but it may not be practical. As a result, some oncology programs, particularly those with moderate volumes, have developed colorectal care models that offer the benefits of coordination without the required investment of a comprehensive clinic with dedicated space (8).

Three possible models are described in Table 3.2.

■ OVERVIEW OF THE PROGRAM

Referral/Intake

The navigation program is based on a structured program of care with a nurse navigator in the coordination role for the CRC patient population. Intake can occur by physician, outreach navigator from the colorectal team, or patient referral via a referral number (toll-free line) housed in the cancer program. All three models agree on a dedicated intake number with a list of specialists available to review each referring patient, outreach navigator, or clinician.

The nurse navigator can also review pathology reports from the hospital's endoscopy suites as well as colonoscopy reports from pathology. The navigator then calls the primary physician and organizes all materials pertaining to each case in need of cancer care follow up. Finally, any screenings conducted by the health system or private practice office link can be possible cases for the colorectal program. Screenings should be reviewed separately by the colorectal team for effective screenings practices, emerging screening technologies, evaluation of screening tests, and information flow from external referring clinicians to specialists.

Model 1: Prospective Treatment Planning Conference for CRC

Prospective weekly multidisciplinary case conference encourages physician consensus prior to therapy initiation, and identifies patients for multimodality care and clinical trials. It is 90% prospective in conjunction with the American College of Surgeons' requirements for a tumor board/case conference and therefore CMEs can be awarded to participating physicians (9). Nurse navigators dedicates 15% of time to colorectal conference coordination. They collate patient charts, slides, and films prior to conference and they take minutes at each meeting so all clinicians get notes in follow up.

According to specialists at the Hoag Cancer Center who have initiated this prospective conference, the benefits include the educational advantages of collaborative treatment planning among general surgeons, radiation oncology, and medical oncology treating substantial numbers of colorectal patients. Physicians find the conference to be particularly valuable for rectal patients—typically requiring evaluation by all three oncology disciplines—who in the past did not benefit from multidisciplinary case review. The conference has enabled more doctors to appropriately identify candidates for neo-adjuvant therapy and sphincter-sparing surgeries (8).

Model 2: Virtual Colorectal Clinic

Prospective planning alone may not accomplish all the coordination and care aspects patients need. The virtual clinic tries to compensate for this by hiring a full-time nurse navigator who can guide patients through the evaluation and treatment planning process across multiple specialists and clinic locations—essentially creating a "virtual" colorectal clinic.

A patient first meets with the navigator and an identified clinical lead physician based on symptoms and diagnostics completed thus far. The lead then serves as gatekeeper to subsequent specialist visits, and following

■ Table 3.2 Models of Multidisciplinary Care for CRC

Model	Navigation
Prospective Treatment Planning Conference	Access to a nurse navigator—navigator may spend some time coordinating retrospective tumor board Patient has independently scheduled consultations, diagnostics
Virtual Colorectal Clinic	Dedicated nurse navigator Coordination of consults/diagnostics Portions of tumor board cases are prospective
Comprehensive Colorectal Clinic	Dedicated navigation staff to disease site Seamless evaluation completed in one visit or virtually in 2 to 3 days Formal method for determining case inclusion in prospective treatment planning conferences or 100% of cases presented Database for patient tracking including entry to system, diagnostic workup, and care coordination including survivorship

From (8).

the initial visit, the navigator schedules visits with the additional oncologist as needed. Cases are brought to the prospective case conference for discussion. Arrangements may also be made by the navigator for the patient to meet with other supportive care services as needed.

Upon referral, the clinical navigator may determine enough information exists to bring the patient right to the colorectal clinic where all the discipline sees the patient in a coordinated time slot. This represents a step beyond the virtual clinic model, where patients meet with different specialists individually across multiple visits and get facilitated care.

The virtual program's success is largely attributed to the navigator's triage training and coordination with a team of disease specific clinicians. Evaluation is accomplished by both patient and physician customer satisfaction surveys (8).

Model 3: Comprehensive Prospective Colorectal Clinic

The final example is the most complex and comes from the Dana Farber Cancer Center. Dana Farber developed a GI center in 1996. The center includes an eight-exam room clinic, where patients are seen 3 days a week from 1 to 5 PM. Patients with untreated, nonmetastatic disease (40% of clinic patients) meet consecutively with a surgeon, medical oncologist, and radiation oncologist. The specialists first meet to review the patient's medical history, films and slides, with the option of requesting the on-staff radiologist to review films "real-time" to ensure consensus in interpretation. Then each specialist meets with the patients individually, both to examine them and to discuss treatment recommendations. Sixty percent of clinic patients with metastatic disease are typically scheduled only with a medical oncologist for clinical evaluation. See Table 3.3 for flow process.

■ NURSE NAVIGATOR PLACEMENT—LOCATION, LOCATION, LOCATION!

An oncology nurse navigator is hired to work in a plethora of settings including but not limited to private practices such as gastroenterology; hospital cancer programs; inpatient or outpatient settings including radiology, pathology, gastroenterology, medical oncology, surgery, radiation oncology, clinical trial office; or free standing clinics. The location of placement is based on first point of entry or barrier/difficult to navigate area within the multidisciplinary program. Some roles may include triage whereby review of pathology takes place to code the patients based on level of diagnosis and metastatic disease.

Once intake has occurred, the patient would be a classified into one of two groups, either single specialty review alone or multidisciplinary review. Depending on the extent of disease, patients may be in need of case management services or other support services to help them through their treatment regimen. Treating physicians working in conjunction with the nurse navigator will coordinate the plan of action with the navigator who will function in a case management mode during the patients care. Other duties of the navigator are described in Table 3.4 (10).

■ NAVIGATION ROLE IN COLORECTAL QUALITY CARE

As CRC multidisciplinary clinics are developed, the navigator plays an integral role in identifying barriers,

■ Table 3.3 Dana Farber Patient Care Process for Colorectal Clinic

Patient Preparation	Collaborative Treatment Planning	"Round Robin" Clinic Exams	Communication of Treatment Plans
Navigator telephones patient, takes medical history, diagnosis	Three specialists review patient information	Three specialists see patient individually	In addition to verbal communication, a written plan is sent to the patient, referring physician
Arranges for delivery of pathology reports and imaging studies	Formulate treatment plan	Explain treatment recommendations, answer questions	
	Time for conference approximately 20 min	Time for exams approximately 90 min	

From (8).

Table 3.4 Example: JOB DESCRIPTION—Fox Chase Cancer Center Colorectal Nurse Navigator

PRIMARY FUNCTION:

The Colorectal Navigator functions with the goal of providing quality care to cancer patients and their families. This is accomplished through expert oncology nursing practice in the areas of care coordination, consultation, education, and research.

The Colorectal Navigator in collaboration with the multidisciplinary cancer team (physicians, support staff, administration, marketing, and outreach) develops, maintains, and coordinates the colorectal care program which includes a multidisciplinary colorectal evaluation service, colorectal health and cancer education, and promotion of the program to physicians, patients, consumers, payors, co-workers, community, and outside organizations.

ACCOUNTABILITIES

I. Clinician

- A. Plans, implements, coordinates, and evaluates the care of colorectal cancer patients
  1. Demonstrates an understanding of basic principles of physical and psychosocial assessment related to adult development.
  2. Confers with appropriate team members regarding actual/potential health care needs.
  3. Provides direct care for patients with complex needs in collaboration with staff.
  4. Follows patient/families through/across departmental lines as appropriate to that individual's care needs (eg, inpatient, outpatient, gastroenterology, radiation therapy, home care, palliative care, etc.).
  5. Accepts and initiates referrals to appropriate departments in the institution or outside as appropriate for follow-up care.
- B. Schedules interdisciplinary assessments, offers decision-making support, provides one-on-one counseling as needed, conducts pre- and postoperative education.
- C. Acts as a change agent through formulation of new standards and policies.
- D. Formulates, interprets, and implements policy, procedures, and standards related to colorectal cancer patients
- E. Facilitates Colorectal Cancer Support Group.
- F. Functions as a mentor to nursing staff.
- G. Assures that all patients are treated with respect and consideration, that their right to treatment or service is respected, that confidentiality, privacy, and security are maintained, and that they are involved in all aspects of their care.
- H. Maintains confidentiality, security, and integrity of data and information, according to HIPAA standards.
- I. Adheres to ANA Code of Ethics for Registered Nurses.
- J. Demonstrates appropriate interpersonal skills, utilizing principles of Emotional Intelligence to promote effective teamwork.
- K. Demonstrates ability to assess, interpret, and provide interventions based on age specific data.
- L. Demonstrates knowledge for all ages of patient care including geriatric and adult patients:
  1. of skills to provide appropriate patient care
  2. of principles of growth and development over the life span
  3. of mandated reporting laws
  4. of ethnic, religious, and cultural impact in the diagnosis and treatment of chronic illness.

II. Education

- A. Works both independently and with other health care disciplines/departments in developing, implementing, and evaluating colorectal programs for patients, nursing, and community education.
  1. Provides education to patients and families.
  2. Maximizes opportunities in the clinical setting for informal education of staff, patients, and families.
  3. Acts as a resource person for staff to problem-solve potential complications that might arise in relation to specific therapies.
  4. Acts as a resource person for outside institutions and patients following discharge.
  5. Assesses learning needs, plans, implements, and evaluates nursing education programs within the institution.
  6. Provides continuing education outside the institution as requested.
- B. Introduces nursing practice innovations as it relates to colorectal cancer care and educates staff and other disciplines (as appropriate) re: same.
- C. Seeks opportunities to participate in related community educational activities.
- D. Serves as a clinical preceptor to new colorectal navigators from outside institutions.
- E. Develops and maintains a colorectal health resource center.

III. Coordination/Administrative Activities

- A. Participates in development of practice standards for the colorectal cancer program.
- B. Participates in the development and evaluation of colorectal program quality improvement metrics.

(Continued)

■ **Table 3.4** *(Continued)*

C. Collaborates with Oncology Program Director to maintain colorectal program operations within fiscal parameters.
D. Fosters a patient-centered care approach to colorectal program development.
E. Collaborate with marketing and public relations departments to develop and design materials for entire customer base from physicians to consumers.
F. Evaluate potential funding opportunities to support the mission and goals of the colorectal program.

IV. Researcher

A. Establishes regular time period to review current nursing literature/research.
B. Promotes understanding of oncology clinical trials–clinical, behavioral, and prevention studies to physicians and nursing staff as related to colorectal diseases.
C. Interprets, evaluates, and communicates pertinent research findings to nursing staff which should be integrated into nursing care.
D. Participates in Nursing Evidence-Based Practice Council.
E. Collaborates with Director of Nursing Research in proposal development, data collection, analysis, and interpretation as needed as it relates to colorectal disease.

V. Consultant

A. Collaborates with nursing councils on decisions affecting patient care as it relates to colorectal cancer patients and in establishing goals and priorities of clinical practice.
B. Participates as requested on nursing and multidisciplinary committees.
C. Accepts appropriate consultative requests for assistance to nursing staff, patients, and other disciplines within home institution as well as outside institutions as deemed appropriate by administration.

VI. Professional Growth

A. Maintains and updates personal competency and continuing education through attendance at CE programs.
B. Participates in related professional and/or community organizations.
C. Strongly recommended certification as an oncology nurse.
D. Strives to contribute to nursing literature through submission of at least one article/year for publication.

enhancements, and strategies to support the customers including referring clinicians, the colorectal team, and patients and families. As the colorectal team begins the quality improvement process, several key national groups should be considered for their expertise in developing quality metrics that the navigator can support and in some instances facilitate. They include:

- National Comprehensive Cancer Network
- Oncology Roundtable/Health Care Advisory Board
- Oncology Nursing Society—Colorectal Oncology Consortium
- American College of Surgeons/Commission on Cancer
- American Society of Clinical Oncology
- American College of Radiation Oncology
- American Academy of Oncology Administrators

Each colorectal team needs to select outcome quality metrics that are most important to the quality of care in their institution as well as the long-term sustainability of the multidisciplinary disease management team. These include patient-focused measures such as retention rate, physician-focused measures such as clinical trial discussion with patients, and clinical quality-focused measures such as compliance with guidelines and pathways.

Customer satisfaction is the one major driving force and patient demand for navigation services. Several institutions have developed satisfaction tools to not only look at patient satisfaction but also referring clinician satisfaction (Tables 3.4 and 3.5 A and B; 11).

As accountable care programs are increasingly mandated, navigation offers a "must have" service to any multidisciplinary CRC program. There are multiple resources available to the colorectal multidisciplinary team to support the development of a nurse navigator role. Oncology Nursing Society's *Breast Cancer, Site Specific Cancer* series, second edition highlights resources appropriate for any navigation program to consider (12).

In conclusion, the multidisciplinary team approach for CRC care finds navigation as an imperative to success. Navigation is not a person but a process. Utilizing navigators in various roles such as outreach navigator, clinical trials navigator, clinical navigator, quality navigator, and survivorship navigator gives the team a passing of the baton in colorectal care that is seamless to the patients and their families, and supportive to the health care clinical teams they serve.

Table 3.5A Breast Health Patient Navigator

Please give your overall rating of the Navigator Program. Would you say you were...

Very Dissatisfied Neutral Very Satisfied

How would you rate your overall experience with the navigator? Would you say you were...

Very Dissatisfied Neutral Very Satisfied

Please circle your response; please add comments for choice of 3 or below.

Physician Survey	VERY DISSATISFIED		NEUTRAL		VERY SATISFIED
1. I am satisfied with navigator's awareness of appropriate resources.	1	2	3	4	5
2. I am satisfied with the navigator's timeliness in coordination of care.	1	2	3	4	5
3. The navigator was helpful providing education to my patient.	1	2	3	4	5
4. The navigator worked in conjunction with me to address patient concerns.	1	2	3	4	5
5. I was satisfied with the navigator's overall responsiveness.	1	2	3	4	5
6. The navigator was thorough and kept me informed.	1	2	3	4	5
7. I feel the navigator worked well with my office staff.	1	2	3	4	5
8. Overall, I value the navigation service to my practice.	1	2	3	4	5
9. I would recommend this service to other patients.	1	2	3	4	5

Suggestions or comments: ______________________________

____

____

Name (optional) ______________________________

■ Table 3.5B Breast Health Patient Navigator

Please give your overall rating of the Navigator Program. Would you say you were...

Very Dissatisfied Neutral Very Satisfied

How would you rate your overall experience with the navigator? Would you say you were...

Very Dissatisfied Neutral Very Satisfied

Please circle your response; please add comments for choice of 3 or below.

Patient Survey	VERY DISSATISFIED		NEUTRAL		VERY SATISFIED
1. I received adequate information pertaining to education.	1	2	3	4	5
2. My calls were returned in a timely manner.	1	2	3	4	5
3. I felt the navigator knew about my case.	1	2	3	4	5
4. The navigator provided me with helpful information during my care.	1	2	3	4	5
5. Support services referrals met my needs˙	1	2	3	4	5
6. I was satisfied with instructions and had responsive answers to questions.	1	2	3	4	5
7. The navigator was thorough and kept me informed.	1	2	3	4	5
8. I valued working with the navigator.	1	2	3	4	5
9. I found the patient journey binder materials helpful.	1	2	3	4	5
10. I would recommend this service to others.	1	2	3	4	5

Suggestions or comments: ____________________

____

____

Name (optional) ____________________

Did having a navigator and being part of this program keep you from seeking care elsewhere?

____

■ REFERENCES

1. Freund KM, Battaglia TA, Calhoun E, et al.; Patient Navigation Research Program Group. National Cancer Institute Patient Navigation Research Program: methods, protocol, and measures. *Cancer.* 2008; 113(12):3391–3399.
2. National Cancer Institute. NCI's patient navigator research program: Fact Sheet. http://www.cancer.gov/cancertopics/factsheet/PatientNavigator. Accessed April 2, 2005.
3. Freeman HP. A model patient navigation program. *Oncol Issues.* September/October, 2004;19:44–46.
4. Association of Community Cancer Centers. Patient Navigation Program Pre-Assessment Tool, Cancer Care Patient Navigation: A practical guide for community cancer centers, © *ACCC*, 2009.
5. Carroll JK, Winters PC, Purnell JQ, Devine K, Fiscella K. Do navigators' estimates of navigation intensity predict navigation time for cancer care? *J Cancer Educ.* 2011;26(4):761–766.
6. Lebwohl B, Neugut AI, Stavsky E, et al. Effect of a patient navigator program on the volume and quality of colonoscopy. *J Clin Gastroenterol.* 2011; 45(5):e47–e53.
7. Ma GX, Shive S, Tan Y, et al. Community-based colorectal cancer intervention in underserved Korean Americans. *Cancer Epidemiol.* 2009; 33(5):381–386.
8. Oncology Round Table, *Advisory Board* Interviews, February 18, 2005. Oncology Roundtable, Colorectal Resource Grid, *Advisory Board,* January 2009.
9. Commission on Cancer Standards. Cancer Program Standards 2009 Revised Edition (released March 2009). American College of Surgeons© 2003, 2006, 2009.
10. Sein E, Keeley P, Miller B, et al. eds. Fox Chase Cancer Center Partners Breast Care Coordinators/Navigators Orientation Manual. Philadelphia, PA: Fox Chase Cancer Center Partners, 2009.
11. Fox Chase Cancer Center/Virtua Health Customer Satisfaction Surveys. Published on the web via the Association of Community Cancer Centers, 2011.
12. Sein E. Building breast centers of excellence through patient navigation and care coordination. In: Mahon SM, eds. *Site specific cancer* series: *Breast cancer.* 2nd ed. Pittsburgh, PA: Oncology Nursing Society. 2011; 213–229.

4 Assessment and Management of Colorectal Polyps and Cancer Precursor Lesions

REID M. NESS

■ INTRODUCTION

Colorectal cancer (CRC) is the second leading cause of cancer death in the United States and the fourth leading cause of cancer death in the world (1). Fortunately, research over the last 40 years has greatly increased our knowledge of the process of carcinogenesis in the colon and its progression through precursor lesions to cancer. This has allowed for interventions not only to discover CRC early, before they can metastasize, but also to prevent cancer development through the identification and removal of precursor lesions. These strategies have contributed to the decrease in CRC incidence that has occurred in the United States almost every year since 1985 (1). Despite such success, CRC claimed over 51,000 lives in 2012 (1). In this chapter, we discuss CRC progression through intermediary precursor lesions, their identification, and removal. We will also discuss the prognostic information provided through the identification of such lesions and their implications for further surveillance.

■ MOLECULAR PATHOGENESIS OF CRC

Currently, there are believed to be three distinct molecular pathways through which CRC can arise: the chromosomal instability (CIN) pathway, the DNA mismatch repair (MMR) pathway, and the CpG island hypermethylation phenotype (CIMP) pathway.

Chromosomal Instability Pathway

CIN results from mutations that either activate growth promoting molecular pathways or diminish the activities of tumor suppressor genes (2). Tumors arising from this pathway are characterized by deletions, insertions, loss of herterozygosity, and other gross chromosomal abnormalities. The most critical gene to carcinogenesis by this pathway is the adenomatous polyposis coli (APC) gene. The recognition of the importance of the *APC* gene began with studies linking its mutations to the inheritance of the familial adenomatous polyposis (FAP) syndrome (2; see Table 4.1). This syndrome usually arises in individuals inheriting a single dysfunctional copy of the *APC* gene. The loss of the functional allele through deletion or somatic mutation leads to the development of adenomatous polyps (3,4). The presence of hundreds to thousands of these lesions in the colon is the hallmark of FAP and leads to the 100% risk of CRC in these patients. Attenuated FAP is the term applied to a less vigorous polyposis (10 to 100 adenomas) that also leads to a substantially increased risk of CRC. Many of the patients with attenuated FAP also have mutations in the *APC* gene (5–9). Importantly, somatic mutations in both *APC* alleles have been identified in 80% of nonfamilial or "sporadic" CRC (10).

The *APC* gene product is vital to cellular control over the Wnt signaling pathway through its ability to phosphorylate the signaling molecule beta-catenin that marks it for degradation (11–13). Mutations in the *APC* gene lead to truncated, dysfunctional proteins that are incapable of beta-catenin regulation, the accumulation of beta-catenin in the nucleus, and the activation of transcription factor TCF-4 (14–16). TCF-4 is responsible for the activation of cellular proliferation pathways and the inhibition of cellular differentiation and apoptosis (17–19). This is believed to create aberrant crypt foci, which are the smallest precursors of colorectal adenomas (3,20). These collections of cells with CIN are now predisposed to other somatic mutations leading to carcinogenesis. A good example of a commonly acquired mutation is in the *K-ras* oncogene (21–23). *Ras* oncogenes encode a family of small proteins that regulate the transmission of extracellular growth signals to the nucleus (24). *K-ras* mutations are the most frequently mutated in CRC, up to 50%. These mutations have been shown to be rare in small adenomas but are found in 50% of adenomas greater than 1 cm in size (21,25; see Table 4.1).

DNA Mismatch Repair Pathway

Mismatch repair genes are responsible for correcting the common single nucleotide base mispairings that occur

Table 4.1 Classification of Molecular Pathways for Colorectal Carcinogenesis

	Chromosomal Instability Pathway	Mismatch Repair Pathway	Serrated Pathway	
	Hereditary (FAP) and Sporadic	Hereditary (HNPCC)	Hereditary (SPS) and Sporadic	
Precursor lesion	Adenoma	Adenoma	SSA/Ps	SSA/Ps and TSA
Chromosomal instability	Present	Absent	Absent	Absent
MSI status	MSS	MSI-H	MSI-H	MSI-L
CIMP status	Negative	Negative	High	High
K-ras mutation	Present	±	Absent	Absent
BRAF mutation	Absent	Absent	Present	Present
MLH1 status	Normal	Mutated	Methylated	Partially methylated
MGMT methylation	Absent	Absent	±	Present

FAP, familial adenomatous polyposis; HNPCC, hereditary nonpolyposis CRC syndrome; SPS, serrated polyposis syndrome; SSA, sessile serrated adenomas/polyps; TSA, traditional serrated adenomas; MSI, microsatellite instability; MSS, microsatellite stable; MSI-H, high-level microsatellite instability; MSI-L, low-level microsatellite instability; ±, may or may not be present; CIMP, CpG island methylator phenotype; *K-ras, BRAF*, oncogenes; *MLH1*, mismatch repair gene; MGMT, O-6-methylguanine DNA methyltransferase.

during DNA replication (26–28). Affected cells accumulate DNA errors throughout the genome. The accumulation of these errors specifically affects the length of microsatellites, short sequences of nucleotide bases that are repeated tens to hundreds of times within specified areas of the genome and tend to be of stable length within a given person. The length of certain sentinel microsatellites can be assessed and graded as microsatellite stable (MSS) or microsatellite instability (MSI) low, high, and indeterminate (29,30). MSI is the phenotypic expression of MMR dysfunction within a given CRC (31–34; see Table 4.1). Several genes are important to this process including *MLH1, MSH2, PMS2*, and *MSH6*. Germline mutations in any one of these genes has been shown to be the genetic defect underlying the hereditary nonpolyposis CRC (HNPCC) syndrome (35). Patients with this syndrome do not develop increased numbers of colorectal adenomas. Nonetheless, they have a lifetime risk of CRC that may range from 25%–75% (36,37). The loss of MMR gene expression, usually *MLH1*, can also be found in approximately 15% of sporadic CRC (29,38,39). Interestingly, these sporadic tumors usually do not contain MMR gene mutations but rather have epigenetic changes that silence MMR gene expression (40).

CpG Island Hypermethylation Phenotype Pathway

Certain CRCs contain a high frequency of hypermethylation in the promoter regions of certain genes. This hypermethylation most often occurs at CpG dinucleotides referred to as a CpG island (40–42). Methylated CpG is bound by certain proteins called methyl-CpG binding domain proteins that act to block gene transcription (43–45). Colorectal tumors that have a high frequency of CpG methylation are said to have the CpG island hypermethylation phenotype or CIMP. These events often occur in the promoter regions of MMR genes (especially *MLH1*) leading to a silencing of their expression. Activating mutations in the *BRAF* gene are almost always present in sporadic CRCs with MSI-high (MSI-H) and may be the underlying cause of the CIMP (40; see Table 4.1). In contrast, HNPCC-related CRCs do not carry *BRAF* mutations and are more likely to contain *K-ras* mutations (46,47). There is now evidence that CRC with MSI and *BRAF* mutations may progress from lesions termed sessile serrated adenomas/polyps (SSA/Ps; 48–50). A presumed inherited syndrome called serrated polyposis syndrome (SPS) has been defined by the endoscopic identification of serrated polyps either in large numbers or in the proximal colon with or without a definite family association (51). Although the CIMP phenotype is present in most of these lesions, no definite genetic mutation has been identified.

PRECANCEROUS COLORECTAL NEOPLASMS

Adenomatous Polyps

Colorectal adenomas are the most common polypoid lesions occurring in the colon, making up 1/2 to 2/3 of all polyps identified at colonoscopy (52–55). As previously discussed, there is ample evidence from our knowledge of FAP, observational and molecular biologic studies in sporadic CRC to conclude that adenomatous polyps are precursor lesions for CRC. Furthermore, we have shown that removal of these lesions decreases the subsequent risk of CRC in specific and general populations (56–68).

As previously discussed, these lesions are thought to represent intermediary lesions along the CIN pathway for FAP-related and sporadic CRCs and along the MMR pathway in patients with HNPCC. The problem is that adenomatous polyps are common lesions occurring in greater than 25% of individuals at age 50 and over 50% above age 70 (69–74). Because these lesions are so prevalent in the population, there has been controversy concerning the risk posed by their identification in a given person and the modality and frequency of surveillance thereafter (75).

Adenoma Epidemiology

As noted above, colorectal adenomas are common lesions. Studies show that the main determinant of adenoma prevalence in the population is age. We have long known from autopsy studies, that colorectal adenomas increase in frequency with age (69). We are now confirming these findings in studies of asymptomatic individuals using high-quality colonoscopy and other imaging modalities (76–78). Of note, adenomas become preferentially more prevalent in the right colon compared to the left colon with increasing age (79). Colorectal adenomas are more prevalent in men compared to women in both autopsy and endoscopic studies (69,74,80,81). Race has also been shown to affect colorectal adenoma prevalence and distribution in the colon. Studies suggest that colorectal adenomas are more likely to be large and right sided in African Americans compared to Caucasians (82,83).

Adenoma Natural History

Because colorectal adenomas are such common lesions and CRC are much less common, only a small fraction of colorectal adenomas are thought to have any significant probability of becoming CRC. Observational studies suggest that as adenomas progress in size, their risk of containing foci of malignant transformation also increases (84). Yet even in lesions greater than 1 cm in diameter, the risk of cancerous transformation has only been observed to be ~1% per year (85). Overall, modeling studies suggest that to fit existing adenoma prevalence and CRC incidence data, the time for adenoma transformation to cancer in those lesions that become cancer averages 20 to 30 years (86). It is this long window of opportunity that allows for CRC prevention through screening for colorectal adenomas. Adenomas must be screened for because they are rarely symptomatic. Only large adenomas are even possibly associated with iron deficiency and they seldom if ever lead to obstruction.

Adenoma Classification

All adenomas are considered to be dysplastic but they can be grouped into low- and high-grade categories. Low-grade dysplasia is used to describe the usual degree of crypt distortion and cellular atypia associated with adenomas in general. High-grade dysplasia is used to describe tissue in which hyperproliferation extends into the base of the crypt and cellular atypia has reached a level to commensurate with carcinoma but without breaching of the muscularis mucosa (84). Adenomas are further differentiated based on their crypt depth and architecture. Adenomatous tissue with fairly shallow, heavily arborized crypts is described as tubular, while tissue with extension of crypts deep toward the center of the lesion is described as villous. Adenomas are classified as tubular if 75% of their mass can be described as tubular. Adenomas are described as tubulovillous if 26%–75% of their mass can be described as tubular. Adenomas are described as villous if 25% or less of their mass can be described as tubular. These classifications account for 80%, 15%, and 5% of prevalent adenomas (84). This classification system is important as studies have shown that an increasing villous component correlates with the likelihood of finding high-grade dysplasia or invasive cancer with the adenomatous lesion (84). As we will discuss, certain morphologic and pathologic features of adenomas are predictors of future adenoma formation and CRC development. This has led to a grouping of lesions with an increased risk both of cancer in the initial lesion and of metachronous colonic neoplasms labeled “advanced adenomas.” These lesions are described as adenomas having: (a) an endoscopic diameter greater than 1 cm; and/or (b) villous or tubulovillous histology; and/or (c) high-grade dysplasia (87).

Serrated Polyps

Serrated polyps are common colonic lesions characterized histologically by a serrated (saw-toothed) appearance of the crypt epithelium. Until recently, these lesions were thought to have little or no propensity to evolve into CRC. Serrated polyps are present in 25%–50% of individuals at autopsy (69,88–94) and at only a slightly lower prevalence in colonoscopic studies (95–99). They can be divided into three subtypes based on histology: hyperplastic polyps, SSA/Ps, and traditional serrated adenoma (TSA) (100). SSA/Ps have now been identified as the probable precursor lesion of CRCs that arise via the CIMP pathway (101–109).

Hyperplastic Polyps

Hyperplastic polyps are a type of serrated polyp characterized histologically by straight crypts that penetrate to the muscularis mucosa with minimal distortion. Hyperplastic polyps display only minimal cytosolic or nuclear atypia (100). Hyperplastic polyps are the most prevalent non-neoplastic polypoid lesions of the colon and comprise 70%–95% of all serrated adenomas. They are predominantly left-sided and usually less than 5 mm in diameter

(50,110–113). Their overall prevalence increases only minimally with age in adulthood (69,88–94,98,99,114) and is generally believed to be higher in men (50,69,88, 90,92,94,99,111,114,115). Data support the supposition that small, left-sided hyperplastic polyps are neither markers for CRC nor for proximal noncancerous lesions (62,84,116–120).

Sessile Serrated Adenoma/Polyps and Traditional Serrated Adenomas

SSA/Ps are serrated lesions characterized by disorganized and distorted crypts. In contrast to hyperplastic polyps, SSA/Ps often exhibit various degrees of cytosolic and nuclear atypia (100,121,122). The crypts themselves are often dilated with mucin that also coats the luminal surface of the lesion (100). Most SSA/Ps the CpG island hypermethylation phenotype and *BRAF* mutations (48–50,123–127). SSA/Ps with foci of adenoma-like dysplasia often demonstrate MSI and have hypermethylation of *MLH1* within the foci. SSA/Ps with dysplasia are thought to represent a further progression toward CRC (128).

TSAs have long complex crypt architecture giving the lesion a villous appearance. There is also a characteristic pattern of ectopic crypts oriented perpendicular to the villous structures of the lesion. The predominant epithelial cells typically have an abundant eosinophilic cytoplasm with bland nuclei and an open chromatin pattern (100,122). TSAs are more genetically diverse than SSA/Ps. They may be CIMP high or low and have either *BRAF* or *K-ras* mutations or neither (129,130). Although hypermethylation of *MLH1* and resulting MSI are rare, hypermethylation of the DNA repair gene 6-methylguanine-DNA methyltransferase (MGMT) is commonly identified in these lesions (131).

SSA/Ps and TSA Epidemiology

In the general population, SSA/Ps comprise approximately 5%–25% of serrated lesions and are preferentially distributed to the right colon. TSAs are uncommon lesions in comparison and tend to be found in the rectum and sigmoid colon (50,110–113,132–134).

SSA/Ps and TSA Natural History

Observational studies indicate that CRC can arise from SSA/Ps especially those with cytological dysplasia (133). Overall there is the suggestion of at least a 15-year interval for the progression of a nondysplastic SSA/Ps through a dysplastic SSA/Ps intermediate state to CRC (133, 135–138). SSA/Ps are strongly associated with synchronous CRCs in the proximal colon especially those with the MSI-high phenotype (139,140). Likewise MSI-high cancers are more likely to be discovered with synchronous SSA/Ps than MSS cancers (141). This provides strong evidence supporting the theory that SSA/Ps are the precursor lesion for CIMP positive CRCs.

SCREENING FOR POLYPS AND PRECURSOR LESIONS

Screening for CRC has been recommended since 1980 (142). Since then, the accumulation of data on carcinogenesis and our experience with screening have led to numerous iterations of screening recommendations from various countries and agencies. The most quoted currently are those from the U.S. Multi-Society Taskforce on CRC (143). CRC screening has been proven to decrease CRC mortality by 15%–33% when testing for occult blood in the stool was employed (54,144,145) and 43% when one-time sigmoidoscopy was employed between 55 and 64 years of age (146). Perhaps more importantly, screening for CRC has been shown to decrease CRC incidence, by 20% for fecal occult blood testing (FOBT; 147) and 33% for one-time sigmoidoscopy (146). The results from these randomized, controlled studies have been confirmed in the U.S. general population by a progressive decrease in CRC incidence and mortality since the mid-1980s (1).

Diagnostic modalities used for CRC screening basically either detect blood in spontaneously voided stool or seek to detect the cancer or precursor lesions either directly using endoscopy or indirectly using radiographic imaging. Older testing for blood in stool used guaiac-based chemical testing, which had poor sensitivity for cancer and little or no sensitivity for cancer precursor lesions (148–150). Newer guaiac-based screening tests and immunohistochemical tests that quantitatively detect human hemoglobin have improved sensitivity for CRC to 64%–82% (151). Unfortunately, their sensitivity for adenomatous polyps is much lower, 30%–41% for advanced adenomas (151). In contrast, the sensitivity of colonoscopy and CT colonography is in the range of 84%–100% for CRC and greater than 80% for advanced adenomas (78,152–158). This has led to the current U.S. Multi-Society Taskforce on CRC recommendations for screening in persons at standard risk as they appear in Table 4.2 (143).

Certain demographic traits and conditions have been determined to pose a substantially increased risk of CRC leading to special considerations in the screening guidelines (143). The germline syndromes FAP and HNPCC have very specialized screening guidelines related to the extreme risk for CRC development. Likewise, patients with long-standing and extensive inflammatory bowel disease (IBD) of the colon have specialized screening regimen. The most common predictive factor for CRC is having an affected first-degree family member diagnosed before age 60. Adenomas and CRC diagnosed at such a young age have been found to

Table 4.2 Current U.S. Multi-Society Task Force on Colorectal Cancer Screening Guidelines

Screening Group	Age to Start Screening	Test Modality	Screening Interval
Average-risk	50	gFOBT with high sensitivity for cancer	Annual
		FIT with high sensitivity for cancer	Annual
		FSIG	Every 5 years
		Colonoscopy	Every 10 years
		DCBE	Every 5 years
		CTC	Every 5 years
Family history: CRC or adenomas in a first-degree relative before age 60 or in ≥ 2 first-degree relatives of any age	40 or 10 years before youngest case in immediate family	Colonoscopy	
Family history: CRC or adenomas in a first-degree relative after age 60 or ≥ 2 second-degree relatives with CRC	40	Colonoscopy	

gFOBT, guiac-based fecal occult blood test; FIT, fecal immunochemical test; FSIG, flexible sigmoidoscopy; DCBE, double-contrast barium enema; CTC, CT colonography; CRC, colorectal cancer.

Levin B, et al. Screening and surveillance for the early detection of CRC and adenomatous polyps, 2008: a joint guideline from the American Cancer Society, the US Multi-Society Task Force on CRC, and the American College of Radiology. *Gastroenterology*, 2008;134(5):1570–1595.

pose an approximately 2- and 4-fold increased risk of CRC development, respectively (159). Also, CRC occurs at an earlier age in these patients (160,161). For this reason, screening is recommended to begin at age 40 or younger in these patients and to employ colonoscopy every 5 years (143).

POLYP AND PRECURSOR LESION DETECTION AND REMOVAL

As has already been discussed, only endoscopy and external imaging using CT or MRI have sufficient sensitivity for detecting CRC precursor lesions to be useful in CRC prevention. The main determinant of the ability of any of these modalities to detect a specific precursor lesion is the size of the lesion. The sensitivity of colonoscopy for adenomas in a study where two colonoscopies were performed the same day found a first colonoscopy per lesion sensitivity of 94% for lesions greater than or equal to 10 mm, 87% for lesions 6 to 9 mm, and 73% for lesions less than or equal to 5 mm (152). Similar results have been found for CT colonography (78) and sigmoidoscopy in the distal colon (52,53,162). The other characteristic of a given precursor lesion that can affect detection is its endoscopic morphology or shape. Not all precursor lesions have a classic polypoid shape. Shape can be classified as:

- *Pedunculated*: a lesion having the neoplastic tissue at the end of a muscular stalk producing a mushroom-like shape
- *Sessile*: elevated lesions that do not have a stalk and are completely attached to the colon wall
- *Flat*: minimally elevated lesions (less than half the diameter of the lesion)
- *Depressed*: having a portion of the lesion surface below the level of the surrounding mucosa

The morphology of superficial neoplastic lesions or type 0 lesions has been further defined by guidelines that group pedunculated and sessile lesions as type 1 or protruding and flat or depressed lesions as type 2 or nonprotruding (see Table 4.3; 163). As might be expected, flat and depressed lesions are harder to identify than lesions with higher relief and their detection more affected by factors influencing quality of colonoscopy (164–167). This fact is important as approximately 27%–36% of adenomas and almost all serrated adenomas can be classified as flat (168–171). Depressed lesions, though rare (less than 1% of adenomas), are thought to harbor high-grade dysplasia and CRC at a higher rate than other lesion morphologies (168–171). Lesion location can also affect detectability.

Table 4.3 The Macroscopic Classification of Superficial Digestive-Tract Lesions

Endoscopic Appearance		Classification
Protruding	Pedunculated	Ip
	Sessile	Is
Nonprotruding/nonexcavated	Slightly elevated	IIa
	Completely flat	IIb
	Slightly depressed	IIc
	Elevated with some depression	IIc + IIa
		IIa + IIc
Excavated	Ulcer	III
	Excavated and depressed	IIc + III
		III + IIc

Endoscopic Classification Review, Update on the Paris classification of superficial neoplastic lesions in the digestive tract. *Endoscopy*, 2005;37(6):570–578.

Community studies show a reduction in CRC among individuals having undergone previous colonoscopy by 67%–84% in the left colon but only 1%–54% in the right colon (172–176). Many of these missed right-sided lesions are now believed to be SSA/Ps with flat morphology (100).

The resection of precursor lesions is performed endoscopically using one of several endoscopic devices and techniques. Previously, it was believed that endoscopic resection was adequate to remove most target lesions in their entirety. Recent studies cast some doubt on that assumption. Of interval cancers following colonoscopic polypectomy, 19%–27% have been shown to occur in the same colon segments as the resected lesions (177–179). This may be explained by a finding of residual tissue following the resection of sessile/flat adenomas greater than 2 cm in size in over 17% of cases in one study (180).

The quality of the screening endoscopy may be the best determinant of the overall effectiveness of precursor lesion detection and removal. Factors such as inadequate colon preparation (which compromises visibility) and inadequate time of withdrawal can affect the effectiveness of a given colonoscopy regarding cancer prevention (164–167). These data have led to the quality guidelines for the performance of colonoscopy and the reporting of results (81,181,182). Despite these guidelines, the endoscopists themselves remain perhaps the most significant variable in determining colonoscopic quality (134,167,183–185). A well-publicized study has shown that interval CRCs occur at much higher rates among cases performed by endoscopists who discover adenomas in less than 20% of individuals presenting for initial screening compared to their peers who discover adenomas in greater than 20% of their screening patients (186).

Surveillance Following Polyp and Precursor Lesion Identification and Removal

In the parlance of CRC prevention: Screening is the process of seeking to identify neoplasms for the first time in an individual, while surveillance is the process of seeking to identify missed or new neoplasms in an individual in whom they have been previously found. In most cases, following the identification of a precursor lesion, the interval to the next surveillance colonoscopy is determined by the exact nature of the neoplasms discovered during the preceding endoscopy (75,87).

Studies have shown that patients with no neoplasms found on initial colonoscopy have only a 1.3%–2.4% of finding advanced adenomas within 5 years versus the 4%–10% rate of advanced adenoma discovery at screening (187–192). Likewise, observational and case control studies have shown a decreased risk of CRC following colonoscopy for at least 10 years (172,174–176,190). A recent trial of one-time sigmoidoscopy revealed a decreased risk of CRC incidence and mortality in the distal colon 10 years after negative sigmoidoscopic screening (146). For this reason, colonoscopic screening has been set at a 10-year frequency (75,143).

Certain characteristics of identified neoplasms indicate an increased risk of finding advanced adenomas and CRC during surveillance. Adenoma number (greater than or equal to 3 vs 1–2 adenomas), size (greater than or equal to 1 cm vs less than 1 cm), histology (villous and tubulovillous vs tubular) and the presence of high-grade dysplasia all indicate a mild to moderately increased risk of advanced adenoma on surveillance (64,68,87,187,191–195). These findings are now classified as high-risk adenomas (HRA) and indicate a need for colonoscopic surveillance 3 years following colonoscopy as part of screening according to the Multi-Society Task Force (MSTF; see Table 4.4; 75). Conversely, the finding of 1 to 2 tubular adenomas, less than 1 cm in diameter, are now classified as low-risk adenomas (LRA; 75). The finding of such lesions has not been shown to substantially increase the risk of advanced adenomas or CRC above the standard population for 5 years following initial colonoscopy (64,68,87,187,191–195). For this reason, the period to the first surveillance colonoscopy is recommended to be 5 to 10 years in patients with

Table 4.4 Current U.S. Multi-Society Task Force on CRC Colonoscopic Screening and Surveillance Guidelines in Individuals with an Average Risk at Baseline

Baseline Colonoscopy: Most Advanced Finding(s)	Recommended Surveillance Interval (Years)
No polyps	10
Small (< 10 mm) hyperplastic polyps in rectum or sigmoid	10
1 to 2 small (< 10 mm) tubular adenomas	5 to 10
3 to 10 tubular adenomas	3
> 10 adenomas	< 3
One or more tubular adenomas ≥ 10 mm	3
One or more villous adenomas	3
Adenoma with HGD	5
Sessile serrated adenoma/polyp(s) < 10 mm with no dysplasia	3
Sessile serrated adenoma/polyp(s) ≥ 10 mm or sessile serrated adenoma/ polyp(s) with dysplasia	3
Traditional serrated adenoma	3
Serrated polyposis syndrome	3

The recommendations assume that the baseline colonoscopy was complete and adequate and that all visible polyps were completely removed.

Lieberman DA, et al. Guidelines for colonoscopy surveillance after screening and polypectomy: a consensus update by the US Multi-Society Task Force on CRC. *Gastroenterology*, 2012;143(3):844–857.

LRA findings, similar to the screening recommendation (75). Of special note, any known or likely incomplete adenoma resection should result in consideration of early endoscopic follow-up (2–6 months; 51,75).

The finding of more than 10 adenomas at baseline examination represents a small but important group that may have FAP (greater than 100 adenomas) or attenuated FAP (10–100 adenomas). Although FAP is usually inherited with an autosomal dominant pattern through mutations in the *APC* gene, some families are noted to exhibit an autosomal recessive pattern of inheritance. In these families, the polyposis phenotype has been determined to arise from mutations in the mutY homolog (*MUTYH*) gene (196). This syndrome has been termed *MUTYH* associated polyposis or MAP. FAP may also arise through de novo mutations in as many as 25% of patients (197). The National Comprehensive Cancer Network (NCCN) currently recommends genetic testing for *APC* and *MUTYH* mutation in persons with more than 10 adenomas identified at colonoscopy (51).

Hyperplastic polyps are not thought to be CRC precursor lesions and in general do not alter the screening frequency (75). As stated previously, SSA/Ps greater than 1 cm are felt to be the precursor lesion for the 20%–30% of CRCs that arise through the CIMP pathway. Recent studies have shown that serrated polyps greater than 1 cm in size or located proximal to the sigmoid colon are markers for synchronous advanced adenomas and CRC at screening colonoscopy and metachronous advanced neoplasms during surveillance (140,198). One study also showed that small proximal serrated polyps unto themselves only predicted a risk of adenomas during surveillance similar to adenoma findings grouped as LRAs by the MSTF (198). For this reason the MSTF recommendations for SSA/Ps greater than 1 cm in diameter or containing dysplasia are the same as for HRAs. Conversely, the recommendation for SSA/Ps less than 1 cm in diameter and without dysplasia is the same as for LRAs (see Table 4.4; 75). TSAs in the absence of any real significant data on their association with advanced colonic neoplasms on surveillance are treated as HRAs also (75).

As stated earlier, a presumed genetic syndrome labeled the SPS has been described that is characterized by the finding of multiple serrated polyps at endoscopy. It is defined by the WHO in a person meeting any of the following criteria: (a) greater than 5 serrated polyps proximal to the sigmoid colon with 2 or more greater than or equal to 1 cm in diameter; (b) any serrated polyps proximal to the sigmoid colon with a first-degree family member with SPS; or (c) greater than 20 serrated polyps of any size anywhere in the colon. The risk of CRC in SPS is uncertain but the early age of onset and commonly reported family history of colorectal polyps and cancer suggests some unidentified inherited mutation. One study reported a 7% risk of CRC after 5 years of surveillance (199). The MSTF recommendation for screening in SPS is annual colonoscopy following diagnosis (75).

Recent cohort studies have indicated that although the finding of an HRA or an equivalent serrated polyp is an important predictor of advanced adenomas for the next subsequent colonoscopy, this risk does not necessarily carry over to all future colonoscopies. The findings of the surveillance colonoscopy itself best predict the risk of advanced adenomas on the next surveillance colonoscopy (200–202). Thus LRAs and their serrated polyp equivalents should be surveyed again in 5 years and HRAs and their serrated polyp equivalents in 3 years (see Table 4.5). The findings of no adenomas following a baseline LRA were found to have a very low risk of

Table 4.5 Current U.S. Multi-Society Task Force on CRC Colonoscopic Surveillance Guidelines Following First Surveillance Colonoscopy

Baseline Colonoscopy Finding	First Surveillance Colonoscopy Finding	Interval to Second Surveillance Colonoscopy (Years)
LRA (low-risk adenoma)	HRA	3
	LRA	5
	No adenoma	10
HRA (high-risk adenoma)	HRA	3
	LRA	5
	No adenoma	5

Lieberman DA, et al. Guidelines for colonoscopy surveillance after screening and polypectomy: a consensus update by the US Multi-Society Task Force on CRC. *Gastroenterology*, 2012;143(3):844–857.

subsequent advanced adenomas and are now recommended for follow-up in 10 years by the MTSF (75).

CRC is both a common cancer in developed nations and a common cause of death. Despite this fact, the well-characterized precursor lesions and their ease of identification with colonoscopy and imaging make CRC a prime target for secondary cancer prevention. The decrease in CRC incidence and prevalence over the past 30 years is one of the medical community's few success stories in the endeavor of cancer prevention. Nonetheless, secondary prevention can be optimized and improved through the careful, high-quality use of current screening/surveillance modalities and the development of improved noninvasive screening modalities. Hopefully, in the near future, CRC will become a rare and uncommon source of morbidity and mortality.

REFERENCES

1. Siegel R, Naishadham D, Jemal A. Cancer statistics, 2012. *CA Cancer J Clin.* 2012;62(1):10–29.
2. Fearon ER, Vogelstein B. A genetic model for colorectal tumorigenesis. *Cell.* 1990;61(5):759–767.
3. Lamlum H, Ilyas M, Rowan A, et al. The type of somatic mutation at APC in familial adenomatous polyposis is determined by the site of the germline mutation: a new facet to Knudson's 'two-hit' hypothesis. *Nat Med.* 1999; 5(9):1071–1075.
4. Lamlum H, Papadopoulou A, Ilyas M, et al. APC mutations are sufficient for the growth of early colorectal adenomas. *Proc Natl Acad Sci USA.* 2000;97(5):2225–2228.
5. Lynch HT, Smyrk T, McGinn T, et al. Attenuated familial adenomatous polyposis (AFAP). A phenotypically and genotypically distinctive variant of FAP. *Cancer.* 1995;76(12):2427–2433.
6. Spirio L, Olschwang S, Groden J, et al. Alleles of the APC gene: an attenuated form of familial polyposis. *Cell.* 1993;75(5):951–957.
7. Brensinger JD, Laken SJ, Luce MC, et al. Variable phenotype of familial adenomatous polyposis in pedigrees with 3' mutation in the APC gene. *Gut.* 1998;43(4):548–552.
8. Burt RW, Leppert MF, Slattery ML, et al. Genetic testing and phenotype in a large kindred with attenuated familial adenomatous polyposis. *Gastroenterology.* 2004;127(2):444–451.
9. Sieber OM, Segditsas S, Knudsen AL, et al. Disease severity and genetic pathways in attenuated familial adenomatous polyposis vary greatly but depend on the site of the germline mutation. *Gut.* 2006;55(10):1440–1448.
10. Rowan AJ, Lamlum H, Ilyas M, et al. APC mutations in sporadic colorectal tumors: A mutational "hotspot" and interdependence of the "two hits". *Proc Natl Acad Sci USA.* 2000;97(7):3352–3357.
11. Bienz M, Clevers H. Linking colorectal cancer to Wnt signaling. *Cell.* 2000;103(2):311–320.
12. Fearnhead NS, Britton MP, Bodmer WF. The ABC of APC. *Hum Mol Genet.* 2001;10(7):721–733.
13. Uthoff SM, Eichenberger MR, McAuliffe TL, Hamilton CJ, Galandiuk S. Wingless-type frizzled protein receptor signaling and its putative role in human colon cancer. *Mol Carcinog.* 2001;31(1):56–62.
14. Goss KH, Groden J. Biology of the adenomatous polyposis coli tumor suppressor. *J Clin Oncol.* 2000;18(9):1967–1979.
15. Morin PJ, Sparks AB, Korinek V, et al. Activation of beta-catenin-Tcf signaling in colon cancer by mutations in beta-catenin or APC. *Science.* 1997;275(5307):1787–1790.
16. Korinek V, Barker N, Morin PJ, et al. Constitutive transcriptional activation by a beta-catenin-Tcf complex in APC-/- colon carcinoma. *Science.* 1997;275(5307):1784–1787.
17. Kim PJ, Plescia J, Clevers H, Fearon ER, Altieri DC. Survivin and molecular pathogenesis of colorectal cancer. *Lancet.* 2003;362(9379):205–209.
18. Shih IM, Wang TL, Traverso G, et al. Top-down morphogenesis of colorectal tumors. *Proc Natl Acad Sci USA.* 2001;98(5):2640–2645.
19. van de Wetering M, Sancho E, Verweij C, et al. The beta-catenin/TCF-4 complex imposes a crypt progenitor phenotype on colorectal cancer cells. *Cell*, 2002;111(2):241–250.
20. Spirio LN, Samowitz W, Robertson J, et al. Alleles of APC modulate the frequency and classes of mutations that lead to colon polyps. *Nat Genet.* 1998;20(4):385–388.
21. Takayama T, Ohi M, Hayashi T, et al. Analysis of K-ras, APC, and beta-catenin in aberrant crypt foci in sporadic adenoma, cancer, and familial adenomatous polyposis. *Gastroenterology.* 2001;121(3):599–611.
22. Tortola S, Marcuello E, González I, et al. p53 and K-ras gene mutations correlate with tumor aggressiveness but are not of routine prognostic value in colorectal cancer. *J Clin Oncol.* 1999;17(5):1375–1381.
23. Shibata D, Schaeffer J, Li ZH, Capella G, Perucho M. Genetic heterogeneity of the c-K-ras locus in colorectal adenomas but not in adenocarcinomas. *J Natl Cancer Inst.* 1993;85(13):1058–1063.
24. Bourne HR, Sanders DA, McCormick F. The GTPase superfamily: conserved structure and molecular mechanism. *Nature.* 1991;349(6305):117–127.
25. Vogelstein B, Fearon ER, Hamilton SR, et al. Genetic alterations during colorectal-tumor development. *N Engl J Med.* 1988; 319(9):525–532.

26. Chung DC, Rustgi AK. DNA mismatch repair and cancer. *Gastroenterology.* 1995;109(5):1685–1699.
27. Papadopoulos N, Nicolaides NC, Liu B, et al. Mutations of GTBP in genetically unstable cells. *Science.* 1995;268(5219):1915–1917.
28. Papadopoulos N, Nicolaides NC, Wei YF, et al. Mutation of a mutL homolog in hereditary colon cancer. *Science.* 1994;263(5153):1625–1629.
29. Boland CR, Thibodeau SN, Hamilton SR, et al. A National Cancer Institute Workshop on Microsatellite Instability for cancer detection and familial predisposition: development of international criteria for the determination of microsatellite instability in colorectal cancer. *Cancer Res.* 1998;58(22):5248–5257.
30. Hatch SB, Lightfoot HM Jr, Garwacki CP, et al. Microsatellite instability testing in colorectal carcinoma: choice of markers affects sensitivity of detection of mismatch repair-deficient tumors. *Clin Cancer Res.* 2005;11(6):2180–2187.
31. Ionov Y, Peinado MA, Malkhosyan S, Shibata D, Perucho M. Ubiquitous somatic mutations in simple repeated sequences reveal a new mechanism for colonic carcinogenesis. *Nature.* 1993;363(6429):558–561.
32. Fujiwara T, Stolker JM, Watanabe T, et al. Accumulated clonal genetic alterations in familial and sporadic colorectal carcinomas with widespread instability in microsatellite sequences. *Am J Pathol.* 1998;153(4):1063–1078.
33. de la Chapelle A, Hampel H. Clinical relevance of microsatellite instability in colorectal cancer. *J Clin Oncol.* 2010;28(20): 3380–3387.
34. Mueller J, Gazzoli I, Bandipalliam P, Garber JE, Syngal S, Kolodner RD. Comprehensive molecular analysis of mismatch repair gene defects in suspected Lynch syndrome (hereditary nonpolyposis colorectal cancer) cases. *Cancer Res.* 2009;69(17): 7053–7061.
35. Koessler T, Oestergaard MZ, Song H, et al. Common variants in mismatch repair genes and risk of colorectal cancer. *Gut.* 2008;57(8):1097–1101.
36. Quehenberger F, Vasen HF, van Houwelingen HC. Risk of colorectal and endometrial cancer for carriers of mutations of the hMLH1 and hMSH2 gene: correction for ascertainment. *J Med Genet.* 2005;42(6):491–496.
37. Vasen HF, Möslein G, Alonso A, et al. Guidelines for the clinical management of Lynch syndrome (hereditary non-polyposis cancer). *J Med Genet.* 2007;44(6):353–362.
38. Shibata D, Peinado MA, Ionov Y, Malkhosyan S, Perucho M. Genomic instability in repeated sequences is an early somatic event in colorectal tumorigenesis that persists after transformation. *Nat Genet.* 1994;6(3):273–281.
39. Syngal S, Weeks JC, Schrag D, Garber JE, Kuntz KM. Benefits of colonoscopic surveillance and prophylactic colectomy in patients with hereditary nonpolyposis colorectal cancer mutations. *Ann Intern Med.* 1998;129(10):787–796.
40. Weisenberger DJ, Siegmund KD, Campan M, et al. CpG island methylator phenotype underlies sporadic microsatellite instability and is tightly associated with BRAF mutation in colorectal cancer. *Nat Genet.* 2006;38(7):787–793.
41. Das PM, Singal R. DNA methylation and cancer. *J Clin Oncol.* 2004;22(22):4632–4642.
42. van Engeland M, Derks S, Smits KM, Meijer GA, Herman JG. Colorectal cancer epigenetics: complex simplicity. *J Clin Oncol.* 2011;29(10):1382–1391.
43. Baylin SB, Esteller M, Rountree MR, Bachman KE, Schuebel K, Herman JG. Aberrant patterns of DNA methylation, chromatin formation and gene expression in cancer. *Hum Mol Genet.* 2001;10(7):687–692.
44. Baylin S. DNA methylation and epigenetic mechanisms of carcinogenesis. *Dev Biol (Basel).* 2001;106:85–7; discussion 143.
45. Herman JG, Baylin SB. Gene silencing in cancer in association with promoter hypermethylation. *N Engl J Med.* 2003;349(21): 2042–2054.
46. Rajagopalan H, Bardelli A, Lengauer C, Kinzler KW, Vogelstein B, Velculescu VE. Tumorigenesis: RAF/RAS oncogenes and mismatch-repair status. *Nature.* 2002;418(6901):934.
47. Domingo E, Niessen RC, Oliveira C, et al. BRAF-V600E is not involved in the colorectal tumorigenesis of HNPCC in patients with functional MLH1 and MSH2 genes. *Oncogene.* 2005;24(24):3995–3998.
48. Chan TL, Zhao W, Leung SY, Yuen ST; Cancer Genome Project. BRAF and K-ras mutations in colorectal hyperplastic polyps and serrated adenomas. *Cancer Res.* 2003;63(16):4878–4881.
49. Noffsinger AE. Serrated polyps and colorectal cancer: new pathway to malignancy. *Annu Rev Pathol.* 2009;4:343–364.
50. Spring KJ, Zhao ZZ, Karamatic R, et al. High prevalence of sessile serrated adenomas with BRAF mutations: a prospective study of patients undergoing colonoscopy. *Gastroenterology.* 2006;131(5):1400–1407.
51. Burt RW, Barthel JS, Dunn KB, et al.; NCCN. NCCN clinical practice guidelines in oncology. Colorectal cancer screening. *J Natl Compr Canc Netw.* 2010;8(1):8–61.
52. Imperiale TF, Wagner DR, Lin CY, Larkin GN, Rogge JD, Ransohoff DF. Risk of advanced proximal neoplasms in asymptomatic adults according to the distal colorectal findings. *N Engl J Med.* 2000;343(3):169–174.
53. Lieberman DA, Weiss DG, Bond JH, Ahnen DJ, Garewal H, Chejfec G. Use of colonoscopy to screen asymptomatic adults for colorectal cancer. Veterans Affairs Cooperative Study Group 380. *N Engl J Med.* 2000;343(3):162–168.
54. Mandel JS, Bond JH, Church TR, et al. Reducing mortality from colorectal cancer by screening for fecal occult blood. Minnesota Colon Cancer Control Study. *N Engl J Med.* 1993;328(19):1365–1371.
55. Schoenfeld P, Cash B, Flood A, et al.; CONCeRN Study Investigators. Colonoscopic screening of average-risk women for colorectal neoplasia. *N Engl J Med.* 2005;352(20):2061–2068.
56. Atkin WS, Morson BC, Cuzick J. Long-term risk of colorectal cancer after excision of rectosigmoid adenomas. *N Engl J Med.* 1992;326(10):658–662.
57. Bertario L, Russo A, Sala P, et al. Predictors of metachronous colorectal neoplasms in sporadic adenoma patients. *Int J Cancer.* 2003;105(1):82–87.
58. Citarda F, Tomaselli G, Capocaccia R, Barcherini S, Crespi M; Italian Multicentre Study Group. Efficacy in standard clinical practice of colonoscopic polypectomy in reducing colorectal cancer incidence. *Gut.* 2001;48(6):812–815.
59. Newcomb PA, Norfleet RG, Storer BE, Surawicz TS, Marcus PM. Screening sigmoidoscopy and colorectal cancer mortality. *J Natl Cancer Inst.* 1992;84(20):1572–1575.
60. Newcomb PA, Storer BE, Morimoto LM, Templeton A, Potter JD. Long-term efficacy of sigmoidoscopy in the reduction of colorectal cancer incidence. *J Natl Cancer Inst.* 2003;95(8):622–625.
61. Selby JV, Friedman GD, Quesenberry CP Jr, Weiss NS. A case-control study of screening sigmoidoscopy and mortality from colorectal cancer. *N Engl J Med.* 1992;326(10):653–657.
62. Thiis-Evensen E, Hoff GS, Sauar J, Langmark F, Majak BM, Vatn MH. Population-based surveillance by colonoscopy: effect on the incidence of colorectal cancer. Telemark Polyp Study I. *Scand J Gastroenterol.* 1999;34(4):414–420.
63. Winawer SJ, Zauber AG, Ho MN, et al. Prevention of colorectal cancer by colonoscopic polypectomy. The National Polyp Study Workgroup. *N Engl J Med.* 1993;329(27):1977–1981.
64. Cottet V, Jooste V, Fournel I, Bouvier AM, Faivre J, Bonithon-Kopp C. Long-term risk of colorectal cancer after adenoma removal: a population-based cohort study. *Gut.* 2012;61(8):1180–1186.
65. Loeve F, van Ballegooijen M, Boer R, Kuipers EJ, Habbema JD. Colorectal cancer risk in adenoma patients: a nation-wide study. *Int J Cancer.* 2004;111(1):147–151.
66. Jonkers D, Ernst J, Pladdet I, Stockbrügger R, Hameeteman W. Endoscopic follow-up of 383 patients with colorectal adenoma:

an observational study in daily practice. *Eur J Cancer Prev.* 2006;15(3):202–210.
67. Lund JN, Scholefield JH, Grainge MJ, et al. Risks, costs, and compliance limit colorectal adenoma surveillance: lessons from a randomised trial. *Gut.* 2001;49(1):91–96.
68. Martínez ME, Baron JA, Lieberman DA, et al. A pooled analysis of advanced colorectal neoplasia diagnoses after colonoscopic polypectomy. *Gastroenterology.* 2009;136(3):832–841.
69. Williams AR, Balasooriya BA, Day DW. Polyps and cancer of the large bowel: a necropsy study in Liverpool. *Gut.* 1982;23(10):835–842.
70. Heitman SJ, Ronksley PE, Hilsden RJ, Manns BJ, Rostom A, Hemmelgarn BR. Prevalence of adenomas and colorectal cancer in average risk individuals: a systematic review and meta-analysis. *Clin Gastroenterol Hepatol.* 2009;7(12):1272–1278.
71. Pendergrass CJ, Edelstein DL, Hylind LM, et al. Occurrence of colorectal adenomas in younger adults: an epidemiologic necropsy study. *Clin Gastroenterol Hepatol.* 2008;6(9):1011–1015.
72. Rex DK, Lehman GA, Hawes RH, Ulbright TM, Smith JJ. Screening colonoscopy in asymptomatic average-risk persons with negative fecal occult blood tests. *Gastroenterology.* 1991;100(1):64–67.
73. Rex DK, Lehman GA, Ulbright TM, et al. Colonic neoplasia in asymptomatic persons with negative fecal occult blood tests: influence of age, gender, and family history. *Am J Gastroenterol.* 1993;88(6):825–831.
74. Rex DK. Colonoscopy: a review of its yield for cancers and adenomas by indication. *Am J Gastroenterol.* 1995;90(3):353–365.
75. Lieberman DA, Rex DK, Winawer SJ, Giardiello FM, Johnson DA, Levin TR; United States Multi-Society Task Force on Colorectal Cancer. Guidelines for colonoscopy surveillance after screening and polypectomy: a consensus update by the US Multi-Society Task Force on Colorectal Cancer. *Gastroenterology.* 2012;143(3):844–857.
76. Rex DK, Helbig CC. High yields of small and flat adenomas with high-definition colonoscopes using either white light or narrow band imaging. *Gastroenterology.* 2007;133(1):42–47.
77. Kahi CJ, Anderson JC, Waxman I, et al. High-definition chromocolonoscopy vs. high-definition white light colonoscopy for average-risk colorectal cancer screening. *Am J Gastroenterol.* 2010;105(6):1301–1307.
78. Johnson CD, Chen MH, Toledano AY, et al. Accuracy of CT colonography for detection of large adenomas and cancers. *N Engl J Med.* 2008;359(12):1207–1217.
79. Patel K, Hoffman NE. The anatomical distribution of colorectal polyps at colonoscopy. *J Clin Gastroenterol.* 2001;33(3): 222–225.
80. Nguyen SP, Bent S, Chen YH, Terdiman JP. Gender as a risk factor for advanced neoplasia and colorectal cancer: a systematic review and meta-analysis. *Clin Gastroenterol Hepatol.* 2009;7(6):676–81.e1.
81. Rex DK, Petrini JL, Baron TH, et al.; ASGE/ACG Taskforce on Quality in Endoscopy. Quality indicators for colonoscopy. *Am J Gastroenterol.* 2006;101(4):873–885.
82. Lieberman DA, Holub JL, Moravec MD, Eisen GM, Peters D, Morris CD. Prevalence of colon polyps detected by colonoscopy screening in asymptomatic black and white patients. *JAMA.* 2008;300(12):1417–1422.
83. Ozick LA, Jacob L, Donelson SS, Agarwal SK, Freeman HP. Distribution of adenomatous polyps in African-Americans. *Am J Gastroenterol.* 1995;90(5):758–760.
84. O'Brien MJ, Winawer SJ, Zauber AG, et al. The National Polyp Study. Patient and polyp characteristics associated with high-grade dysplasia in colorectal adenomas. *Gastroenterology.* 1990;98(2):371–379.
85. Stryker SJ, Wolff BG, Culp CE, Libbe SD, Ilstrup DM, MacCarty RL. Natural history of untreated colonic polyps. *Gastroenterology.* 1987;93(5):1009–1013.
86. Ness RM, Holmes AM, Klein R, Dittus R. Cost-utility of one-time colonoscopic screening for colorectal cancer at various ages. *Am J Gastroenterol.* 2000;95(7):1800–1811.
87. Winawer SJ, Zauber AG, Fletcher RH, et al.; US Multi-Society Task Force on Colorectal Cancer; American Cancer Society. Guidelines for colonoscopy surveillance after polypectomy: a consensus update by the US Multi-Society Task Force on Colorectal Cancer and the American Cancer Society. *Gastroenterology.* 2006;130(6):1872–1885.
88. Correa P, Strong JP, Reif A, Johnson WD. The epidemiology of colorectal polyps: prevalence in New Orleans and international comparisons. *Cancer.* 1977;39(5):2258–2264.
89. Eide TJ, Stalsberg H. Polyps of the large intestine in Northern Norway. *Cancer.* 1978;42(6):2839–2848.
90. Vatn MH, Stalsberg H. The prevalence of polyps of the large intestine in Oslo: an autopsy study. *Cancer.* 1982;49(4):819–825.
91. Stemmermann GN, Yatani R. Diverticulosis and polyps of the large intestine. A necropsy study of Hawaii Japanese. *Cancer.* 1973;31(5):1260–1270.
92. Clark JC, Collan Y, Eide TJ, et al. Prevalence of polyps in an autopsy series from areas with varying incidence of large-bowel cancer. *Int J Cancer.* 1985;36(2):179–186.
93. Johannsen LG, Momsen O, Jacobsen NO. Polyps of the large intestine in Aarhus, Denmark. An autopsy study. *Scand J Gastroenterol.* 1989;24(7):799–806.
94. Jass JR, Young PJ, Robinson EM. Predictors of presence, multiplicity, size and dysplasia of colorectal adenomas. A necropsy study in New Zealand. *Gut.* 1992;33(11):1508–1514.
95. Provenzale D, Garrett JW, Condon SE, Sandler RS. Risk for colon adenomas in patients with rectosigmoid hyperplastic polyps. *Ann Intern Med.* 1990;113(10):760–763.
96. DiSario JA, Foutch PG, Mai HD, Pardy K, Manne RK. Prevalence and malignant potential of colorectal polyps in asymptomatic, average-risk men. *Am J Gastroenterol.* 1991;86(8):941–945.
97. Bariol C, Hawkins NJ, Turner JJ, Meagher AP, Williams DB, Ward RL. Histopathological and clinical evaluation of serrated adenomas of the colon and rectum. *Mod Pathol.* 2003;16(5):417–423.
98. Lieberman DA, Prindiville S, Weiss DG, Willett W; VA Cooperative Study Group 380. Risk factors for advanced colonic neoplasia and hyperplastic polyps in asymptomatic individuals. *JAMA.* 2003;290(22):2959–2967.
99. Hassan C, Pickhardt PJ, Marmo R, Choi JR. Impact of lifestyle factors on colorectal polyp detection in the screening setting. *Dis Colon Rectum.* 2010;53(9):1328–1333.
100. Rex DK. Does the use of sedation, or the level of sedation, affect detection during colonoscopy? *Am J Gastroenterol.* 2012;107(12):1849–1851.
101. Cooper HS, Patchefsky AS, Marks G. Adenomatous and carcinomatous changes within hyperplastic colonic epithelium. *Dis Colon Rectum.* 1979;22(3):152–156.
102. Sumner HW, Wasserman NF, McClain CJ. Giant hyperplastic polyposis of the colon. *Dig Dis Sci.* 1981;26(1):85–89.
103. Urbanski SJ, Kossakowska AE, Marcon N, Bruce WR. Mixed hyperplastic adenomatous polyps–an underdiagnosed entity. Report of a case of adenocarcinoma arising within a mixed hyperplastic adenomatous polyp. *Am J Surg Pathol.* 1984;8(7): 551–556.
104. Jass JR. Metaplastic polyps and polyposis of the colorectum. *Histopathology.* 1980;4(5):579.
105. Jass JR. Relation between metaplastic polyp and carcinoma of the colorectum. *Lancet.* 1983;1(8314–5):28–30.
106. Fenoglio-Preiser CM. Hyperplastic polyps, adenomatous polyps, and mixed hyperplastic adenomatous polyps of the colon: definitions. *Prog Clin Biol Res.* 1988;279:3–12.
107. Longacre TA, Fenoglio-Preiser CM. Mixed hyperplastic adenomatous polyps/serrated adenomas. A distinct form of colorectal neoplasia. *Am J Surg Pathol.* 1990;14(6):524–537.

108. Torlakovic E, Snover DC. Serrated adenomatous polyposis in humans. *Gastroenterology.* 1996;110(3):748–755.
109. Torlakovic E, Skovlund E, Snover DC, Torlakovic G, Nesland JM. Morphologic reappraisal of serrated colorectal polyps. *Am J Surg Pathol.* 2003;27(1):65–81.
110. Higuchi T, Sugihara K, Jass JR. Demographic and pathological characteristics of serrated polyps of colorectum. *Histopathology.* 2005;47(1):32–40.
111. Carr NJ, Mahajan H, Tan KL, Hawkins NJ, Ward RL. Serrated and non-serrated polyps of the colorectum: their prevalence in an unselected case series and correlation of BRAF mutation analysis with the diagnosis of sessile serrated adenoma. *J Clin Pathol.* 2009;62(6):516–518.
112. Lu FI, van Niekerk de W, Owen D, Tha SP, Turbin DA, Webber DL. Longitudinal outcome study of sessile serrated adenomas of the colorectum: an increased risk for subsequent right-sided colorectal carcinoma. *Am J Surg Pathol.* 2010;34(7):927–934.
113. Pai RK, Hart J, Noffsinger AE. Sessile serrated adenomas strongly predispose to synchronous serrated polyps in non-syndromic patients. *Histopathology.* 2010;56(5):581–588.
114. Omata F, Brown WR, Tokuda Y, et al. Modifiable risk factors for colorectal neoplasms and hyperplastic polyps. *Intern Med.* 2009;48(3):123–128.
115. Hoffmeister M, Schmitz S, Karmrodt E, et al. Male sex and smoking have a larger impact on the prevalence of colorectal neoplasia than family history of colorectal cancer. *Clin Gastroenterol Hepatol.* 2010;8(10):870–876.
116. Bensen SP, Cole BF, Mott LA, Baron JA, Sandler RS, Haile R. Colorectal hyperplastic polyps and risk of recurrence of adenomas and hyperplastic polyps. Polyps Prevention Study. *Lancet.* 1999;354(9193):1873–1874.
117. Laiyemo AO, Murphy G, Sansbury LB, et al. Hyperplastic polyps and the risk of adenoma recurrence in the polyp prevention trial. *Clin Gastroenterol Hepatol.* 2009;7(2):192–197.
118. Lin OS, Gerson LB, Soon MS, Schembre DB, Kozarek RA. Risk of proximal colon neoplasia with distal hyperplastic polyps: a meta-analysis. *Arch Intern Med.* 2005;165(4):382–390.
119. Rex DK, Smith JJ, Ulbright TM, Lehman GA. Distal colonic hyperplastic polyps do not predict proximal adenomas in asymptomatic average-risk subjects. *Gastroenterology.* 1992;102(1):317–319.
120. Dave S, Hui S, Kroenke K, Imperiale TF. Is the distal hyperplastic polyp a marker for proximal neoplasia? *J Gen Intern Med.* 2003;18(2):128–137.
121. East JE, Saunders BP, Jass JR. Sporadic and syndromic hyperplastic polyps and serrated adenomas of the colon: classification, molecular genetics, natural history, and clinical management. *Gastroenterol Clin North Am.* 2008;37(1):25–46, v.
122. Torlakovic EE, Gomez JD, Driman DK, et al. Sessile serrated adenoma (SSA) vs. traditional serrated adenoma (TSA). *Am J Surg Pathol.* 2008;32(1):21–29.
123. Goldstein NS, Bhanot P, Odish E, Hunter S. Hyperplastic-like colon polyps that preceded microsatellite-unstable adenocarcinomas. *Am J Clin Pathol.* 2003;119(6):778–796.
124. Jass JR, Iino H, Ruszkiewicz A, et al. Neoplastic progression occurs through mutator pathways in hyperplastic polyposis of the colorectum. *Gut.* 2000;47(1):43–49.
125. Park SJ, Rashid A, Lee JH, Kim SG, Hamilton SR, Wu TT. Frequent CpG island methylation in serrated adenomas of the colorectum. *Am J Pathol.* 2003;162(3):815–822.
126. Velho S, Moutinho C, Cirnes L, et al. BRAF, K-ras and PIK3CA mutations in colorectal serrated polyps and cancer: primary or secondary genetic events in colorectal carcinogenesis? *BMC Cancer.* 2008;8:255.
127. O'Brien MJ, Yang S, Mack C, et al. Comparison of microsatellite instability, CpG island methylation phenotype, BRAF and K-ras status in serrated polyps and traditional adenomas indicates separate pathways to distinct colorectal carcinoma end points. *Am J Surg Pathol.* 2006;30(12):1491–1501.
128. Sheridan TB, Fenton H, Lewin MR, et al. Sessile serrated adenomas with low- and high-grade dysplasia and early carcinomas: an immunohistochemical study of serrated lesions "caught in the act". *Am J Clin Pathol.* 2006;126(4):564–571.
129. Leggett B, Whitehall V. Role of the serrated pathway in colorectal cancer pathogenesis. *Gastroenterology.* 2010;138(6):2088–2100.
130. Ngo NT, Tan E, Tekkis P, Peston D, Cohen P. Differential expression of p53 and p504s in hyperplastic polyp, sessile serrated adenoma and traditional serrated adenoma. *Int J Colorectal Dis.* 2010;25(10):1193–1200.
131. Whitehall VL, Walsh MD, Young J, Leggett BA, Jass JR. Methylation of O-6-methylguanine DNA methyltransferase characterizes a subset of colorectal cancer with low-level DNA microsatellite instability. *Cancer Res.* 2001;61(3):827–830.
132. Gurudu SR, Heigh RI, De Petris G, et al. Sessile serrated adenomas: demographic, endoscopic and pathological characteristics. *World J Gastroenterol.* 2010;16(27):3402–3405.
133. Lash RH, Genta RM, Schuler CM. Sessile serrated adenomas: prevalence of dysplasia and carcinoma in 2139 patients. *J Clin Pathol.* 2010;63(8):681–686.
134. Hetzel JT, Huang CS, Coukos JA, et al. Variation in the detection of serrated polyps in an average risk colorectal cancer screening cohort. *Am J Gastroenterol.* 2010;105(12):2656–2664.
135. Tanaka M, Kusumi T, Sasaki Y, et al. Colonic intra-epithelial carcinoma occurring in a hyperplastic polyp via a serrated adenoma. *Pathol Int.* 2001;51(3):215–220.
136. Yamauchi T, Watanabe M, Hasegawa H, et al. Serrated adenoma developing into advanced colon cancer in 2 years. *J Gastroenterol.* 2002;37(6):467–470.
137. Oono Y, Fu K, Nakamura H, et al. Progression of a sessile serrated adenoma to an early invasive cancer within 8 months. *Dig Dis Sci.* 2009;54(4):906–909.
138. García-Solano J, Pérez-Guillermo M, Conesa-Zamora P, et al. Clinicopathologic study of 85 colorectal serrated adenocarcinomas: further insights into the full recognition of a new subset of colorectal carcinoma. *Hum Pathol.* 2010;41(10):1359–1368.
139. Messick CA, Church J, Casey G, Kalady MF. Identification of the methylator (serrated) colorectal cancer phenotype through precursor serrated polyps. *Dis Colon Rectum.* 2009;52(9):1535–1541.
140. Hiraoka S, Kato J, Fujiki S, et al. The presence of large serrated polyps increases risk for colorectal cancer. *Gastroenterology.* 2010;139(5):1503–10, 1510.e1.
141. Hawkins NJ, Ward RL. Sporadic colorectal cancers with microsatellite instability and their possible origin in hyperplastic polyps and serrated adenomas. *J Natl Cancer Inst.* 2001;93(17):1307–1313.
142. Eddy D. ACS report on the cancer-related health checkup. *CA Cancer J Clin.* 1980;30(4):193–240.
143. Levin B, Lieberman DA, McFarland B, et al.; American Cancer Society Colorectal Cancer Advisory Group; US Multi-Society Task Force; American College of Radiology Colon Cancer Committee. Screening and surveillance for the early detection of colorectal cancer and adenomatous polyps, 2008: a joint guideline from the American Cancer Society, the US Multi-Society Task Force on Colorectal Cancer, and the American College of Radiology. *Gastroenterology.* 2008;134(5):1570–1595.
144. Hardcastle JD, Chamberlain JO, Robinson MH, et al. Randomised controlled trial of faecal-occult-blood screening for colorectal cancer. *Lancet.* 1996;348(9040):1472–1477.
145. Kronborg O, Fenger C, Olsen J, Jørgensen OD, Søndergaard O. Randomised study of screening for colorectal cancer with faecal-occult-blood test. *Lancet.* 1996;348(9040):1467–1471.
146. Atkin WS, Edwards R, Kralj-Hans I, et al.; UK Flexible Sigmoidoscopy Trial Investigators. Once-only flexible sigmoidoscopy screening in prevention of colorectal cancer: a multicentre randomised controlled trial. *Lancet.* 2010;375(9726):1624–1633.

147. Mandel JS, Church TR, Bond JH, et al. The effect of fecal occult-blood screening on the incidence of colorectal cancer. *N Engl J Med.* 2000;343(22):1603–1607.
148. Lieberman DA, Weiss DG; Veterans Affairs Cooperative Study Group 380. One-time screening for colorectal cancer with combined fecal occult-blood testing and examination of the distal colon. *N Engl J Med.* 2001;345(8):555–560.
149. Imperiale TF, Ransohoff DF, Itzkowitz SH, Turnbull BA, Ross ME; Colorectal Cancer Study Group. Fecal DNA versus fecal occult blood for colorectal-cancer screening in an average-risk population. *N Engl J Med.* 2004;351(26):2704–2714.
150. Allison JE, Tekawa IS, Ransom LJ, Adrain AL. A comparison of fecal occult-blood tests for colorectal-cancer screening. *N Engl J Med.* 1996;334(3):155–159.
151. Allison JE, Sakoda LC, Levin TR, et al. Screening for colorectal neoplasms with new fecal occult blood tests: update on performance characteristics. *J Natl Cancer Inst.* 2007;99(19):1462–1470.
152. Rex DK, Cutler CS, Lemmel GT, et al. Colonoscopic miss rates of adenomas determined by back-to-back colonoscopies. *Gastroenterology.* 1997;112(1):24–28.
153. Bressler B, Paszat LF, Vinden C, Li C, He J, Rabeneck L. Colonoscopic miss rates for right-sided colon cancer: a population-based analysis. *Gastroenterology.* 2004;127(2):452–456.
154. Pickhardt PJ, Choi JR, Hwang I, et al. Computed tomographic virtual colonoscopy to screen for colorectal neoplasia in asymptomatic adults. *N Engl J Med.* 2003;349(23):2191–2200.
155. Pickhardt PJ, Nugent PA, Mysliwiec PA, Choi JR, Schindler WR. Location of adenomas missed by optical colonoscopy. *Ann Intern Med.* 2004;141(5):352–359.
156. Cotton PB, Durkalski VL, Pineau BC, et al. Computed tomographic colonography (virtual colonoscopy): a multicenter comparison with standard colonoscopy for detection of colorectal neoplasia. *JAMA.* 2004;291(14):1713–1719.
157. Van Gelder RE, Nio CY, Florie J, et al. Computed tomographic colonography compared with colonoscopy in patients at increased risk for colorectal cancer. *Gastroenterology.* 2004;127(1):41–48.
158. Rockey DC, Paulson E, Niedzwiecki D, et al. Analysis of air contrast barium enema, computed tomographic colonography, and colonoscopy: prospective comparison. *Lancet.* 2005;365(9456):305–311.
159. Winawer S, Fletcher R, Rex D, et al.; Gastrointestinal Consortium Panel. Colorectal cancer screening and surveillance: clinical guidelines and rationale-Update based on new evidence. *Gastroenterology.* 2003;124(2):544–560.
160. Fuchs CS, Giovannucci EL, Colditz GA, Hunter DJ, Speizer FE, Willett WC. A prospective study of family history and the risk of colorectal cancer. *N Engl J Med.* 1994;331(25):1669–1674.
161. Winawer SJ, Zauber AG, Gerdes H, et al. Risk of colorectal cancer in the families of patients with adenomatous polyps. National Polyp Study Workgroup. *N Engl J Med.* 1996;334(2): 82–87.
162. Levin TR, Palitz A, Grossman S, et al. Predicting advanced proximal colonic neoplasia with screening sigmoidoscopy. *JAMA.* 1999;281(17):1611–1617.
163. Endoscopic Classification Review Group. Update on the paris classification of superficial neoplastic lesions in the digestive tract. *Endoscopy.* 2005;37(6):570–578.
164. Harewood GC, Sharma VK, de Garmo P. Impact of colonoscopy preparation quality on detection of suspected colonic neoplasia. *Gastrointest Endosc.* 2003;58(1):76–79.
165. Froehlich F, Wietlisbach V, Gonvers JJ, Burnand B, Vader JP. Impact of colonic cleansing on quality and diagnostic yield of colonoscopy: the European Panel of Appropriateness of Gastrointestinal Endoscopy European multicenter study. *Gastrointest Endosc.* 2005;61(3):378–384.
166. Parra-Blanco A, Nicolas-Perez D, Gimeno-Garcia A, et al. The timing of bowel preparation before colonoscopy determines the quality of cleansing, and is a significant factor contributing to the detection of flat lesions: a randomized study. *World J Gastroenterol.* 2006;12(38):6161–6166.
167. Kahi CJ, Hewett DG, Rex DK. Relationship of non-polypoid colorectal neoplasms to quality of colonoscopy. *Gastrointest Endosc Clin N Am.* 2010;20(3):407–415.
168. Rembacken BJ, Fujii T, Cairns A, et al. Flat and depressed colonic neoplasms: a prospective study of 1000 colonoscopies in the UK. *Lancet.* 2000;355(9211):1211–1214.
169. Saitoh Y, Waxman I, West AB, et al. Prevalence and distinctive biologic features of flat colorectal adenomas in a North American population. *Gastroenterology.* 2001;120(7):1657–1665.
170. O'brien MJ, Winawer SJ, Zauber AG, et al.; National Polyp Study Workgroup. Flat adenomas in the National Polyp Study: is there increased risk for high-grade dysplasia initially or during surveillance? *Clin Gastroenterol Hepatol.* 2004;2(10):905–911.
171. Soetikno RM, Kaltenbach T, Rouse RV, et al. Prevalence of non-polypoid (flat and depressed) colorectal neoplasms in asymptomatic and symptomatic adults. *JAMA.* 2008;299(9):1027–1035.
172. Singh H, Turner D, Xue L, Targownik LE, Bernstein CN. Risk of developing colorectal cancer following a negative colonoscopy examination: evidence for a 10-year interval between colonoscopies. *JAMA.* 2006;295(20):2366–2373.
173. Bressler B, Paszat LF, Chen Z, Rothwell DM, Vinden C, Rabeneck L. Rates of new or missed colorectal cancers after colonoscopy and their risk factors: a population-based analysis. *Gastroenterology.* 2007;132(1):96–102.
174. Lakoff J, Paszat LF, Saskin R, Rabeneck L. Risk of developing proximal versus distal colorectal cancer after a negative colonoscopy: a population-based study. *Clin Gastroenterol Hepatol.* 2008;6(10):1117–21; quiz 1064.
175. Baxter NN, Goldwasser MA, Paszat LF, Saskin R, Urbach DR, Rabeneck L. Association of colonoscopy and death from colorectal cancer. *Ann Intern Med.* 2009;150(1):1–8.
176. Brenner H, Chang-Claude J, Seiler CM, Rickert A, Hoffmeister M. Protection from colorectal cancer after colonoscopy: a population-based, case-control study. *Ann Intern Med.* 2011; 154(1):22–30.
177. Pabby A, Schoen RE, Weissfeld JL, et al. Analysis of colorectal cancer occurrence during surveillance colonoscopy in the dietary Polyp Prevention Trial. *Gastrointest Endosc.* 2005; 61(3):385–391.
178. Robertson DJ, Greenberg ER, Beach M, et al. Colorectal cancer in patients under close colonoscopic surveillance. *Gastroenterology.* 2005;129(1):34–41.
179. Farrar WD, Sawhney MS, Nelson DB, Lederle FA, Bond JH. Colorectal cancers found after a complete colonoscopy. *Clin Gastroenterol Hepatol.* 2006;4(10):1259–1264.
180. Khashab M, Eid E, Rusche M, Rex DK. Incidence and predictors of "late" recurrences after endoscopic piecemeal resection of large sessile adenomas. *Gastrointest Endosc.* 2009;70(2):344–349.
181. Rex DK, Bond JH, Winawer S, et al.; U.S. Multi-Society Task Force on Colorectal Cancer. Quality in the technical performance of colonoscopy and the continuous quality improvement process for colonoscopy: recommendations of the U.S. Multi-Society Task Force on Colorectal Cancer. *Am J Gastroenterol.* 2002;97(6):1296–1308.
182. Lieberman D, Nadel M, Smith RA, et al. Standardized colonoscopy reporting and data system: report of the Quality Assurance Task Group of the National Colorectal Cancer Roundtable. *Gastrointest Endosc.* 2007;65(6):757–766.
183. Baxter NN, Sutradhar R, Forbes SS, Paszat LF, Saskin R, Rabeneck L. Analysis of administrative data finds endoscopist quality measures associated with postcolonoscopy colorectal cancer. *Gastroenterology.* 2011;140(1):65–72..
184. Barclay RL, Vicari JJ, Doughty AS, Johanson JF, Greenlaw RL. Colonoscopic withdrawal times and adenoma detection during screening colonoscopy. *N Engl J Med.* 2006;355(24): 2533–2541.

185. Kahi CJ, Hewett DG, Norton DL, Eckert GJ, Rex DK. Prevalence and variable detection of proximal colon serrated polyps during screening colonoscopy. *Clin Gastroenterol Hepatol.* 2011;9(1):42–46.
186. Kaminski MF, Regula J, Kraszewska E, et al. Quality indicators for colonoscopy and the risk of interval cancer. *N Engl J Med.* 2010;362(19):1795–1803.
187. Lieberman DA, Weiss DG, Harford WV, et al. Five-year colon surveillance after screening colonoscopy. *Gastroenterology.* 2007;133(4):1077–1085.
188. Imperiale TF, Glowinski EA, Lin-Cooper C, Larkin GN, Rogge JD, Ransohoff DF. Five-year risk of colorectal neoplasia after negative screening colonoscopy. *N Engl J Med.* 2008;359(12):1218–1224.
189. Leung WK, Lau JY, Suen BY, et al. Repeat-screening colonoscopy 5 years after normal baseline-screening colonoscopy in average-risk Chinese: a prospective study. *Am J Gastroenterol.* 2009;104(8):2028–2034.
190. Brenner H, Haug U, Arndt V, Stegmaier C, Altenhofen L, Hoffmeister M. Low risk of colorectal cancer and advanced adenomas more than 10 years after negative colonoscopy. *Gastroenterology.* 2010;138(3):870–876.
191. Miller HL, Mukherjee R, Tian J, Nagar AB. Colonoscopy surveillance after polypectomy may be extended beyond five years. *J Clin Gastroenterol.* 2010;44(8):e162–e166.
192. Chung SJ, Kim YS, Yang SY, et al. Five-year risk for advanced colorectal neoplasia after initial colonoscopy according to the baseline risk stratification: a prospective study in 2452 asymptomatic Koreans. *Gut.* 2011;60(11):1537–1543.
193. Saini SD, Kim HM, Schoenfeld P. Incidence of advanced adenomas at surveillance colonoscopy in patients with a personal history of colon adenomas: a meta-analysis and systematic review. *Gastrointest Endosc.* 2006;64(4):614–626.
194. Laiyemo AO, Murphy G, Albert PS, et al. Postpolypectomy colonoscopy surveillance guidelines: predictive accuracy for advanced adenoma at 4 years. *Ann Intern Med.* 2008;148(6):419–426.
195. Miller J, Mehta N, Feldman M, et al. Findings on serial surveillance colonoscopy in patients with low-risk polyps on initial colonoscopy. *J Clin Gastroenterol.* 2010;44(3):e46–e50.
196. Russell AM, Zhang J, Luz J, et al. Prevalence of MYH germline mutations in Swiss APC mutation-negative polyposis patients. *Int J Cancer.* 2006;118(8):1937–1940.
197. Bisgaard ML, Fenger K, Bülow S, Niebuhr E, Mohr J. Familial adenomatous polyposis (FAP): frequency, penetrance, and mutation rate. *Hum Mutat.* 1994;3(2):121–125.
198. Schreiner MA, Weiss DG, Lieberman DA. Proximal and large hyperplastic and nondysplastic serrated polyps detected by colonoscopy are associated with neoplasia. *Gastroenterology.* 2010;139(5):1497–1502.
199. Boparai KS, Mathus-Vliegen EM, Koornstra JJ, et al. Increased colorectal cancer risk during follow-up in patients with hyperplastic polyposis syndrome: a multicentre cohort study. *Gut.* 2010;59(8):1094–1100.
200. Pinsky PF, Schoen RE, Weissfeld JL, et al. The yield of surveillance colonoscopy by adenoma history and time to examination. *Clin Gastroenterol Hepatol.* 2009;7(1):86–92.
201. Laiyemo AO, Pinsky PF, Marcus PM, et al. Utilization and yield of surveillance colonoscopy in the continued follow-up study of the polyp prevention trial. *Clin Gastroenterol Hepatol.* 2009;7(5):562–7; quiz 497.
202. Robertson DJ, Burke CA, Welch HG, et al. Using the results of a baseline and a surveillance colonoscopy to predict recurrent adenomas with high-risk characteristics. *Ann Intern Med.* 2009;151(2):103–109.

5 Preoperative Staging: Imaging and Endoscopic Approaches

Multimodality Imaging of Colorectal Cancer

ROHIT WALIA

Imaging plays a vital role in conjunction with endoscopy for the screening, staging, surveillance, and restaging of colorectal cancer (CRC).

SCREENING

Colon cancers can be detected on imaging when they cause symptoms or can even be sometimes identified on routine imaging for another purpose. In some cases diverticulitis can appear similar to colon cancers. Even though symptomatology varies for these two conditions, colonoscopy is recommended after the acute phase to exclude a perforated colon cancer and not simple diverticulitis (Figure 5.1).

While screening is still primarily done with optical endoscopy, CT colonography (CTC) or virtual colonography (VC) is playing an increasing role and as an adjunct in incomplete colonoscopy. Double contrast barium enema (DCBE) has fallen out of favor due to low sensitivity. DCBE can detect only about 46% of polyps larger than 1 cm. CTC, in contrast, can identify polyps as small as 5 mm in size, and, indeed, the ability or need to identify polyps below 5 to 6 mm in size remains controversial since the chance that these represent precancerous adenomas or malignancy is very low (1). Recommended screening interval for CTC is 5 to 10 years when there are no polyps equal to or larger than 6 mm (1).

For larger polyps, the recommendations vary depending on size or number. Solitary polyps 6 to 9 mm in size found on CTC could be referred to colonoscopy or could be followed after 3 years with CTC, since the chance that they harbor an invasive carcinoma is 1% or less. These may even regress on follow-up exam, as can sometimes be expected in inflammatory or hyperplastic polyps. However, if there are multiple small polyps, the patient should get a colonoscopy. Patients with 1 cm or larger polyps should get a colonoscopy, as the chance of these being an adenoma are higher. CTC has a sensitivity of up to 90% for detection of lesions this size (2).

PET does not have a good sensitivity for polyp detection, but the lesions detected by PET do have a high chance of being adenomas or of harboring invasive malignancy. Hyperplastic polyps are usually not fluoro-deoxyglucose (FDG) avid.

When evaluating CTC accuracy, optical colonoscopy is used to confirm or dismiss the polyps seen on CTC. Thus, we assume the optical colonoscopy as the standard against which the sensitivity of CTC is assessed. It is, however, difficult to confirm that the polyp seen on the CTC is indeed the same polyp seen on the colonoscopy since anatomic landmarks to identify the segment of colon are not as helpful as on CTC.

A meta-analysis by Halligan et al (3) showed high per patient sensitivity (93%) and high specificity (97%) for detecting polyps 1 cm or over in size on CTC. The sensitivity and specificity dropped to 86% and 86% when all polyps 6 mm and larger in size were included.

In a landmark multicenter study in the *New England Journal of Medicine* in 2008 (4), the sensitivity of CTC for lesions 1 cm or larger was 90%. When lesions 6 mm and larger were included, the sensitivity dropped to 78%. When 5 mm lesions were included, there was a significant drop in sensitivity to 65%.

Safety of CTC Compared to Optical Colonoscopy

CTC does not require sedation, with its attendant risks, and the risk of perforation is slightly lower compared to a colonoscopy. In a study from Israel with a large number of patients, the perforation rate for CTC was 0.06%. However, these were cases of staff-controlled air insufflations rather than CO_2, which may have increased the incidence of perforation. That is, older age and underlying colonic disease were the associated risk factors for perforation in this study (5). Risk of perforation with

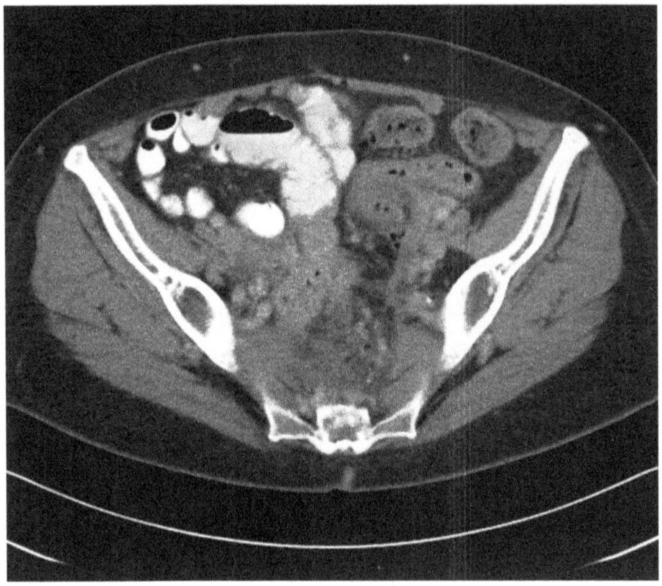

FIGURE 5.1 Perforated diverticulitis simulating a carcinoma.

conventional screening colonoscopy has been difficult to determine due to variability in reporting, but is accepted to be slightly higher at 0.13%–0.2% (6). With polypectomy the incidence of perforation increases.

Use of CTC involves use of radiation. However, the dose of radiation is nearly half of that for a conventional abdominal CT examination. Extrapolating from studies on atomic bomb survivors in Japan in 1945, it has been concluded that risk of cancer-related death from one conventional abdominal CT scan is anywhere from 0.06%–0.02% depending on the age of exposure with increasing age associated with decreased risk.

Cost effectiveness compared to optical colonoscopy is controversial, but a recent American College of Radiology Imaging Network (ACRIN) study in 2011 comparing CTC to "guideline concordant" screening colonoscopy as well as fecal occult blood testing with sigmoidoscopy showed that CTC was the most expensive, but still beneficial compared to a no-screening model (7).

Bowel Preparation for CTC

Patients should be on a clear liquid diet the day before the exam, with no oral intake after midnight. Magnesium citrate or sodium phosphate could be used the evening before for colon cleansing with equal efficacy (8). These can be used with oral bisacodyl. Some preprepared kits for CTC are preferable since these result in a dryer colon compared to a conventional colonoscopy preparation. Feces can also be tagged by oral iodine and/or barium-containing preparation, administered the night before the exam. On the day of the exam, air or CO_2 is used to insufflate the colon. Some patients may experience pain and cramping during insufflation, however, this is temporary. Smooth muscle relaxants like glucagon are not generally administered. Supine and decubitus CT images are then acquired to ensure optimal distension of different segments of the colon. CTC is reviewed as 2D images as well as 3D reconstructed endoluminal "fly through" with the help of a software program. Interpretation and reporting by the radiologist include polyp size, attenuation if relevant (eg, in identifying a lipoma), morphology if relevant (eg, flat lesions), location, and any significant extracolonic findings. As a general consensus, polyps equal or less than 5 mm in size are generally not reported by radiologists.

■ LOCAL STAGING

The radiologist's perspective depends on the part of the large bowel imaged. Rectal carcinoma is different anatomically than the colon and is evaluated differently. Portions of the colon completely enveloped by peritoneum, that is, transverse colon and sigmoid colon, need to be assessed in a different way compared to the portions that are retroperitoneal, that is, the cecum, ascending and descending colon. Different imaging modalities are used in conjunction, depending on the stage of diagnosis. MRI is used mainly for local staging and for identifying and enumerating liver lesions as part of surgical or treatment planning in metastatic disease. CT and PET CT are used for staging as part of the treatment-planning process as well as for evaluating response to therapy and restaging.

It is convenient to divide the discussion of these segments of the colon and imaging characteristics of tumor involving them.

Rectum

Staging of rectal carcinomas can be achieved with an MRI, which has good contrast resolution and can identify layers of the rectal wall. Phased array body surface coil is preferred over an endorectal coil since there are certain restrictions with the endorectal coil. These include difficulty in evaluating high lesions and lesions that are very constricting. The reliability may be compromised by coil migration. Lastly, the small field of view with an endorectal coil may not include some perirectal tissue that may potentially be involved by tumor. The most useful sequence is a T2-weighted, high-resolution matrix, small field of view, turbo spin echo sequence. This optimally demonstrates the contrast between the layers of bowel and the tumor itself. The tumor is intermediate in signal. The mucosa and submucosa appear similar in appearance as a hyperintense inner layer. The muscularis propria in the middle, comprising circular and longitudinal layers, is hypointense and the perirectal fat appears hyperintense. CT is not used for local staging, since it has poor contrast resolution with resulting poor differentiation of the bowel wall layers and low accuracy for T staging.

The T staging of rectal tumor can be determined on MRI as stage T1, limited to the submucosa, stage T2, involving the muscularis propria and stage T3 tumor invading into perirectal fat. Invasion of surrounding organs or peritoneal perforation constitute a stage T4 tumor.

Endorectal ultrasound is also very helpful for differentiating T1, T2, and T3 tumors and reportedly has a slightly higher accuracy than MRI in evaluating depth of tumor invasion. However, it is operator dependent and suffers from a low field of view, which makes it difficult to evaluate the perirectal extent and resectability of higher stage tumors. It is also difficult to distinguish normal or reactive nodes on the ultrasound from metastatic lymph nodes when compared to CT or MRI. The ability with ultrasound to sample the nodes at the time of evaluation is, however, useful.

The rectum is surrounded by perirectal fat, which is in turn enveloped by perirectal fascia (Figure 5.2)—a plane that can be identified on MRI and used by the surgeon to be able to remove the rectum and the perirectal fat along with the contained lymph nodes and vessels as an "en bloc" resection, in effect a total mesorectal excision (TME). This plane is called the circumferential resection margin (CRM). Anteriorly and superiorly, the peritoneal reflection forms the anterior margin of the CRM in rectal cancer resection. It is important for the radiologist to identify preoperative involvement of the CRM, since its involvement is associated with an increased risk of local recurrence after surgery. MRI can accurately predict a close or positive CRM. If there does appear to be CRM involvement, neoadjuvant treatment can be provided to "shrink" the tumor away from the CRM in order to obtain negative resection margins at surgery.

Predicting lymph node involvement on the MRI is more challenging as the involved nodes can be as small as 3 mm. Reactive lymph nodes may also be difficult to distinguish from metastatic nodes. A PET scan is also of limited value for local staging, as these nodes can be below PET resolution. FDG activity in the primary tumor may also obscure activity in nodes that are in proximity to the tumor mass. Heterogeneous signal intensity and irregular node margins are more reliable markers of node involvement but may not always be present. In the future, imaging with super paramagnetic iron oxide (SPIO) particles holds promise for identifying involved nodes.

Lymph node drainage of the rectum is mainly along the superior hemorrhoidal vessels to the nodes around the inferior mesenteric vasculature. Lateral spread can occur in middle and lower rectal tumors along the middle hemorrhoidal vasculature to the internal iliac chain and can be responsible for recurrent disease. Lymph node spread along the inferior hemorrhoidal vessels is rare.

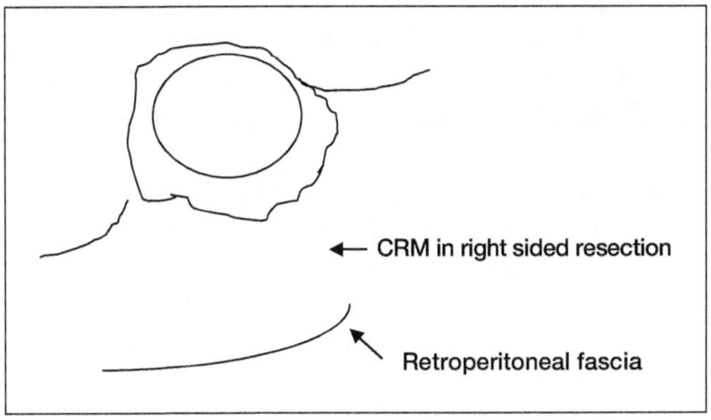

FIGURE 5.2

Carcinoma in Colon Proximal to the Rectum

Currently, CT and MRI are more helpful in detecting metastatic disease in colon carcinoma, since local staging by imaging does not affect the surgical management. CT is, however, useful to identify tumor complications such as obstruction, fistula, or pericolic abscess.

MRI can be used the same way as in the rectum for local staging, due to its ability to resolve colonic wall layers.

Due to poor contrast resolution, CT is not very useful for local staging of early tumors. Also, it can potentially overstage the tumor due to inflammation or desmoplastic reaction around the tumor mimicking the peritumoral fat stranding and nodularity described in T3 tumors. Lastly, severe cachexia causing loss of fat planes between tumor and an adjacent structure can erroneously stage the tumor as T4 with organ involvement (Table 5.1).

CT can be helpful for nodal staging. A 1-cm cutoff is used to identify potential metastatic nodes. The sensitivity of CT for detection of nodal metastasis is in the range of 45%–87%. No status implies there are no nodes greater than 1 cm and no abnormal clustering. N1 status implies that there are 1 to 3 nodes greater than 1 cm or there is clustering of at least 3 nodes less than 1 cm. N2 disease means that there are greater than 3 nodes larger than 1 cm.

Ascending and Descending Colon

These segments are covered by peritoneum anteriorly, and are thus retroperitoneal. T4 disease in these segments would be constituted by perforation through the peritoneum (anteriorly) or invasion of adjacent organs (in retroperitoneal spread). Gross peritoneal perforation is obvious on MRI, but care has to be taken to identify more subtle nodular extension of tumor beyond the peritoneal margin. The CRM in these colonic segments includes the mesentery, which contains the draining lymph nodes. This mesentery attaches to the posterior abdominal wall during embryologic development. Thus,

Table 5.1 T Staging of Colonic Tumors by CT

T Stage	CT Appearance
T1	Intraluminal lesion without distortion of wall
T2	Asymmetric thickening of the colonic wall projecting into the lumen. Smooth muscularis propria, without suggestion of tumor penetration. No pericolonic fat stranding
T3	Peritumoral stranding or nodularity, or tumor beyond the region of the muscularis propria
T4	Irregular elevation of the peritoneum or nodular penetration through the peritonealized surface. Loss of fat planes between colon and adjacent organ or frank invasion of tumor edge into the surrounding structure

the resection margin in these segments extends to the retroperitoneal parietal fascia. Involvement of this resection margin could potentially be a poor prognostic indicator, associated with increased risk of recurrence, especially in right-sided tumors. Involvement of this potential surgical resection margin can be identified on MRI or even CT, as tumor within 1 mm of the retroperitoneal parietal fascia (Figure 5.2).

Transverse and Sigmoid Colon

These segments of colon are completely invested in a peritonealized (serosal) layer, except at the mesenteric border. Thus, any tumor that penetrates through the wall on the antimesenteric side technically constitutes peritoneal involvement. Resection of these segments involves resection of the mesocolon at the root of the vascular pedicle along with the invested lymph nodes within. As the CRM extends all the way to the mesenteric root, the chance of recurrence at the resection margin is low, since tumor uncommonly extends this far. If tumor is at the antimesenteric border, this margin is less clinically significant (Figure 5.3).

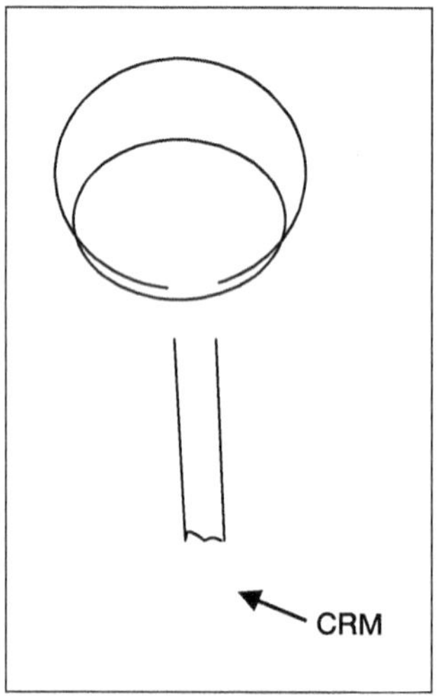

FIGURE 5.3

■ EVALUATION OF METASTATIC DISEASE

Metastatic disease usually occurs within 3 years of surgical resection, most commonly to the liver and lungs. Besides these hematogeneous routes of spread, tumor can also spread through the lymphatics to lymph nodes along the route of drainage or transperitoneal spread, including the ovaries. It is important to detect solitary or low volume disease, as resection of these metastases can affect survival and can even be curative. Imaging is used in conjunction with CEA for this purpose.

Lung metastasis present as small nodules less than a centimeter on a chest CT scan. Due to dual drainage of low rectal tumors, these can present with lung metastasis without liver involvement.

The liver is the most common site of metastasis. Liver disease can be solitary and resection can be curative. PET CT has been reported to be the most sensitive exam for detecting liver metastasis on a meta-analysis (9). Sensitivity of PET CT is as high as 90%. However, the higher sensitivity is per patient, not per lesion (10); that is, PET CT detects more patients with liver metastasis but is less effective for identifying all the metastasis in a single patient.

CT or MRI can identify small multisegmental liver disease and assist in surgical planning. In patients with limited disease in the liver being considered for resection, MRI is the exam of choice for evaluating number and resectability of lesions. In addition, tumor involvement of the potential liver resection margin can be assessed by CT or MRI.

MRI can be used as a problem-solving tool when there are lesions on the CT that are probably benign, but cannot be characterized as such due to their small size. Most commonly, these lesions turn out to be cysts or hemangiomas on the MRI. Very small metastatic lesions or highly necrotic or mucinous lesions that appear innocuous on a CT can be identified on the MRI as metastasis.

Serial imaging is required where there are lesions too small to be characterized by either modality. The use of liver specific contrast agents such as superparamagnetic iron oxide (SPIO) particles may also increase sensitivity and specificity of MRI. Experience with these contrast agents is, however, limited at many centers.

Extrahepatic disease can be detected by CT. However, PET CT has been shown to upstage patients who appear to be resectable on CT and thus significantly alter management in up to 16% of cases (11). PET CT is especially more sensitive than contrast enhanced CT for post-treatment surveillance. However, small lesions (less than 1 cm) or peripheral disease in the liver and low volume peritoneal disease will be hard to detect on a PET CT. Tumors with mucinous histology are also poorly detected. PET CT may show hypermetabolism in extrahepatic inflammatory processes and lung granulomas, leading to false-positive upstaging.

Bone and brain metastasis are unusual. The latter may require an MRI to confirm the disease as well as the number of lesions in the brain parenchyma.

Response to Therapy

Contrast enhanced CT or PET CT can be used to assess treatment response. On the contrast-enhanced CT, response can be identified by decrease in size of the metastatic lesions or by the presence of necrosis within them. The primary lesion, if still present, can also be seen to be decreasing in size. However, it is not always possible to measure the degree of change due to decreased ability of a CT to distinguish residual tumor from post-treatment change. PET CT can also be used to detect metabolic response to therapy even though the CT shows no change in size of the lesions. This property has been advocated as a method of early response to chemotherapy.

■ *Endoscopic Approaches to Colon Cancer*

KIRAN BIDARI
SRINADH KOMANDURI

■ DIAGNOSTIC CONSIDERATIONS FOR COLON CANCER: COLONOSCOPY

Since the vast majority of colonic neoplasms are adenocarcinomas, this section focuses on colorectal adenocarcinoma. Other histological types are uncommon (Table 5.2). CRCs arise from adenomas or flat dysplasia and subsequently evolve into different morphologic patterns, including polypoid, exophytic, circumferential, or flat infiltrating masses (Figures 5.4–5.6). For these malignancies, colonoscopy provides the ability to localize the lesion, obtain tissue confirmation of diagnosis, and evaluate for the presence of synchronous CRC and colonic adenomas.

Synchronous CRC and Adenomas

Synchronous CRC is defined as two or more distinct primary tumors detected simultaneously, separated by normal bowel and not related to direct extension or metastasis. Because the incidence of synchronous CRC and synchronous adenomas is high (approximately 2%–11% and 14%–80% [12–17], respectively), all patients should undergo complete colonoscopy prior to surgical resection.

Detection of synchronous carcinomas changes the surgical approach in 20%–88% of patients and failure to detect synchronous lesions prior to surgery may lead to added morbidity and mortality from a second surgical procedure (18). Removal of synchronous adenomatous polyps has been shown to reduce the number of metachronous tumors (18–20), which are nonanastomotic new tumors developing at least 6 months after the initial diagnosis.

■ Table 5.2 World Health Organization Classification of Carcinomas of the Colon and Rectum

Adenocarcinoma Mucinous adenocarcinoma
Signet-ring cell carcinoma
Small cell carcinoma
Squamous cell carcinoma
Adenosquamous carcinoma
Medullary carcinoma
Undifferentiated carcinoma

The risk of synchronous neoplasm is higher in patients with obstructing cancers versus nonobstructing cancers (21). In these cases malignant colonic obstruction may preclude the ability to perform a full colonoscopy to evaluate for synchronous CRC and alternative methods such as preoperative or postoperative barium enema examination, intraoperative colon palpation, intraoperative or postoperative colonoscopy, CT, PET/CT, MR colonography, and self-expandable metal stent (SEMS) placement with preoperative colonoscopy have been employed with mixed results (22–27).

Endoscopic Confirmation of Diagnosis

Colonoscopy is essential for obtaining tissue for pathologic confirmation of the diagnosis of colon cancer. When CRC is suspected, colonoscopy should be performed and tissue should be obtained when encountering polyps, mass lesions, or colonic strictures. The role of biopsy is to exclude the presence of benign lesions that may mimic malignancy clinically and to determine the histologic type if malignancy is present. In general, polypoid lesions found at the time of colonoscopy should be removed, with the possible exception of small, hyperplastic-appearing polyps in the rectosigmoid region (28). The finding of a colonic adenoma greater than 1 cm by rigid or flexible sigmoidoscopy is an indication for examination of the entire colon, since 30%–50% of these patients will have synchronous adenomas (29,30).

Larger lesions not amenable to endoscopic resection should be biopsied in different areas, including the edges

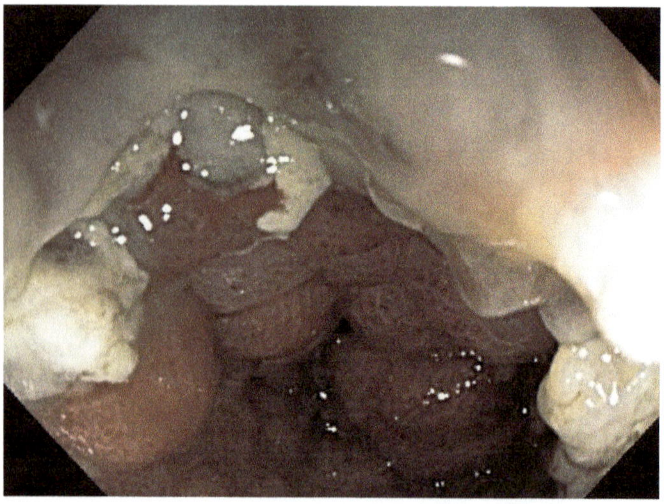

FIGURE 5.4 Circumferential colonic adenocarcinoma.

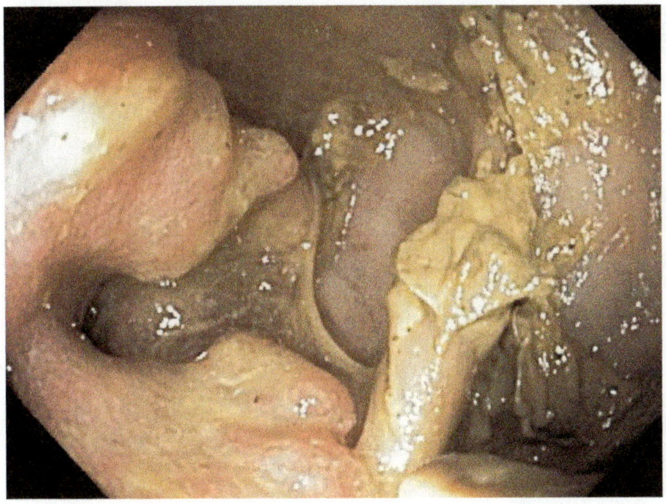

FIGURE 5.5 Exophytic colonic adenocarcinoma.

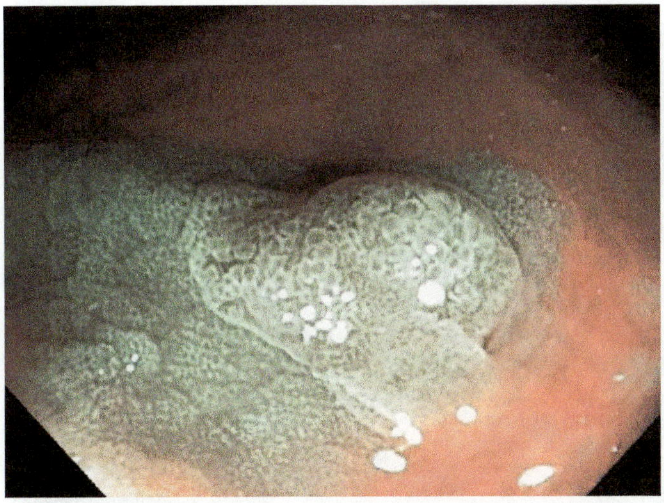

FIGURE 5.6 Flat, infiltrating colonic adenocarcinoma.

and center of the lesion (31). Several studies have demonstrated that the addition of cytology brushings may be complementary to biopsy and may improve the diagnostic yield, particularly, in areas of colonic stricture or obstruction where biopsy may be difficult (32–37). The optimal number of biopsy specimens has not been well studied, but one prospective study of 60 patients showed that the combination of cytology and 4 to 6 biopsies had the greatest diagnostic yield (34). However, the addition of cytology has not yet been adopted into practice as the standard of care. In about 8%–10% of cases of malignancy (38), biopsy may be nondiagnostic, especially if the lesion is extensively ulcerated or otherwise necrotic and viable tumor tissue is not obtained on sampling. When biopsy specimens are nondiagnostic and cancer is highly suspected, clinicians should consider obtaining a second opinion from an expert pathologist and/or performing a repeat colonoscopy for additional tissue sampling. Surgery is indicated for suspicious lesions with nondiagnostic biopsy specimens (31).

In about 5% of patients, colonoscopy may not be able to reach the tumor for technical reasons (eg, malignant obstruction, tortuous colon, poor bowel prep, poor patient tolerability). In these circumstances, double-contrast barium enema or CTC can provide a radiographic diagnosis but lacks the capability of biopsy (22,39–41).

Localization of Malignant Lesions

Colonoscopy has an important role in the localization of malignant lesions for subsequent identification at the time of surgery. Several studies have reported difficulty identifying colonic tumors resulting in removal of the wrong segment of bowel during surgery, emphasizing the need for accurate localization (42,43). For patients undergoing laparoscopic-assisted surgical colonic resection, the colon cannot be palpated, so it is important to have an easily visible marker that can be seen through the lens of the laparoscope.

Endoscopic tattooing is the most reliable method for lesion localization and can localize tumors in 88%–100% of cases (44–47). Other methods, such as colonoscopic localization, CT, barium enema, endoscopic clip placement, and intraoperative colonoscopy have limitations (48–52). Many dyes are available for endoscopic tattooing, but most are rapidly absorbed making them inappropriate for tumor localization. Only India ink and SPOT (GI Supply, Camp Hill, Pennsylvania, USA) should be used in the purposes of tumor localization. SPOT is a prepackaged sterile dilute suspension, whereas India ink must be diluted and sterilized before being injected into the colonic wall.

The technique for tattooing involves injecting the dye directly into the colon wall a few centimeters away from the lesion to avoid the risk of tumor seeding (53). Some studies have demonstrated that a saline test injection method, which involves injecting 1 mL of sterile saline into the submucosa, followed by injection of dye using a second syringe, improves visualization of the dye to 98%, compared to rates of 80% after direct single injection (44,54). The colon wall should be injected at three or four sites circumferentially to improve visualization during surgery.

The incidence of complications after endoscopic tattooing is not well studied. There are few studies assessing the incidence of complications with SPOT. The incidence of clinically relevant complications with India Ink is low (0.22%; 55). Intraperitoneal spillage is relatively common and has been reported in up to 14% of cases but is rarely of clinical significance.

■ ENDOSCOPIC MANAGEMENT OF MALIGNANT COLON POLYPS AND POLYPS WITH HIGH GRADE DYSPLASIA

CRC is defined as the presence of dysplastic glands below the muscularis mucosa, that is, invading the submucosa. Polyps with dysplastic elements confined to the epithelium or lamina propria of the mucosa are, by definition, benign adenomas. It is generally accepted that about 90%–95% of CRCs arise from benign adenomas (adenoma-carcinoma sequence; 56). Adenomas may be classified as either tubular (approximately 70%–85%), tubulovillous (10%–25%) or villous (less than 5%) (Figures 5.7–5.9) and may have either high-grade dysplasia (HGD) or low-grade dysplasia. Approximately, 5%–10% of patients with adenomas have HGD at the time of diagnosis (57–62). Increasing dysplasia and malignant potential correlates with increasing adenoma size, villous component, and patient age (63).

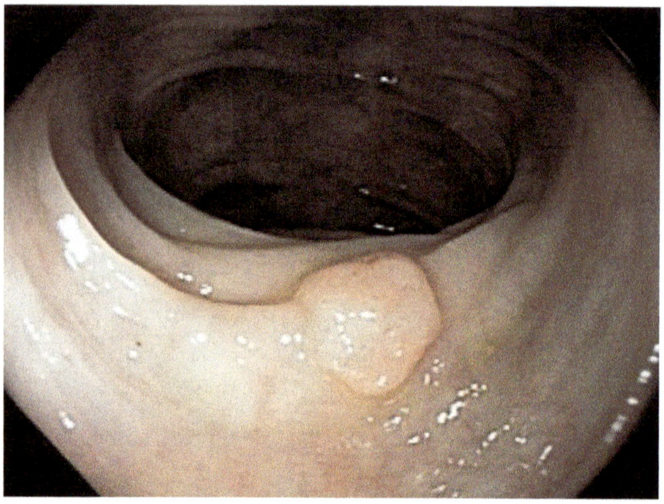

FIGURE 5.7 Tubular adenoma.

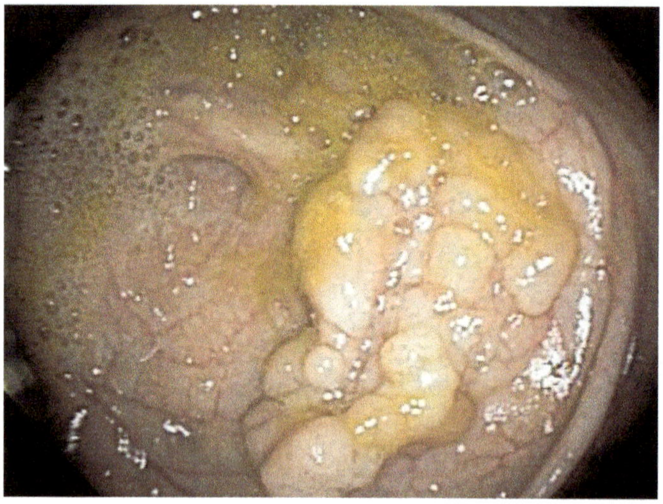

FIGURE 5.8 Tubulo-villous adenoma.

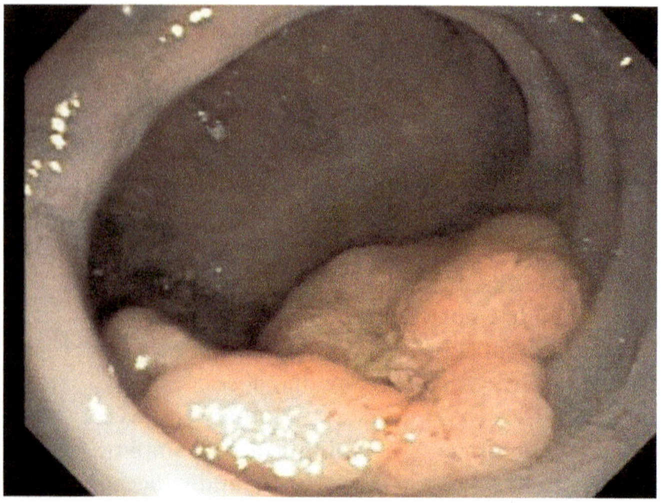

FIGURE 5.9 Villous adenoma.

Management of Polyps With High Grade Dysplasia

HGD is defined as dysplastic, neoplastic tissue confined within the mucosal wall layers without invasion into the submucosa (64). It includes the histological changes previously called "carcinoma in situ," "intramucosal carcinoma," or "focal carcinoma." Abandonment of these terms has been recommended by expert panels because they are misleading, since these lesions do not invade into the submucosa and are, therefore, benign. For pedunculated lesions with HGD, polypectomy or endoscopic mucosal resection (EMR) are curative if final pathology demonstrates complete resection, and these patients should have a repeat colonoscopy in 3 years (31,65). In cases of large sessile lesions, lesions removed in piecemeal fashion or when the endoscopist is unsure of the completeness of resection, repeat colonoscopy should be performed within 3 to 6 months to rule out residual neoplastic tissue at the polypectomy site (29,66). If residual tissue is identified, this should be removed and a second follow-up examination should be performed within 3 to 6 months to verify complete resection. If complete resection is not possible after two to three examinations, the patient should usually be referred for surgical therapy (67).

Management of Malignant Colon Polyps

A malignant polyp (Figure 5.10) is a neoplasm that contains cancerous cells that penetrate through the muscularis mucosa into the submucosa (68). The risk of local lymph-node metastases for these neoplasms varies widely (68–71), but there are several histologic features that are associated with a higher risk of lymph-node metastasis and local cancer recurrence. These features include: incomplete resection, cancer involvement of the resection margin, poorly differentiated histology, vascular and lymphatic invasion (69,71,72).

Many clinicians advocate that endoscopic resection alone is adequate for malignant polyps confined to the submucosa without unfavorable histopathologic features since numerous studies have demonstrated excellent long-term results, often approaching 100% 5-year cancer-free survival rates (73–80). In general, endoscopic resection can be considered adequate if the following criteria are met: (a) the polyp is considered to be completely excised by the endoscopist and is submitted in toto for pathologic examination; (b) the polyp is fixed and sectioned so that it is possible to accurately determine the depth of invasion, grade of differentiation, and completeness of excision of the carcinoma; (c) the cancer is not poorly differentiated; (d) there is no vascular or lymphatic involvement; and (e) the margin of excision is not involved (67,69,73–75,81). In these instances, the risk for local recurrence or for lymph node metastasis is likely less than the risk of death from colonic surgery.

Patients with malignant pedunculated polyps confined to the submucosa with favorable prognostic criteria have a 0.3% 5-year risk of cancer recurrence or lymph node metastasis after endoscopic resection, whereas patients with similar sessile polyps have a 4.8% 5-year risk of recurrence (74). Therefore, patients with malignant sessile polyps should have a follow-up colonoscopy in 3 months to check for residual abnormal tissue at the polypectomy site. After one negative follow-up examination, care can revert to standard surveillance as performed for patients with benign adenomas (67).

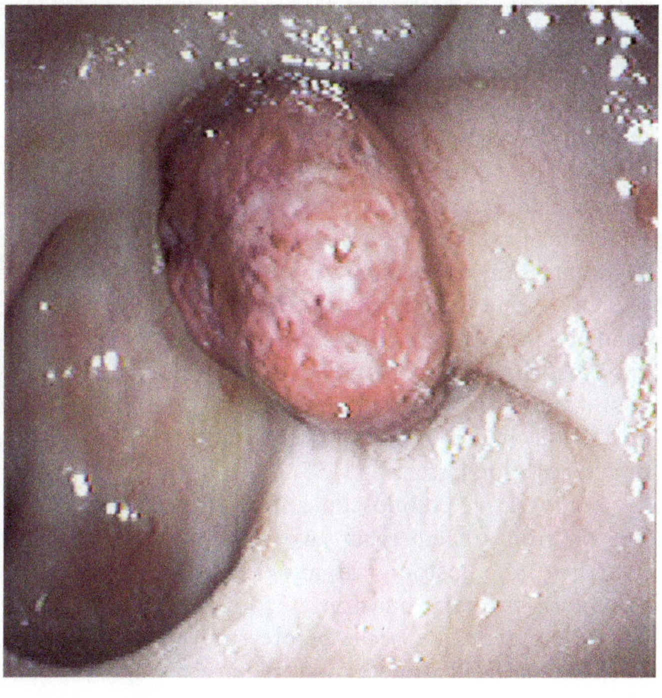

FIGURE 5.10 Polypoid colonic adenocarcinoma (malignant polyp).

In cases where malignant polyps have unfavorable histologic features or extend through the submucosa into the deeper wall layers, surgical resection is recommended.

EMR and Other Advanced Techniques

There are numerous methods for polypectomy including cold biopsy, hot biopsy, snare excision, fulguration, piecemeal excision, EMR, and endoscopic mucosal dissection (ESD). Standard polypectomy techniques are often inadequate to sufficiently treat large sessile and flat colonic lesions, which are associated with a higher incidence of HGD and adenocarcinoma. For these lesions, EMR is often considered the standard of care.

The technique of EMR (Figures 5.11 and 5.12) involves the use of a submucosal injection solution to permit complete resection of the mucosa through the mid and deep

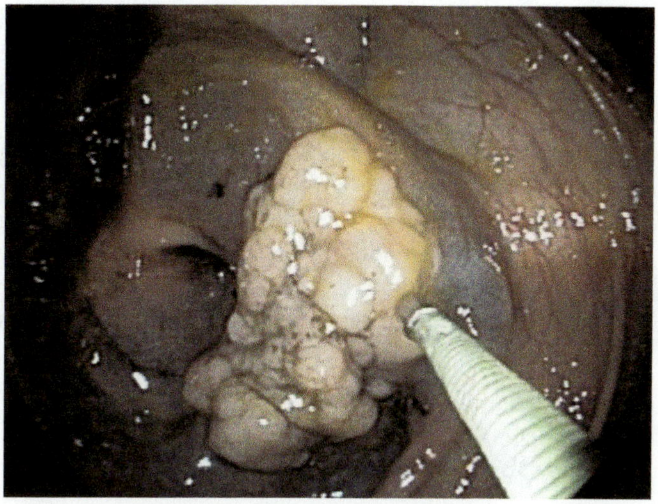

FIGURE 5.11 EMR submucosal injection.

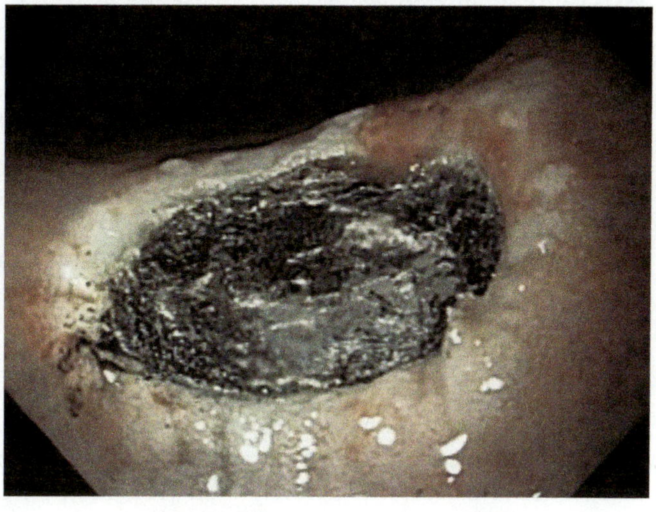

FIGURE 5.12 Appearance after EMR.

submucosa. The inability to raise the base of a polyp after submucosal solution injection, the so-called "non-lifting sign," can indicate the presence of malignancy invading into the submucosa and precludes endoscopic resection of the lesion (82–87).

En bloc removal of large polyps is preferable to piecemeal excision because it provides more accurate histologic assessment and reduces the risk of local recurrence, but it is often not possible for large polyps (88–91). The high frequency of recurrence (up to 46%) for large colorectal polyps mandates close endoscopic follow up (91–96). The use of ablative therapies, such as argon plasma coagulation (APC) to eradicate residual foci of adenomatous tissue has been shown to decrease the rate of recurrence (92–94). The most frequent complications associated with EMR are bleeding (1%–45%), perforation (0.7%–4%), and postpolypectomy syndrome (0%–7.6%; 91–99).

An extension of the EMR technique, ESD allows en bloc excision of large colorectal polyps, thereby providing more accurate pathological assessment and lower recurrence rates, but requires significant expertise and is limited to only a few centers in the United States. The procedure is associated with a high perforation rate (up to 6%; 89,100). Newer technologies such as chromoendoscopy, magnification endoscopy, narrow band imaging optical colonoscopy, and confocal endomicroscopy may have roles for improving CRC detection and determining which lesions can be endoscopically resected. Preliminary research into these modalities is promising, but further studies are needed before they can be recommended as standard of care.

Endoscopic Management of Malignant Colonic Obstruction

Malignant obstruction of the colon is the initial presentation of CRC in 7%–29% of patients (101–107). Acute malignant obstruction can be managed with emergent surgery, with a single-stage primary resection and anastomosis or a two-stage surgery that involves creation of a diverting colostomy to decompress the colon with subsequent colostomy closure at a later date (101,108–110). Various nonoperative approaches to decompress the obstructed colon and such as dilation, cryotherapy, electrocoagulation, percutaneous tube cecostomy, decompression tubes, have been reported with mixed results (111–119).

Laser therapy with a neodymium-yttrium aluminum garnet laser (Nd:YAG) has a high success rate ranging from 80%–90% of patients for obstructing rectosigmoid tumors, but requires significant expertise and often several treatment sessions (116–118,120–122). Given its high incidence of complications including perforation, bleeding, pain, fistula formation, and abscess formation occur in up to 10%–15% of cases, it is rarely used (122,123). APC can be useful in patients with obstructing rectosigmoid tumors and may offer comparable results to laser therapy at reduced costs and much greater availability. It is, however, limited by the need for several treatment sessions and often the need for repeat therapy for recurrent obstruction due to tumor regrowth (119,124,125).

The placement of SEMS has recently evolved into the most widely used nonsurgical option for colonic decompression given its high success rate and low complication rate and is now considered the standard of care (126–128). Several studies have demonstrated the safety and efficacy of SEMS for malignant colonic obstruction. A systematic review focusing on 88 studies that employed SEMS found the following: (a) technical success was achieved 96% of patients (range, 66%–100%) and clinical success (defined as clinical and radiologic evidence of colonic decompression) was achieved in 92%; (b) median duration of patency was 106 days; (c) median rate of reintervention was 20%; (d) median stent migration rate was 11%; (e) median perforation rate was 4.5% and (f) median rate of reobstuction was 12% (129). SEMS placement for definitive palliation for inoperable obstructing tumors has nearly equivalent technical and clinical success rates when compared to preoperative SEMS without the need for a permanent colostomy (126,127,129–132).

Many types of colonic stents are available including fully covered, partially covered, and uncovered metal stents. In the United States, all SEMS specifically designed for use within the colon are uncovered. Some studies have demonstrated no difference in the technical or clinical success rates among different stent types, but have shown that covered stents have a greater tendency to migrate, while uncovered stents have a higher likelihood of reobstruction (127,133,134). An uncovered stent should provide adequate and effective decompression when placed as a bridge to surgery, but the decision regarding stent type for definitive palliation is more challenging.

Currently, there are two main indications for endoscopic management of colonic obstruction with colonic stenting: preoperative decompression as a bridge to surgery and palliation of patients who are poor surgical candidates or have advanced disease (135–139). Preoperative decompression with colonic stenting can be performed in patients with partial obstruction of the colon or complete obstruction, provided there are no signs of systemic toxicity. Emergent surgery is warranted for patients with complete colonic obstruction with signs of systemic toxicity, due to the higher risk of ischemia and perforation that precludes colonic stenting (135).

Preoperative colonoscopic stenting permits: (a) conversion from an emergent two-step surgical procedure including a colostomy to an elective one-step resection with primary anastomosis; (b) evaluation of the patient's extent of disease before surgery; (c) optimization of comorbid illnesses before surgery; and (d) complete colonoscopy to evaluate for synchronous lesions, the incidence of which is higher in obstructing cancers (21,27,140). Many studies have demonstrated that emergent surgery in a patient with an unprepared colon leads to significant morbidity and mortality (141,142). When compared to open surgery, preoperative colonic stenting followed by elective surgery is associated with lower mortality, shorter hospital stay, fewer medical complications, and decreased likelihood of stoma formation at any point during management (136,143–147). Moreover, there has been no difference in long-term survival between patients undergoing preoperative colonic decompression with stent placement compared to those who undergo emergent surgery (136,143). Approximately, 32%–76% of patients who do undergo emergent surgery with diverting colostomy are unable to undergo colostomy closure due to comorbidities or refusal to undergo further surgery (101,110,141). The creation of a colostomy not only has an adverse effect on patient quality of life, but its closure is also associated with substantial morbidity and mortality (101,148). Several studies have shown that SEMS are cost effective when compared with open surgery (138,144,147).

SEMS are usually placed with endoscopic guidance, either through the scope (TTS) or over a guidewire, with the aid of fluoroscopy (Figure 5.13). A water-soluble or barium enema examination or rectal contrast CT may be helpful prior to SEMS placement to evaluate the anatomy, stricture length, and degree of malignant obstruction. In patients with distal colonic obstruction, a few cleansing enemas is sufficient bowel preparation, whereas patients with more proximal lesions should undergo cautious standard colonoscopy bowel preparation. Generally, prophylactic antibiotics are not indicated with the exception of patients who have a markedly dilated colon, who have an increased risk of perforation and clinically significant bacteremia during insufflation. Balloon dilation of a malignant stricture before SEMS placement is not necessary and may be associated with a higher risk of perforation (140,149). The stent should be deployed under direct endoscopic visualization and fluoroscopy with at least 2 cm exposed distal and proximal to the obstructing lesion, such that there is a "waist" where the stent traverses the tumor with a flare at the proximal and distal ends of the stent (Figure 5.14). If this is not the case, additional stents can be used to completely traverse the stricture. After SEMS placement in the left colon, stools should be maintained at a soft consistency to avoid fecal impaction, which can usually be achieved by advising patient to take mineral oil supplements or laxatives and consume a low residue diet. Patients who have SEMS placed for more proximal lesions may consume a general diet as stool is of a softer consistency in this region.

The major complications associated with colonic stenting include perforation, bleeding, abdominal pain, reobstruction, and stent migration. Perforation occurs in less than 5% of patients, may be immediate or delayed, and is more likely to occur in the distal colon where stent deployment is more challenging. Stent migration occurs in about 11% of cases, usually within 1 week of insertion, and the risk may be increased in patients who subsequently receive chemotherapy or radiation and in those who receive covered stents. Stent reobstruction is often secondary to fecal impaction, tumor ingrowth or tumor overgrowth. Reobstruction due to tumor ingrowth or overgrowth is often managed by placing additional stents through the original stent (140).

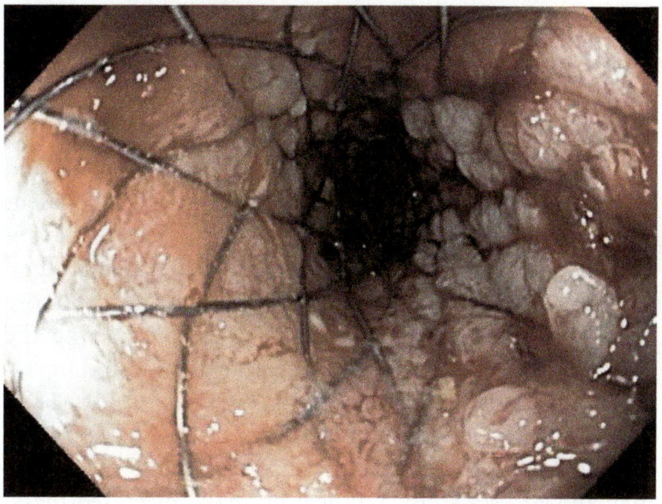

FIGURE 5.13 Placement of a self-expandable metal stent.

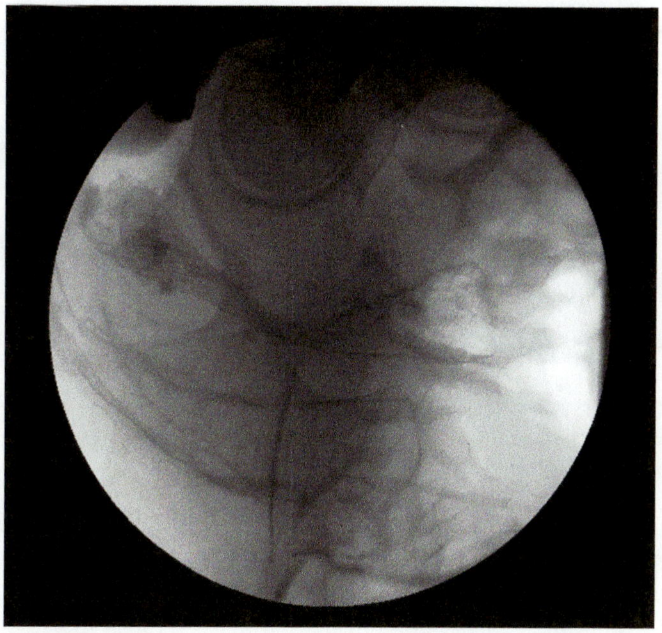

FIGURE 5.14 Fluoroscopic image of a self-expandable metal stent.

Other Primary Malignancies of the Colon

As mentioned previously, the vast majority of colonic neoplasms are adenocarcinomas. Aside from adenocarcinomas, other malignancies that are primary to the large bowel include carcinoid tumors, lymphomas, and Kaposi's sarcoma. Colonic carcinoid tumors often present at a younger age and occur predominantly in the appendix, ileum, and rectum. Generally, appendiceal and rectal carcinoids appear as submucosal nodules and are more indolent (Figure 5.15), whereas carcinoids involving the cecum and ileum are usually symptomatic and frequently metastatic at the time of diagnosis (Figure 5.16; 150–152). Primary non-Hodgkin's lymphoma of the large bowel often arises in the cecum, rectum, or sigmoid colon and may appear as a solitary fungating mass, ulcerated mass, or multiple colonic polyps (Figure 5.17; 153). Disseminated Kaposi's sarcoma is typically found in patients with AIDS and is manifested as characteristic violaceous macules or nodules (Figure 5.18; 154). Metastases from other cancers, most commonly ovarian cancer, can mimic a primary large bowel malignancy. For these malignancies, colonoscopy provides the ability to visualize the lesion and obtain pathologic confirmation of diagnosis.

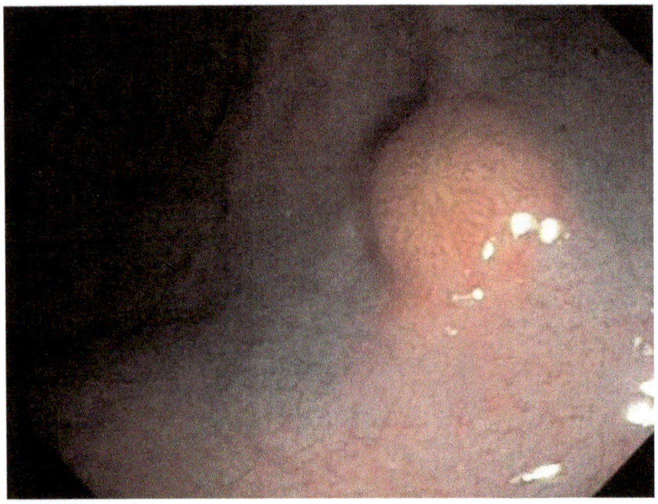

FIGURE 5.15 Rectal carcinoid.

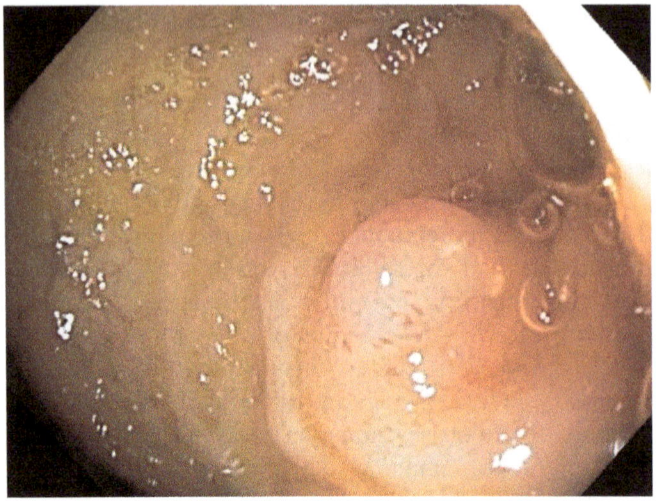

FIGURE 5.16 Ileal carcinoid.

■ ENDOSCOPIC APPROACHES TO RECTAL CANCER

Diagnostic Considerations for Rectal Cancer

When the diagnosis of rectal cancer is suspected, endoscopy should be performed to obtain pathologic

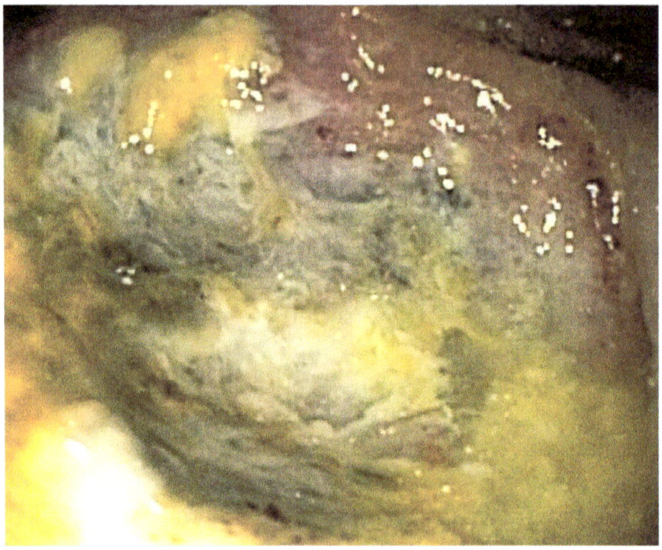

FIGURE 5.17 Primary colonic non-Hodgkin's lymphoma.

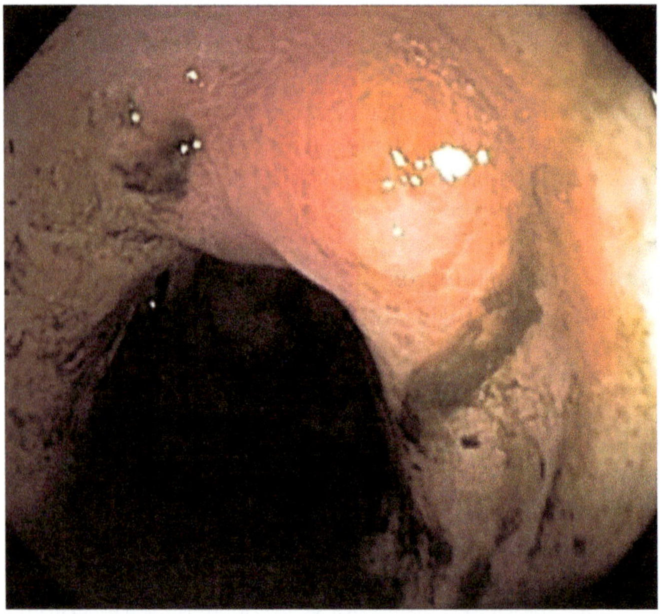

FIGURE 5.18 Kaposi's sarcoma of the colon.

confirmation of diagnosis, assess the location of the malignancy and evaluate for the presence of synchronous CRC. Prior to endoscopy, the performance of digital rectal examination (DRE) is important to assess tumor mobility (mobile, tethered, or fixed), consistency (hard, soft, or nodular), morphology, ulceration, and location (anterior, posterior, lateral), as well as its relationship to adjacent structures (prostate, vagina, and sphincter complex). However, the accuracy of DRE for evaluating penetration of the bowel wall in distal rectal cancers is poor, ranging from 39%–92%, and should therefore only be used in conjunction with other staging modalities (155–159). Rigid, rather than flexible sigmoidoscopy, can most accurately define the distances between the anal verge, distal tumor margin, top of the anorectal ring and dentate line, and helps determine the orientation of the tumor within the rectum. It is, therefore, often recommended for purposes of tumor localization (160,161).

Overview of Endorectal Ultrasound in the Imaging and Staging of CRC

Preoperative Staging

CRC is staged according to the TNM system established by the American Joint Committee on Cancer and the International Union against Cancer (Table 5.3). Despite major advances in chemotherapy, radiation therapy, and surgical technique, the primary determinant of outcome is the pathologic stage of the tumor and its associated lymph node status. For rectal cancer, major decisions about neoadjuvant therapy and the type of operation offered to a patient depend upon accurate evaluation of the depth of tumor invasion and the nodal status of a given lesion. Assessment of the cancer invasion through the bowel wall (T stage) remains the primary and most important factor in the treatment of patients with rectal cancer.

The ultimate goals of surgery are to improve local control and overall survival and maintain quality of life by preserving sphincter, genitourinary, and sexual function. To this end, some superficially invasive, small cancers (selected Stage T1 N0) may be effectively managed with local excision (LE), including transanal excision and transanal endoscopic microsurgery, which offer minimal morbidity and long-term functional problems compared to radical resection (ie, abdominoperineal resection [APR] or low anterior resection [LAR]). However, evidence suggests that those patients treated with LE have higher local recurrence rates than those treated with radical resection (162–165). The decision to perform LE for early cancers is based on knowledge of the risk of lymph node metastases for a given tumor stage (Table 5.4; 166–169). After final pathology is available from a LE, factors associated with a significantly increased risk of lymph node metastases, and therefore local recurrence, include poor differentiation, lymphovascular invasion, and size greater than 3 cm (170,171). Subsequent radical resection should be considered in these patients. Clearly, accurate preoperative staging is necessary to carefully select candidates for LE.

The decision for neoadjuvant therapy is also heavily reliant upon accurate preoperative staging. Neoadjuvant therapy is generally considered in the following circumstances: (a) T3/4 tumors; (b) clinically node-positive T1/2 tumors; (c) distal rectal tumors (within 5 cm of the anal verge); and (d) tumors that appear to invade or are in close proximity to the mesorectal fascia. The National Comprehensive Cancer Network (NCCN) recommends

Table 5.3 TNM Staging for Colorectal Cancer

Primary Tumor (T)	
TX	Primary tumor cannot be assessed
T0	No evidence of primary tumor
Tis	Carcinoma in situ: intraepithelial or invasion of lamina propria
T1	Tumor invades submucosa
T2	Tumor invades muscularis propria
T3	Tumor invades through the muscularis propria into pericolorectal tissues
T4a	Tumor penetrates to the surface of the visceral peritioneum
T4b	Tumor directly invades or is adherent to other organs or structures
Regional Lymph Node (N)	
NX	Regional lymph nodes cannot be assessed
N0	No regional lymph node metastasis
N1	Metastasis in one to three regional lymph nodes
N1a	Metastasis in one regional lymph node
N1b	Metastasis in two to three regional lymph nodes
N1c	Tumor deposit(s) in the subserosa, mesentery, or nonperitonealized pericolic or perirectal tissues without regional nodal metastasis
N2	Metastasis in four or more regional lymph nodes
N2a	Metastasis in four to six regional lymph nodes
N2b	Metastasis in seven or more regional lymph nodes
Distant Metastasis (M)	
M0	No distant metastasis
M1	Distant metastasis
M1a	Metastasis confined to one organ or site
M1b	Metastases in more than one organ/site or the peritoneum

Table 5.4 Risk of Lymph Node Metastases in Rectal Cancer Based on Tumor (T) Stage

Tumor Stage	Risk of Lymph Node Metastasis (%)
T1	10–18
T2	17–47
T3	66
T4	79

treatment with neoadjuvant therapy in patients with T3/4, N0 and any T, N1/2 tumors (172). For patients with T3/4 tumors, clear benefits of neoadjuvant therapy include significant downstaging, higher rates of sphincter preservation and reduction in local recurrence and long-term treatment toxicity (166,173–180). For patients with distal rectal tumors, preoperative therapy may enable conversion of the surgical procedure from an APR to a sphincter-preserving operation (181–184). Neoadjuvant therapy may also be considered if a tumor invades or is in close proximity of the mesorectal fascia, which is the CRM when TME is performed. This finding is highly predictive of residual tumor at the CRM, which places the patient at high risk of local recurrence. These patients have a decreased likelihood of achieving a tumor-free CRM with upfront surgery and neoadjuvant therapy may help downstage the tumor and reduce the rate of local recurrence.

In general, transrectal endoscopic ultrasound (TEUS) and MRI can both be used for primary tumor staging and are more accurate than axial CT scans for assessing depth of tumor invasion and nodal status. Limitations of TEUS include interobserver variability and a significant learning curve. The performance of TEUS is considered to be the standard of care in the preoperative staging of rectal cancer.

Preoperative Staging With Transrectal Endoscopic Ultrasound

Prior to TEUS, a few cleansing enemas are usually sufficient to cleanse the bowel, although a standard colonoscopy preparation could optimize imaging so that it is free of artifacts. Sigmoidoscopy should be performed prior to TEUS to ensure the lumen is clear of debris. During TEUS, the echoendoscope is inserted approximately 30 cm. The mesorectum is then assessed for evidence of nodal metastases and the rectal wall and periluminal structures are carefully inspected for abnormalities while slowly withdrawing the echoendoscope. Endosonographically, the bowel wall is seen as five alternating hyperechoic and hypoechoic layers. Although TEUS can be performed with rigid instruments, flexible fiberoptic echoendoscopes may facilitate traversal of malignant strictures and improve

Table 5.5 Staging of Rectal Cancer by Transrectal Endoscopic Ultrasound

Primary Tumor (T)	
uT0	Confined to mucosa
uT1	Tumor invades up to, but not through, the submucosa
uT2	Tumor invades into, but not through, the muscularis propria
uT3	Tumor invades through the bowel wall into perirectal fat
uT4a	Tumor involves adjacent structures
Regional Lymph Node (N)	
uN0	No definable lymph nodes by ultrasound
uN1	Ultrasonographically apparent lymph nodes

the ability to assess for lymphadenopathy. The ultrasonagraphic staging of tumors is denoted by the prefix "u" and corresponds to the TNM classification (Table 5.5).

Primary Tumor (T) Staging

Carcinomas are hypoechoic and the degree to which they disrupt and penetrate the rectal wall layers suggests the local stage (Figures 5.19–5.21; 185). The accuracy of TEUS for primary tumor (T) staging ranges from 80%–95%, compared to 65%–75% for CT and 75%–85% for MRI (159,186–190). MRI has been compared to TEUS in several smaller series of patients and appears to have similar accuracy for T staging except in differentiating between T1 and T2 tumors, where EUS may be superior (191–193). A recent meta-analysis evaluating all TEUS studies from 1990 to 2008 showed that accuracy was high for all T stages (Table 5.6; 194). TEUS tends to overstage rather than understage tumors because it cannot always reliably distinguish between tumor and peri-tumor inflammation. One large meta-analysis demonstrated that rates of overstaging and understaging were 13% and 7% for CT, 13% and 13% for MRI, and 11% and 5% for TEUS (195). Interestingly, one study has demonstrated that the improved accuracy of TEUS compared to CT and MRI translated into a change in management in 31% of patients (196).

Regional Lymph Node (N) Staging

Accurate regional lymph node (N) staging is essential because the presence of nodal metastasis (Figure 5.22) correlates with higher local recurrence rates, shortened survival, and worsened prognosis and indicates the need for neoadjuvant therapy (197,198). The accuracy for assessment for nodal metastases with TEUS ranges from

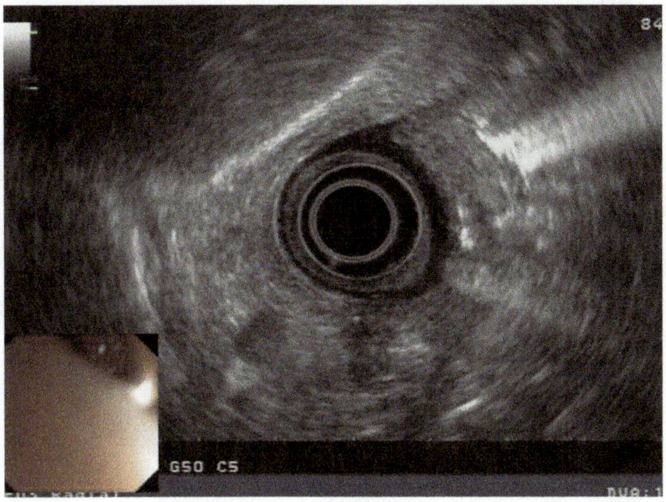

FIGURE 5.19 T2 stage rectal cancer.

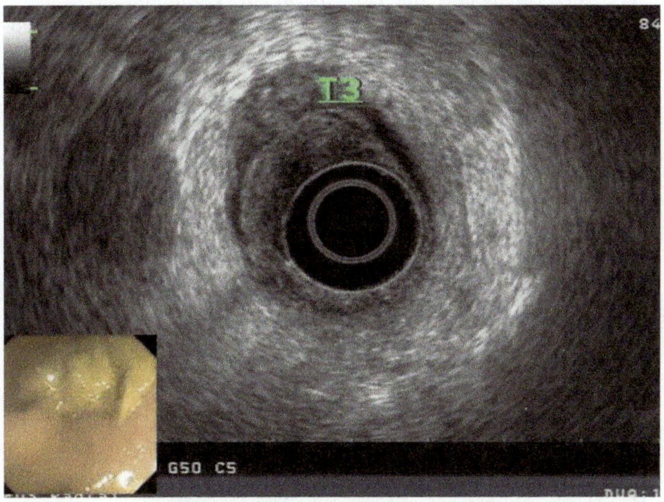

FIGURE 5.20 T3 stage rectal cancer.

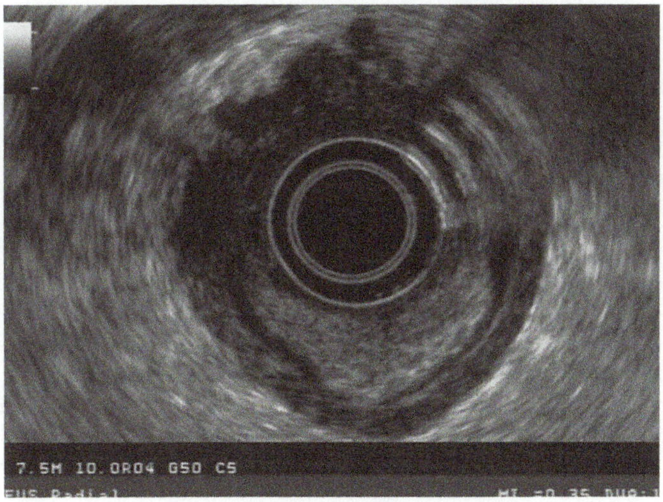

FIGURE 5.21 T4 stage rectal cancer.

Table 5.6 Accuracy of Transrectal Endoscopic Ultrasound for Primary Tumor (T) Staging

	Pooled Sensitivity	Pooled Specificity
T0	87.8% (85.3%–90.0%)	98.3% (97.8%–98.7%)
T1	80.5% (77.9%–82.9%)	95.6% (94.9%–96.3%)
T2	96.4% (95.4%–97.2%)	90.6% (89.5%–91.7%)
T3	95.4% (92.4%–97.5%)	98.3% (97.8%–98.7%)

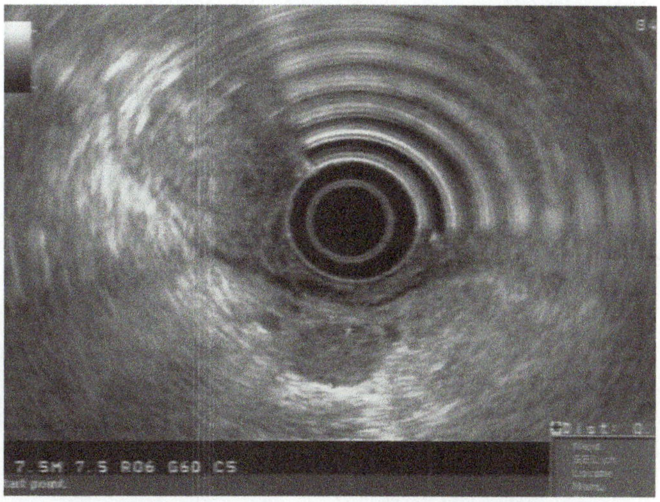

FIGURE 5.22 Nodal metastasis on TEUS.

70%–75%, compared to 55%–65% for CT and 60%–65% for MRI (199–201). A meta-analysis of 35 studies estimated that the pooled sensitivity and specificity for TEUS in diagnosing nodal involvement by rectal cancers were 73% and 76%, respectively (199,201–204). In general, TEUS is better at detecting lymph nodes in the middle and distal thirds of the rectum (205,206). Assessment for nodal metastases is difficult because the majority of metastatic lymph nodes are less than 5 mm and are located within 3 cm of the primary tumor (207). Among lymph nodes less than 5 mm, 18% harbor metastases (208).

Discrepancies in accuracy may be partially due to the lack of established criteria used for defining nodal metastases (186). One study sought to determine if the conventional EUS nodal echo features used to predict nodal metastasis in patients with esophageal cancer (hypoechoic echogenicity, round shape, smooth border, and size greater than 10 mm) applied to patients with rectal cancer (186). They found these features to be predictive of malignant pathology only when all four features were present, which occurred in only 23% of lymph nodes. Nodal hypoechogenicity and short axis greater than 5 mm were independent factors for malignancy, while a long axis length greater than 9 mm was 95% specific for the presence of malignancy. Prior TEUS studies identified a nodal size of greater than 7 mm as an optimal size cutoff for predicting nodal metastases, with an accuracy of 83% compared with surgical pathology (209).

Given the lack of established criteria to define nodal metastases, some experts suggest that fine needle aspiration biopsy (FNA) may be performed to help verify nodal status (186). One study failed to demonstrate an improvement in nodal staging with FNA, finding that accuracy for TEUS alone was comparable to TEUS-FNA, but more studies are needed (196). FNA may not add significant value to TEUS alone because perirectal lymph nodes are often too small to visualize unless they harbor metastatic disease. Therefore, biopsy would not be expected to improve accuracy when compared to visual criteria alone. Generally, it is most reasonable to perform FNA in patients with early T-stage disease with lymphadenopathy, where the decision for neoadjuvant therapy may be affected by nodal status.

Preoperative staging is also important to determine whether a tumor invades or is in close proximity of the CRM, since neoadjuvant therapy is considered in these instances. Generally, for anterior tumors, the status of the CRM can be predicted by either TEUS or MRI, while for posterior or posterolateral tumors, MRI is the preferred strategy.

In summary, the gastroenterologist has a crucial role in the management of CRC. Endoscopy provides the ability to localize and tattoo malignant lesions for intraoperative identification, obtain tissue confirmation of the diagnosis of malignancy, evaluate for the presence of synchronous CRCs, resect malignant polyps and polyps with HGD, and relieve malignant colonic obstruction through the placement of SEMS, while transrectal endoscopic ultrasound plays an integral role in the preoperative staging of rectal cancer.

■ REFERENCES

1. Zalis ME, Barish MA, Choi JR, et al.; Working Group on Virtual Colonoscopy. CT colonography reporting and data system: a consensus proposal. Radiology. 2005;236(1):3–9.
2. Dachman AH. Diagnostic performance of virtual colonoscopy. Abdom Imaging. 2002;27(3):260–267.
3. Halligan S, Altman DG, Taylor SA, et al. CT colonography in the detection of colorectal polyps and cancer: systematic review, meta-analysis, and proposed minimum data set for study level reporting. Radiology. 2005;237(3):893–904.
4. Johnson CD, Chen MH, Toledano AY, et al. Accuracy of CT colonography for detection of large adenomas and cancers. N Engl J Med. 2008;359(12):1207–1217.
5. Sosna J, Blachar A, Amitai M, et al. Colonic perforation at CT colonography: assessment of risk in a multicenter large cohort. Radiology. 2006;239(2):457–463.
6. Gatto NM, Frucht H, Sundararajan V, Jacobson JS, Grann VR, Neugut AI. Risk of perforation after colonoscopy and sigmoidoscopy: a population-based study. *J Natl Cancer Inst.* 2003;95(3):230–236.
7. Vanness DJ, Knudsen AB, Lansdorp-Vogelaar I, et al. Comparative economic evaluation of data from the ACRIN National CT Colonography Trial with three cancer intervention and surveillance modeling network microsimulations. *Radiology.* 2011; 261(2):487–498.
8. Borden ZS, Pickhardt PJ, Kim DH, Lubner MG, Agriantonis DJ, Hinshaw JL. Bowel preparation for CT colonography: blinded comparison of magnesium citrate and sodium phosphate for catharsis. *Radiology.* 2010;254(1):138–144.
9. Kinkel K, Lu Y, Both M, Warren RS, Thoeni RF. Detection of hepatic metastases from cancers of the gastrointestinal tract by using noninvasive imaging methods (US, CT, MR imaging, PET): a meta-analysis. *Radiology.* 2002;224(3):748–756.
10. Bipa C, Maarten S, et al. Colorectal liver metastases: CT, MR imaging, and PET for diagnosis—meta-analysis. *Radiology.* 2005; 237:123–131.
11. Rohren EM, Paulson EK, Hagge R, et al. The role of F-18 FDG positron emission tomography in preoperative assessment of the liver in patients being considered for curative resection of hepatic metastases from colorectal cancer. *Clin Nucl Med.* 2002; 27(8):550–555.
12. Langevin JM, Nivatvongs S. The true incidence of synchronous cancer of the large bowel. A prospective study. *Am J Surg.* 1984;147(3):330–333.
13. Masvidal Calpe R, Codina Cazador A, Farrés Coll R, Alcobilla Ferrara E, Gómez Castella F, Gironés Vila J. Synchronous colonic and rectal carcinomas. *Rev Esp Enferm Dig.* 1993;84(4):231–234.
14. Nikoloudis N, Saliangas K, Economou A, et al. Synchronous colorectal cancer. *Tech Coloproctol.* 2004;8 Suppl 1:s177–s179.
15. Kimura T, Iwagaki H, Fuchimoto S, Hizuta A, Orita K. Synchronous colorectal carcinomas. *Hepatogastroenterology.* 1994;41(5): 409–412.
16. Takeuchi H, Toda T, Nagasaki S, et al. Synchronous multiple colorectal adenocarcinomas. *J Surg Oncol.* 1997;64(4):304–307.
17. Barillari P, Ramacciato G, De Angelis R, et al. Effect of preoperative colonoscopy on the incidence of synchronous and metachronous neoplasms. *Acta Chir Scand.* 1990;156(2):163–166.
18. Dasmahapatra KS, Lopyan K. Rationale for aggressive colonoscopy in patients with colorectal neoplasia. *Arch Surg.* 1989;124(1):63–66.
19. Tate JJ, Rawlinson J, Royle GT, Brunton FJ, Taylor I. Pre-operative or postoperative colonic examination for synchronous lesions in colorectal cancer. *Br J Surg.* 1988;75(10):1016–1018.
20. Nava HR, Pagana TJ. Postoperative surveillance of colorectal carcinoma. *Cancer.* 1982;49(5):1043–1047.
21. Bat L, Neumann G, Shemesh E. The association of synchronous neoplasms with occluding colorectal cancer. *Dis Colon Rectum.* 1985;28(3):149–151.
22. Fenlon HM, McAneny DB, Nunes DP, Clarke PD, Ferrucci JT. Occlusive colon carcinoma: virtual colonoscopy in the preoperative evaluation of the proximal colon. *Radiology.* 1999;210(2): 423–428.
23. Neri E, Giusti P, Battolla L, et al. Colorectal cancer: role of CT colonography in preoperative evaluation after incomplete colonoscopy. *Radiology.* 2002;223(3):615–619.
24. Hartmann D, Bassler B, Schilling D, et al. Incomplete conventional colonoscopy: magnetic resonance colonography in the evaluation of the proximal colon. *Endoscopy.* 2005;37(9):816–820.
25. Veit P, Kühle C, Beyer T, et al. Whole body positron emission tomography/computed tomography (PET/CT) tumour staging with integrated PET/CT colonography: technical feasibility and first experiences in patients with colorectal cancer. *Gut.* 2006;55(1):68–73.
26. Sollenberger LL, Eisenstat TE, Rubin RJ, Salvati EP. Is preoperative colonoscopy necessary in carcinoma of the colon and rectum? *Am Surg.* 1988;54(2):113–115.
27. Vitale MA, Villotti G, d'Alba L, Frontespezi S, Iacopini F, Iacopini G. Preoperative colonoscopy after self-expandable metallic stent placement in patients with acute neoplastic colon obstruction. *Gastrointest Endosc.* 2006;63(6):814–819.
28. Rex DK, Bond JH, Winawer S, et al.; U.S. Multi-Society Task Force on Colorectal Cancer. Quality in the technical performance

of colonoscopy and the continuous quality improvement process for colonoscopy: recommendations of the U.S. Multi-Society Task Force on Colorectal Cancer. *Am J Gastroenterol.* 2002;97(6): 1296–1308.

29. Guidelines for colorectal cancer screening and surveillance. Gastrointest Endosc, 2000. 51(6): 777–782.
30. Winawer SJ, O'Brien MJ, Waye JD, et al. Risk and surveillance of individuals with colorectal polyps. Who Collaborating Centre for the Prevention of Colorectal Cancer. *Bull World Health Organ.* 1990;68(6):789–795.
31. Davila RE, Rajan E, Adler D, et al.; ASGE. ASGE guideline: the role of endoscopy in the diagnosis, staging, and management of colorectal cancer. *Gastrointest Endosc.* 2005;61(1):1–7.
32. Jeevanandam V, Treat MR, Forde KA. A comparison of direct brush cytology and biopsy in the diagnosis of colorectal cancer. *Gastrointest Endosc.* 1987;33(5):370–371.
33. Kontzoglou K, Moulakakis KG, Alexiou D, et al. The role of liquid-based cytology in the investigation of colorectal lesions: a cytohistopathological correlation and evaluation of diagnostic accuracy. *Langenbecks Arch Surg.* 2007;392(2):189–195.
34. Marshall JB, Diaz-Arias AA, Barthel JS, King PD, Butt JH. Prospective evaluation of optimal number of biopsy specimens and brush cytology in the diagnosis of cancer of the colorectum. *Am J Gastroenterol.* 1993;88(9):1352–1354.
35. Geramizadeh B, Hooshmand F, Kumar PV. Brush cytology of colorectal malignancies. *Acta Cytol.* 2003;47(3):431–434.
36. Brouwer R, MacDonald A, Matthews R, Gunn J, Monson JR, Hartley JE. Brush cytology for the diagnosis of colorectal cancer. *Dis Colon Rectum.* 2009;52(4):598–601.
37. Mortensen NJ, Eltringham WK, Mountford RA, Lever JV. Direct vision brush cytology with colonoscopy: an aid to the accurate diagnosis of colonic strictures. *Br J Surg.* 1984;71(12):930–932.
38. Winawer SJ, Leidner SD, Hajdu SI, Sherlock P. Colonoscopic biopsy and cytology in the diagnosis of colon cancer. *Cancer.* 1978;42(6):2849–2853.
39. Morrin MM, Farrell RJ, Raptopoulos V, McGee JB, Bleday R, Kruskal JB. Role of virtual computed tomographic colonography in patients with colorectal cancers and obstructing colorectal lesions. *Dis Colon Rectum.* 2000;43(3):303–311.
40. Kim JH, Kim WH, Kim TI, et al. Incomplete colonoscopy in patients with occlusive colorectal cancer: usefulness of CT colonography according to tumor location. *Yonsei Med J.* 2007;48(6):934–941.
41. Levin B, Lieberman DA, McFarland B, et al.; American Cancer Society Colorectal Cancer Advisory Group; US Multi-Society Task Force; American College of Radiology Colon Cancer Committee. Screening and surveillance for the early detection of colorectal cancer and adenomatous polyps, 2008: a joint guideline from the American Cancer Society, the US Multi-Society Task Force on Colorectal Cancer, and the American College of Radiology. *Gastroenterology.* 2008;134(5):1570–1595.
42. Cho YB, Lee WY, Yun HR, Lee WS, Yun SH, Chun HK. Tumor localization for laparoscopic colorectal surgery. *World J Surg.* 2007;31(7):1491–1495.
43. Wexner SD, Cohen SM, Ulrich A, Reissman P. Laparoscopic colorectal surgery–are we being honest with our patients? *Dis Colon Rectum.* 1995;38(7):723–727.
44. Park JW, Sohn DK, Hong CW, et al. The usefulness of preoperative colonoscopic tattooing using a saline test injection method with prepackaged sterile India ink for localization in laparoscopic colorectal surgery. *Surg Endosc.* 2008;22(2):501–505.
45. Arteaga-González I, Martín-Malagón A, Fernández EM, et al. The use of preoperative endoscopic tattooing in laparoscopic colorectal cancer surgery for endoscopically advanced tumors: a prospective comparative clinical study. *World J Surg.* 2006;30(4):605–611.
46. Fu KI, Fujii T, Kato S, et al. A new endoscopic tattooing technique for identifying the location of colonic lesions during laparoscopic surgery: a comparison with the conventional technique. *Endoscopy.* 2001;33(8):687–691.
47. Feingold DL, Addona T, Forde KA, et al. Safety and reliability of tattooing colorectal neoplasms prior to laparoscopic resection. *J Gastrointest Surg.* 2004;8(5):543–546.
48. Stanciu C, Trifan A, Khder SA. Accuracy of colonoscopy in localizing colonic cancer. *Rev Med Chir Soc Med Nat Iasi.* 2007;111(1):39–43.
49. Solon JG, Al-Azawi D, Hill A, Deasy J, McNamara DA. Colonoscopy and computerized tomography scan are not sufficient to localize right-sided colonic lesions accurately. *Colorectal Dis.* 2010;12(10 Online):e267–e272.
50. Piscatelli N, Hyman N, Osler T. Localizing colorectal cancer by colonoscopy. *Arch Surg.* 2005;140(10):932–935.
51. Rockey DC, Paulson E, Niedzwiecki D, et al. Analysis of air contrast barium enema, computed tomographic colonography, and colonoscopy: prospective comparison. *Lancet.* 2005;365(9456):305–311.
52. Ellis KK, Fennerty MB. Marking and identifying colon lesions. Tattoos, clips, and radiology in imaging the colon. *Gastrointest Endosc Clin N Am.* 1997;7(3):401–411.
53. Kang HJ, Lee BI, Kim BW, et al. Potential cancer cell inoculation of tattoo site through use of a contaminated needle. *Gastrointest Endosc.* 2006;63(6):884–886.
54. Sawaki A, Nakamura T, Suzuki T, et al. A two-step method for marking polypectomy sites in the colon and rectum. *Gastrointest Endosc.* 2003;57(6):735–737.
55. Nizam R, Siddiqi N, Landas SK, Kaplan DS, Holtzapple PG. Colonic tattooing with India ink: benefits, risks, and alternatives. *Am J Gastroenterol.* 1996;91(9):1804–1808.
56. Muto T, Bussey HJ, Morson BC. The evolution of cancer of the colon and rectum. *Cancer.* 1975;36(6):2251–2270.
57. Rembacken BJ, Fujii T, Cairns A, et al. Flat and depressed colonic neoplasms: a prospective study of 1000 colonoscopies in the UK. *Lancet.* 2000;355(9211):1211–1214.
58. Saitoh Y, Waxman I, West AB, et al. Prevalence and distinctive biologic features of flat colorectal adenomas in a North American population. *Gastroenterology.* 2001;120(7):1657–1665.
59. Tsuda S, Veress B, Tóth E, Fork FT. Flat and depressed colorectal tumours in a southern Swedish population: a prospective chromoendoscopic and histopathological study. *Gut.* 2002;51(4):550–555.
60. Konishi K, Kaneko K, Kurahashi T, et al. A comparison of magnifying and nonmagnifying colonoscopy for diagnosis of colorectal polyps: A prospective study. *Gastrointest Endosc.* 2003;57(1):48–53.
61. Kiesslich R, von Bergh M, Hahn M, Hermann G, Jung M. Chromoendoscopy with indigocarmine improves the detection of adenomatous and nonadenomatous lesions in the colon. *Endoscopy.* 2001;33(12):1001–1006.
62. Gschwantler M, Kriwanek S, Langner E, et al. High-grade dysplasia and invasive carcinoma in colorectal adenomas: a multivariate analysis of the impact of adenoma and patient characteristics. *Eur J Gastroenterol Hepatol.* 2002;14(2):183–188.
63. O'Brien MJ, Winawer SJ, Zauber AG, et al. The National Polyp Study. Patient and polyp characteristics associated with high-grade dysplasia in colorectal adenomas. *Gastroenterology.* 1990;98(2):371–379.
64. Pascal RR. Dysplasia and early carcinoma in inflammatory bowel disease and colorectal adenomas. *Hum Pathol.* 1994;25(11):1160–1171.
65. Winawer SJ, Zauber AG, Fletcher RH, et al. Guidelines for colonoscopy surveillance after polypectomy: a consensus update by the US Multi-Society Task Force on Colorectal Cancer and the American Cancer Society. *CA Cancer J Clin.* 2006;56(3):143–59; quiz 184.
66. Cohen LB, Waye JD. Treatment of colonic polyps–practical considerations. *Clin Gastroenterol.* 1986;15(2):359–376.
67. Bond JH. Polyp guideline: diagnosis, treatment, and surveillance for patients with colorectal polyps. Practice Parameters Committee of the American College of Gastroenterology. *Am J Gastroenterol.* 2000;95(11):3053–3063.

68. Cooper HS. Surgical pathology of endoscopically removed malignant polyps of the colon and rectum. *Am J Surg Pathol.* 1983; 7(7):613–623.
69. Morson BC, Whiteway JE, Jones EA, Macrae FA, Williams CB. Histopathology and prognosis of malignant colorectal polyps treated by endoscopic polypectomy. *Gut.* 1984;25(5): 437–444.
70. Coverlizza S, Risio M, Ferrari A, Fenoglio-Preiser CM, Rossini FP. Colorectal adenomas containing invasive carcinoma. Pathologic assessment of lymph node metastatic potential. *Cancer.* 1989; 64(9):1937–1947.
71. Nascimbeni R, Burgart LJ, Nivatvongs S, Larson DR. Risk of lymph node metastasis in T1 carcinoma of the colon and rectum. *Dis Colon Rectum.* 2002;45(2):200–206.
72. Muller S, Chesner IM, Egan MJ, et al. Significance of venous and lymphatic invasion in malignant polyps of the colon and rectum. *Gut.* 1989;30(10):1385–1391.
73. Haggitt RC, Glotzbach RE, Soffer EE, Wruble LD. Prognostic factors in colorectal carcinomas arising in adenomas: implications for lesions removed by endoscopic polypectomy. *Gastroenterology.* 1985;89(2):328–336.
74. Cranley JP, Petras RE, Carey WD, Paradis K, Sivak MV. When is endoscopic polypectomy adequate therapy for colonic polyps containing invasive carcinoma? *Gastroenterology.* 1986; 91(2):419–427.
75. Waye JD, Haggitt RC. Controversies, dilemmas, and dialogues. When is colonoscopic resection of an adenomatous polyp containing a "malignancy" sufficient? *Am J Gastroenterol.* 1990; 85(12):1564–1568.
76. Christie JP. Malignant colon polyps–cure by colonoscopy or colectomy? *Am J Gastroenterol.* 1984;79(7):543–547.
77. Cooper HS, Deppisch LM, Gourley WK, et al. Endoscopically removed malignant colorectal polyps: clinicopathologic correlations. *Gastroenterology.* 1995;108(6):1657–1665.
78. Seitz U, Bohnacker S, Seewald S, et al. Is endoscopic polypectomy an adequate therapy for malignant colorectal adenomas? Presentation of 114 patients and review of the literature. *Dis Colon Rectum.* 2004;47(11):1789–96; discussion 1796.
79. Volk EE, Goldblum JR, Petras RE, Carey WD, Fazio VW. Management and outcome of patients with invasive carcinoma arising in colorectal polyps. *Gastroenterology.* 1995; 109(6):1801–1807.
80. Ueno H, Mochizuki H, Hashiguchi Y, et al. Risk factors for an adverse outcome in early invasive colorectal carcinoma. *Gastroenterology.* 2004;127(2):385–394.
81. Wilcox GM, Anderson PB, Colacchio TA. Early invasive carcinoma in colonic polyps. A review of the literature with emphasis on the assessment of the risk of metastasis. *Cancer.* 1986;57(1):160–171.
82. Ferrara F, Luigiano C, Ghersi S, et al. Efficacy, safety and outcomes of 'inject and cut' endoscopic mucosal resection for large sessile and flat colorectal polyps. *Digestion.* 2010;82(4):213–220.
83. Ahlawat SK, Gupta N, Benjamin SB, Al-Kawas FH. Large colorectal polyps: endoscopic management and rate of malignancy: does size matter? *J Clin Gastroenterol.* 2011;45(4):347–354.
84. Kato H, Haga S, Endo S, et al. Lifting of lesions during endoscopic mucosal resection (EMR) of early colorectal cancer: implications for the assessment of resectability. *Endoscopy.* 2001;33(7):568–573.
85. Uno Y, Munakata A. The non-lifting sign of invasive colon cancer. *Gastrointest Endosc.* 1994;40(4):485–489.
86. Ishiguro A, Uno Y, Ishiguro Y, Munakata A, Morita T. Correlation of lifting versus non-lifting and microscopic depth of invasion in early colorectal cancer. *Gastrointest Endosc.* 1999;50(3):329–333.
87. Kobayashi N, Saito Y, Sano Y, et al. Determining the treatment strategy for colorectal neoplastic lesions: endoscopic assessment or the non-lifting sign for diagnosing invasion depth? *Endoscopy.* 2007;39(8):701–705.
88. Tanaka S, Haruma K, Oka S, et al. Clinicopathologic features and endoscopic treatment of superficially spreading colorectal neoplasms larger than 20 mm. *Gastrointest Endosc.* 2001;54(1):62–66.
89. Saito Y, Fukuzawa M, Matsuda T, et al. Clinical outcome of endoscopic submucosal dissection versus endoscopic mucosal resection of large colorectal tumors as determined by curative resection. *Surg Endosc.* 2010;24(2):343–352.
90. Katsinelos P, Kountouras J, Paroutoglou G, Zavos C, Rizos C, Beltsis A. Endoscopic mucosal resection of large sessile colorectal polyps with submucosal injection of hypertonic 50 percent dextrose-epinephrine solution. *Dis Colon Rectum.* 2006; 49(9):1384–1392.
91. Su MY, Hsu CM, Ho YP, et al. Endoscopic mucosal resection for colonic non-polypoid neoplasms. *Am J Gastroenterol.* 2005;100(10):2174–2179.
92. Zlatanic J, Waye JD, Kim PS, Baiocco PJ, Gleim GW. Large sessile colonic adenomas: use of argon plasma coagulator to supplement piecemeal snare polypectomy. *Gastrointest Endosc.* 1999;49(6):731–735.
93. Brooker JC, Saunders BP, Shah SG, Thapar CJ, Suzuki N, Williams CB. Treatment with argon plasma coagulation reduces recurrence after piecemeal resection of large sessile colonic polyps: a randomized trial and recommendations. *Gastrointest Endosc.* 2002;55(3):371–375.
94. Regula J, Wronska E, Polkowski M, et al. Argon plasma coagulation after piecemeal polypectomy of sessile colorectal adenomas: long-term follow-up study. *Endoscopy.* 2003;35(3):212–218.
95. Walsh RM, Ackroyd FW, Shellito PC. Endoscopic resection of large sessile colorectal polyps. *Gastrointest Endosc.* 1992; 38(3):303–309.
96. Kanamori T, Itoh M, Yokoyama Y, Tsuchida K. Injection-incision–assisted snare resection of large sessile colorectal polyps. *Gastrointest Endosc.* 1996;43(3):189–195.
97. Yoshikane H, Hidano H, Sakakibara A, et al. Endoscopic resection of laterally spreading tumours of the large intestine using a distal attachment. *Endoscopy.* 1999;31(6):426–430.
98. Bergmann U, Beger HG. Endoscopic mucosal resection for advanced non-polypoid colorectal adenoma and early stage carcinoma. *Surg Endosc.* 2003;17(3):475–479.
99. Bories E, Pesenti C, Monges G, et al. Endoscopic mucosal resection for advanced sessile adenoma and early-stage colorectal carcinoma. *Endoscopy.* 2006;38(3):231–235.
100. Fujishiro M, Yahagi N, Kakushima N, et al. Outcomes of endoscopic submucosal dissection for colorectal epithelial neoplasms in 200 consecutive cases. *Clin Gastroenterol Hepatol.* 2007;5(6):678–83; quiz 645.
101. Deans GT, Krukowski ZH, Irwin ST. Malignant obstruction of the left colon. *Br J Surg.* 1994;81(9):1270–1276.
102. Devon KM, Vergara-Fernandez O, Victor JC, McLeod RS. Colorectal cancer surgery in elderly patients: presentation, treatment, and outcomes. *Dis Colon Rectum.* 2009;52(7):1272–1277.
103. Smothers L, Hynan L, Fleming J, Turnage R, Simmang C, Anthony T. Emergency surgery for colon carcinoma. *Dis Colon Rectum.* 2003;46(1):24–30.
104. Phillips RK, Hittinger R, Fry JS, Fielding LP. Malignant large bowel obstruction. *Br J Surg.* 1985;72(4):296–302.
105. Mella J, Biffin A, Radcliffe AG, Stamatakis JD, Steele RJ. Population-based audit of colorectal cancer management in two UK health regions. Colorectal Cancer Working Group, Royal College of Surgeons of England Clinical Epidemiology and Audit Unit. *Br J Surg.* 1997;84(12):1731–1736.
106. Serpell JW, McDermott FT, Katrivessis H, Hughes ES. Obstructing carcinomas of the colon. *Br J Surg.* 1989;76(9):965–969.
107. Umpleby HC, Williamson RC. Survival in acute obstructing colorectal carcinoma. *Dis Colon Rectum.* 1984;27(5):299–304.
108. Lopez-Kostner F, Hool GR, Lavery IC. Management and causes of acute large-bowel obstruction. *Surg Clin North Am.* 1997;77(6):1265–1290.

109. Hsu TC. Comparison of one-stage resection and anastomosis of acute complete obstruction of left and right colon. *Am J Surg.* 2005;189(4):384–387.
110. Villar JM, Martinez AP, Villegas MT, et al. Surgical options for malignant left-sided colonic obstruction. *Surg Today.* 2005;35(4):275–281.
111. Oz MC, Forde KA. Endoscopic alternatives in the management of colonic strictures. *Surgery.* 1990;108(3):513–519.
112. Barr H, Bown SG, Krasner N, Boulos PB. Photodynamic therapy for colorectal disease. *Int J Colorectal Dis.* 1989;4(1):15–19.
113. Hoekstra HJ, Verschueren RC, Oldhoff J, van der Ploeg E. Palliative and curative electrocoagulation for rectal cancer. Experience and results. *Cancer.* 1985;55(1):210–213.
114. Morrison MC, Lee MJ, Stafford SA, Saini S, Mueller PR. Percutaneous cecostomy: controlled transperitoneal approach. *Radiology.* 1990;176(2):574–576.
115. Tanaka T, Furukawa A, Murata K, Sakamoto T. Endoscopic transanal decompression with a drainage tube for acute colonic obstruction: clinical aspects of preoperative treatment. *Dis Colon Rectum.* 2001;44(3):418–422.
116. Tai LS, Chia YW. Endoscopic Nd:YAG laser treatment of inoperable lower gastrointestinal cancer. *Ann Acad Med Singap.* 1996;25(5):712–716.
117. Rao VS, Al-Mukhtar A, Rayan F, Stojkovic S, Moore PJ, Ahmad SM. Endoscopic laser ablation of advanced rectal carcinoma–a DGH experience. *Colorectal Dis.* 2005;7(1):58–60.
118. Jakobs R, Miola J, Eickhoff A, Adamek HE, Riemann JF. Endoscopic laser palliation for rectal cancer–therapeutic outcome and complications in eighty-three consecutive patients. *Z Gastroenterol.* 2002;40(8):551–556.
119. Eickhoff A, Jakobs R, Schilling D, et al. Prospective nonrandomized comparison of two modes of argon beamer (APC) tumor desobstruction: effectiveness of the new pulsed APC versus forced APC. *Endoscopy.* 2007;39(7):637–642.
120. Brunetaud JM, Maunoury V, Cochelard D. Lasers in rectosigmoid tumors. *Semin Surg Oncol.* 1995;11(4):319–327.
121. Loizou LA, Grigg D, Boulos PB, Bown SG. Endoscopic Nd:YAG laser treatment of rectosigmoid cancer. *Gut.* 1990;31(7):812–816.
122. Gevers AM, Macken E, Hiele M, Rutgeerts P. Endoscopic laser therapy for palliation of patients with distal colorectal carcinoma: analysis of factors influencing long-term outcome. *Gastrointest Endosc.* 2000;51(5):580–585.
123. Frech EJ, Adler DG. Endoscopic therapy for malignant bowel obstruction. *J Support Oncol.* 2007;5(7):303–10, 319.
124. Ramadori, G., A. Lindhorst, and T. Armbrust, Colorectal tumors with complete obstruction—endoscopic recovery of passage replacing emergency surgery? A report of two cases. BMC Gastroenterol, 2007. 7: p. 14.
125. Baumhoer D, Armbrust T, Ramadori G. Nonsurgical treatment of the primary tumor in four consecutive cases of metastasized colorectal carcinoma. *Endoscopy.* 2005;37(12):1232–1236.
126. Khot UP, Lang AW, Murali K, Parker MC. Systematic review of the efficacy and safety of colorectal stents. *Br J Surg.* 2002; 89(9):1096–1102.
127. Sebastian S, Johnston S, Geoghegan T, Torreggiani W, Buckley M. Pooled analysis of the efficacy and safety of self-expanding metal stenting in malignant colorectal obstruction. *Am J Gastroenterol.* 2004;99(10):2051–2057.
128. García-Cano J, González-Huix F, Juzgado D, et al. Use of self-expanding metal stents to treat malignant colorectal obstruction in general endoscopic practice (with videos). *Gastrointest Endosc.* 2006;64(6):914–920.
129. Watt AM, Faragher IG, Griffin TT, Rieger NA, Maddern GJ. Self-expanding metallic stents for relieving malignant colorectal obstruction: a systematic review. *Ann Surg.* 2007;246(1):24–30.
130. Lee HJ, Hong SP, Cheon JH, et al. Long-term outcome of palliative therapy for malignant colorectal obstruction in patients with unresectable metastatic colorectal cancers: endoscopic stenting versus surgery. *Gastrointest Endosc.* 2011;73(3):535–542.
131. Small AJ, Coelho-Prabhu N, Baron TH. Endoscopic placement of self-expandable metal stents for malignant colonic obstruction: long-term outcomes and complication factors. *Gastrointest Endosc.* 2010;71(3):560–572.
132. Vrazas JI, Ferris S, Bau S, Faragher I. Stenting for obstructing colorectal malignancy: an interim or definitive procedure. *ANZ J Surg.* 2002;72(6):392–396.
133. Lee KM, Shin SJ, Hwang JC, et al. Comparison of uncovered stent with covered stent for treatment of malignant colorectal obstruction. *Gastrointest Endosc.* 2007;66(5):931–936.
134. Park S, Cheon JH, Park JJ, et al. Comparison of efficacies between stents for malignant colorectal obstruction: a randomized, prospective study. *Gastrointest Endosc.* 2010;72(2):304–310.
135. Baron TH, Harewood GC. Enteral self-expandable stents. *Gastrointest Endosc.* 2003;58(3):421–433.
136. Saida Y, Sumiyama Y, Nagao J, Uramatsu M. Long-term prognosis of preoperative "bridge to surgery" expandable metallic stent insertion for obstructive colorectal cancer: comparison with emergency operation. *Dis Colon Rectum.* 2003;46(10 Suppl):S44–S49.
137. Carne PW, Frye JN, Robertson GM, Frizelle FA. Stents or open operation for palliation of colorectal cancer: a retrospective, cohort study of perioperative outcome and long-term survival. *Dis Colon Rectum.* 2004;47(9):1455–1461.
138. Xinopoulos D, Dimitroulopoulos D, Theodosopoulos T, et al. Stenting or stoma creation for patients with inoperable malignant colonic obstructions? Results of a study and cost-effectiveness analysis. *Surg Endosc.* 2004;18(3):421–426.
139. Ng KC, Law WL, Lee YM, Choi HK, Seto CL, Ho JW. Self-expanding metallic stent as a bridge to surgery versus emergency resection for obstructing left-sided colorectal cancer: a case-matched study. *J Gastrointest Surg.* 2006;10(6):798–803.
140. Baron TH, Dean PA, Yates MR 3rd, Canon C, Koehler RE. Expandable metal stents for the treatment of colonic obstruction: techniques and outcomes. *Gastrointest Endosc.* 1998; 47(3):277–286.
141. Leitman IM, Sullivan JD, Brams D, DeCosse JJ. Multivariate analysis of morbidity and mortality from the initial surgical management of obstructing carcinoma of the colon. *Surg Gynecol Obstet.* 1992;174(6):513–518.
142. Tekkis PP, Kinsman R, Thompson MR, Stamatakis JD; Association of Coloproctology of Great Britain, Ireland. The Association of Coloproctology of Great Britain and Ireland study of large bowel obstruction caused by colorectal cancer. *Ann Surg.* 2004;240(1):76–81.
143. Tilney HS, Lovegrove RE, Purkayastha S, et al. Comparison of colonic stenting and open surgery for malignant large bowel obstruction. *Surg Endosc.* 2007;21(2):225–233.
144. Targownik LE, Spiegel BM, Sack J, et al. Colonic stent vs. emergency surgery for management of acute left-sided malignant colonic obstruction: a decision analysis. *Gastrointest Endosc.* 2004;60(6):865–874.
145. Martinez-Santos C, Lobato RF, Fradejas JM, Pinto I, Ortega-Deballón P, Moreno-Azcoita M. Self-expandable stent before elective surgery vs. emergency surgery for the treatment of malignant colorectal obstructions: comparison of primary anastomosis and morbidity rates. *Dis Colon Rectum.* 2002;45(3):401–406.
146. Siddiqui A, Khandelwal N, Anthony T, Huerta S. Colonic stent versus surgery for the management of acute malignant colonic obstruction: a decision analysis. *Aliment Pharmacol Ther.* 2007;26(10):1379–1386.
147. Binkert CA, Ledermann H, Jost R, Saurenmann P, Decurtins M, Zollikofer CL. Acute colonic obstruction: clinical aspects and cost-effectiveness of preoperative and palliative treatment with self-expanding metallic stents–a preliminary report. *Radiology.* 1998;206(1):199–204.
148. Nugent KP, Daniels P, Stewart B, Patankar R, Johnson CD. Quality of life in stoma patients. *Dis Colon Rectum.* 1999; 42(12):1569–1574.

149. Mauro MA, Koehler RE, Baron TH. Advances in gastrointestinal intervention: the treatment of gastroduodenal and colorectal obstructions with metallic stents. *Radiology.* 2000;215(3):659–669.
150. Marshall JB, Bodnarchuk G. Carcinoid tumors of the gut. Our experience over three decades and review of the literature. *J Clin Gastroenterol.* 1993;16(2):123–129.
151. Orloff MJ. Carcinoid tumors of the rectum. *Cancer.* 1971; 28(1):175–180.
152. Caldarola VT, Jackman RJ, Moertel CG, Dockerty MB. Carcinoid Tumors of the Rectum. *Am J Surg.* 1964;107:844–849.
153. Wong MT, Eu KW. Primary colorectal lymphomas. *Colorectal Dis.* 2006;8(7):586–591.
154. Sánchez del Monte J, Hernández Guerrero A, Sobrino Cossio S, et al. Clinical manifestations and endoscopic characteristics of Kaposi's sarcoma in patients with acquired immunodeficiency syndrome. *Rev Gastroenterol Mex.* 2005;70(4):416–423.
155. Rafaelsen SR, Kronborg O, Fenger C. Digital rectal examination and transrectal ultrasonography in staging of rectal cancer. A prospective, blind study. *Acta Radiol.* 1994;35(3):300–304.
156. Glaser F, Schlag P, Herfarth C. Endorectal ultrasonography for the assessment of invasion of rectal tumours and lymph node involvement. *Br J Surg.* 1990;77(8):883–887.
157. Hildebrandt U, Feifel G. Preoperative staging of rectal cancer by intrarectal ultrasound. *Dis Colon Rectum.* 1985;28(1):42–46.
158. Starck M, Bohe M, Fork FT, Lindström C, Sjöberg S. Endoluminal ultrasound and low-field magnetic resonance imaging are superior to clinical examination in the preoperative staging of rectal cancer. *Eur J Surg.* 1995;161(11):841–845.
159. Beynon J. An evaluation of the role of rectal endosonography in rectal cancer. *Ann R Coll Surg Engl.* 1989;71(2):131–139.
160. Baatrup G, Bolstad M, Mortensen JH. Rigid sigmoidoscopy and MRI are not interchangeable in determining the position of rectal cancers. *Eur J Surg Oncol.* 2009;35(11):1169–1173.
161. Schoellhammer HF, Gregorian AC, Sarkisyan GG, Petrie BA. How important is rigid proctosigmoidoscopy in localizing rectal cancer? *Am J Surg.* 2008;196(6):904–8; discussion 908.
162. Paty PB, Nash GM, Baron P, et al. Long-term results of local excision for rectal cancer. *Ann Surg.* 2002;236(4):522–29; discussion 529.
163. Madbouly KM, Remzi FH, Erkek BA, et al. Recurrence after transanal excision of T1 rectal cancer: should we be concerned? *Dis Colon Rectum.* 2005;48(4):711–9; discussion 719.
164. Endreseth BH, Myrvold HE, Romundstad P, Hestvik UE, Bjerkeset T, Wibe A; Norwegian Rectal Cancer Group. Transanal excision vs. major surgery for T1 rectal cancer. *Dis Colon Rectum.* 2005;48(7):1380–1388.
165. Mellgren A, Sirivongs P, Rothenberger DA, Madoff RD, García-Aguilar J. Is local excision adequate therapy for early rectal cancer? *Dis Colon Rectum.* 2000;43(8):1064–71; discussion 1071.
166. Sitzler PJ, Seow-Choen F, Ho YH, Leong AP. Lymph node involvement and tumor depth in rectal cancers: an analysis of 805 patients. *Dis Colon Rectum.* 1997;40(12):1472–1476.
167. Brodsky JT, Richard GK, Cohen AM, Minsky BD. Variables correlated with the risk of lymph node metastasis in early rectal cancer. *Cancer.* 1992;69(2):322–326.
168. Mellgren A, Sirivongs P, Rothenberger DA, Madoff RD, García-Aguilar J. Is local excision adequate therapy for early rectal cancer? *Dis Colon Rectum.* 2000;43(8):1064–71; discussion 1071.
169. Minsky BD, Rich T, Recht A, Harvey W, Mies C. Selection criteria for local excision with or without adjuvant radiation therapy for rectal cancer. *Cancer.* 1989;63(7):1421–1429.
170. Chambers WM, Khan U, Gagliano A, Smith RD, Sheffield J, Nicholls RJ. Tumour morphology as a predictor of outcome after local excision of rectal cancer. *Br J Surg.* 2004;91(4): 457–459.
171. Nascimbeni R, Burgart LJ, Nivatvongs S, Larson DR. Risk of lymph node metastasis in T1 carcinoma of the colon and rectum. *Dis Colon Rectum.* 2002;45(2):200–206.
172. Engstrom PF, Arnoletti JP, Benson AB 3rd, et al.; National Comprehensive Cancer Network. NCCN Clinical Practice Guidelines in Oncology: rectal cancer. *J Natl Compr Canc Netw.* 2009;7(8):838–881.
173. Janjan NA, Crane C, Feig BW, et al. Improved overall survival among responders to preoperative chemoradiation for locally advanced rectal cancer. *Am J Clin Oncol.* 2001;24(2):107–112.
174. Janjan NA, Khoo VS, Abbruzzese J, et al. Tumor downstaging and sphincter preservation with preoperative chemoradiation in locally advanced rectal cancer: the M. D. Anderson Cancer Center experience. *Int J Radiat Oncol Biol Phys.* 1999;44(5):1027–1038.
175. Garcia-Aguilar J, Pollack J, Lee SH, et al. Accuracy of endorectal ultrasonography in preoperative staging of rectal tumors. *Dis Colon Rectum.* 2002;45(1):10–15.
176. Påhlman L, Glimelius B. Pre- or postoperative radiotherapy in rectal and rectosigmoid carcinoma. Report from a randomized multicenter trial. *Ann Surg.* 1990;211(2):187–195.
177. Frykholm GJ, Glimelius B, Påhlman L. Preoperative or postoperative irradiation in adenocarcinoma of the rectum: final treatment results of a randomized trial and an evaluation of late secondary effects. *Dis Colon Rectum.* 1993;36(6):564–572.
178. van Gijn W, Marijnen CA, Nagtegaal ID, et al.; Dutch Colorectal Cancer Group. Preoperative radiotherapy combined with total mesorectal excision for resectable rectal cancer: 12-year follow-up of the multicentre, randomised controlled TME trial. *Lancet Oncol.* 2011;12(6):575–582.
179. Cammà C, Giunta M, Fiorica F, Pagliaro L, Craxì A, Cottone M. Preoperative radiotherapy for resectable rectal cancer: A meta-analysis. *JAMA.* 2000;284(8):1008–1015.
180. Improved survival with preoperative radiotherapy in resectable rectal cancer. Swedish Rectal Cancer Trial. *N Engl J Med*, 1997. 336(14): p. 980–7.
181. Sauer R, Becker H, Hohenberger W, et al.; German Rectal Cancer Study Group. Preoperative versus postoperative chemoradiotherapy for rectal cancer. *N Engl J Med.* 2004;351(17):1731–1740.
182. Allal AS, Bieri S, Pelloni A, et al. Sphincter-sparing surgery after preoperative radiotherapy for low rectal cancers: feasibility, oncologic results and quality of life outcomes. *Br J Cancer.* 2000;82(6):1131–1137.
183. Minsky BD. Sphincter preservation for rectal cancer: fact or fiction? *J Clin Oncol.* 2002;20(8):1971–1972.
184. Wagman R, Minsky BD, Cohen AM, Guillem JG, Paty PP. Sphincter preservation in rectal cancer with preoperative radiation therapy and coloanal anastomosis: long term follow-up. *Int J Radiat Oncol Biol Phys.* 1998;42(1):51–57.
185. Karantanas AH, Yarmenitis S, Papanikolaou N, Gourtsoyiannis N. Preoperative imaging staging of rectal cancer. *Dig Dis.* 2007;25(1):20–32.
186. Gleeson FC, Clain JE, Papachristou GI, et al. Prospective assessment of EUS criteria for lymphadenopathy associated with rectal cancer. *Gastrointest Endosc.* 2009;69(4):896–903.
187. Saitoh N, Okui K, Sarashina H, Suzuki M, Arai T, Nunomura M. Evaluation of echographic diagnosis of rectal cancer using intrarectal ultrasonic examination. *Dis Colon Rectum.* 1986;29(4):234–242.
188. Orrom WJ, Wong WD, Rothenberger DA, Jensen LL, Goldberg SM. Endorectal ultrasound in the preoperative staging of rectal tumors. A learning experience. *Dis Colon Rectum.* 1990;33(8):654–659.
189. Herzog U, von Flüe M, Tondelli P, Schuppisser JP. How accurate is endorectal ultrasound in the preoperative staging of rectal cancer? *Dis Colon Rectum.* 1993;36(2):127–134.
190. Savides TJ, Master SS. EUS in rectal cancer. *Gastrointest Endosc.* 2002;56(4 Suppl):S12–S18.
191. Zagoria RJ, Schlarb CA, Ott DJ, et al. Assessment of rectal tumor infiltration utilizing endorectal MR imaging and comparison with endoscopic rectal sonography. *J Surg Oncol.* 1997;64(4):312–317.

192. Gualdi GF, Casciani E, Guadalaxara A, d'Orta C, Polettini E, Pappalardo G. Local staging of rectal cancer with transrectal ultrasound and endorectal magnetic resonance imaging: comparison with histologic findings. *Dis Colon Rectum.* 2000;43(3):338–345.
193. Meyenberger C, Huch Böni RA, Bertschinger P, Zala GF, Klotz HP, Krestin GP. Endoscopic ultrasound and endorectal magnetic resonance imaging: a prospective, comparative study for preoperative staging and follow-up of rectal cancer. *Endoscopy.* 1995;27(7):469–479.
194. Puli SR, Bechtold ML, Reddy JB, Choudhary A, Antillon MR, Brugge WR. How good is endoscopic ultrasound in differentiating various T stages of rectal cancer? Meta-analysis and systematic review. *Ann Surg Oncol.* 2009;16(2):254–265.
195. Kwok H, Bissett IP, Hill GL. Preoperative staging of rectal cancer. *Int J Colorectal Dis.* 2000;15(1):9–20.
196. Harewood GC, Wiersema MJ, Nelson H, et al. A prospective, blinded assessment of the impact of preoperative staging on the management of rectal cancer. *Gastroenterology.* 2002;123(1):24–32.
197. Kim NK, Baik SH, Seong JS, et al. Oncologic outcomes after neoadjuvant chemoradiation followed by curative resection with tumor-specific mesorectal excision for fixed locally advanced rectal cancer: Impact of postirradiated pathologic downstaging on local recurrence and survival. *Ann Surg.* 2006;244(6):1024–1030.
198. Das P, Skibber JM, Rodriguez-Bigas MA, et al. Clinical and pathologic predictors of locoregional recurrence, distant metastasis, and overall survival in patients treated with chemoradiation and mesorectal excision for rectal cancer. *Am J Clin Oncol.* 2006;29(3):219–224.
199. Puli SR, Reddy JB, Bechtold ML, Choudhary A, Antillon MR, Brugge WR. Accuracy of endoscopic ultrasound to diagnose nodal invasion by rectal cancers: a meta-analysis and systematic review. *Ann Surg Oncol.* 2009;16(5):1255–1265.
200. Guinet C, Buy JN, Ghossain MA, et al. Comparison of magnetic resonance imaging and computed tomography in the preoperative staging of rectal cancer. *Arch Surg.* 1990;125(3):385–388.
201. Rifkin MD, Ehrlich SM, Marks G. Staging of rectal carcinoma: prospective comparison of endorectal US and CT. *Radiology.* 1989;170(2):319–322.
202. Hildebrandt U, Klein T, Feifel G, Schwarz HP, Koch B, Schmitt RM. Endosonography of pararectal lymph nodes. *In vitro* and *in vivo* evaluation. *Dis Colon Rectum.* 1990;33(10):863–868.
203. Tio TL, Coene PP, van Delden OM, Tytgat GN. Colorectal carcinoma: preoperative TNM classification with endosonography. *Radiology.* 1991;179(1):165–170.
204. Guinet C, Buy JN, Ghossain MA, et al. Comparison of magnetic resonance imaging and computed tomography in the preoperative staging of rectal cancer. *Arch Surg.* 1990;125(3):385–388.
205. Muthusamy VR, Chang KJ. Optimal methods for staging rectal cancer. *Clin Cancer Res.* 2007;13(22 Pt 2):6877s–6884s.
206. Bhutani MS. Recent developments in the role of endoscopic ultrasonography in diseases of the colon and rectum. *Curr Opin Gastroenterol.* 2007;23(1):67–73.
207. Bipat S, Glas AS, Slors FJ, Zwinderman AH, Bossuyt PM, Stoker J. Rectal cancer: local staging and assessment of lymph node involvement with endoluminal US, CT, and MR imaging–a meta-analysis. *Radiology.* 2004;232(3):773–783.
208. Skandarajah AR, Tjandra JJ. Preoperative loco-regional imaging in rectal cancer. *ANZ J Surg.* 2006;76(6):497–504.
209. Heneghan JP, Salem RR, Lange RC, Taylor KJ, Hammers LW. Transrectal sonography in staging rectal carcinoma: the role of gray-scale, color-flow, and Doppler imaging analysis. *AJR Am J Roentgenol.* 1997;169(5):1247–1252.

6 Pathology and Molecular Diagnostics

STANLEY R. HAMILTON

The pathology of colon and rectal neoplasia provides key information for the multidisciplinary management of patients with these diseases. In those patients who have developed colorectal carcinoma (CRC), pathologic diagnosis and characterization are the starting point for decisions about treatment, and the stage of the disease that portends prognosis informs the options that are considered by the gastroenterologist, surgeon, and radiation oncologist. In addition, pathology provides information about the setting of the carcinoma that has implications for the approach to the patient (eg, CRC in the setting of a chronic inflammatory bowel disease such as ulcerative colitis or Crohn's disease), but also to the patient's family members (eg, CRC in a hereditary syndrome). The pathologic types of precursor lesions for CRC influence strategies for risk assessment, screening, and surveillance. In addition to the contributions to patient management made by the anatomical/gastrointestinal pathologist, the subspecialty of molecular pathology is fulfilling ever-increasing roles in multidisciplinary care as the pathogenesis of the molecular alterations, and especially their implications for tumor biology, are understood and applied clinically. This chapter addresses the pathology and molecular pathology of epithelial tumors of the colon and rectum, including malignant tumors and their precursor lesions.

■ PATHOLOGY OF COLON AND RECTAL CARCINOMA

Macroscopic Pathology

Anatomical Site

Colorectal carcinoma can occur anywhere from the cecum and ileocecal valve region to the distal rectum at the anal canal (Table 6.1; 1,2). The distribution within patient populations is variable, however, with colon carcinoma being far more common in Western and developed populations with the most frequent site in the sigmoid colon, but a predominance of rectal carcinoma in less-developed countries, often at relatively young age before the fifth decade of life (3,4). Gender differences also occur, with rectal carcinoma more frequent in men than women.

Tumor Size

The size of colon or rectal carcinomas is dependent upon the timing of their detection and their rate of growth, with smaller tumors generally having a shorter duration than larger tumors. Their detection, however, is influenced by factors other than size, such as the development of symptoms and signs (eg, evident bleeding due to ulceration) anatomical location that influences symptoms that call attention to the mass, and compliance with screening and surveillance recommendations (5). Carcinomas in the right colon may remain asymptomatic for long periods of time due to the distance from the anus so that fecal blood is not evident and the large circumference of the right colon and presence of liquid feces so that obstructive symptoms do not occur. The size of the mass does not necessarily reflect the size of the carcinoma; other histopathologic components can be present, as evidenced by large tumors that can consist predominantly of villous adenoma with only a small area of carcinoma.

Configuration

CRC have widely variable appearances. The exophytic/fungating type grows predominantly into the colorectal lumen, whereas the endophytic type grows predominantly within the wall. Ulceration can occur in both types, but is more evident in the endophytic variety that usually lacks an intraluminal component (5). The growth relative to the circumference of the bowel can be annular with involvement of the majority of the circumference, often leading to stenosis of the lumen. Rare tumors have a diffusely infiltrative pattern like that commonly seen in "linitis plastica" carcinoma of the stomach, with only subtle visible mucosal alterations.

As is the case for tumor size, the configuration of a tumor can be influenced by the presence of a precursor lesion.

Table 6.1 Topography of Colon and Rectal Carcinoma

Site	ICD-O-3 Code
Ileocecal valve	–
Cecum	C18.0
Ascending colon/right (ascending) colon	C18.2
Hepatic flexure of colon	C18.3
Transverse colon	C18.4
Splenic flexure of colon	C18.5
Descending colon/left (descending) colon	C18.6
Sigmoid colon	C18.7
Overlapping lesion of colon	C18.8
Colon, NOS*	C18.9
Rectosigmoid junction	C19.9
Rectum, NOS*	C20.9
Other	–

*NOS, not otherwise specified.
Modified from (1,2).

Carcinomas can occur in pedunculated adenomas that have a stalk of nonneoplastic mucosa and submucosa of variable length. There is a tendency for macroscopic appearance to associate with anatomical site: carcinomas in the left colon are more frequently endophytic, whereas those in the right colon proximal to the splenic flexure are more often exophytic. On cut section of the mass, the mucinous histopathologic type and mucinous areas within other histopathologic types have a gelatinous appearance (5). The macroscopic appearances have implications for detection by radiographic procedures and endoscopy, which address the wall and lumen as contrasted with the luminal surface respectively.

Perforation

Ulceration or fistula formation through the necrotic portion of colon carcinomas located above the peritoneal reflection and on the portion of the circumference covered by serosa can lead to transmural perforation into the peritoneal cavity. When the tumor becomes adherent to other organs, fistula tracts can develop into other anatomical sites in the GI tract in the case of colon carcinoma, and into pelvic organs in the case of rectal carcinoma. Fistula formation can also occur into pericolic fibroadipose tissue of the mesentery or retroperitoneum, depending upon anatomic location. Perforation can occur through nonneoplastic colonic wall due to ischemia or obstruction.

Obstruction

Stricture of the lumen due to tumor constriction of the colorectal wall, development of a large exophytic mass, or kinking of the lumen due to adhesion to other intraabdominal structures can lead to obstruction of passage of feces. The colorectum proximal to the site of obstruction is usually dilated as compared to the more distal lumen, although poststenotic dilatation can occur. Inflammation of the mucosa, often with the histopathologic findings of ischemic injury, can occur as a result of obstructive colitis (6).

Distant Metastasis

The most common site of distant metastasis is the liver, followed by the lungs (5). The size and appearance of the metastasis are influenced by pathologic factors analogous to the primary tumor, including duration, vascular supply, anatomic location, and surrounding structures.

Context

Evaluation of the bowel away from the colon or rectal carcinoma is important in determining the context in which the tumor developed. For example, mucosal changes of chronic inflammatory bowel disease that was a predisposing condition can be detected, but must be distinguished from obstructive colitis in patients whose tumor produces obstruction (6). The presence of large numbers of polyps raises the question of a polyposis syndrome, and the histopathologic classification of the polyps is the starting point for diagnosis. The histopathology of mural abnormalities is also important. Ureterosigmoidostomies are evident.

Histopathology of Colon and Rectal Carcinoma

Definition of Carcinoma

The term "carcinoma" should be applied in the colorectum to only those epithelial tumors that have invaded through the muscularis mucosae into the submucosa because a tumor with this characteristic has potential for metastasis and resultant mortality of the patient (5). By contrast, a tumor with the histopathologic characteristics of carcinoma that has invaded only the muscularis mucosae and/or lamina propria, sometimes termed "intramucosal carcinoma" because it has invasion that is a hallmark of malignancy, has essentially no propensity for metastasis (1,2,5). The same holds true for those lesions that have the architectural and cytologic features of carcinoma but are confined to the epithelium ("in situ carcinoma" or "intraepithelial carcinoma"). The role of histopathologic sampling of the lesion is obviously crucial, as failure to detect submucosal involvement can explain the very rare cases that have metastasis but appear to violate the definition of carcinoma in the colorectum that is based upon breaching of the muscularis mucosae.

The term "high-grade dysplasia" is often used for those CRC-like lesions that have not invaded beyond the muscularis mucosae (5), but the term "carcinoma in situ" is also used (1,2). This inconsistent terminology that is unique to the colorectum is the source of confusion in clinical management, because "intramucosal carcinoma" in other anatomical sites in the GI tract (eg, esophagus and stomach) can lead to metastasis and mortality in a small subset of patients, as contrasted to the colorectum. The explanation of this unusual discordance between histopathology and tumor biology is unknown. The historical explanation that lymphatic vessels are not present in the colorectal mucosa is incorrect, as evidenced by the presence of lymphoid nodules and associated lymphatics. Regardless of the explanation, use of the terminology "high-grade dysplasia" despite evidence of mucosal invasion helps to limit overtreatment of benign-behaving lesions.

Types of Carcinoma

By far, the vast majority (more than 90%) of colon and rectal carcinoma is adenocarcinoma (5). There is also a variety of other histopathologic subtypes that can be seen, as summarized in Table 6.2.

Adenocarcinoma

The glandular features of adenocarcinomas can vary from architectural findings of well-formed glands to histopathologic findings of subtle intracytoplasmic mucin vacuoles to expression of antigens such as villin and mucoprotein backbones. "Dirty necrosis" (7) in topographic regions is often seen in colon and rectal adenocarcinoma without high levels of microsatellite instability (MSI-H).

Subtypes of Adenocarcinoma (5)

Mucinous adenocarcinoma is applied to tumors with more than 50% of the lesion consisting of extracellular mucin, usually in pools containing detached malignant cells, or with malignant epithelium lining the pools. These tumors often have MSI-H, and molecular characterization is important in determining prognosis. MSI-H mucinous adenocarcinomas are low-grade whereas mucinous adenocarcinomas without MSI-H are often highly aggressive (5,8,9). Mucinous areas comprising less than 50% of the carcinoma are seen commonly.

Signet ring cell carcinoma is characterized by more than 50% of the tumor cells with a prominent intracytoplasmic mucin vacuole that displaces and alters the configuration of the nucleus. This type of tumor can occur as a diffusely infiltrating type, like linitis plastica of the stomach with poorly cohesive tumor cells infiltrating through the mural structures with relatively little host reaction, in the desmoplastic stroma, or with the signet ring cells situated within mucin pools, often in clusters, as a component of mucinous adenocarcinoma. The term "globoid cells" is sometimes used to refer to prominent mucin vacuoles that are substantially larger than the nucleus of the tumor cell. As in mucinous adenocarcinoma as described above, microsatellite instability status is associated with the biological behavior.

Medullary carcinoma has sheets of large tumor cells that have large, vesicular nuclei, prominent nucleoli, abundant eosinophilic cytoplasm, often with little or no gland formation (10). A striking feature is the occurrence of numerous tumor-infiltrating lymphocytes that represent host immunologic response to this type of tumor that nearly always has MSI-H.

Serrated adenocarcinomas have saw-tooth configuration to the malignant glands. These tumors often have MSI-H, BRAF mutation, and CpG island methylation (see Molecular Pathology section below).

Table 6.2 Histopathologic Classification of Carcinoma of the Colon and Rectum

Type	Subtype	ICD-O code
Adenocarcinoma		8140/3
	Mucinous adenocarcinoma (>50% mucinous)	8480/3
	Signet-ring/globoid cell carcinoma (>50% signet-ring)	8490/3
	Cribriform comedo-type adenocarcinoma	8201/3
	Micropapillary carcinoma	8265/3
	Serrated adenocarcinoma	8213/3
	Adenocarcinoma in situ*	8510/3
Medullary carcinoma		8510/3
Adenosquamous carcinoma		8560/3
Squamous cell carcinoma		8070/3
Spindle cell carcinoma		8032/3
Neuroendocrine carcinoma		8246/3
	Large cell neuroendocrine carcinoma	8013/3
	Small cell neuroendocrine carcinoma	8041/3
Mixed adenoneuroendocrine carcinoma		8244/3
Undifferentiated carcinoma		8020/3
Carcinoma, not otherwise specified (NOS)		8010/3
Other rare variants (see text)		

* The terms "high-grade dysplasia" and "severe dysplasia" are preferable as synonyms for in situ adenocarcinoma and in situ carcinoma (2).
Modified from (1,2,5).

Cribriform comedo-type carcinoma resembles comedocarcinoma of the breast in having "Roman bridge" architecture with bands of tumor cells across the gland lumina. There is a strong association of this histologic type with CpG island methylation (see Molecular Pathology below).

Micropapillary adenocarcinoma has small clusters of malignant cells within stromal spaces that sometimes have the appearance of vascular channels.

Adenosquamous carcinoma has squamous areas and gland-forming areas, or admixtures of the cell types within the topography of the tumor.

Other Types of Carcinoma (5)

Pure squamous cell carcinoma is exceedingly uncommon in the colon and rectum.

Spindle cell carcinoma has a sarcomatoid appearance but retains keratin expression, resulting in its classification as carcinoma rather than sarcoma.

Undifferentiated carcinoma represents a diagnosis of exclusion due to the absence of other types of differentiation. Occasional tumors of this type have MSI-H.

Rare variants include poorly cohesive carcinoma in which the tumor cells resemble macophages without signet ring cells, Paneth cell-rich papillary adenocarcinoma, clear-cell carcinoma, and choriocarcinoma.

Neuroendocrine Tumors

This type of tumor is uncommon in the colon and rectum, but is generally classified as in other areas of the GI tract (Table 6.3).

Tumor Grade

In adenocarcinomas, differentiation is based upon the extent of glandular architecture, although cytologic features are often taken into consideration (Table 6.4).

The glandular pattern in adenocarcinomas is strikingly heterogeneous in size and shape, and is influenced by desmoplastic host reaction. Poor differentiation at the invasive front of some gland-forming adenocarcinomas is characterized by invasion of individual or small clusters of cancer cells and has been termed "tumor budding" (5,11,12).

Histopathologic Features of Colon and Rectal Carcinoma (5)

A hallmark of colon and rectal carcinoma is invasion from the mucosa into the deeper layers of the large bowel. The extent and site of invasion are important, and when invasion occurs through the muscularis propria, the anatomy dictates the structures that become involved. Extension to the serosal surface provides access of the cancer to the peritoneal cavity (13) or into other peritonealized organs when adherence of the two surfaces occurs due to peritoneal reaction. Invasion into the perirectal fibroadipose tissue or the retroperitoneum of the areas of the colon that are covered by fibroadipose tissue, for example, the cecum, occurs in nonperitonealized sites.

Invasion provides access to mural structures that in turn provide routes for metastasis: lymphatic vessels that drain into lymph nodes; capillaries that on the venous side drain into the portal tract initially to the liver from the colon or into the caval system from the rectum; and perineural spaces and nerves. Host response is manifested by tumor-infiltrating lymphocytes and peritumoral lymphoid nodules that have been dubbed "Crohn-like lymphoid response" (14–16) despite no association with the inflammatory bowel disease, as well as by desmoplastic connective tissue that can be highly variable in amount. Metastasis to lymph nodes is related to anatomical site of the carcinoma (Table 6.5).

Metastasis in lymph nodes may replace the nodal tissue, involve only small areas, often in the subcapsular sinuses, or occur as individual tumor cells (ITCs) that are difficult to detect by light microscopy alone. Discontinuous extranodal tumor deposits that develop from vascular involvement can mimic obliterated lymph nodes (17,18).

The number of lymph nodes that are harvested and examined by histopathology is important in evaluating the quality of surgery and of pathologic examination (19–23). A minimum of 12 lymph nodes is required, but preoperative therapy reduces the number of lymph nodes that can be found so that the size of the examined lymph nodes is also a quality indicator. Small lymph nodes of 1 to 2 mm in size should be present in the histopathologic sections.

Surgical margins of resection are the regions of colon and rectal resection specimens that are transected by the surgeon, or gastroenterologist in the case of snare polypectomy and endoscopic mucosal or submucosal resection (24–28). These margins must be distinguished from anatomic structures, for example, the serosal surface, for purposes of staging. The use of tattoo powder or colored tattoo ink is especially helpful in the subsequent histopathologic distinction of margins and anatomical structures. The distance of the carcinoma from the resection margins and the integrity of those margins, especially the circumferential margin in total mesorectal excision of rectal carcinoma, are important in assessing the quality of surgical technique and providing indicators of prognosis (Table 6.6).

Effects of Therapy

With the advent of routine preoperative neoadjuvant chemoradiation for rectal cancer and initial efforts at preoperative neoadjuvant chemotherapy for colon cancer, the histopathology of the resected or re-biopsied tumor is often altered by the treatment effects when the therapy is effective (29–32). Manifestation includes the absence of residual tumor with replacement by fibrosis, often with hemosiderin deposition and cholesterol clefts; large areas of necrosis; and bizarre nuclear cytology. Residual tumor/regression after therapy is now graded (Table 6.7).

Table 6.3 Classification of Neuroendocrine Tumors of the Colon and Rectum

Classification	Subtype	Criteria	ICD-O code
Neuroendocrine tumor, grade 1 (NET G1, carcinoid)		Less than 2 mitotic figures/10 high power fields and/or ≤ 2% Ki67 labeling index	8240/3
	EC cell, serotonin-producing neuroendocrine tumor*		8241/3
	L cell, glucagon-like peptide and PP/PYY-producing NETs*		8152/1
Neuroendocrine tumor, grade 2 (NET G2)		2–20 mitotic figures/10 high power fields and/or 3%–20% Ki67 labeling index	8249/3
Neuroendocrine carcinoma (NEC)		Greater than 20 mitotic figures/10 high power fields and/or > 20% Ki67 labeling index	8246/3
	Large cell NEC		8013/3
	Small cell NEC		8041/3
Mixed adenoneuroendocrine carcinoma (MANEC)		Component of adenocarcinoma and neuroendocrine carcinoma	8244/3

* These subtypes are occasionally grade 2.
Modified from (1,5).

Table 6.4 Criteria for Histopathologic Grading of Colon and Rectal Adenocarcinomas

Criterion	Differentiation	Grade*	Description
Greater than 95% glands	Well differentiated	1	Low-grade
50%–95% glands	Moderately differentiated	2	Low-grade
Greater than 0–49% glands	Poorly differentiated	3	High-grade*
No glands	Undifferentiated	3 (6), 4 (1)	High-grade*

* MSI-H is associated with better prognosis despite the threatening histopathologic appearance. As a result, MSI-H carcinomas are classified as low-grade with the molecular features overriding the histopathologic findings.
Modified from (1,5).

Table 6.5 Regional Lymph Nodes of the Colon and Rectum

Segment	Regional Lymph Nodes*
Cecum	Pericolic, anterior cecal, posterior cecal, ileocolic, right colic
Ascending colon	Pericolic, ileocolic, right colic, middle colic
Hepatic flexure	Pericolic, middle colic, right colic
Transverse colon	Pericolic, middle colic
Splenic flexure	Pericolic, middle colic, left colic, inferior mesenteric
Descending colon	Pericolic, left colic, inferior mesenteric, sigmoid
Sigmoid colon	Pericolic, inferior mesenteric, superior rectal (hemorrhoidal), sigmoidal, sigmoid mesenteric
Rectosigmoid	Pericolic, perirectal, left colic, sigmoid mesenteric, sigmoidal, inferior mesenteric, superior rectal (hemorrhoidal), middle rectal (hemorrhoidal)
Rectum	Perirectal, sigmoid mesenteric, inferior mesenteric, lateral sacral, presacral, internal iliac, sacral promontory, superior rectal (hemorrhoidal), middle rectal (hemorrhoidal), inferior rectal (hemorrhoidal)

*Metastasis to lymph node outside of these sites is distant metastasis.
Modified from (1,2).

Table 6.6 Categorization of Surgical Margins of Resection for Residual Tumor (AJCC, 7th Edition)

R0	Complete resection, margins histologically negative, no residual tumor left after resection (primary tumor, regional nodes)
R1	Incomplete resection, margins histologically involved, microscopic tumor remains after resection of gross disease (primary tumor, regional nodes)
R2	Incomplete resection, margins macroscopically involved or gross disease remains after resection (eg, primary tumor, regional nodes, or liver metastasis)

Modified from (1).

Table 6.7 Tumor Regression Grade After Preoperative Neoadjuvant Therapy

Description	Tumor Regression Grade/Residual Tumor
No viable cancer cells/no residual tumor	0 (Complete response)
Single cells or small groups of cancer cells	1 (Moderate response /minimal residual tumor)
Residual cancer outgrown by fibrosis	2 (Minimal response)
Minimal or no tumor kill; extensive residual cancer	3 (Poor response /no definite response)

Modified from (1,2).

Table 6.8 Primary Tumor (T Categories) for TNM Staging of Colon and Rectal Carcinoma (AJCC, 7th Edition)

TX	Primary tumor cannot be assessed
T0	No evidence of primary tumor
Tis	Carcinoma in situ: Intraepithelial or invasion of lamina propria*
T1	Tumor invades through the muscularis mucosae into submucosa
T2	Tumor invades into, but not through, muscularis propria
T3	Tumor invades through the muscularis propria into pericolic/perirectal tissues
T4a	Tumor penetrates to the surface of the visceral peritoneum**
T4b	Tumor directly invades or is adherent to other organs or structures**,***

* Tis includes cancer confined within the crypt basement membrane (intraepithelial) or lamina propria of the mucosa (intramucosal) with no invasion through the muscularis mucosae into the submucosa.

** Direct invasion in T4 includes invasion of other organs or other segments of the colorectum as a result of direct extension through the serosa, as confirmed on microscopic examination or, for cancers in a retroperitoneal or subperitoneal location, direct invasion of other organs or structures by virtue of extension beyond the muscularis propria.

*** Tumor that is adherent to other organs or structures on visual examination or imaging, is classified as cT4b. However, if no tumor is present in the adhesion on histopathology, the classification is pT1–4a depending on the anatomical depth of wall invasion.
Modified From (1).

Staging and Prognosis

Many of the macroscopic and histopathologic features of colon and rectal cancer as already discussed above are indicators of prognosis. Beginning in the late 1920s, pathologic classifications that grouped cases and then compared the survival outcome of the patients in the groups were reported. The best known from that era is the Dukes classifications proposed in a series of papers by Cuthbert Dukes of St. Mark's Hospital in London. This classification of patients who underwent curative resection of rectal carcinoma without evident residual or metastatic disease was based upon depth of invasion and status of regional lymph nodes. These features remain as the key elements in the TNM (Tumor, Nodes, Metastasis) classification that is in use today for colon and rectal carcinoma and that has expanded the categories to patients with residual and metastatic disease. The American Joint Committee on Cancer (AJCC) in collaboration with the World Health Organization (WHO) and International Union Against Cancer (UICC) has created and repeatedly updated the TNM system that is in world-wide use for staging (1,5,6,33–35). The criteria of the AJCC seventh edition from 2010 with minor descriptive modifications are shown in Tables 6.8 to 6.10.

Prefixes are used in these categories to provide additional details: p for pathologic staging; c for clinical staging including use of diagnostic imaging; y for staging after neoadjuvant therapy and surgical resection; and r for recurrent tumor staged after a disease-free interval (1). The TNM categories are grouped into stage groupings as shown in Table 6.11.

In addition to TNM stage, which has been linked to survival data to provide survival rates for patients in the stage groupings (1), additional prognostic pathologic factors are recognized to contribute to the estimation of patient outcome (Table 6.12).

The AJCC staging system for neuroendocrine tumors of the colon and rectum differs from that for carcinomas. In the T category, no "in situ" (Tis) category is included, although the category appears in the anatomic stage/prognostic groups, and tumor size is a criterion in addition to depth of invasion (Table 6.13). The lymph node (N) and distant metastasis categories, and therefore the anatomic stage/prognostic groups, are less complex than that for carcinomas (Tables 6.14 to 6.16).

Histopathologic Manifestations of Predisposing Conditions

In addition to the emphasis on histopathologic examination of the tumor in specimens of colon and rectal

Table 6.9 Regional Lymph Nodes (N Categories) for TNM Staging of Colon and Rectal Carcinoma (AJCC, 7th Edition)

NX	Regional lymph nodes cannot be assessed
N0	No regional lymph node metastasis
N1	Metastasis in 1 to 3 regional lymph nodes
N1a	Metastasis in 1 regional lymph node
N1b	Metastasis in 2 to 3 regional lymph nodes
N1c	Tumor deposit(s) in the subserosa, mesentery, or nonperitonealized pericolic or perirectal tissues without identified regional nodal metastasis
N2	Metastasis in 4 or more regional lymph nodes
N2a	Metastasis in 4 to 6 regional lymph nodes
N2b	Metastasis in 7 or more regional lymph nodes

Modified from (1).

Table 6.10 Distant Metastasis (M Categories) for TNM Staging of Colon and Rectal Carcinoma (AJCC, 7th Edition)

M0	No distant metastasis
M1	Distant metastasis
M1a	Metastasis confined to one organ or site (eg., liver, lung, ovary, nonregional node)
M1b	Metastases in more than one organ/site or the peritoneum

Modified from (1).

Table 6.11 Anatomic Stage/Prognostic Groups of Colon and Rectal Carcinoma (AJCC, 7th Edition)

Stage	T	N	M
0	Tis	N0	M0
I	T1	N0	M0
	T2	N0	M0
IIA	T3	N0	M0
IIB	T4a	N0	M0
IIC	T4b	N0	M0
IIIA	T1-T2	N1/N1c	M0
	T1	N2a	M0
IIIB	T3-T4a	N1/N1c	M0
	T2-T3	N2a	M0
	T1-T2	N2b	M0
IIIC	T4a	N2a	M0
	T3-T4a	N2b	M0
	T4b	N1-N2	M0
IVA	Any T	Any N	M1a
IVB	Any T	Any N	M1b

Modified from (1).

Table 6.12 Prognostic (Site-Specific) Pathologic Factors

Discontinuous extranodal tumor deposits (17,18)*
Circumferential resection margin (28)*
Perineural invasion*
Tumor regression grade after neo-adjuvant therapy (30–32)
Tumor budding (5,11,12)

*Quality indicator (BMJ Open 2013;3:e002818)
Modified from (1).

Table 6.13 Primary Tumor (T) Categories for TNM Staging of Colon and Rectal Neuroendocrine Tumors (AJCC, 7th Edition)

TX	Primary tumor cannot be assessed
T0	No evidence of primary tumor
T1	Tumor invades lamina propria or submucosa and size 2 cm or less
T1a	Tumor size less than 1 cm in greatest dimension
T1b	Tumor size 1 to 2 cm in greatest dimension
T2	Tumor invades muscularis propria or size more than 2 cm with invasion of lamina propria or submucosa
T3	Tumor invades through the muscularis propria into the subserosa, or into nonperitonealized pericolic or perirectal tissues
T4	Tumor invades peritoneum or other organs

The prefix m is added for multiple tumors due to the higher frequency of multiplicity of neuroendocrine tumors than carcinomas.
Modified from (1).

Table 6.14 Regional Lymph Node (N) Categories for TNM Staging of Colon and Rectal Neuroendocrine Tumors (AJCC, 7th Edition)

NX	Regional lymph nodes cannot be assessed
N0	No regional lymph node metastasis
N1	Regional lymph node metastasis

Modified from (1).

Table 6.15 Distant Metastasis (M) Categories for TNM Staging of Colon and Rectal Neuroendocrine Tumors (AJCC, 7th Edition)

M0	No distant metastasis
M1	Distant metastasis

Modified from (1).

Table 6.16 Anatomic Stage/Prognostic Groups of Colon and Rectal Neuroendocrine Tumors (AJCC, 7th Edition)

Stage	T	N	M
0	Tis	N0	M0
I	T1	N0	M0
IIA	T2	N0	M0
IIB	T3	N0	M0
IIIA	T4	N0	M0
IIIB	Any T	N1	M0
IV	Any T	Any N	M1

Stage III includes cases without lymph node metastasis, in contrast to the colon and rectal carcinoma groups.
Modified from (1).

carcinoma, the context in which the tumor developed can sometimes be identified. Chronic inflammatory bowel diseases predispose to colon and rectal cancer, and the histopathologic manifestations of ulcerative colitis, Crohn disease, and schistosomiasis can be recognized, sometimes in patients who have no antecedent diagnosis of the conditions. Polyposis syndromes (see Chapter 2) can be recognized by the presence of multiple polyps, and the classification of the syndromes that directs genetic testing begins with the histopathology of the polyps.

The histopathologic characteristics of colon and rectal carcinomas that arise through the microsatellite instability pathway can provide a clue to the presence of Lynch syndrome (see Chapter 6). These findings can impact the surveillance of the patient who has developed a colon or rectal cancer, and direct attention to family members who may be at risk for inherited syndromes.

Pathology Reporting

The quality of pathology reporting is important to estimation of patient prognosis. As a result, a variety of pathology professional organizations around the world have addressed standardization and quality control/quality assurance of reporting on colon and rectal carcinomas (33). In the United States, the College of American Pathologists (CAP) as part of the International Collaboration on Cancer Reporting (ICCR) has created a protocol for the examination of specimens that includes required data elements. The protocol, along with those for other cancer types, is available on the organization's website at www.CAP.org. The protocol is coordinated with the American Joint Committee on Cancer and International Union Against Cancer classification. The protocol addresses excisional biopsy/polypectomy specimens and resection specimens including transanal disk excision of rectal neoplasms. The delineation of required data elements provides a benchmark for the quality of pathology reports and specific data elements to be included. For example, the Case Summary for resection specimens requires:

- Specimen type
- Surgical procedure
- Tumor site
- Tumor size
- Macroscopic tumor perforation
- Histologic type
- Histologic grade
- Microscopic tumor extension
- Margin status for all applicable margins
- Treatment effects
- Lymphovascular invasion
- Perineural invasion
- Discontinuous extramural tumor deposits
- TNM pathologic stage

■ PATHOLOGY OF PRECURSOR LESIONS AND CONDITIONS

Adenoma

The most common precursor lesion to colon and rectal carcinoma is the colorectal adenoma. The vast majority of the carcinomas that develop in an adenoma is adenocarcinoma, but neuroendocrine carcinoma is found on occasion. The benign adenoma is characterized by dysplastic epithelium that has a spectrum of changes from low-grade to high-grade as defined by architectural complexity, nuclear stratification, and nuclear morphology. The adenoma is commonly polypoid with elevation into the colorectal lumen and can be on a stalk of non-neoplastic mucosa and submucosa. The lesion can be sessile or flat with little elevation above the mucosal surface, or depressed, sometimes making recognition difficult. Characteristics of adenomas associated with increased occurrence of carcinoma are larger size, the presence of villous architecture, and high-grade epithelial dysplasia, features that define the "advanced adenoma" (36). The microscopic precursor to adenoma is easily defined in familial adenomatous polyposis (FAP) as dysplastic aberrant crypt foci (dACF), but these lesions are uncommonly found in patients with sporadic colorectal neoplasia (37).

Serrated Lesions

The hallmark of serrated lesions is a stellate or sawtooth architecture of the gland lumina because of the configuration of the epithelium. The lesions that manifest serration, however, are diverse, including their molecular pathogenesis (38–42).

The serrated lesion of greatest interest is the sessile serrated adenoma/polyp (SSA/P) that most commonly occurs in the right colon and is now recognized as one of the precursor lesions to colon and rectal carcinomas with MSI-H. Dysplasia occurs in some SSA/Ps and is the precursor to the invasive carcinoma.

The traditional serrated adenoma is uncommon, usually occurs in the left colon, and has a distinctive syncytial eosinophilic epithelium.

The hyperplastic polyp is most frequent in the distal colon and rectum and was the earliest recognized serrated polyp. This lesion has an association with colon, and especially rectal, carcinoma but is not thought to be a precursor lesion from which cancer arises.

Hamartomatous Polyps

This category of precursor is also diverse. Hamartomatous polyps associated with colon and rectal carcinoma include the juvenile polyp with dilated glands and abundant inflamed stroma in the setting of juvenile polyposis syndrome (JPS), but not in the sporadic setting, and unusual branched polyps in patients with JPS; Peutz-Jeghers hamartomas with characteristic smooth muscle arborization that is sometimes subtle, making classification difficult; and Cowden's syndrome (PTEN deficiency syndrome) polyps. The latter are remarkably heterogeneous in their histopathology and can resemble juvenile polyps with dilatation of crypts and inflamed stroma but also can be ganglioneuromas, lipomas, and polypoid lymphoid hyperplasia.

Although the hamartomatous polyposis syndromes are associated with increased risk of CRC, epithelial dysplasia within the hamartomas themselves is relatively uncommon. Pseudo-carcinomatous epithelial entrapment/pseudoinvasion is a hallmark of Peutz-Jeghers polyps and can be mistaken for invasive carcinoma.

Dysplasia Complicating Chronic Inflammatory Bowel Diseases

Dysplasia that often resembles adenomatous epithelium can be found in patients with ulcerative colitis, Crohn's disease, and schistosomiasis.

MOLECULAR PATHOLOGY OF COLON AND RECTAL CARCINOMA

The understanding of the molecular underpinnings of colorectal neoplasia has evolved over more than three decades with the application of advancing genetic and genomic technologies. The pathways that participate in the development of colon and rectal cancer are well-elucidated (5,8). The striking molecular heterogeneity among tumors and the differences in the molecular characteristics of cancers from different geographic, racial, and ethnic patient populations are now clear and highlight the difficulty in making further progress in the treatment and prevention of the disease, due to the occurrence of numerous molecular subtypes.

Three main molecular subtypes have been defined: the chromosomal instability pathway, the microsatellite instability pathway, and the CpG island hypermethylation pathway (Table 6.17).

Chromosomal Instability Pathway (CIN)

This pathway is characterized by alterations at the level of chromosomes, including amplifications, deletions, and rearrangements. The initiating molecular basis is abnormality in *Wnt/APC/beta-catenin* pathway genes that result in beta-catenin transcription factor migration to the cell nucleus and loss of regulation of a large number of genes. The inherited form of colon and rectal cancers in this pathway occurs in FAP in which there is a germline mutation in the *APC* gene followed by somatic inactivation or loss of the second allele through loss of the long arm of chromosome 5, methylation of the promoter region of *APC*, or inactivating mutation of the second previously wild type allele. In the sporadic setting, inactivation of the pathway occurs via a variety of mechanisms. Ninety-four percent of colon and rectal cancers in The Cancer Genome Atlas (TCGA) study (43) have a mutation in one or more members of the Wnt signaling pathway, including a total of 16 different genes, for example, *beta-catenin, SOX9, ARID1A, FAM123B*, the *DKK* family, and *TCF7L2*. Progression events in this pathway include the acquisition of rearrangements, deletions, and amplifications of chromosomes manifested as allelic imbalances, and frequent mutations in *K-ras, TP53*, and *PIK3CA* and *SMAD4*.

Table 6.17 Molecular Pathways in Colorectal Neoplasia

Pathway	Molecular Basis	Progression Events
Chromosomal instability (CIN)	*APC-beta catenin* genes in Wnt pathway Inherited type: FAP	Allelic imbalances and gene mutations
Microsatellite instability (MSI-H)	Nucleotide mismatch repair genes Inherited form: Lynch (HNPCC) Sporadic type: Hypermethylation of *MLH1*	Gene mutations
Microsatellite instability (MSI-L)	Uncertain	Gene mutations and allelic imbalances
CpG island methylation (CIMP)	Dysregulation of DNA methyltransferases	Transcriptional silencing, chromatin alterations,
MUTYH	*MutYH* base excision repair gene Inherited (recessive)	G→T mutations, 18q, etc. LOH
Ultramutated	Multiple mismatch repair genes or DNA polymerase gene	Allelic imbalances and gene mutations
Non-coding RNA (ncRNA)	Dysregulation of ncRNAs	Altered gene expression

Microsatellite Instability Pathway (MSI)

In contrast to the chromosomal instability pathway, the microsatellite instability pathway is characterized by infrequent chromosomal-level alterations but numerous mutations in repeated nucleotide sequences, termed microsatellites, and in individual nucleotides (8,43–45). The hallmark is lengthening and shorting of microsatellites due to failure of mismatch repair after DNA replication errors as a result of alterations in nucleotide mismatch repair gene function. The inherited form of the disease is Lynch syndrome due to an inherited alteration, most commonly in *MSH2* or *MLH1*, followed by inactivation of the second copy of the gene (see Chapter 2). In the sporadic setting, hypermethylation of the promoter of the *MLH1* gene is responsible. The progression events are characterized by numerous gene mutations, with a different pattern of mutations as compared to CIN, especially numerous frameshift mutations, including the *APC* gene that is frequently mutated in the *TCGA* set. The differences in the mutation profiles are illustrated in Table 6.18.

A subset of tumors with alteration in the length of microsatellites has infrequent changes, and is termed microsatellite instability-low (MSI-L). The molecular basis of this subset, as well as the clinical implications, are not yet well explained.

CpG Island Methylation (CIMP)

This pathway is characterized by acquired hypermethylation of the promoter region and initial exons of a large number of genes in the genome that have CpG dinucleotide islands in their sequence (8,46,47). The molecular basis is the transcriptional silencing of genes that acquire hypermethylation accompanied by alterations in chromatin structure. Subtypes in this group in the *TCGA* set are characterized by hypermethylation of the *MLH1* gene that leads to MSI-H with extensive methylation referred to as CIMP-high; lower levels of hypermethylation termed CIMP-low; and two clusters with infrequent methylation distinguished by different patterns of involved genes (43).

MutYH Pathway

This rare pathway involves germline abnormality of the *MutYH* base excision repair gene, with the phenotype manifested when both copies of the gene are inactivated in the child of parents, each with a germline abnormality in the gene. The resulting phenotype is similar to attenuated FAP in having small numbers of adenomas and late onset of colon or rectal carcinoma. The molecular progression includes high frequency of G-to-T mutations in genes and frequent allelic losses, for example, chromosome 18q (5).

Ultramutated Pathway

This small subset of colon and rectal cancers found in the *TCGA* set has an extremely high rate of mutations in the genome, often more than 100 per 10^6 bases, in the absence of MSI-H (43). These tumors are characterized by multiple mutations in mismatch repair genes, including *MLH1, MLH3, MSH2, MSH3, MSH6*, and *PMS2*, or mutation in DNA polymerase genes, especially POLE (epsilon). Subsequent alterations are similar to those in microsatellite-stable CRC (48).

Table 6.18 Comparison of Ranked Frequency in *TCGA* of Mutated and Expressed Genes in Nonhypermutated (Mainly Chromosomal Instability Type) and Hypermutated (Mainly Microsatellite Instability Type) Colon and Rectal Carcinomas

Gene	Rank in Non-Hypermutated CRC (% of Tumors)	Rank in Hypermutated CRC (% of Tumors)
APC	1 (81)	2 (51)
TP53	2 (60)	–
K-ras	3 (43)	–
TTN	4 (31)	–
PIK3CA	5 (18)	–
FBXW7	6 (11)	–
SMAD4	7 (10)	–
NRAS	8 (9)	–
TCF7L2	9 (9)	8 (31)
ACVR2A	–	1 (63)
TGFBR2	–	3 (51)
BRAF	–	4 (46)
MSH3	–	5 (40)
MSH6	–	6 (40)
MYO1B	–	7 (31)
CASP8	–	9 (29)

From (43).

Non-Coding RNA Pathway

Non-coding RNAs include small and long types that are important in gene regulation (49–56). The small non-coding microRNAs (miRNAs) have been much better characterized than the long ones and are known to be overexpressed and underexpressed, and in turn to result in up- or down-regulation of gene expression, including numerous genes known to be important in colorectal tumorigenesis. These have potential as biomarkers (see next section).

■ CLINICAL-PATHOLOGIC CORRELATIONS WITH MOLECULAR PATHWAYS

The molecular pathways that are altered in colon and rectal cancers have loose associations with pathologic features. Non-hypermutated colon and rectal carcinomas had no significant differences in the *TCGA* set (43). The presence of *K-ras* mutation has been associated with a polypoid growth pattern (57), and MSI-H with right-sided location, poor differentiation including mucinous and signet-ring cell types, variegated histopathologic patterns, frequent tumor-infiltrating lymphocytes and Crohn-like lymphoid nodules, absence of "dirty necrosis," and association with SSA/P as a frequent precursor lesion (15,16,58,59).

Clinical characteristics are also associated with molecular pathways and have potential as biomarkers. The overall survival of patients with *BRAF* mutation in their colon and rectal cancer varies with the context; those with MSI-H have survival similar to patients with MSI-H who lack the *BRAF* mutation (60–62), whereas cancers that are microsatellite-stable or MSI-L and have *BRAF* mutation are associated with poor prognosis (61,62). The responses of colon carcinomas to adjuvant chemotherapy are influenced by MSI status. MSI-H cancers have little or no improved outcome after therapy with 5-fluorouracil (5-FU; 63), but survival may be improved by a combination of 5-FU with irinotecan (64,65) or with oxaliplatin (66,67). These results may be explained by MSI-H associated mutation of *MRE11A* or *hRAD50* that regulate double-strand breaks and sensitize the cell to irinotecan, or the lack of recognition of the bulky adducts of oxaliplatin by mismatch repair proteins. Preclinical studies have identified methotrexate as an active agent in MSI-H cell lines (68). Overexpression of miR155 or miR-21 is associated with down-regulation of MLH1 and MSH2 and may reduce 5-FU efficacy (69). On the other hand, mutation of heat shock protein 110 or MSH3 in MSI-H cells sensitizes to 5-FU and oxaliplatin or poly(ADP-ribose) polymerase (PARP) inhibitors (70–72). The absence of chromosomal instability is associated with taxane sensitivity. Selective inhibition of the PI3K/AKT/mTOR pathway has potential for benefit (73–75), and the high frequency of *BRAF* mutation in MSI-H cancers suggests a role for *BRAF* inhibitors. Translation of these preclinical leads into therapies requires clinical studies.

Gene expression profiling has drawn substantial attention in attempts to produce signatures for the clinical behavior of CRC (76–78), but at the present time, clinical utility of microsatellite instability status, *K-ras* mutation, *BRAF* mutation, *PI3CA* mutation, *PTEN* expression, and *MLH1* methylation has been reported. As shown in Table 6.18, these molecular alterations can be useful in evaluation of patients for the presence of Lynch syndrome (79–81); in estimating prognosis; in consideration of use of postoperative adjuvant chemotherapy; and in use of epithermal growth factor receptor (EGFR)-inhibiting antibodies (82–85). Loss of mismatch repair proteins (86) or polymerase chain reaction analysis of mono- or dinucleotide repeat sequences can indicate the presence of MSI-H (Table 6.19).

In the presence of loss in carcinoma cells of *MLH1* expression (in concert with loss of its *PMS2* binding partner) by immunohistochemistry, the presence of *BRAF* V600E protein by immunohistochemistry (87) or *BRAF* mutation and *MLH1* hypermethylation indicate that the patient has developed the colon or rectal cancer on an acquired, somatic basis. In the absence of *BRAF* mutation and *MLH1* hypermethylation, Lynch syndrome is likely, and sequencing of *MLH1* in the germline can result in the identification of the responsible alteration that can be used in management of at-risk family members. This approach is applicable to all stages of CRC, and universal testing is advocated in the guidelines of the Evaluation of Genomic Applications in Practice and Prevention (EGAPP) Working Group (88) and the National Society of Genetic Counselors and the Collaborative Group of the Americas on Inherited CRC (CGA-ICC; 89).

The stage-specific prognosis of MSI-H CRC in Stage I through Stage IV is more favorable than that of MSI-L and microsatellite-stable carcinomas. This finding can influence decisions about use of postoperative adjuvant therapy in patients with Stage II or III disease, as the risks for patients with a MSI-H carcinoma may outweigh the benefits, especially in Stage II disease (90). By contrast, the adverse outcome of *BRAF*-mutated microsatellite-stable or MSI-L carcinoma can dictate aggressive therapy.

In the selection of patients with Stage IV or recurrent carcinoma for inhibition of the EGFR pathway, abundant data indicate that again? mutation, and probably *BRAF* mutation, *PIK3CA* mutation, and loss of *PTEN* expression, identify patients who are unlikely to respond (63,83,84). The selection of molecular tests to be used is influenced by the stage of the patient's disease.

Table 6.19 Clinical Uses of Molecular Diagnostics in Patients With Colon and Rectal Carcinoma

	Clinical Use				Stage of Colon or Rectal Cancer Patient			
Biomarker*	Lynch syndrome	Prognostic indicator	Chemotherapy decision	EGFRi decision**	I	II	III	IV or Recurrence
MSI by IHC and PCR	X				X	X	X	X
MSI by IHC and PCR		X			X	X	X	X
MSI by IHC and PCR			X			X	X	
K-ras mutation				X				X
BRAF mutation and IHC for V600E				X				X
BRAF mutation and IHC for V600E		X (MSS)***			X	X	X	X
BRAF mutation and IHC for V600E	X (*MLH1* loss)				X	X	X	X
PIK3CA mutation				X				X
PTEN IHC				X				X
MLH1 methylation	X (*MLH1* loss)				X	X	X	X

*MSI, microsatellite instability status. IHC, immunohistochemistry. For MSI IHC evaluation, mismatch repair gene products MSH2, MLH1, MSH6, and PMS2 are used. PCR, polymerase chain reaction amplification of panel of dinucleotide and mononucleotide repeat sequences.

**Epidermal growth factor receptor inhibitor therapy (cetuximab, panitumumab).

***MSS, microsatellite-stable.

CONCLUSIONS

High-quality pathologic examination is essential to high-quality multidisciplinary care of patients with colon or rectal carcinoma. The use of molecular biomarkers based on understanding of the pathogenesis of the malignant disease and its precursor lesions and predisposing conditions has potential to lead to molecular mechanism-based prevention strategies and to targeted therapies. Intra- and intertumoral heterogeneity pose the greatest challenges, as TCGA data show that each carcinoma is unique, representing an "N of 1." Identification of the ever-growing number of molecular subtypes based upon the drivers that dictate tumor biology, and their implications for therapeutic responses, are key (91). Substantial additional research is needed to close the wide gap between the remarkable current understanding of the molecular pathology of colon and rectal carcinoma and the clinical applications of that understanding to improve the outcome of patients with the disease.

REFERENCES

1. Edge SB, Byrd DR, Compton CC, Fritz AG, Greene FK, Trotti A, eds. AJCC Cancer Staging Manual. 17th ed. New York, NY: Springer; 2010, 143–164.
2. Washington K, Berlin F, Branton P, et al. Protocol for the Examination of Specimens from Patients with Primary Carcinoma of the Colon and Rectum. ColoRectum 3.2.0.0, College of American Pathologists, 2012.
3. Soliman AS, Bondy ML, Raouf AA, Makram MA, Johnston DA, Levin B. Cancer mortality in Menofeia, Egypt: comparison with US mortality rates. *Cancer Causes Control.* 1999;10(5):349–354.
4. Freedman LS, Edwards BK, Ries LAG, Young JL. Cancer incidence in four member countries (Cyprus, Egypt, Israel, and Jordon) of the Middle East Cancer Consortium (MECC) Compared with US SEER. MECC Monograph. National Cancer Institute, NIH Pub. No. 06–5873, Bethesda, MD, 41–50.
5. Hamilton SR, Nakamura S-I, Bosman FT, et al. Carcinoma of the colon and rectum. Chapter 8 in WHO Classification of Tumours of the Digestive System. In: Bosman FT, Carneiro F, Hruban RH, Theise ND, eds. International Agency for Research on Cancer, Lyon; 2010:134–146.
6. Lu CC, Chen HH, Lin SE. Ischemic versus non-ischemic obstructive ileocolitis secondary to colorectal cancer: a review of 393 cases. *Jpn J Clin Oncol.* 2010;40(10):927–932.
7. Greenson JK, Huang SC, Herron C, et al. Pathologic predictors of microsatellite instability in colorectal cancer. *Am J Surg Pathol.* 2009;33(1):126–133.
8. Markowitz SD, Bertagnolli MM. Molecular origins of cancer: Molecular basis of colorectal cancer. *N Engl J Med.* 2009;361(25):2449–2460.
9. Kang H, O'Connell JB, Maggard MA, Sack J, Ko CY. A 10-year outcomes evaluation of mucinous and signet-ring cell carcinoma of the colon and rectum. *Dis Colon Rectum.* 2005;48(6):1161–1168.
10. Wick MR, Vitsky JL, Ritter JH, Swanson PE, Mills SE. Sporadic medullary carcinoma of the colon: a clinicopathologic comparison with nonhereditary poorly differentiated enteric-type adenocarcinoma and neuroendocrine colorectal carcinoma. *Am J Clin Pathol.* 2005;123(1):56–65.
11. Mitrovic B, Schaeffer DF, Riddell RH, Kirsch R. Tumor budding in colorectal carcinoma: time to take notice. *Mod Pathol.* 2012;25(10):1315–1325.
12. Karamitopoulou E, Zlobec I, Kölzer V, et al. Proposal for a 10-high-power-fields scoring method for the assessment of tumor budding in colorectal cancer. *Mod Pathol.* 2013;26(2):295–301.
13. Shepherd NA, Baxter KJ, Love SB. The prognostic importance of peritoneal involvement in colonic cancer: a prospective evaluation. *Gastroenterology.* 1997;112(4):1096–1102.
14. Jass JR. Pathology of hereditary nonpolyposis colorectal cancer. *Ann N Y Acad Sci.* 2000;910(Jun):62–73; discussion 73.
15. Alexander J, Watanabe T, Wu TT, Rashid A, Li S, Hamilton SR. Histopathological identification of colon cancer with microsatellite instability. *Am J Pathol.* 2001;158(2):527–535.

16. Greenson JK, Bonner JD, Ben-Yzhak O, et al. Phenotype of microsatellite unstable colorectal carcinomas: Well-differentiated and focally mucinous tumors and the absence of dirty necrosis correlate with microsatellite instability. *Am J Surg Pathol.* 2003;27(5):563–570.
17. Puppa G, Maisonneuve P, Sonzogni A, et al. Pathological assessment of pericolonic tumor deposits in advanced colonic carcinoma: relevance to prognosis and tumor staging. *Mod Pathol.* 2007;20(8):843–855.
18. Lo DS, Pollett A, Siu LL, Gallinger S, Burkes RL. Prognostic significance of mesenteric tumor nodules in patients with stage III colorectal cancer. *Cancer.* 2008;112(1):50–54.
19. Cserni G, Vinh-Hung V, Burzykowski T. Is there a minimum number of lymph nodes that should be histologically assessed for a reliable nodal staging of T3N0M0 colorectal carcinomas? *J Surg Oncol.* 2002;81(2):63–69.
20. Goldstein NS. Lymph node recoveries from 2427 pT3 colorectal resection specimens spanning 45 years: recommendations for a minimum number of recovered lymph nodes based on predictive probabilities. *Am J Surg Pathol.* 2002;26(2):179–189.
21. Chang GJ, Rodriguez-Bigas MA, Skibber JM, Moyer VA. Lymph node evaluation and survival after curative resection of colon cancer: systematic review. *J Natl Cancer Inst.* 2007;99(6):433–441.
22. Görög D, Nagy P, Péter A, Perner F. Influence of obesity on lymph node recovery from rectal resection specimens. *Pathol Oncol Res.* 2003;9(3):180–183.
23. Wijesuriya RE, Deen KI, Hewavisenthi J, Balawardana J, Perera M. Neoadjuvant therapy for rectal cancer down-stages the tumor but reduces lymph node harvest significantly. *Surg Today.* 2005;35(6):442–445.
24. Arbman G, Nilsson E, Hallböök O, Sjödahl R. Local recurrence following total mesorectal excision for rectal cancer. *Br J Surg.* 1996;83(3):375–379.
25. Coverlizza S, Risio M, Ferrari A, Fenoglio-Preiser CM, Rossini FP. Colorectal adenomas containing invasive carcinoma. Pathologic assessment of lymph node metastatic potential. *Cancer.* 1989;64(9):1937–1947.
26. Cooper HS, Deppisch LM, Gourley WK, et al. Endoscopically removed malignant colorectal polyps: clinicopathologic correlations. *Gastroenterology.* 1995;108(6):1657–1665.
27. Cooper HS. Pathology of endoscopically removed malignant colorectal polyp. *Curr Diagn Pathol.* 2007;13(6):423–437.
28. Birbeck KF, Macklin CP, Tiffin NJ, et al. Rates of circumferential resection margin involvement vary between surgeons and predict outcomes in rectal cancer surgery. *Ann Surg.* 2002;235(4):449–457.
29. Kapiteijn E, Marijnen CA, Nagtegaal ID, et al.; Dutch Colorectal Cancer Group. Preoperative radiotherapy combined with total mesorectal excision for resectable rectal cancer. *N Engl J Med.* 2001;345(9):638–646.
30. Gavioli M, Luppi G, Losi L, et al. Incidence and clinical impact of sterilized disease and minimal residual disease after preoperative radiochemotherapy for rectal cancer. *Dis Colon Rectum.* 2005;48(10):1851–1857.
31. Ruo L, Tickoo S, Klimstra DS, et al. Long-term prognostic significance of extent of rectal cancer response to preoperative radiation and chemotherapy. *Ann Surg.* 2002;236(1):75–81.
32. Ryan R, Gibbons D, Hyland JM, et al. Pathological response following long-course neoadjuvant chemoradiotherapy for locally advanced rectal cancer. *Histopathology.* 2005;47(2):141–146.
33. Blenkinsopp WK, Stewart-Brown S, Blesovsky L, Kearney G, Fielding LP. Histopathology reporting in large bowel cancer. *J Clin Pathol.* 1981;34(5):509–513.
34. Di Fabio F, Nascimbeni R, Villanacci V, et al. Prognostic variables for cancer-related survival in node-negative colorectal carcinomas. *Dig Surg.* 2004;21(2):128–133.
35. Fujita S, Shimoda T, Yoshimura K, Yamamoto S, Akasu T, Moriya Y. Prospective evaluation of prognostic factors in patients with colorectal cancer undergoing curative resection. *J Surg Oncol.* 2003;84(3):127–131.
36. Martínez ME, Baron JA, Lieberman DA, et al. A pooled analysis of advanced colorectal neoplasia diagnoses after colonoscopic polypectomy. *Gastroenterology.* 2009;136(3):832–841.
37. Lance P, Hamilton SR. Sporadic aberrant crypt foci are not a surrogate endpoint for colorectal adenoma prevention. *Cancer Prev Res (Phila).* 2008;1(1):4–8.
38. Snover DC, Ahnen DJ, Burt RW, Odze RD. Serrated polyps of the colon and rectum and serrated polyposis. In: Bosman FT, Carneiro F, Hruban RH, Theise ND, eds. WHO Classification of Tumours of the Digestive System. Geneva, Switzerland: WHO Press; 2010: 160–165.
39. Snover DC, Jass JR, Fenoglio-Preiser C, Batts KP. Serrated polyps of the large intestine: a morphologic and molecular review of an evolving concept. *Am J Clin Pathol.* 2005;124(3):380–391.
40. Bettington M, Walker N, Clouston A, Brown I, Leggett B, Whitehall V. The serrated pathway to colorectal carcinoma: current concepts and challenges. *Histopathology.* 2013;62(3):367–386.
41. Burnett-Hartman AN, Newcomb PA, Potter JD, et al. Genomic aberrations occurring in subsets of serrated colorectal lesions but not conventional adenomas. *Cancer Res.* 2013; 73(9):2863–2872.
42. Patai AV, Molnár B, Tulassay Z, Sipos F. Serrated pathway: alternative route to colorectal cancer. *World J Gastroenterol.* 2013;19(5):607–615.
43. The Cancer Genome Atlas Network. Comprehensive molecular characterization of human colon and rectal cancer. *Nature.* 2012;487:330–337.
44. Boland CR, Thibodeau SN, Hamilton SR, et al. A National Cancer Institute Workshop on Microsatellite Instability for cancer detection and familial predisposition: development of international criteria for the determination of microsatellite instability in colorectal cancer. *Cancer Res.* 1998;58(22): 5248–5257.
45. Umar A, Boland CR, Terdiman JP, et al. Revised Bethesda Guidelines for hereditary nonpolyposis colorectal cancer (Lynch syndrome) and microsatellite instability. *J Natl Cancer Inst.* 2004;96(4):261–268.
46. Bae JM, Kim JH, Kang GH. Epigenetic alterations in colorectal cancer: the CpG island methylator phenotype. *Histol Histopathol.* 2013; 28(5):585–595.
47. Hammoud SS, Cairns BR, Jones DA. Epigenetic regulation of colon cancer and intestinal stem cells. *Curr Opin Cell Biol.* 2013;25(2):177–183.
48. Donehower LA, Creighton CJ, Schultz N, et al. MLH1-silenced and non-silenced subgroups of hypermutated colorectal carcinomas have distinct mutational landscapes. *J Pathol.* 2013;229(1): 99–110.
49. Okayama H, Schetter AJ, Harris CC. MicroRNAs and inflammation in the pathogenesis and progression of colon cancer. *Dig Dis.* 2012;30(Suppl 2):9–15.
50. Rossi S, Di Narzo AF, Mestdagh P, et al. microRNAs in colon cancer: a roadmap for discovery. *FEBS Lett.* 2012;586(19): 3000–3007.
51. Hong L, Han Y, Zhou Y, Nita A. Angiogenesis-related microRNAs in colon cancer. *Expert Opin Biol Ther.* 2013;13(1): 77–84.
52. Bartley AN, Yao H, Barkoh BA, et al. Complex patterns of altered MicroRNA expression during the adenoma-adenocarcinoma sequence for microsatellite-stable colorectal cancer. *Clin Cancer Res.* 2011;17(23):7283–7293.
53. Tokarz P, Blasiak J. The role of microRNA in metastatic colorectal cancer and its significance in cancer prognosis and treatment. *Acta Biochim Pol.* 2012;59(4):467–474.
54. Kunte DP, DelaCruz M, Wali RK, et al. Dysregulation of microRNAs in colonic field carcinogenesis: implications for screening. *PLoS ONE.* 2012;7(9):e45591.
55. Gaedcke J, Grade M, Camps J, et al. The rectal cancer microRNAome–microRNA expression in rectal cancer and matched normal mucosa. *Clin Cancer Res.* 2012;18(18):4919–4930.

56. Yamamoto H, Adachi Y, Taniguchi H, et al. Interrelationship between microsatellite instability and microRNA in gastrointestinal cancer. *World J Gastroenterol.* 2012;18(22):2745–2755.
57. Chen H, Lefferts JA, Schwab MC, Suriawinata AA, Tsongalis GJ. Correlation of polypoid colorectal adenocarcinoma with preexisting adenomatous polyps and K-ras mutation. *Cancer Genet.* 2011;204(5):245–251.
58. Al-Sohaily S, Biankin A, Leong R, Kohonen-Corish M, Warusavitarne J. Molecular pathways in colorectal cancer. *J Gastroenterol Hepatol.* 2012;27(9):1423–1431.
59. Yim KL. Microsatellite instability in metastatic colorectal cancer: a review of pathology, response to chemotherapy and clinical outcome. *Med Oncol.* 2012;29(3):1796–1801.
60. Gavin PG, Colangelo LH, Fumagalli D, et al. Mutation profiling and microsatellite instability in stage II and III colon cancer: an assessment of their prognostic and oxaliplatin predictive value. *Clin Cancer Res.* 2012;18(23):6531–6541.
61. Lochhead P, Kuchiba A, Imamura Y, et al. Microsatellite instability and BRAF mutation testing in colorectal cancer prognostication. *J Natl Cancer Inst.* 2013 July 22 [Epub ahead of print].
62. Samowitz WS, Sweeney C, Herrick J, et al. Poor survival associated with the BRAF V600E mutation in microsatellite-stable colon cancers. *Cancer Res.* 2005;65(14):6063–6069.
63. Dietel M, Jöhrens K, Laffert M, et al. Predictive molecular pathology and its role in targeted cancer therapy: a review focusing on clinical relevance. *Cancer Gene Ther.* 2013;20(4):211–221.
64. Vilar E, Scaltriti M, Balmaña J, et al. Microsatellite instability due to hMLH1 deficiency is associated with increased cytotoxicity to irinotecan in human colorectal cancer cell lines. *Br J Cancer.* 2008;99(10):1607–1612.
65. Bertagnolli MM, Niedzwiecki D, Compton CC, et al. Microsatellite instability predicts improved response to adjuvant therapy with irinotecan, fluorouracil, and leucovorin in stage III colon cancer: Cancer and Leukemia Group B Protocol 89803. *J Clin Oncol.* 2009;27(11):1814–1821.
66. Zaanan A, Fléjou JF, Emile JF, et al. Defective mismatch repair status as a prognostic biomarker of disease-free survival in stage III colon cancer patients treated with adjuvant FOLFOX chemotherapy. *Clin Cancer Res.* 2011;17(23):7470–7478.
67. Han SW, Lee HJ, Bae JM, et al. Methylation and microsatellite status and recurrence following adjuvant FOLFOX in colorectal cancer. *Int J Cancer.* 2013;132(9):2209–2216.
68. Morales C, Ribas M, Aiza G, Peinado MA. Genetic determinants of methotrexate responsiveness and resistance in colon cancer cells. *Oncogene.* 2005;24(45):6842–6847.
69. Valeri N, Gasparini P, Fabbri M, et al. Modulation of mismatch repair and genomic stability by miR-155. *Proc Natl Acad Sci USA.* 2010;107(15):6982–6987.
70. Dorard C, de Thonel A, Collura A, et al. Expression of a mutant HSP110 sensitizes colorectal cancer cells to chemotherapy and improves disease prognosis. *Nat Med.* 2011;17(10):1283–1289.
71. Panza A, Pazienza V, Ripoli M, et al. Interplay between SOX9, ß-catenin and PPAR-gamma activation in colorectal cancer. *Biochim Biophys Acta.* 2013.
72. Takahashi M, Koi M, Balaguer F, Boland CR, Goel A. MSH3 mediates sensitization of colorectal cancer cells to cisplatin, oxaliplatin, and a poly(ADP-ribose) polymerase inhibitor. *J Biol Chem.* 2011;286(14):12157–12165.
73. Baba Y, Nosho K, Shima K, et al. Phosphorylated AKT expression is associated with PIK3CA mutation, low stage, and favorable outcome in 717 colorectal cancers. *Cancer.* 2011;117(7):1399–1408.
74. Pal I, Mandal M. PI3K and Akt as molecular targets for cancer therapy: current clinical outcomes. *Acta Pharmacol Sin.* 2012;33(12):1441–1458.
75. Liao X, Morikawa T, Lochhead P, et al. Prognostic role of PIK3CA mutation in colorectal cancer: cohort study and literature review. *Clin Cancer Res.* 2012;18(8):2257–2268.
76. Black ER, Falzon L, Aronson N. Gene expression profiling for predicting outcomes in stage II colon cancer. [Internet] Agency for Healthcare Research and Quality (US). 2012 Dec. Report No.: 12(13)-EHC143.EF.
77. Akiyoshi T, Kobunai T, Watanabe T. Recent approaches to identifying biomarkers for high-risk stage II colon cancer. *Surg Today.* 2012;42(11):1037–1045.
78. Adams MD, Veigl ML, Wang Z, et al. Global mutational profiling of formalin-fixed human colon cancers from a pathology archive. *Mod Pathol.* 2012;25(12):1599–1608.
79. Bartley AN, Luthra R, Saraiya DS, Urbauer DL, Broaddus RR. Identification of cancer patients with Lynch syndrome: clinically significant discordances and problems in tissue-based mismatch repair testing. *Cancer Prev Res (Phila).* 2012;5(2):320–327.
80. Domingo E, Niessen RC, Oliveira C, et al. BRAF-V600E is not involved in the colorectal tumorigenesis of HNPCC in patients with functional MLH1 and MSH2 genes. *Oncogene.* 2005;24(24):3995–3998.
81. Bessa X, Ballesté B, Andreu M, et al.; Gastrointestinal Oncology Group of Spanish Gastroenterological Association. A prospective, multicenter, population-based study of BRAF mutational analysis for Lynch syndrome screening. *Clin Gastroenterol Hepatol.* 2008;6(2):206–214.
82. Lièvre A, Bachet JB, Le Corre D, et al. K-ras mutation status is predictive of response to cetuximab therapy in colorectal cancer. *Cancer Res.* 2006;66(8):3992–3995.
83. Amado RG, Wolf M, Peeters M, et al. Wild-type K-ras is required for panitumumab efficacy in patients with metastatic colorectal cancer. *J Clin Oncol.* 2008;26(10):1626–1634.
84. Benson AB 3rd, Bekaii-Saab T, Chan E, et al. Metastatic colon cancer, version 3.2013: featured updates to the NCCN Guidelines. *J Natl Compr Canc Netw.* 2013;11(2):141–52; quiz 152.
85. Arrington AK, Heinrich EL, Lee W, et al. Prognostic and predictive roles of K-ras mutation in colorectal cancer. *Int J Mol Sci.* 2012;13(10):12153–12168.
86. Taliano RJ, LeGolvan M, Resnick MB. Immunohistochemistry of colorectal carcinoma: current practice and evolving applications. *Hum Pathol.* 2013;44(2):151–163.
87. Capper D, Voigt A, Bozukova G, et al. BRAF V600E-specific immunohistochemistry for the exclusion of Lynch syndrome in MSI-H colorectal cancer. *Int J Cancer.* 2013.
88. Palomaki GE, McClain MR, Melillo S, Hampel HL, Thibodeau SN. EGAPP supplementary evidence review: DNA testing strategies aimed at reducing morbidity and mortality from Lynch syndrome. *Genet Med.* 2009;11(1):42–65.
89. Weissman SM, Burt R, Church J, et al. Identification of individuals at risk for Lynch syndrome using targeted evaluations and genetic testing: National Society of Genetic Counselors and the Collaborative Group of the Americas on Inherited Colorectal Cancer joint practice guideline. *J Genet Couns.* 2012;21(4):484–493.
90. Sargent DJ, Marsoni S, Monges G, et al. Defective mismatch repair as a predictive marker for lack of efficacy of fluorouracil-based adjuvant therapy in colon cancer. *J Clin Oncol.* 2010;28(20):3219–3226.
91. Ogino S, Fuchs CS, Giovannucci E. How many molecular subtypes? Implications of the unique tumor principle in personalized medicine. *Expert Rev Mol Diagn.* 2012;12(6):621–628.

7 Management of Nonmetastatic Colon Cancer

■ Surgical Considerations

ALLISON GOLDBERG
ADAM C. BERGER

■ HISTORY OF SURGERY FOR COLON CANCER

Colostomy

Prior to advent of anesthesia, the best that could be offered to patients with colon cancer was proximal diversion via stoma creation in order to relieve obstruction. The first attempt at this was performed by Pillore of Rouen in 1776 in a patient with a large tumor at the colorectal junction. In this operation, the distended cecum was exposed through a transverse incision, opened, and fixed to the margins of the wound with a couple of sutures. This operation produced great relief of the obstruction; however, the patient died 28 days later because of jejunal necrosis secondary to the large amounts of mercury that were given to the patient in a conservative attempt to relieve the obstruction (1). Pierre Fine of Geneva carried out the first successful transverse colostomy in 1797 in a patient with a rectosigmoid obstructing growth; she lived for 3.5 months before dying of ascites (1).

Colonic Resection

Jean Francis Reybard of Lyon performed the first successful resection of a sigmoid colonic growth with anastomosis of the ends of the bowel in 1823 (without anesthesia!). The patient lived for 1 year. In 1879, Vincenz Czerny successfully resected a colonic growth with end-to-end anastomosis, and in the same year Theodor Billroth performed a colonic resection and brought the proximal end of the bowel out as a colostomy (1). By the end of 1899, the number of reported colon resections had risen to 57 with a mortality rate of 37% with most deaths due to peritonitis secondary to intestinal leakage or necrosis of the suture line. Two-stage procedures, popularized by Johannes von Mikulicz-Radecki and Frank Thomas Paul, were able to reduce mortality rates to around 12.5%. In these procedures, the loop of colon containing the tumor was brought out in one stage, resected at a second stage with formation of a colostomy, and finally the colostomy was closed at the third stage (1). Safe modern surgery consisting of primary resection with immediate anastomosis of the colon depended on the development of better techniques of bowel suture, enhanced knowledge of the importance of blood supply at the anastomosis, and the importance of operating on decompressed bowel (1).

■ EPIDEMIOLOGY OF COLON CANCER

The incidence and mortality of colon cancer varies significantly throughout the world, with Australia, New Zealand, Europe, and North America having much higher incidence rates than Africa and South Central Asia. Worldwide, there were 1.2 million new cases and 608,700 deaths in 2008, with CRC being the third most common cancer in males, and the second most common in females (2). In the United States, both incidence and mortality from colon cancer have been decreasing, while incidence rates in many other Western countries have increased or remained stable. In the United States in 2010, approximately 102,900 new cases of colon cancer were diagnosed, and 51,000 people died from the disease (3). Both in the United States and worldwide, there has been a shift to more right-sided colon cancers, with a relative increase in cecal primary tumors (4). This shift in anatomic distribution may be due to improvements in screening, with flexible sigmoidoscopy finding more adenomatous polyps, challenges of colonoscopy in the right colon secondary to poor preparation or incomplete colonoscopy, or may be a true change in incidence of cecal cancers.

The most common locations for colon cancers are typically the right colon followed by the sigmoid colon.

In a large (N = 3411) prospective adjuvant therapy trial for colon cancer done in the 1990s, the most common site was the right colon (41%), followed by the sigmoid colon (37%). Other sites in the colon were relatively rare: transverse colon—7.6%; descending colon—6.3%; and splenic flexure—5.2% (5).

Basic Anatomy

The arterial, venous, and lymphatic anatomy of the colon is of critical importance when planning a surgical resection for colon cancer. The main arterial supply to the colon comes from the superior mesenteric artery (SMA) and inferior mesenteric artery (IMA). The SMA branches directly off the aorta, descends posterior to the pancreas, crosses anterior to the left renal vein and gives off three main branches. The first, the ileocolic artery, supplies the terminal ileum, the cecum, and the appendix. The second, the right colic artery, supplies the ascending colon and hepatic flexure, however, its exact anatomy is variable. It is absent in 2%–18% of people, and when present can arise directly from the SMA or as a branch of the ileocolic or middle colic artery. The third artery, the middle colic, gives off a right and left branch. The right branch supplies the proximal transverse colon while the left branch supplies the distal transverse colon. The middle colic artery also has anatomic variations; it is absent in 4%–20% of people and up to 10% of people are found to have an accessory, or additional, middle colic artery.

The IMA arises 3 to 4 cm superior to the aortic bifurcation. Its major branches to the colon include the left colic artery and two to six sigmoid branches. The left colic artery supplies the distal transverse colon, the splenic flexure, and the descending colon. The sigmoid branches supply the sigmoid colon and collateralize with the left colic artery to form arcades.

There are two main arteries that connect the blood supply of the SMA and IMA. The first is the marginal artery, a large collateral vessel that forms a continuous arcade along the mesenteric border of the colon. It receives contributions from the ileocolic, right colic, middle colic, left colic, and sigmoidal arteries. The second is known as the Arc of Riolan or the meandering mesenteric artery. This vessel is highly variable in size and can have anterograde or retrograde flow depending on stenoses or obstructions in the SMA or IMA. Of note, up to 50% of specimens lack clearly defined arterial supply to a small segment of colon at the splenic flexure. Therefore, in practice, surgeons attempt to avoid creating anastomoses using the splenic flexure to avoid a tenuous or insufficient blood supply.

Venous drainage of the colon is via two main veins, the superior mesenteric vein (SMV) and the inferior mesenteric vein (IMV). The SMV drains the cecum, appendix, ascending colon and most of the transverse colon. The IMV drains the distal transverse colon, the descending colon, the sigmoid colon, and most of the rectum. It empties into the splenic vein to the left of the aorta.

The lymphatic drainage of the colon follows the arterial supply. Lymphatic drainage is crucial for surgical planning, as it will help define appropriate margins. Additionally, accurate staging of colon cancer depends on sufficient lymph node (LN) removal. The epicolic nodes can be found along the bowel wall and in the epiploicae. The paracolic nodes are adjacent to the marginal artery. The intermediate nodes are found along the main branches of the large blood vessels, and primary nodes are found along the SMA and IMA. The ascending and transverse colon ultimately drain to the superior mesenteric LNs and communicate with the adjacent celiac and upper lumbar nodes. The distal transverse colon, descending colon, and sigmoid colon drain to the inferior mesenteric LNs and communicate with the lumbar nodes along the aorta. Both the superior and inferior mesenteric LNs eventually drain to the cisterna chyli.

Bowel Prep

Traditionally, a mechanical bowel preparation and oral antibiotics were administered to any nonobstructed patient prior to an elective colon resection. It was felt that these measures would decrease anastomotic failure. Mechanical bowel preps include 2 to 4 L of polyethylene glycol, 90 mL of sodium phosphate, or sodium phosphate pills. Preoperative antibiotic regimens often include neomycin and erythromycin, metronidazole, or ciprofloxacin (6). Today, however, multiple studies have shown that preoperative bowel preparation may not be necessary. In a multicenter randomized trial, Contant et al showed that mechanical bowel prep did not influence the rate of anastomotic leakage (4.8% with bowel prep vs 5.4% without). Of note, in the patients that did leak, those who had a mechanical bowel prep were less likely to form an abscess (0.3% with bowel prep vs 2.5% without; 7). An updated meta-analysis of mechanical bowel prep by Slim et al showed that bowel prep did not significantly affect the rate of anastomotic leak and further showed that bowel prep did not significantly affect rate of abdominal or pelvic abscesses or wound sepsis. Additionally, the bowel prep group was shown to have significantly more surgical site infections (8). The need for preoperative mechanical bowel prep is an ongoing debate among surgeons.

There is more agreement about the need for preoperative parenteral antibiotics. As elective colon resections are considered "clean contaminated" cases, there is benefit from a single dose of intravenous antibiotics 30 minutes prior to incision. Additional intraoperative doses at 4 hours intervals are appropriate if needed, but postoperative antibiotics of any sort are not generally recommended. Suggested regimens include a second- or third-generation cephalosporin or a fluoroquinolone with metronidazole or clindamycin.

Preoperative Workup

Before proceeding with surgical removal of a colon cancer, a full preoperative workup should be performed. Laboratory studies including a complete blood count, liver function tests, and a carcinoembryonic antigen should be obtained. Most surgeons prefer to also obtain a chest x-ray and CT scan of the abdomen to evaluate for locally advanced or metastatic disease, which is ultimately found in approximately 20% of patients. Locally advanced or metastatic disease does not rule out the possibility of proceeding with a primary resection, but knowledge of its existence allows for more complete preoperative planning. If a patient is found to have a strong family history or early onset of disease, genetic testing may also be appropriate. Whenever possible, all patients scheduled for an elective colectomy should also undergo a complete colonoscopy. This test can evaluate for synchronous cancers, which are found 3%–5% of the time, as well as allow for tattooing of the index lesion (9,10). Finally, PET scan or PET-CT is being used with increasing frequency, but at this time is not cost effective for routine use, and is felt to be more appropriate for staging patients before resection of liver metastases or assessing a patient's response to chemotherapy (11).

Standard Surgical Resections

There are three main goals to all surgical resections of colon cancers. The first goal is removal of the index lesion with 5 cm margins, as well as resection of the lesion's vascular supply and lymphatic drainage. This ensures sufficient margins and adequate lymphadenectomy. Second, an appropriate surgical resection includes an en bloc resection of any structures contiguous with the lesion. Finally, continuity of the bowel must be reestablished. All surgical procedures begin with a thorough exploration of the abdomen and all abdominal organs, with special attention paid to the liver, omentum, all peritoneal surfaces, and nodal basins to fully evaluate for metastatic disease. Intraoperative ultrasound can also be useful to further evaluate the liver. Anastomoses should adhere to the ideals of maintaining a good blood supply and avoiding tension. This requires preservation of vascular pedicles and adequate mobilization of the colon. Randomized trials have demonstrated no significant differences in outcomes regarding hand-sewn or stapled anastomosis.

Right Hemicolectomy (Figures 7.1 and 7.2)

A right colectomy is an appropriate procedure for tumors of the cecum and ascending colon. In this procedure, the terminal ileum, cecum, and ascending colon are resected, and the ileocolic artery, right colic artery, and the right branch of the middle colic artery are ligated at their origins. Approximately 5 to 10 cm of distal small intestine should be resected along with the right colon to ensure adequate blood supply at the stapled edge of the ileum. An anastomosis is then performed between the terminal ileum and transverse colon. This anastomosis can be hand-sewn or stapled.

For lesions of the proximal and mid transverse colon, an extended right colectomy is usually performed. In addition to the resection performed in a standard right colectomy, the hepatic flexure, transverse colon, and the splenic flexure are removed, and the middle colic artery is ligated as its origin, rather than the origin of its right branch. In this procedure, the terminal ileum is anastomosed to the proximal left colon (Figure 7.2). The blood supply to the colon (and anastomosis) is based on the ascending branch of the left colic artery. Anastomosis between the hepatic and splenic flexures is to be avoided due to concerns over the adequacy of the blood supply. Additionally, this type of anastomosis is associated with increased tension due to the natural tendency of ascending and descending colons to migrate to and lie in their anatomic position within the lateral gutters. Again, this anastomosis can be hand-sewn or stapled.

Left Hemicolectomy (Figure 7.3)

A left hemicolectomy is performed for lesions of the distal transverse or descending colon. In this procedure, the colon is resected from at least 5-cm proximal to the lesion to the sigmoid colon or to the rectosigmoid junction. The left branch of the middle colic artery, left colic artery, and the sigmoidal pedicle are divided. A hand-sewn or stapled anastomosis can then be fashioned between the distal transverse colon and the sigmoid colon or, if the inferior mesenteric vessels are divided, the anastomosis would be to the rectosigmoid junction. This generally requires full mobilization of splenic flexure to avoid undue tension on the anastomosis.

Sigmoid Colectomy (Figure 7.4)

A sigmoid colectomy is appropriate for lesions in the sigmoid colon. The sigmoid colon is resected and the arterial pedicle just distal to the left colic takeoff from the IMA is divided. An anastomosis is created (hand-sewn or stapled) between the descending colon and the rectosigmoid junction.

Special Cases

Patients who present with perforated colon lesions offer a particular challenge. The perforations are most often seen either at the lesion itself or proximal to the lesion with the perforation secondary increased intraluminal pressure. Because of fecal contamination, these patients will likely require a stoma. They can either undergo resection with end colostomy or resection with re-anastomosis

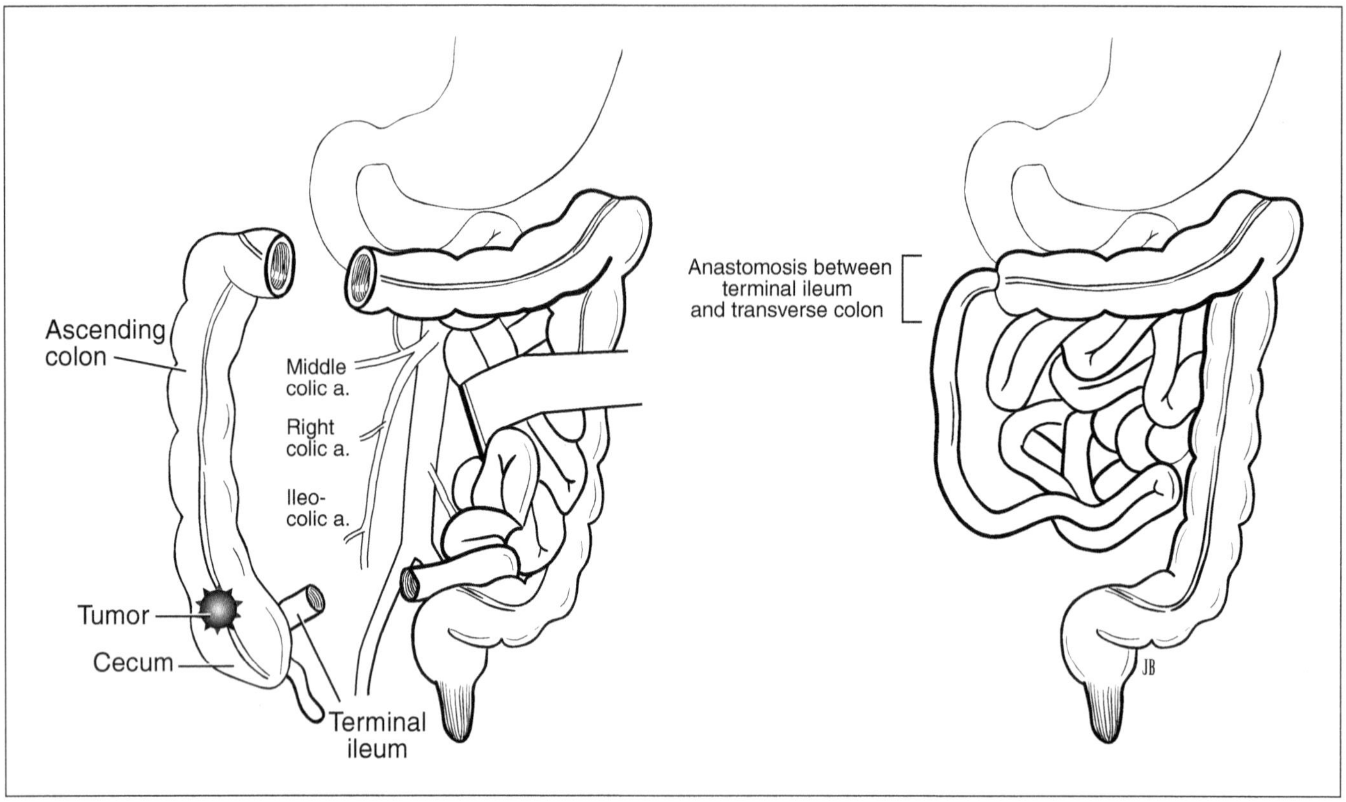

FIGURE 7.1 Anatomic demonstration of resection for right hemicolectomy in which the ileocolic, right colic, and right branch of the middle colic vessels are all ligated. The transection points are in the transverse colon distal to the hepatic flexure and in the terminal ileum. Anastomosis is between the terminal ileum and proximal transverse colon. (Illustration by Jennifer Brumbaugh, MA.)

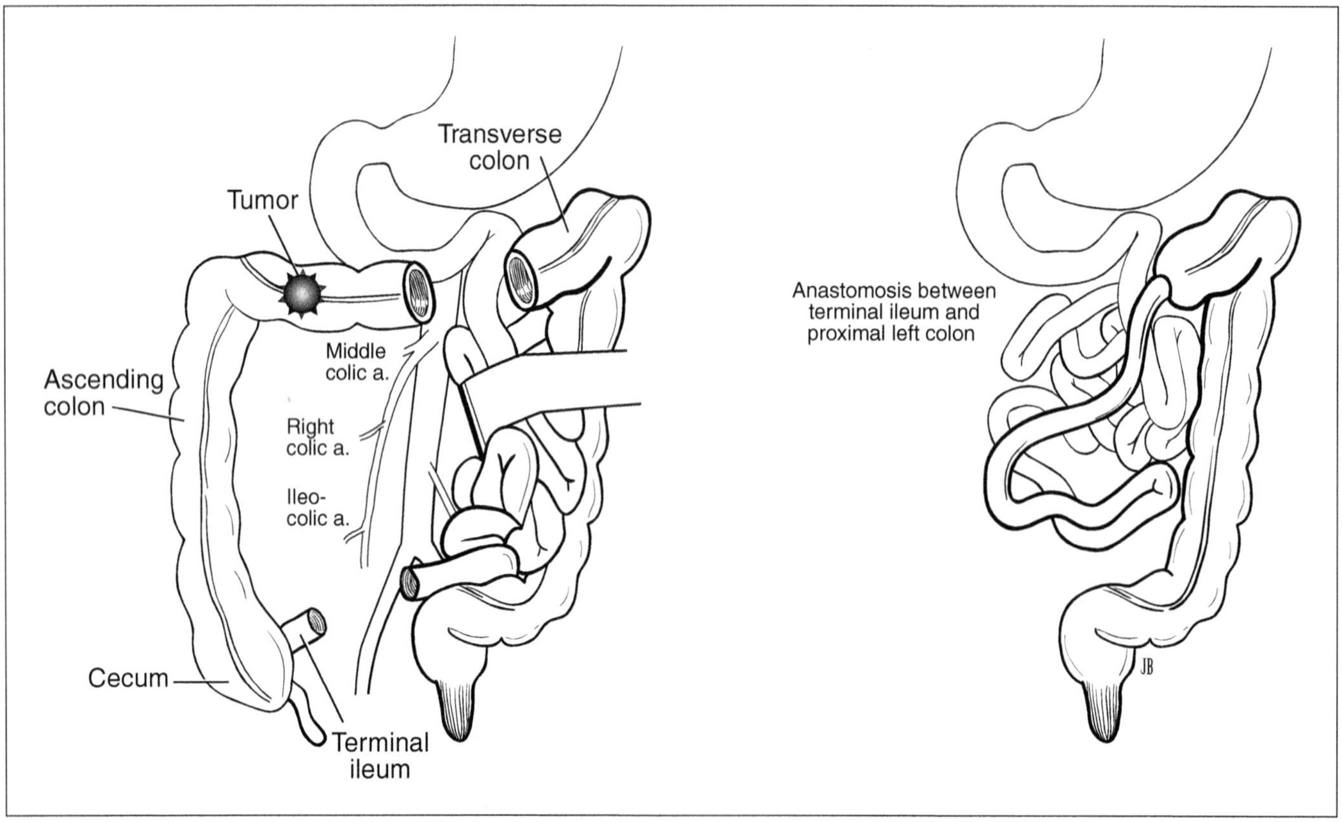

FIGURE 7.2 For tumors at the hepatic flexure, an extended right hemicolectomy is performed, which also includes division of the middle colic artery and anastomosis between terminal ileum and distal transverse colon or descending colon. (Illustration by Jennifer Brumbaugh, MA.)

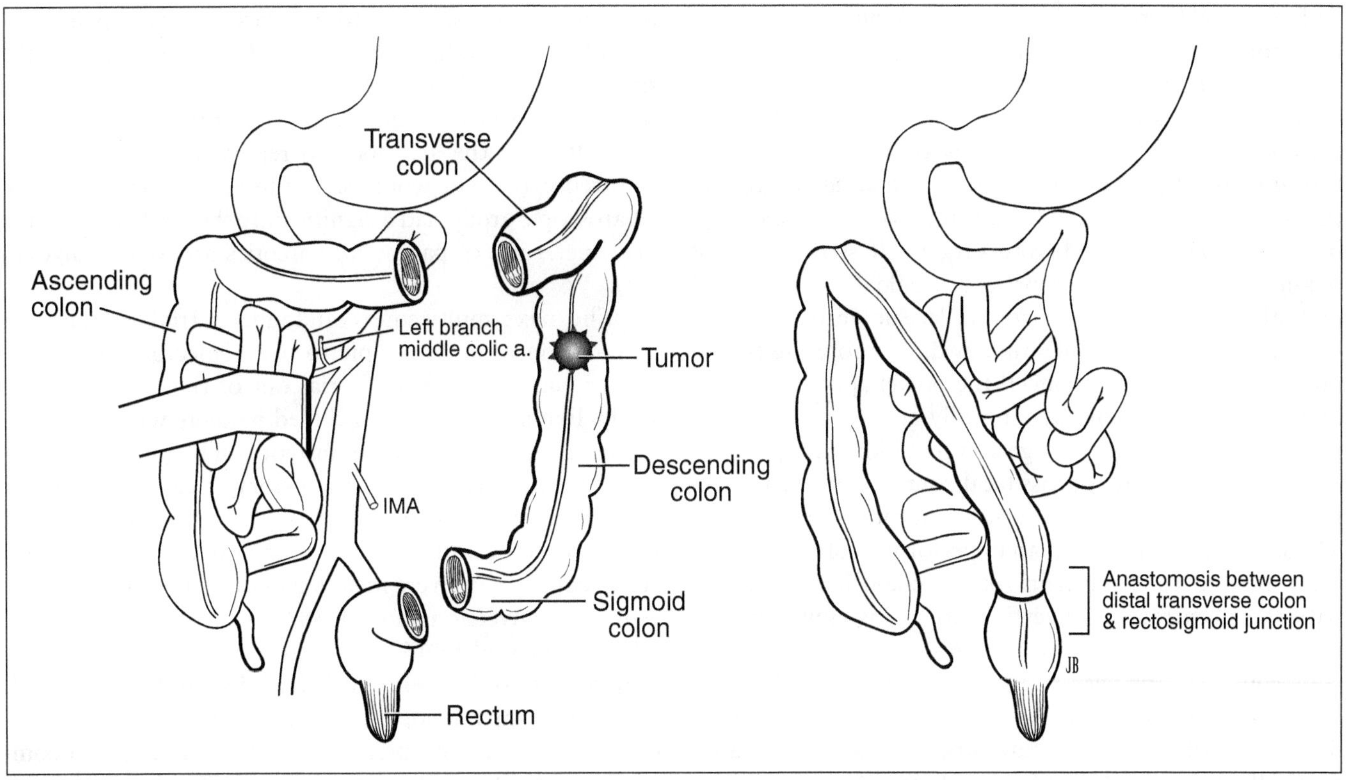

FIGURE 7.3 For tumors of the left (descending) colon, the left branch of the middle colic, the left colic, and the IMA are divided. The colon is transected at the mid transverse colon and the rectum and anastomosis is performed between transverse colon and rectum. (Illustration by Jennifer Brumbaugh, MA.)

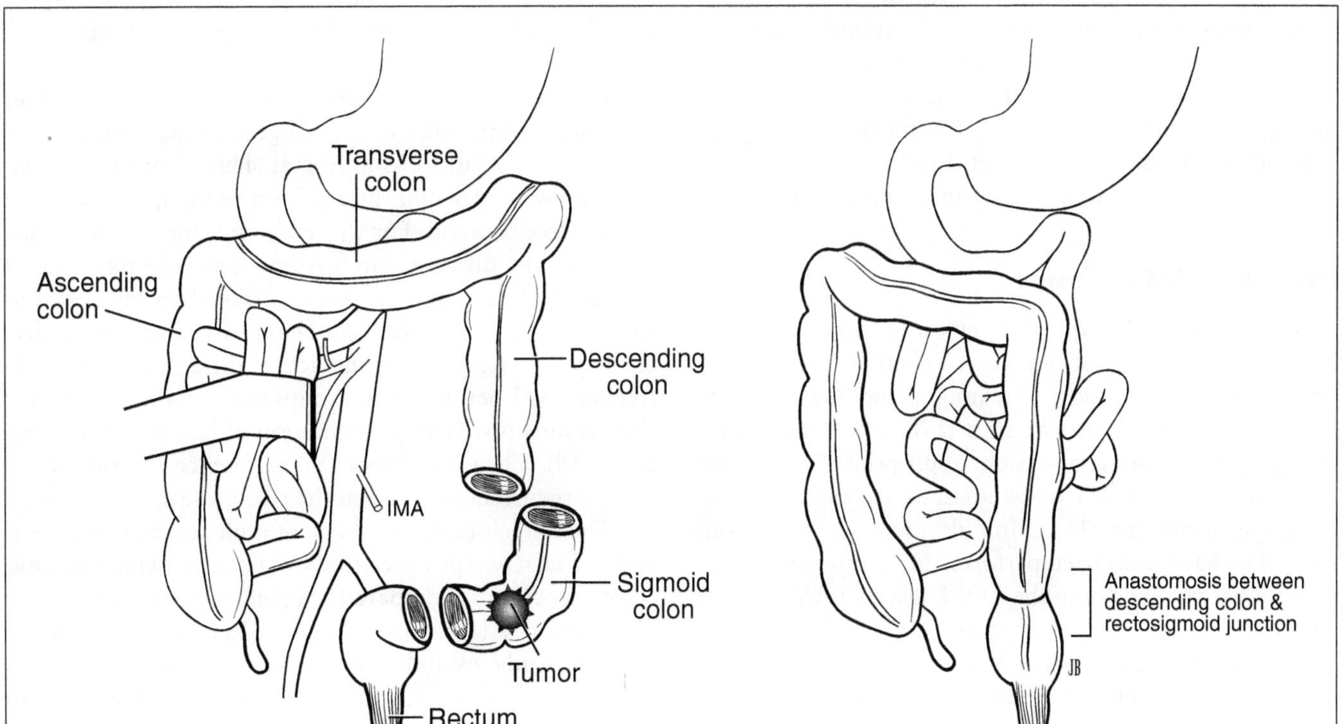

FIGURE 7.4 For lesions confined to the sigmoid colon, a sigmoid colectomy can be performed. Again, the IMA is divided, and an anastomosis is created between the descending colon and the rectum. Depending on the redundancy of the descending colon, this may require a mobilization of the splenic flexure in order to perform a tension-free anastomosis. (Illustration by Jennifer Brumbaugh, MA.)

and proximal loop colostomy depending on the severity of fecal contamination and patient status.

Obstructing colon lesions also require unique management. These lesions are particularly problematic because the colon proximal to the lesion is generally dilated and full of stool. If possible, preoperative stenting can relieve the obstruction and allow for a full preoperative workup, including colonoscopy, before surgery. If stenting is not possible or available, the patient should be resuscitated and taken to the operating room. Patient status and level of fecal contamination determines the appropriate procedure in the operating room. If the bowel appears healthy and the patient is hemodynamically stable, it is possible to perform an on-table lavage and resection with primary anastomosis. If there is gross fecal contamination, a resection with end colostomy is the most appropriate procedure. The surgeon should then plan to perform a colonoscopy in the future to rule out synchronous colon lesions. If the patient is in extremis, a diverting loop colostomy proximal to the lesion can decompress the obstruction. A colonoscopy could later be performed via that stoma to allow for appropriate preoperative planning for a definitive procedure. Regardless, the ultimate procedure should be anatomically determined based on the location of the lesion.

In a review of 243 patients who underwent emergency operations for obstructing colon cancers, Lee et al demonstrated that 233 patients (92%) underwent primary resection with primary anastomosis possible in 197 patients. Of the 101 patients with left-sided lesions who underwent primary anastomoses, segmental resection with on-table lavage was performed in 75 patients and subtotal colectomy in the other 26 patients. Operative mortality rate was 9.4% for those undergoing primary resection and 8% for those undergoing anastomosis. Leak rates were not different based on right- versus left-sided lesions or type of anastomosis (12).

Laparoscopic Colectomy

Laparoscopic colectomy for colon cancer was first described in 1990 (13). However, a variety of concerns arose immediately, most alarming being high rates of tumor recurrence at trocar sites (14) as well as worries over proper oncologic resection, appropriate LN staging, and altered tumor cell dissemination secondary to laparoscopic technique (15). Multiple prospective randomized trials have since been performed to address these and other concerns, including the COST trial, CLASICC trial, COLOR trial, and Barcelona trial.

The COST trial was the first major prospective, randomized, multi-center, noninferiority trial comparing laparoscopic and open colectomy for colon cancer. The trial excluded patients with locally advanced or metastatic disease, disease of the transverse colon and rectum, and patients with acute bowel obstruction or perforation. Its primary endpoint was time to tumor recurrence, and the authors reported a conversion rate from laparoscopic to open resection of 21% overall. In the report of long-term results, the study shows no difference in disease-free or overall 5-year survival, as well as no difference in overall recurrence rates (16). Of note, the authors also reported no difference in recurrence rates in wounds. Furthermore, they show the laparoscopic group had a significantly shorter length of stay and briefer use of parenteral narcotics and oral analgesics (15).

The next multicenter randomized trial to report a comparison of laparoscopic to open colectomy for colon cancer was the CLASICC trial out of the UK (17). This study, like many others, excluded patients with cancer of the transverse colon, acute obstruction secondary to cancer, synchronous lesions, or a history of cancer in the last 5 years. Notably, while most of the major comparisons of laparoscopic and open colectomy exclude patients with rectal cancer, they were included in this study. The authors report a conversion rate of 38% in year 1 of the trial, which improved to 16% by year 6 (17). In their results, they report no difference in 3-year disease free or overall survival for laparoscopic treatment of colon or rectal cancer, as compared to open surgery. The authors also comment on quality of life scores, seeing no major differences in quality of life for patients who underwent laparoscopic compared to open colon resection.

The other major randomized multicenter trial comparing laparoscopic to open colectomy was the COLOR trial from Europe. Like the COST trial, this was a noninferiority trial, and the study excluded patients with locally advanced or metastatic disease, disease of the transverse colon or rectum or obstructing disease (18). However, they also excluded patients with BMI greater than 30, perhaps making their results less universal. Their reported conversion rate was 19% and their primary endpoint was 3-year disease-free survival. For this endpoint, the authors could not rule out a difference in favor of open colectomy unless moving the patients who were assigned to laparoscopic treatment but preoperatively changed to the open colectomy group. Regardless, the actual difference in disease-free survival between the groups was small, so they felt their results justify implementation of laparoscopic colectomy (18). They also report no difference in port site or wound recurrences between the two groups.

The Barcelona trial, while not multicenter, was important in that it was powered to show a benefit of laparoscopic colon resection as compared to open resection, rather than noninferiority (19). Just like the COST and COLOR trials, the study excluded patients with locally advanced or metastatic disease, disease of the transverse colon or rectum, and obstructing disease. Of note, this study had a median follow up of 95 months, much longer than the other mentioned trials. The primary endpoint for this study was cancer related survival, and the authors found a trend toward improved cancer related and overall survival for the laparoscopic group (P = .07 and .06, respectively). When subgroup analysis was performed and patients were stratified by tumor stage, the authors found that for Stage III tumors, laparoscopic colectomy was associated with statistically significantly improved overall survival and cancer-related survival (19). Furthermore, if they analyzed the data based on actual surgery rather than on an intention-to-treat analysis, they found laparoscopic colectomy was associated with improved overall survival and cancer-free survival for all patients. The authors argue that their improved survival rates with laparoscopic surgery are perhaps related to the single center aspect of this trial. They feel the larger, multicenter trials likely had surgeons of more varied experience, and by performing their trial in a single dedicated laparoscopic center, they were able to lower complication rates and tumor handling, leading to an attenuated stress and inflammatory response, and therefore, a better outcome. Of course, their results are then only applicable to other dedicated laparoscopic centers, rather than the surgical community as a whole.

Together these trials (Table 7.1), and others like them, have shown that laparoscopic colectomy is, at least, not inferior to open colectomy for resection of nonobstructing, nondisseminated colon cancers in terms of survival. Furthermore, these trials have refuted the worry that laparoscopic colectomy would lead to increased port site recurrences, and have shown decreased length of stay and shorter duration for use of narcotics in the laparoscopic group. More work is needed to evaluate if there are subgroups of patients for whom laparoscopic colectomy would be of particular benefit when compared to open resection.

Importance of LN Examination and Yield

There has been increasing evidence that the number of LNs evaluated by the pathologist has an important impact on survival (5). The prevailing theory is that a thorough LN evaluation results in more accurate staging and, thus, better determination of prognosis. This concept of stage migration was first described by Feinstein et al in 1985 and was termed the Will Rogers phenomenon (20). In general, there are two opposing views regarding the role of lymphadenectomy, particularly in breast cancer. The traditional Halstedian view claims that lymphadenectomy is important for staging and survival. Others feel that cancer is a systemic disease and that lymphadenectomy is useful only as a staging tool and does not affect survival. Many factors may contribute to the increasing number of LNs examined by the pathologist and its effect on survival. These may include a more extensive lymphadenectomy performed by the surgeon or a more thorough examination of the specimen by the pathologist that helps determine the nodal stage. In colon cancer operations, improved staging may be seen because the surgeon who performs a meticulous and extensive node dissection is usually one who thoroughly stages the patient preoperatively and intraoperatively, extensively inspects for peritoneal implants and liver metastases, and performs a better technical operation with a complete en-bloc resection of involved structures.

In 2002, a pathologist published a large study (N = 2,427) of patients with T3 tumors. In this study of patients with Stage II colon cancer, patients who had less

Table 7.1 Comparison of Various Laparoscopic Colectomy Trials

Trial	COST: 2004, 2007	Barcelona: 2008	COLOR: 2009 (Long Term)	CLASICC: 2005, 2007
Type	Prospective, randomized, multicenter, noninferiority	Prospective, randomized, single center	Prospective, randomized, multicenter, noninferiority	Multicenter, randomized
Number of patients	428 open 435 lap	108 open 111 lap	542 open 534 lap	268 open 526 lap
Primary endpoint	Time to tumor recurrence	Cancer-related survival	3-year disease-free survival	3-year overall survival, 3 year disease-free survival, 3-year local recurrence
Conversion rate	21%	11%	19%	38% in year 1, 16% in year 6
Findings	Lap—significantly longer OR time, shorter LOS, shorter total analgesic use No difference in primary endpoint at 5 years	Tendency toward higher cancer-related survival and overall survival in lap group (P = .07 and .06)	3-year disease-free survival difference was small	3-year survival and disease-free survival no worse for lap than open
Port site recurrences	Two in lap, one in open			No difference
Follow-up	At least 5 years	Median 95 months	Median 53 months	Median 36.8 months

Lap, laparoscopic colectomy; open, open colectomy.

than or equal to 7 LN evaluated had a 5-year survival of 62.5% compared to 75.8% for those patients with greater than or equal to 17 LN examined. He also noted that an increasing number of recovered LNs was significantly associated with an increasing percentage of specimens with LN metastases. This number increased from 52%–74% when LN recovery went from 12 to 25 nodes. One of the most interesting findings of this study was that the mean number of LNs per specimen significantly increased when pathology assistants replaced pathologists in the grossing room (21). In another study, Law et al demonstrated that patients with Stage II colon cancer (T3/T4) who had less than or equal to 6 LN examined had a 5-year survival of 62%, which was significantly lower than those with greater than 6 LN examined (86% 5-year survival; 22).

In another large study of patients with colon cancer, LeVoyer et al evaluated LN yields in a secondary analysis of INT-0089, which evaluated adjuvant chemotherapy in patients with resected colon cancer. These authors demonstrated that increasing numbers of nodes analyzed had a significant impact on prognosis in both node-negative and node-positive colon cancer. For node-negative patients, 5-year survival was 80% in those with 1 to 10 LN evaluated, compared to 92% for those with greater than 20 LNs analyzed (5). For patients with N1 disease, 5-year survival increased from 74% for those with 1 to 10 nodes analyzed to 93% for those with greater than 40 LN evaluated.

Finally, there is also very good evidence now that LN ratio (the ratio of positive LNs to total LNs removed) is an important prognostic factor for patients with colon cancer. In a secondary analysis of INT-0089, Berger et al demonstrated that increasing LN ratio was a significant, independent prognostic factor for overall, disease-specific, and cancer-specific survival in patients with colon cancer after resection and adjuvant therapy. This factor was important for patients with positive LNs and greater than 10 LNs harvested but lost its effect for patients with less than 10 lymph removed (23). This effect was most dramatic for patients with N2 disease with a ratio between 5% and 19% who had a 73% 5-year survival, which was improved compared to N1 patients with a ratio greater than 20% (23). Therefore, it has become clear in the last few years that the number of examined LNs and the ratio of positive to total LNs are important prognostic factors for patients with resected CRC.

■ The Role of Chemotherapy

REBECCA A. MOSS

■ INTRODUCTION

With modern multidisciplinary management, overall mortality from CRC has overall decreased from almost 50% in the 1970s to only 35% in recent years. In this section, we review the factors surrounding adjuvant therapy that most influence survival. We review the evidence that made the addition of oxaliplatin to chemotherapy the standard of care in patients with Stage III disease, and will examine current trends, the hope for personalized medicine, and discuss how multidisciplinary coordination of care may improve outcomes, such as the earlier initiation of adjuvant therapy in the postoperative period.

As colon cancer screening becomes more widely available and accepted, appropriate multidisciplinary management of localized disease to decrease mortality takes on more importance. More than two decades after screening colonoscopy in asymptomatic individuals was initially advocated to save lives from colon cancer (24), we finally have definitive evidence from a prospective study that colonoscopicpolypectomy results in reduced mortality from CRC (25).

Encouragingly, some authors have also found evidence that adenocarcinoma is being diagnosed at an earlier stage (26,27). This stage migration likely reflects the more widespread availability and use of appropriate endoscopic procedures. Investigators from different regions have described changes in the anatomical distribution of colon cancer over the past several decades, with an increasing proportion of proximal cancers reported as a common trend (27), which might be attributed to screening modalities.

■ DECREASE IN MORTALITY WITH ADJUVANT CHEMOTHERAPY

While screening and improved surgical technique contribute to the improved survival from CRC, chemotherapy has been an important adjunctive measure with significant gains in the past three decades. Adjuvant chemotherapy was first shown to reduce the risk of death from colon cancer by Moertel et al in the *New England Journal of Medicine* in February of 1990. They reported that 1 year of adjuvant chemotherapy with levamisole and fluorouracil (5-FU) for patients with Duke's Stage C colon cancer reduced the risk of cancer recurrence by 41% and reduced the risk of death by 33%, with 3.6 year survival estimates of 71% for the treatment arm and 55% for the observation arm (28,29). The estimated 5-year overall survival on the basis of these results was 63%. Therefore, in the early 1990s, a full year of adjuvant 5-FU plus levamisole was widely recommended for Stage III colon cancer (30).

Long-term follow-up on a similar 1-year adjuvant chemotherapy trial, the adjCCA-01trial demonstrated similar results with leucovorin being superior to levamisole, with median overall survival of 88.9 months versus 78.6 ($P = .003$; 31). In fact, levamisole, which has deleterious side effects (32,33) has been replaced by leucovorin on the basis of a number of trials and meta-analyses (34,35).

In addition to the change to leucovorin, the standard of care was reduced from a full year of chemotherapy to just 6 months on the basis of a number of trials, such the mature results of the Intergroup 0089 trial (36), which showed differences in toxicity but no evidence that longer treatment was statistically superior in disease-free or overall survival. A meta-analysis of three European trials published in 1995 also found that 5-FU given for 6 months can achieve a similar survival benefit to that achieved with a year of therapy (37). At present, 6 months of adjuvant therapy is the standard of care.

Continuous infusion 5-FU can be delivered with less toxicity and has replaced daily bolus 5-FU, based on results of trials such as the Phase III Southwest Oncology Group 9415/Intergroup 0153 Randomized Trial of Fluorouracil, Leucovorin, and Levamisole, which closed in December 1999 after an interim analysis (38).

The success of 5-FU-based chemotherapy creates a challenge for investigating new agents, particularly, if the gold-standard overall survival is used as the primary endpoint in adjuvant chemotherapy trials. For this reason, disease-free survival becomes an attractive surrogate endpoint. An analysis of data from the ACCENT group, assembling individual patient data from 18 phase III adjuvant trials in colon cancer from 1978 to 1999, showed that adjuvant chemotherapy provides significant disease-free survival benefit, primarily by reducing the recurrence rate within the first 2 years of adjuvant therapy, translating into a long-term overall survival for adjuvant chemotherapy (39,40). In fact, this extended benefit suggests that in modern adjuvant trials, 6 or 7 years may be required to demonstrate overall survival improvements, further supporting disease-free survival as the preferred primary end point for future adjuvant colon cancer clinical trials (39).

Benefits and Risks of Oxaliplatin

Oxaliplatin is the first, and to date, the only additional medication to show benefit in the adjuvant setting since 5-FU became the standard of care. A key issue in treating patients with this medication is addressing the neurotoxicity, which ultimately limits the reasonable duration of this therapy.

Oxaliplatin in combination with 5-FU became standard of care for resected Stage III colon cancer when the results of the MOSAIC trial demonstrated that FOLFOX4 significantly extended 5-year disease-free survival from 67.4%–73.3% versus the de Gramont regimen of bimonthly high-dose leucovorin and 5-FU bolus plus a continuous infusion of 5-FU (41). However, these benefits were weighted heavily by the benefit in the Stage III subgroup. In fact, there was no significant benefit shown in a subgroup analysis of those patients with Stage II disease. With these results, 6 months of adjuvant FOLFOX became the standard of care for Stage III disease.

Two other trials have been published since demonstrating similar survival benefit with oxaliplatin added to a fluoropyrimidine regimen: the NSABP C-07 trial of FLOX versus bolus plus continuous-infusion 5-FU plus leucovorin (42) and the NO16968 XELOXA trial (43), comparing capecitabine plus oxaliplatin for resected Stage III colon cancer to the Mayo Clinic regimen of bolus 5-FU and leucovorin, which was the standard of care at the time of study initiation in April, 2003.

Unfortunately, the benefit in disease-free survival shown in all of these trials came at the cost of long-term peripheral sensory neuropathy. In the international XELOXA trial, 78% of patients on the oxaliplatin arm experienced some neurosensory toxicity; the median onset of neuropathy was at 60 days and the toxicity lasted for a median duration of 35 days, with a remarkable range of 18 to 621 days. A reported 11% of patients on this trial experienced grade 3/4 neurosensory toxicity, comparable to the MOSAIC and NSABP C-07 trials (44).

Sensory neuropathy resulting from cumulative oxaliplatin doses is routinely the limiting factor in the duration of treatment (45,46). As with cisplatin and carboplatin, the peripheral neuropathy of oxaliplatin occurs in a cumulative manner. Even after discontinuation of therapy, the symptoms may continue to progress for up to 2 months. Although the mechanism of this toxicity is not fully understood, some authors have proposed that polymorphism in the DNA repair genes may cause individuals to be less proficient in repairing the platinum-induced DNA damage that cause neuronal apoptosis (47).

At the end of treatment on the MOSAIC trial, 3.16% of patients had grade 2 neuropathy, defined as moderate sensory loss and paresthesia and 12.4% had grade 3 neuropathy severe enough to interfere with function. At 1 year, 4.8% of patients had residual grade 2 neuropathy and 1.1% had residual grade 3 neuropathy (41). Other authors have reported that at the cumulative dose of oxaliplatin used in the formal FOLFOX4 regimen, severe grade 3 oxaliplatin-associated neuropathy occurs in up to 30% of patients and that the cumulative form of neuropathy may affect up to 80% of these patients (48).

The NSABP C-07 trial used a lower cumulative target dose of oxaliplatin of 765 mg/m^2. The actual median dose administered was 677 mg/m^2 (range of 320–763 mg/m^2). Time to resolution of neuropathy for those receiving oxaliplatin continued beyond 2 years for more than 10% in the oxaliplatin group (49). Although there is no questions that greater neurotoxicity is experienced during therapy by patients receiving oxaliplatin, published reports of the incidence of this side effect are variable, and may be influenced by reporting methods.

Whatever the definitive incidence of neuropathy, efforts to decrease this toxicity, especially in patients treated adjuvantly, have garnered a significant amount of interest. Calcium and magnesium infusion is becoming the standard of care to minimize this toxicity, both on the basis of individual studies (50) and a meta-analysis comprised of four prospective randomized clinical trials and three retrospective clinical trials involving 1170 CRC patients, which demonstrated that the incidence of grade 3 acute neurotoxicity in those who received calcium and magnesium was significantly lower than that of the control group with no significant differences in median progression-free or overall survival (51).

Substitution of Oral 5-FU: The Efficacy of Capecitabine

Capecitabine is an attractive alternative to continuous infusional 5-FU in terms of patient convenience and as the oral chemotherapies have not been affected by drug shortages that threaten older infusional medications (52). In the adjuvant setting, the X-ACT trial demonstrated that single agent capecitabine resulted in a disease-free survival at least equivalent to 5-FU plus leucovorin (Mayo Clinic regimen) and overall survival that did not differ significantly. The authors also reported significantly lower incidences of neutropenia and stomatitis with capecitabine, although the incidence of grade 3 hand-foot syndrome was significantly higher with capecitabine. The authors attribute a higher number of dose delays and interruptions to the difficulty educating patients to recognize the toxic effects of grade 2 or greater severity (53).

Follow-up presented at the 2012 ASCO Gastrointestinal Cancers Symposium of the NO16968/XELOXA study showed that 7-year disease-free survival rates were 63% for XELOX and 56% for 5-FU and leucovorin. After a median follow-up of 83 months, the hazard ratio for overall survival was 0.83 (95% CI 0.70–0.99; $P = .0367$). The absolute 7-year overall survival rates were 73% with XELOX and 67% with 5-FU and leucovorin.

After adjusting for stratification and prognostic variables, the hazard ratios remained essentially unchanged for both disease-free survival (0.79; 95% CI 0.68–0.91; $P = .0016$) and overall survival (0.84; 95% CI 0.71–1.00; $P= .0477$; 81). This durable benefit of the XELOX therapy supports its use as a standard of care. However, insurance coverage may make the choice of oral chemotherapy prohibitively expensive for many patients (55); for this group of patients, infusional 5-FU may be more affordable.

■ UNREALIZED PROMISE: FAILURE IN THE ADJUVANT SETTING OF OTHER AGENTS APPROVED FOR STAGE IV DISEASE

The adjuvant setting for colon cancer treatment has demonstrated a surprising number of failures for agents that are effective for Stage IV disease (56). Several agents have been repeatedly disappointing as adjuvant treatment in resected colon cancer and should not be prescribed.

Irinotecan

The first such example to emerge was irinotecan. Despite a clear benefit in both progression-free survival and overall survival the metastatic setting (57,58) three phase III studies of adjuvant irinotecan have been negative, PETACC-3 ACCORD-02 trial (58) and CALGB 89803 (59). In the PETACC-3 trial, not only did irinotecan added to 5-FU and leucovorin not confer an improvement in disease-free survival or overall survival in patients with Stage III colon cancer compared with the de Gramontinfusional 5-FU and leucovorin adjuvant regimen alone (60,61), 5-FU and leucovorin was actually found to be superior.

Similar to the disappointing results with adjuvant irinotecan, and despite the clear benefit of targeted agents in the metastatic setting (62–66), after many clinical studies, no clear role for targeted agents in the adjuvant setting for colon cancer has been identified.

Bevacizumab

After the success of bevacizumab in the metastatic setting for colon cancer (62), the NSABP C-08 trial was designed to randomly allocate 2,710 patients with Stages II and III colon cancer to adjuvant mFOLFOX6 with or without bevacizumab (67). Disease-free survival was the primary endpoint of the trial. Patients randomized to bevacizumab had a 3-year disease-free survival of 77.4% versus 75.5% for chemotherapy alone, a nonsignificant 11% reduction of 11% ($P = .15$; 67). The investigators chose to use a 1-year total exposure to bevacizumab (6 months with adjuvant chemotherapy and 6 months as a single agent, on the basis of the adjuvant experience) with trastuzumab therapy in breast cancer.

Wolmark et al presented the results of C-08 at ASCO 2009 demonstrating that bevacizumab for 1 year with mFOLFOX6 does not significantly prolong disease-free survival in Stages II and III colon cancer. There has been much interest in a significant but transient effect demonstrated during bevacizumab exposure that did not translate to sustained improvement in disease-free survival. This observed ephemeral effect does not support the use of bevacizumab in the adjuvant setting.

Similarly, the AVANT trial (68) enrolled 3451 patients with Stage III or high-risk Stage II colon cancer to chemotherapy alone, or either FOLFOX or XELOX chemotherapy with bevacizumab. Unfortunately, and in contrast to the trend observed in the NSABP C-08 trial, both bevacizumab arms had hazard ratios trending toward worse disease-free survival than chemotherapy alone.

Echoing the PETACC3 experience with adjuvant irinotecan, targeting the EGFR with cetuximab added to mFOLFOX-6 in a the NCCTG intergroup phase III trial N0147 resulted in worse disease-free survival in Stage III colon cancer patients with both wild-type and mutated *K-ras* tumors (69). The trial was redesigned in 2008 to incorporate prospective *K-ras* testing, and enrolled patients without mutations in *K-ras* from that point forward, but the addition of cetuximab was ineffective across all subgroups studied and had a 71% grade 3/4 toxicity rate compared to with 51% in the control arm (70). However, after CALGB 89803, PETACC-3, and Accord02 showed no benefit to the irinotecan in adjuvant therapy, the irinotecan arms of N0147 were discontinued. There was, however, no benefit found to the addition of cetuximab on the remaining FOLFOX arm (71), and there is therefore no role for this agent in the adjuvant treatment of patients with colon cancer.

■ CURRENT OPEN QUESTIONS AND AREAS OF DEBATE IN ADJUVANT COLON CANCER

As new evidence emerges, the standard of care will shift. Here, we note 4 areas of active research and indicate possible future directions for treatment: the open question of how to treat Stage II disease; the importance of duration of chemotherapy; the role of timeliness of initiation of chemotherapy; the role of predictive biomarkers in adjuvant colon cancer; and the role of chemotherapy in the adjuvant treatment of elderly patients.

How to Treat Stage II Disease

The role of adjuvant chemotherapy in Stage II colon cancer remains one of the more challenging decisions in oncology (72). There may be subgroups of Stage II colon cancer patients who do have worse prognosis than others, particularly T4bN0 (73), and there is relative uniformity in the available guidelines for offering adjuvant chemotherapy to these patients (74).

However, adjuvant chemotherapy is not the current standard of care in the era of modern chemotherapy for Stage II colon cancer. The most influential adjuvant trial, MOSAIC, did not show an overall survival benefit in Stage II patients with the addition of oxaliplatin to 5-FU, although the authors did report a trend toward improvement in disease-free survival at 5 years (41). Similarly, in a pooled analysis of several studies of 6 months of adjuvant 5-FU and leucovorin with 1025 patients with Duke's Stage B2 cancer in the data set did not reveal a benefit to adjuvant therapy (75).

A recent analysis of outcome data from the SEER—Medicare registry of older patients treated under real-world conditions demonstrated no difference in 5-year survival when comparing those patients with Stage II colon cancer who received postoperative chemotherapy versus those who did not (76). Interestingly, they found a similar lack of benefit for those patients in the subgroup that were defined as "high risk" as per the published guidelines (77,78): diagnosis in the setting of bowel obstruction or perforation, the need for emergent operation, T4 stage, inadequate nodal resection of less than 12 nodes, or peritumoral lymphatic or vascular invasion. Similar criteria are reflected in the current NCCN guidelines (Table 7.2).

Another informative pooled analysis of the NSABP C-07 and C-08 trials evaluating the contribution of oxaliplatin to adjuvant treatment of patients with Stage II CRC demonstrated no significant difference in either disease-free survival of overall survival among the 991 patients treated with oxaliplatin plus 5-FU versus the 2009 patients treated with 5-FU alone (79).

Table 7.2 Guidelines for High-Risk Stage II

ASCO Guidelines

The clinical decision should be based on:

- A discussion with the patient
- Less than 13 LNs examined
- T4 lesion
- Bowel obstruction at presentation, perforation
- Poor histologic grade
- Peritumorallymphovascular involvement
- Poorly differentiated histology
- Questionable surgical margin
- NCCN Guidelines (76)
- Lymphovascular invasion
- Bowel obstruction
- Less than 12 LNs examined
- Perineural invasion
- Perforation
- Close, indeterminate or positive margins

From (77).

This demonstrated lack of benefit to the addition of oxaliplatin in Stage II colon cancer is supported by a Cochrane review of the evidence regarding adjuvant therapy for resected Stage II colon cancer published in 2008. The authors concluded that adjuvant 5-FU carries a real but very small benefit, estimated as a number-needed-to-treat of up to 100 patients in order to save one life, and that the current evidence does not support the use of oxaliplatin in the adjuvant setting for Stage II colon cancer (33).

In contrast to the above results, the QUASAR trial (30) specifically aimed to determine the size and duration of benefit of chemotherapy for patients with Stage II colon and rectal cancer. One thousand six hundred seventeen patients were randomly assigned to observation for their cancer and 1622 were randomly assigned to receive chemotherapy, as 6 months of bolus 5-FU and folinic acid. The investigators found that adjuvant chemotherapy was associated with a significant improvement in survival for patients with Stage II cancer. Of note, the median age in this trial was 53 for both men and women.

Gill et al reported a differential magnitude of benefit with proportional reductions in risk of recurrence and death in a pooled analysis of adjuvant trials of 5-FU-based chemotherapy (34). The risk reduction in node negative disease was 17% reduction of recurrence and 15% reduction of death with the addition a of adjuvant 5-FU-based chemotherapy. The magnitude of benefit was much larger in node-positive disease: 40% and 35%, respectively. On the basis of these and other trials, the Cochrane review (80) did conclude that that adjuvant 5-FU therapy, is associated with a disease-free survival benefit for patients with Stage II colon cancer, but that these benefits are small and not necessarily associated with improved overall survival, and do not support the use of oxaliplatin chemotherapy.

HOW MUCH IS ENOUGH? THE IDEA EFFORT AND EVIDENCE FOR SHORTER DURATION OF CHEMOTHERAPY

A number of trials discussed above demonstrated that 6 months of adjuvant therapy was adequate, with no additional benefit to 12 months of therapy, and therefore 6 months of adjuvant therapy is the current standard of care. Interestingly, an even shorter duration of adjuvant therapy may be equally beneficial. A Cochrane review of available trials found no significant difference in recurrence-free survival or overall survival for a shorter duration of therapy (3 to 6 months) versus a longer duration of chemotherapy (9 to 12 months; 54).

In a study excluded from that Cochrane review, Chau et al demonstrated that 12 weeks of protracted venous infusion of 5-FU was as effective as 6 months of bolus 5-FU and folinic acid as adjuvant treatment of resected colon cancer. This trial had an impressive median followup of greater than 5 years (54).

To answer the question whether 3 months of adjuvant oxaliplatin based chemotherapy is equivalent to 6 months, a noninferiority trial is required. Because of the large number of patients that would be necessary to participate in such a trial (46), an international collaboration of investigators leading individual clinical trials testing the 3 versus 6 months questions has assembled a preplanned IDEA (International Duration Evaluation in Adjuvant Colon Cancer) meta-analysis. This is the largest prospective international collaboration on colon cancer to date. Investigators will collect data on over 10,500 patients with Stage III colon cancer to address the question of 3 versus 6 months duration with a noninferiority margin of 2.5%.

Multidisciplinary Management: Is Promptness More Important Than Duration?

Interestingly, in the Chau trial the benefit was greatest in those patients who initiated CI 5-FU within 8 weeks of surgery (81). There is, in fact, an accumulating body of evidence that time to initiation of adjuvant therapy is in and of itself and extremely important prognostic marker. The benefit in the short-duration therapy group raises the question of whether the time to adjuvant chemotherapy is more important than the duration of adjuvant therapy.

Based on the trials we have discussed here, the standard of care is to initiate postoperative chemotherapy within 8 weeks of surgery. The evidence base for gains from adjuvant chemotherapy in colon cancer Stage III is at level I according to ASCO guidelines, however, only when the treatment started within 5 to 6 weeks after the surgery. Essentially, because most clinical trials mandate that adjuvant chemotherapy is to commence within 6 to 8 weeks after surgery, a routine clinical assumption is that chemotherapy should commence as soon as practical (82). Many authors have examined how the timing of the initiation of postoperative chemotherapy affects overall survival. The relevance of timing of adjuvant chemotherapy can for ethical reasons never be tested in a randomized trial, since a delay beyond what is reasonable for postoperative recovery can only be detrimental (84).

It is interesting that regional chemotherapy, an extreme example of adjuvant chemotherapy given as soon as possible after resection as it can be delivered in the hepatic circulation immediately postoperatively has, in small series, been suggested to have significant benefits in overall survival (33).

In a meta-analysis of five published studies comparing delayed chemotherapy with standard care (83), Des Guetz et al found that delaying chemotherapy more than 8 weeks was associated to worsen overall survival (RR: 1.20; 95% CI 1.15–1.26). In addition, including all studies whatever their cutoff, longer delay was associated to a worse overall survival, although counterintuitively, not a worse relapse-free survival.

Berglund et al (82) published results from a randomized trial of 708 patients with Stage III colon cancer who were randomly assigned to receive surgery alone (N = 364) or surgery plus 5-FU-based chemotherapy (N = 344). An absolute difference in 5-year survival of only 7% favoring the adjuvant group was found in this trial, contrary to the reduction in the death rate of 33% favoring 5-FU plus levamisole found by other authors (5). When data were analyzed, it was found that one-third of the patients in the Swedish trial had started postoperative chemotherapy treatment after 8 weeks. It was speculated that this delay could be one reason why the expected survival gain was not seen. In fact, those patients included in the trial who had their treatment initiated beyond 8 weeks appeared to have no gain from the chemotherapy.

Hershman et al (84) examined the SEER database to describe the overall survival as a function of the timing of initiation of adjuvant chemotherapy in a patient population age greater than 65 years. For overall survival, they described a first significant increase in the hazard ratio when the initiation of chemotherapy after Stage III colon cancer was delayed to the 2-month to 3-month interval. They did find that disease specific survival was found to significantly worsen only after an interval of more than 3 months (HR 1.5; $P < .05$; 84,85).

A recent meta-analysis by Biagi et al (83) demonstrated that a 4-week increase in time to adjuvant chemotherapy was associated with a significant decrease in both overall survival (HR, 1.14; 95% CI, 1.10–1.17) and disease-free survival (HR, 1.14; 95% CI, 1.10–1.18). Applying these findings to a patient who is ready to initiate adjuvant chemotherapy 4 weeks after surgery but is delayed because of logistical rather than medical reasons, that same patient would have a 14% increased risk of mortality if treated at 8 weeks and 30% increased risk at 12 weeks (83).

It is possible, as discussed by Hershman et al (84), that related factors and not the tumor or the interval between surgery and chemotherapy itself may be the reason for the worse outcome observed after an interval of 2 to 3 months. However, given the above evidence supporting timely initiation of adjuvant chemotherapy, and the numerous patient and institutional factors that may delay the initiation of this important measure, timely access to adjuvant chemotherapy is an appropriate clinical quality indicator (86).

The principal take-away point for the clinician from this mounting evidence is that time may be of the essence in starting postsurgical adjuvant chemotherapy. An appropriate goal is to start chemotherapy within 4 weeks when clinically feasible.

PERSONALIZED MEDICINE—UNREALIZED PROMISES IN ADJUVANT COLON CANCER

Predictive and prognostic biomarkers offer the enticing goal of personalizing cancer medicine. However, many reach the marketplace before they have been validated, and their adoption is often hindered by variable clinical evidence. In contrast to the established role of *K-ras* in predicting response to EGFR-targeted agents in metastatic colon cancer (87,88), the clinical evidence supporting biomarker tests in CRC such as mismatch repair (MMR) protein testing, loss of heterozygosity at 18q21 and the Oncotype DX Colon Cancer Assay, have significant variability in the level of clinical evidence associated with these tests (89), and have not been conclusively shown to be predictive of response to chemotherapy.

Oncotype

O'Connell et al reported the application of the quantitative reverse transcription polymerase chain reaction (RT-qPCR) platform developed for the Oncotype DX Breast Cancer Assay in four independent colon cancer studies to generate the 12-gene recurrence score and 11-gene treatment score algorithms. Seven cancer-related genes were selected for consistent association with colon cancer recurrence (90). Three of these genes are associated with activated stroma (*BGN, INHBA,* and *FAP*), and three represent a cell cycle pathway (*MK167, MYBL2* and *MYC*; 91).

In contrast to the Oncotype DX breast cancer assay (92), the Oncotype DX colon cancer assay has not been validated in a prospective, controlled study for adjuvant colon cancer, and has therefore not conclusively been shown to predict benefit from adjuvant chemotherapy.

MARKERS THAT ARE NOT PROGNOSTIC: *K-RAS*, MSS, AND LOH AT 18Q

In metastatic colon cancer, *K-ras* status is predictive of response to *EGFR* targeting agents, but not prognostic (88,93). Ogoni et al analyzed the prognostic significance of the *K-ras* mutation in Stage III colon cancer using a database of Stage III colon cancers from the CALGB89803 trial that compared the weekly Roswell Park regimen of 5-FU and leucovorin to the weekly bolus regimen of irinotecan 5-FU and leucovorin (IFL). Archived formalin-fixed paraffin-embedded tissue was available for 508 patients and the *K-ras* gene was sequenced. They conclude that the *K-ras* mutation did not have a substantial prognostic role in Stage III colon cancer treated with adjuvant chemotherapy (94). However, some authors have interpreted the results of the N0147 trial of mFOLFOX 6 ± cetuximab, which showed disease-free survival to be lower in both *K-ras* mutant arms when compared to *K-ras* WT to suggest a negative prognostic significance for the *K-ras* mutation in Stage III disease (70,71). This is consistent with some earlier meta-analyses (95), which have been criticized for suffering from publication bias (94).

While molecular characteristics of the tumor are not yet ready to predict which patients should be assigned to receive adjuvant chemotherapy, or any particular regimen of 5-FU-based adjuvant chemotherapy, there are several markers that are emerging to be prognostic of response, most notably microsatellite stability and loss of heterozygosity (LOH) at 18q21.

Microsatellite instability (MSI) as a result of the inactivation of the MMR system characterizes approximately 15% of CRC as a result of either germline mutational inactivation of MMR genes in Lynch syndrome or sporadic epigenetic silencing by hypermethylation of the MMR gene promoters. The prognosis of MSI tumors is clearly distinct from other CRCs. There are significant data that patients with these tumors do not benefit from adjuvant 5-FU-based chemotherapy (96), although there remains some controversy as to whether there remains some benefit to chemotherapy even for these better-prognosis patients (97).

Watanabe et al found that among patients with microsatellite stable (MSS) cancer treated with 5-FU-based adjuvant chemotherapy with Stage III disease, retention of the 18q alleles (the site of the *DCC* gene) was prognostic for a favorable outcome with a 5-year disease-free survival rate of 64%, as compared to 44% a month those with LOH at 18q (86). This is concordant with earlier results suggesting that among patients with LOH at 18q21 in primary cancer, an increased rate of tumor recurrence is directly responsible for poor survival (98).

When there is uncertainty about the need to treat Stage II disease, testing for dMMR may provide guidance, understanding that this has not been validated in prospective trials. The most recent prospective trial using this approach was ECOG 5202, in which patients were stratified by MSI-high and 18q LOH and assigned to chemotherapy only if they were considered high risk by 18q LOH with either MSS or MSI-low. Unfortunately, this trial included bevacizumab in the experimental design, and was abandoned after the results of the C-08 and AVANT trials did not show benefit to bevacizumab in the adjuvant setting (67,68).

ELDERLY PATIENTS

Most patients with colon cancer are older than 65 years (99). There are unfortunately limited data on the ability to predict tolerance to anticancer therapy and the appropriate use of treatment modalities in the setting of comorbidity and concurrent frailty. In addition, the low representation of older patients in clinical trials results in very limited evidence to guide oncologists in the appropriate management of this population (99).

Not surprisingly given the limited data on safety in this population, adjuvant chemotherapy for Stage III colon cancer treatment rates decline dramatically with chronologic age (99).

An analysis by O'Conner et al (76) showed that adjuvant chemotherapy did not improve overall survival for elderly patients with Stage II colon cancer with high risk status. Similarly, Jackson McCleary et al examined the data from 10,499 patients younger than 70 years and 2170 patients who were 70 years or older in six phase III adjuvant trials (100) and found that whereas younger patients less than 70 years of age derived significant benefit from oxaliplatin-based therapy, patients more than 70 years of age do not receive the same benefit from combination therapy.

In contrast to the above results in elderly patients treated with combination chemotherapy, a meta-analysis by Sargent et al of seven randomized trials of 5-FU plus levamisole or leucovorin versus surgery alone included a total of 3351 patients, of which 15% were aged 70 years or older. These data showed no significant interaction between age and efficacy of treatment (34).

In the face of these results, it is difficult to recommend oxaliplatin-based chemotherapy in the elderly, but given the overall efficacy of combination chemotherapy, a predictive model developed by Hurria et al (101) may be useful in selecting those elderly patients likely to tolerate chemotherapy without significant grade 3 to 5 toxicity. The model incorporates age as well as a number of important geriatric assessment characteristics. Interestingly, Hurria et al found that in these patients, being treated for a GI malignancy, which would include colon cancer, increased the risk of toxicity (Figure 7.5).

	Prevalence		Grades 3 to 5 Toxicity				
Risk Factor	No.	%	No.	%	OR	95% CI	Score
Age ≥ 72 years	270	54	163	60	1.85	1.22 to 2.82	2
Cancer type GI or GU	185	37	120	65	2.13	1.39 to 3.24	2
Chemotherapy dosing, standard dose	380	76	204	54	2.13	1.29 to 3.52	2
No. of chemotherapy drugs, polychemotherapy	351	70	192	55	1.69	1.08 to 2.65	2
Hemoglobin < 11 g/dL (male), < 10 g/dL (female)	62	12	46	74	2.31	1.15 to 4.64	3
Creatinine clearance (Jelliffe, ideal weight) < 34 mL/min	44	9	34	77	2.46	1.11 to 5.44	3
Hearing, fair or worse	123	25	76	62	1.67	1.04 to 2.69	2
No. of falls in last 6 months, 1 or more	91	18	61	67	2.47	1.43 to 4.27	3
IADL: Taking medications, with some help/unable	39	8	28	72	1.50	0.66 to 3.38	1
MOS: Walking 1 block, somewhat limited/very limited	109	22	69	63	1.71	1.02 to 2.86	2
MOS: Decreased social activity because of physical/emotional health, limited at least sometimes	218	44	126	58	1.36	0.90 to 2.06	1

GU, genitourinary; IADL, instrumental activities of daily living; MOS, Medical Outcomes Study; OR, odds ratio.

FIGURE 7.5 Predictive model.

■ CONCLUSIONS

While surgical resection remains the cornerstone of management for patients with Stages I–III disease, a considerable proportion of patients will ultimately relapse and die from colon cancer. Adjuvant chemotherapy for Stage III disease is the standard of care based on trials such as that conducted by Chau et al (54) who have found a significant survival advantage for patients in whom adjuvant chemotherapy was initiated within 8 weeks of surgery (*P* = .044). However, even with the addition of oxaliplatin to adjuvant chemotherapy, the 6-year overall survival rates for resected Stage III colon cancer is only 78.5% (18).

The cumulative toxicity associated with the current standard of care in Stage III colon cancer of 6 months of oxaliplatin-containing chemotherapy points to a need to conclusively address the issue of adjuvant treatment duration to ensure that the toxicity is balanced by benefit in terms of disease-free survival and overall survival. This question is currently being addressed by an international collaboration that is planned to include the over 10,000 patients necessary to complete a noninferiority study to answer the duration question of 6 versus 3 months of therapy (46). In the meantime, evidence is mounting that the duration of adjuvant chemotherapy may not be of as much importance as the timeliness of that therapy, therefore multidisciplinary efforts focused on the timely delivery of care may be of great benefit to patients treated adjuvantly.

Unfortunately, we do not have prospective trials to guide us in the assignment of "high-risk" Stage II patients to adjuvant chemotherapy, but the cumulative evidence is that in this population there is no clear benefit to the addition of oxaliplatin, so it seems reasonable to spare that population of cumulative toxicity associated with that drug. In this setting, testing such as for defects in the MMR pathway may provide guidance, but are not supported by prospective trials.

Similarly, limited data are available to guide us in the treatment of older patients, particularly those who are infirm, but evidence (100) suggests that fit older patients are able to tolerate treatment and derive similar clinical benefits from adjuvant 5-FU as younger patients.

Since 1990, there have been enormous gains in saving lives with the addition of chemotherapy to surgical treatment of localized colon cancer. It is hoped that we will, in the coming decade, develop better predictive biomarkers for response to therapy, a better understanding of both the optimal timing of and duration of therapy, and develop a more sophisticated molecular understanding of what constitutes "high-risk" disease.

REFERENCES

1. Ellis, H. *A History of Surgery*. London, England: Greenwich Medical Media Limited; 2001: pp. 109–110.
2. http://globocan.iarc.fr/factsheets/populations/factsheet.asp?uno=900 Accessed on 23 May 2012.
3. Jemal A, Siegel R, Xu J, Ward E. Cancer Statistics 2010. *Cancer J Clin*. 2010;60(5):277–300.
4. Bendix F, Schmidt U, Mroczkowski P, Gastinger I, Lippert H, Kube R. Colon carcinoma—classification into right and left-side cancer or according to colonic subsite? Analysis of 29,568 patients. *Eur J Surg Oncol*. 2011;37(2):134–139.
5. LeVoyer TE, Sigurdson ER, Hanlon, AL, et al. Colon cancer survival is associated with increasing number of lymph nodes analyzed: a secondary survey of intergroup trial int-0089. *J Clin Oncol*. 2003;21:2912–2919.
6. Nichols RL, Smith JW, Garcia RY, Waterman RS, Holmes JW. Current practices of preoperative bowel preparation among North American colorectal surgeons. *Clin Infect Dis*. 1997;24(4):609–619.
7. Contant CM, Hop WC, Van'tSant HP, Oostvogel HJ et al. Mechanical bowel preparation for elective colorectal surgery: a multicenter randomized trial. *Lancet* 2007;370:2112–2117.
8. Slim K, Vicaut E, Launay-Savary MV, Contant C, Chipponi J. Updated systematic review and meta-analysis of randomized clinical trials on the role of mechanical bowel preparation before colorectal surgery. *Ann Surg*. 2009;249(2):203–209.
9. Kim MS, Park YJ. Detection and treatment of synchronous lesions in colorectal cancer: the clinical implication of perioperative colonoscopy. *World J Gastroenterol*. 2007;13(40):4108–4111.
10. Langevin JM, Nivatvongs S. The true incidence of synchronous cancer of the large bowel. A prospective study. *Am J Surg*. 1984;147(3):330–333.
11. http://www.nccn.org/professionals/physician_gls/pdf/colon.pdf Accessed on 23 May 2012.
12. Lee YM, Law WL, Chu KW et al. Emergency surgery for obstructing colorectal cancer: a comparison between right-sided and left-sided lesions. *J Am Coll Surg*. 2001;192:719
13. Phillips EH, Franklin M, Carroll BJ, Fallas MJ, Ramos R, Rosenthal D. Laparoscopic Colectomy. *Ann Surg*. 1992;216:703–707.
14. Berends FJ, Kazemier G, Bonjer HJ, Lange JF. Subcutaneous metastases after laparoscopic colectomy. *Lancet*. 1994;344–358.
15. Clinical Outcomes of Surgical Therapy Study Group. A comparison of laparoscopically assisted and open colectomy for colon cancer. *N Engl J Med*. 2004;350(20):2050–2059.
16. Fleshman J, Sargent DJ, Green E, et al for The Clinical Outcomes of Surgical Therapy Study Group. Laparoscopic colectomy for cancer is not inferior to open surgery based on 5-year data from the COST Study Group trial. *Ann Surg*. 2007;246(4):655–662; discussion 662–664.
17. Jayne DG, Guillou PJ, Thorpe H, et al. Randomized trial of laparoscopic-assisted resection of colorectal carcinoma: 3-year results of the UK MRC CLASICC Trial Group. *J Clin Oncol*. 2007;25(21):44–52.
18. Veldkamp R, Hop WC, Kuhry E, et al. for the Colon Cancer Laparoscopic or Open Resection Study Group. Survival after laparoscopic surgery versus open surgery for colon cancer: long-term outcome of a randomised clinical trial. *Lancet Oncol*. 2009;10(1):44–52.
19. Lacy AM, Delgado S, Castells A, et al. The long-term results of a randomized clinical trial of laparoscopy-assisted versus open surgery for colon cancer. *Ann Surg*. 2008;248(1):1–7.
20. Feinstein AR, Sosin DM, Wells CK. The Will Rogers phenomenon: stage migration and new diagnostic techniques as a source of misleading statistics for survival in cancer. *N Engl J Med*. 1995;312:1604–1608.
21. Goldstein NS, Lymph node recoveries from 2427 pT3 colorectal resection specimens spanning 45 years: recommendations for a minimum number of recovered lymph nodes based on predictive probabilities. *Am J Surg Path*. 2002:26(2):179–189.
22. Law CH, Wright FC, Rapanos T, et al. Impact of lymph node retrieval and pathological ultra-staging on the prognosis of stage II colon cancer. *J SurgOncol*. 2003;84(3):120–126
23. Neugut AI, Forde KA. Screening colonoscopy: has the time come? *Am J Gastroenterol*. 1988;83(3):295–297.
24. Zauber AG, Winawer SJ, O'Brien MJ, et al. Colonoscopic-polypectomy and long-term prevention of colorectal-cancer deaths. *N Engl J Med*. 2012;366(8):687–696.
25. Proctor MJ, Chrighton E, Richards CH, Mcmillan DC, Horgan PG. The effect of screening on stage of disease and tumor characteristics in patients with operable colorectal cancer. *ASCO Meeting Abstracts*. June 9, 2011;29(15_suppl):3540.
26. Sharma VK, Vasudeva R, Howden CW. Changes in colorectal cancer over a 15-year period in a single United States city. *Am J Gastroenterol*. 2000;95(12):3615–3619.
27. Moertel CG, Fleming TR, Macdonald JS, et al. Levamisole and fluorouracil for adjuvant therapy of resected colon carcinoma. *N Engl J Med*. 1990;322(6):352–358.
28. Moertel CG, Fleming TR, Macdonald JS, et al. Fluorouracil plus levamisole as effective adjuvant therapy after resection of stage III colon carcinoma: a final report. *Ann Intern Med*. 1995;122(5):321–326.
29. Gray R, Barnwell J, McConkey C, Hills RK, Williams NS, Kerr DJ. Adjuvant chemotherapy versus observation in patients with colorectal cancer: a randomised study. *Lancet*. 2007; 370(9604):2020–2029.
30. Arkenau HT, Bermann A, Rettig K, Strohmeyer G, Porschen R. 5-Fluorouracil plus leucovorin is an effective adjuvant chemotherapy in curatively resected stage III colon cancer: long-term follow-up results of the adjCCA-01 trial. *Annals of Oncology*. 2003;14(3):395–399.
31. Chlebowski RT, Lillington L, Nystrom JS, Sayre J. Late mortality and levamisole adjuvant therapy in colorectal cancer. *Br J Cancer*. 1994;69(6):1094–1097.
32. Figueredo A, Coombes ME, Mukherjee S. Adjuvant therapy for completely resected stage II colon cancer. *Cochrane Database Syst Rev*. 2008(3):CD005390.
33. Sargent DJ, Goldberg RM, Jacobson SD, et al. A pooled analysis of adjuvant chemotherapy for resected colon cancer in elderly patients. *N Engl J Med*. 2001;345(15):1091–1097.
34. Gill S, Loprinzi CL, Sargent DJ, et al. Pooled analysis of fluorouracil-based adjuvant therapy for stage II and III colon cancer: who benefits and by how much? *J Clin Oncol*. 2004;22(10): 1797–1806.
35. Haller DG, Catalano PJ, Macdonald JS, et al. Phase III study of fluorouracil, leucovorin, and levamisole in high-risk stage II and III colon cancer: final report of Intergroup 0089. *J Clin Oncol*. 2005;23(34):8671–8678.
36. Efficacy of adjuvant fluorouracil and folinic acid in colon cancer. International Multicentre Pooled Analysis of Colon Cancer Trials (IMPACT) investigators. *Lancet*. 1995;345(8955):939–944.
37. Poplin EA, Benedetti JK, Estes NC, et al. Phase III Southwest Oncology Group 9415/Intergroup 0153 randomized trial of fluorouracil, leucovorin, and levamisole versus fluorouracil continuous infusion and levamisole for adjuvant treatment

of stage III and high-risk stage II colon cancer. *J Clin Oncol.* 2005;23(9):1819–1825.

38. de Gramont A, Hubbard J, Shi Q, et al. Association between disease-free survival and overall survival when survival is prolonged after recurrence in patients receiving cytotoxic adjuvant therapy for colon cancer: simulations based on the 20,800 patient ACCENT data set. *J Clin Oncol.* 2010;28(3): 460–465.
39. Sargent D, Sobrero A, Grothey A, et al. Evidence for cure by adjuvant therapy in colon cancer: observations based on individual patient data from 20,898 patients on 18 randomized trials. *J Clin Oncol.* 2009;27(6):872–877.
40. Andre T, Boni C, Navarro M, et al. Improved overall survival with oxaliplatin, fluorouracil, and leucovorin as adjuvant treatment in stage II or III colon cancer in the MOSAIC trial. *J Clin Oncol.* 2009;27(19):3109–3116.
41. Kuebler JP, Wieand HS, O'Connell MJ, et al. Oxaliplatin combined with weekly bolus fluorouracil and leucovorin as surgical adjuvant chemotherapy for stage II and III colon cancer: results from NSABP C-07. *J Clin Oncol.* 2007;25(16):2198–2204.
42. Haller DG, Tabernero J, Maroun J, et al. Capecitabine plus oxaliplatin compared with fluorouracil and folinic acid as adjuvant therapy for Stage III colon cancer. *J Clin Oncol.* 2011;29(11):1465–1471.
43. Schmoll H-J, Cartwright T, Tabernero J, et al. Phase III trial of capecitabine plus oxaliplatin as adjuvant therapy for Stage III colon cancer: a planned safety analysis in 1,864 patients. *J Clin Oncol.* 2007;25(1):102–109.
44. Raymond E, Chaney SG, Taamma A, Cvitkovic E. Oxaliplatin: a review of preclinical and clinical studies. *Ann Oncol.* 1998;9(10):1053–1071.
45. Hubbard J, Grothey A. Reduced chemotherapy duration: a good idea? *Current Colorectal Cancer Reports.*7(3):241–245.
46. McWhinney SR, Goldberg RM, McLeod HL. Platinum neurotoxicity pharmacogenetics. *Mol Cancer Ther.* 2009;8(1):10–16.
47. Argyriou AA, Velasco R, Briani C, et al. Peripheral neurotoxicity of oxaliplatin in combination with 5-fluorouracil (FOLFOX) or capecitabine (XELOX): a prospective evaluation of 150 colorectal cancer patients. *Ann Oncol.* 2012.
48. Land SR, Kopec JA, Cecchini RS, et al. Neurotoxicity from oxaliplatin combined with weekly bolus fluorouracil and leucovorin as surgical adjuvant chemotherapy for stage II and III colon cancer: NSABP C-07. *J Clin Oncol.* 2007;25(16):2205–2211.
49. Grothey A, Nikcevich DA, Sloan JA, et al. Intravenous calcium and magnesium for oxaliplatin-induced sensory neurotoxicity in adjuvant colon cancer: NCCTG N04C7. *J Clin Oncol.* 2011;29(4):421–427.
50. Wen F, Zhou Y, Wang W, et al. Ca/Mg infusions for the prevention of oxaliplatin-related neurotoxicity in patients with colorectal cancer: a meta-analysis. *Ann Oncol.* 2012.
51. Gatesman ML, Smith TJ. The shortage of essential chemotherapy drugs in the United States. *N Engl J Med.* 2011; 365(18):1653–1655.
52. Twelves C, Wong A, Nowacki MP, et al. Capecitabine as adjuvant treatment for stage III colon cancer. *N Engl J Med.* 2005;352(26):2696–2704.
53. Schmoll H-J, Tabernero J, Maroun JA, et al. Capecitabine plus oxaliplatin (XELOX) versus bolus 5-fluorouracil/leucovorin (5-FU/LV) as adjuvant therapy for stage III colon cancer: Survival follow-up of study NO16968 (XELOXA). *ASCO Meeting Abstracts.* 2012;30(4_suppl):388.
54. Chau I, Norman AR, Cunningham D, et al. A randomised comparisonbetween 6 months of bolus fluorouracil/leucovorin and12 weeks of protracted venous infusion fluorouracil as adjuvant treatment in colorectal cancer. *Ann Oncol.* 2005;16(4):549–557.
55. de Gramont A, Chibaudel B, Bachet JB, et al. From chemotherapy to targeted therapy in adjuvant treatment for stage iii colon cancer. Semin Oncol. Aug;38(4):521–532.
56. Saltz LB, Cox JV, Blanke C, et al. Irinotecan plus fluorouracil and leucovorin for metastatic colorectal cancer. Irinotecan Study Group. *N Engl J Med.* 2000;343(13):905–914.
57. Colucci G, Gebbia V, Paoletti G, et al. Phase III randomized trial of FOLFIRI versus FOLFOX4 in the treatment of advanced colorectal cancer: a multicenter study of the Gruppo Oncologico Dell'Italia Meridionale. *J Clin Oncol.* 2005;23(22):4866–4875.
58. Ychou M, Raoul JL, Douillard JY, et al. A phase III randomised trial of LV5FU2 + irinotecan versus LV5FU2 alone in adjuvant high-risk colon cancer (FNCLCC Accord-02/FFCD9802). *Ann Oncol.* 2009;20(4):674–680.
59. Saltz LB, Niedzwiecki D, Hollis D, et al. Irinotecan fluorouracil plus leucovorin is not superior to fluorouracil plus leucovorin alone as adjuvant treatment for stage iii colon cancer: results of CALGB 89803. J Clin Oncol. 2007;25(23):3456–3461.
60. Van Cutsem E, Labianca R, Bodoky G, et al. Randomized phase III trial comparing biweekly infusional fluorouracil/leucovorin alone or with irinotecan in the adjuvant treatment of stage III colon cancer: PETACC-3. *J Clin Oncol.* 2009;27(19):3117–3125.
61. Hurwitz H, Fehrenbacher L, Novotny W, et al. Bevacizumab plus irinotecan, fluorouracil, and leucovorin for metastatic colorectal cancer. *N Engl J Med.* 2004;350(23):2335–2342.
62. Hochster HS, Hart LL, Ramanathan RK, et al. Safety and efficacy of oxaliplatin and fluoropyrimidine regimens with or without bevacizumab as first-line treatment of metastatic colorectal cancer: results of the TREE Study. *J Clin Oncol.* 2008;26(21):3523–3529.
63. Cunningham D, Humblet Y, Siena S, et al. Cetuximabmonotherapy and cetuximab plus irinotecan in irinotecan-refractory metastatic colorectal cancer. *N Engl J Med.* 2004;351(4):337–345.
64. Giantonio BJ, Catalano PJ, Meropol NJ, et al. Bevacizumab in combination with oxaliplatin, fluorouracil, and leucovorin (FOLFOX4) for previously treated metastatic colorectal cancer: results from the Eastern Cooperative Oncology Group Study E3200. *J Clin Oncol.* 2007;25(12):1539–1544.
65. Van Cutsem E, Peeters M, Siena S, et al. Open-label phase III trial of panitumumab plus best supportive care compared with best supportive care alone in patients with chemotherapy-refractory metastatic colorectal cancer. *J Clin Oncol.* 2007;25(13):1658–1664.
66. Allegra CJ, Yothers G, O'Connell MJ, et al. Phase III trial assessing bevacizumab in stages II and III carcinoma of the colon: results of NSABP protocol C-08. *J Clin Oncol.* 2011;29(1):11–16.
67. De Gramont A, Van Cutsem, E., Tabernero, J et al. AVANT: Results from a randomized, three-arm multinational phase III study to investigate bevacizumab with either XELOX or FOLFOX4 versus FOLFOX4 alone as adjuvant treatment for colon cancer *ASCO 2011.* Vol 29:Supplement 362
68. Huang J, Sargent DJ, Mahoney MR, et al. Adjuvant FOLFIRI with or without cetuximab in patients with resected stage III colon cancer: NCCTG Intergroup phase III trial N0147. *ASCO Meeting Abstracts.* 2011;29(4_suppl):363.
69. Murphy JE, Ryan DP. American Society of Clinical Oncology 2010 colorectal update. *Expert Rev Anticancer Ther.* 2011;10(9):1371–1373.
70. Goldberg RM, Sargent DJ, Thibodeau SN, et al. Adjuvant mFOLFOX6 plus or minus cetuximab (Cmab) in patients (pts) with K-ras mutant (m) resected stage III colon cancer (CC): NCCTG Intergroup Phase III Trial N0147. *ASCO Meeting Abstracts.* 2010;28(15_suppl):3508.
71. Meropol NJ. Ongoing challenge of stage II colon cancer. *J Clin Oncol.* 2011;29(25):3346–3348.
72. Gunderson LL, Jessup JM, Sargent DJ, Greene FL, Stewart AK. Revised TN categorization for colon cancer based on National Survival Outcomes Data. *J Clin Oncol.* 2010;28(2):264–271.
73. Romanus D, Weiser MR, Skibber JM, et al. Concordance with NCCN colorectal cancer guidelines and asco/nccn quality measures: an NCCN institutional analysis. *J Natl Compr Canc Netw.* 2009;7(8):895–904.

74. Efficacy of adjuvant fluorouracil and folinic acid in B2 colon cancer. International Multicentre Pooled Analysis of B2 Colon Cancer Trials (IMPACT B2) Investigators. *J Clin Oncol.* 1999;17(5):1356–1363.
75. O'Connor ES, Greenblatt DY, LoConte NK, et al. Adjuvant chemotherapy for stage ii colon cancer with poor prognostic features. *J Clin Oncol.* 2011;29(25):3381–3388.
76. Engstrom PF, Arnoletti JP, Benson AB, et al. Colon cancer. *J Natl Compr Canc Netw.* 2009;7(8):778–831.
77. Benson AB, Schrag D, Somerfield MR, et al. American society of clinical oncology recommendations on adjuvant chemotherapy for stage ii colon cancer. *J Clin Oncol.* 2004;22(16): 3408–3419.
78. Yothers GA, Allegra CJ, O'Connell MJ, et al. The efficacy of oxaliplatin (Ox) when added to 5-fluorouracil/leucovorin (FU/L) in stage II colon cancer. *ASCO Meeting Abstracts.* 2011;29(15_suppl):3507.
79. Figueredo A, Charette ML, Maroun J, Brouwers MC, Zuraw L. Adjuvant therapy for stage II colon cancer: a systematic review from the Cancer Care Ontario Program in evidence-based care's gastrointestinal cancer disease site group. *J Clin Oncol.* 2004;22(16):3395–3407.
80. Des Guetz G, Uzzan B, Morere JF, Perret G, Nicolas P. Duration of adjuvant chemotherapy for patients with non-metastatic colorectal cancer. *Cochrane Database Syst Rev.* (1):CD007046.
81. Biagi JJ, Raphael MJ, Mackillop WJ, Kong W, King WD, Booth CM. Association between time to initiation of adjuvant chemotherapy and survival in colorectal cancer. *JAMA.* 2011; 305(22):2335–2342.
82. Berglund A, Cedermark B, Glimelius B. Is it deleterious to delay the start of adjuvant chemotherapy in colon cancer stage III? *Ann Oncol.* 2008;19(2):400–402.
83. Des Guetz G, Nicolas P, Perret GY, Morere JF, Uzzan B. Does delaying adjuvant chemotherapy after curative surgery for colorectal cancer impair survival? A meta-analysis. *Eur J Cancer.* 2010;46(6):1049–1055.
84. Hershman D, Hall MJ, Wang X, et al. Timing of adjuvant chemotherapy initiation after surgery for stage III colon cancer. *Cancer.* 2006;107(11):2581–2588.
85. Watanabe T, Wu TT, Catalano PJ, et al. Molecular predictors of survival after adjuvant chemotherapy for colon cancer. *N Engl J Med.* 2001;344(16):1196–1206.
86. Van Cutsem E, Lang, I., D'haens, G, et al. K-ras status and efficacy in the first-line treatment of patients with metastatic colorectal cancer (mCRC) treated with FOLFIRI with or without cetuximab: The CRYSTAL experience. Paper presented at: 2008 *ASCO Annual Meeting* 2008.
87. Amado RG, Wolf M, Peeters M, et al. Wild-type K-ras is required for panitumumab efficacy in patients with metastatic colorectal cancer. *J Clin Oncol.* 2008;26(10):1626–1634.
88. Kelley RK, Van Bebber SL, Phillips KA, Venook AP. Personalized medicine and oncology practice guidelines: a case study of contemporary biomarkers in colorectal cancer. *J Natl Compr Canc Netw.* 2011;9(1):13–25.
89. O'Connell M, Lavery I, Yothers G, et al. Relationship between tumor gene expression and recurrence in four independent studies of stage II/II colon cancer patients treated with surgery alone and surgery plus 5-FU/LV. *J Clin Oncol.* 2010;28:3937–3944.
90. Clark-Langone K, Sangli C, Krishnakumar J, Watson D. Translating tumor biology into personalized treatment planning: analytical performance characteristics of the Oncotype DX(R) Colon Cancer Assay. *BMC Cancer.* 2010;10(1):691.
91. Paik S, Tang G, Shak S, et al. Gene expression and benefit of chemotherapy in women with node-negative, estrogen receptor-positive breast cancer. *J Clin Oncol.* 2006;24(23):3726–3734.
92. Van Cutsem E, Kohne CH, Hitre E, et al. Cetuximab and chemotherapy as initial treatment for metastatic colorectal cancer. *N Engl J Med.* 2009;360(14):1408–1417.
93. Ogino S, Meyerhardt JA, Irahara N, et al. K-ras mutation in stage iii colon cancer and clinical outcome following Intergroup Trial CALGB 89803. *Clin Cancer Res.* 2009;15(23):7322–7329.
94. Andreyev HJ, Norman AR, Cunningham D, et al. Kirsten ras mutations in patients with colorectal cancer: the 'RASCAL II' study. *Br J Cancer.* 2001;85(5):692–696.
95. Ribic CM, Sargent DJ, Moore MJ, et al. Tumor microsatellite-instability status as a predictor of benefit from fluorouracil-based adjuvant chemotherapy for colon cancer. *N Engl J Med.* 2003;349(3):247–257.
96. Tejpar S, Saridaki Z, Delorenzi M, Bosman F, Roth AD. Microsatellite instability, prognosis and drug sensitivity of stage II and III colorectal cancer: more complexity to the puzzle. *J Natl Cancer Inst.* 2011;103(11):841–844.
97. Jernvall P, Makinen MJ, Karttunen TJ, Makela J, Vihko P. Loss of heterozygosity at 18q21 is indicative of recurrence and therefore poor prognosis in a subset of colorectal cancers. *Br J Cancer.* 1999;79(5–6):903–908.
98. Schrag D, Cramer LD, Bach PB, Begg CB. Age and adjuvant chemotherapy use after surgery for stage iii colon cancer. *J Natl Cancer Inst.* 2001;93(11):850–857.
99. Dotan E, Browner I, Hurria A, Denlinger C. Challenges in the management of older patients with colon cancer. *J Natl Compr Canc Netw.* 2012;10(2):213–224; quiz 225.
100. Jackson McCleary NA, Meyerhardt J, Green E, et al. Impact of older age on the efficacy of newer adjuvant therapies in >12,500 patients (pts) with stage II/III colon cancer: Findings from the ACCENT Database. *ASCO Meeting Abstracts.* 2009;27(15S):4010.
101. Hurria A, Togawa K, Mohile SG, et al. Predicting chemotherapy toxicity in older adults with cancer: a prospective multicenter study. *J Clin Oncol.* 2011;29(25):3457–3465.
102. Blum D. Impact of increasing out-of-pocket costs for insured cancerpatients. *Drug Benefit Trends.* 2009;21: 45–153.

8 Nonmetastatic Rectal Cancer: Early and Locally Advanced

Radiation Oncology

WILLIAM A. HALL
ROSHAN S. PRABHU
JEROME C. LANDRY

The objective of this chapter is to provide a review of the role of RT, chemotherapy, and surgery in the management of localized cancers of the rectum.

INTRODUCTION

Colorectal cancer (CRC) is the third most common cancer among men and women in the United States and represents the second most common cause of cancer death. In 2010, there were close to 40,000 new cases of rectal cancer alone (1). Significant advances have been made in the past 10 years in the diagnosis and management of CRC. Incidence rates have decreased, largely as a consequence of improved screening that led to the early detection and eradication of precancerous polyps (2). Along with lower incidence rates, mortality rates from CRC have declined from 30.77 per 100,000 in 1990 to 20.5 per 100,000 in 2006 (1).

Rectal cancer was historically a surgical disease, and surgery is still the only potentially curative option for this disease. However, with improvements in surgical technique, such as the wide adoption of the total mesorectal excision (TME) surgical technique, along with advances in chemotherapy and radiotherapy (RT) delivery, rectal cancer outcomes have improved in recent years (3).

While the surgical management of rectal cancer has progressed substantially, the consistent adoption of surgical guidelines and techniques in both Europe and the United States has not been uniform (4). Similarly, RT techniques including fractionation schedule, sequencing with surgery, and choice of concurrent chemotherapy have remained controversial, with distinct differences existing between practice patterns in the United States and Europe (5). Furthermore, advances in antineoplastic therapy for metastatic CRC are being studied to evaluate their role in earlier disease. These factors have combined to make uniform consensus with regard to surgery, chemotherapy, and RT of rectal cancer difficult to achieve.

STAGING AND WORKUP

As the first principle for any patient with cancer, the clinical staging and workup should begin with a complete history and physical exam. An evaluation of the patient with rectal cancer includes a complete colonoscopy to rule out synchronous primary cancers. If a patient has an obstructing rectal tumor that precludes endoscopic evaluation of the proximal colon, a completion colonoscopy is mandated after the completion of therapy for the rectal cancer. Once an initial pathologic diagnosis is established, further evaluation for the presence of nodal and/or distant metastatic disease should be completed. This typically is done with a CT scan of the chest, abdomen, and pelvis with oral and IV contrast. In addition to evaluation for metastatic disease, the depth of tumor invasion for T staging should be obtained with endoscopic ultrasound, endorectal MRI, or pelvic MRI. The role of PET in CRC is evolving and, while not routinely indicated, may be considered in the evaluation of specific subsets of patients with rectal cancer. Recently, emerging evidence has shown that PET/CT can play an increasingly important role in the management of these patients, with some series showing the largest benefit in patients with low rectal tumors (6–8). Given the substantial dependence of treatment recommendations on accurate staging, consensus on the preoperative stage is critical among members of the multidisciplinary team prior to making any management decisions. Additionally, accurate definition of the extent of tumor involvement is critical for the radiation oncologist in designing accurate and targeted treatment plans to maximize tumor kill and minimize normal tissue damage.

PROGNOSTIC FACTORS

An understanding of the various prognostic factors that impact outcomes is essential to the management of patients with rectal cancer. This understanding is important both in the selection of therapeutic modalities as well as for counseling the patient and family regarding prognosis. The staging of rectal cancer is the most important prognostic factor, and is dependent on both invasion into the bowel wall and the presence or absence of nodal or distant metastasis (9). Not surprisingly, both T and N stage have been closely correlated with patient outcomes and appear to independently influence both disease-specific survival and overall survival (OS; 10,11). In addition to TNM stage, the involvement of the circumferential resection margin (CRM) also strongly influences outcomes (12). A recent meta-analysis confirmed the prognostic value of CRM status in the modern day treatment of rectal cancer. The presence of a positive CRM is a powerful independent predictor for development of both local recurrence and distant metastasis, as well as for OS (13). The largest hazard ratio (HR) for local recurrence is in patients with an involved CRM after neoadjuvant therapy. In general, a positive CRM is tumor 1 mm or less from the margin. There have been numerous studies devoted to the subject of the CRM, and the general conclusion is that the larger the distance of the tumor from the CRM, the better the prognosis (14–18). Along with TNM stage and CRM, the importance of lymphovascular space invasion has been examined in multiple series and has been shown to correlate with risk of both local and distant metastasis, as well as OS (19–22). Additional prognostic factors that should be considered include perineural invasion (23), extranodal tumor deposits (24), tumor response to neoadjuvant therapy (25), and histologic tumor grade (26). Additional information, such as microsatellite instability (MSI) status (27), have prognostic significance. Furthermore, tumor genetics, such as 18q LOH, have emerged as important variables. A more detailed review of these prognostic factors can be found in Chapter 6: Pathology and Molecular Pathology.

ANATOMIC CONSIDERATIONS FOR THE RADIATION ONCOLOGIST

An understanding of the anatomic factors regarding rectal cancer is essential for designing optimal radiation treatment plans. The rectum has been traditionally defined as the terminal segment of the large bowel beginning approximately 12 to 15 cm proximal to the anal verge, with the dentate line dividing the rectum from the anus. The surgical definition of the distal end of the rectum is slightly different, with the puborectalis ring just proximal to the dentate line considered the recto-anal transition. The rectum has also been historically subdivided into proximal and distal portions based on the level of the peritoneal reflection along the anterior surface of the rectum, which is usually around the level of S3 (28,29). The upper third of the rectum is covered with peritoneum on both sides as well as anteriorly. As the rectum continues distally into the pelvis, the peritoneal coverage changes for the middle third of the rectum, with only the anterior aspect covered with peritoneum. This anterior surface makes up the posterior border of the rectouterine pouch in females and the rectovesicular space in males. The lower third of the rectum is devoid of peritoneal covering. In addition to being more difficult to resect given the spatial confines, there is also no natural barrier for invasion of tumor into local adjacent structures. The course of the major vessels that supply the rectum helps to define the lymphatic drainage. The major regional draining lymph nodes, as defined by the seventh edition of the American Joint Committee on Cancer (AJCC) staging handbook, are the perirectal, sigmoid mesenteric, inferior mesenteric, lateral sacral, presacral, internal iliac, sacral promontory, superior rectal, middle rectal, and inferior rectal lymph node groups (9). For T4 rectal cancers, the external iliac nodal chain is considered at increased risk, and is generally included as part of the regional nodal drainage pattern for radiation planning.

EARLY STAGE RECTAL CANCER: POSTOPERATIVE RADIATION IN THE SETTING OF LIMITED SURGICAL RESECTION

Early stage rectal cancer is typically defined as T1-T2 N0 tumors, with either invasion into the submucosa or the muscularis propria and without any evidence of nodal involvement or distant metastasis (Stage I; 9). The mainstay of treatment for early stage rectal cancer is surgical excision alone. A logical question that has been examined in multiple prospective randomized studies is the role of radiation in the management of patients who have undergone limited surgical excision (ie, transanal excision).

In general, TME either via the low anterior approach (LAR) or abdominoperineal approach (APR) is the gold standard in surgical resection (30). As an alternative to more extensive surgery, transanal surgical excision can be attempted in a well-defined group of appropriately informed and compliant low risk patients. The transanal excision approach has been investigated since the 1980s as a less aggressive and less invasive option for patients with early stage low rectal cancers (31). In general, transanal excision has been shown to have inferior oncologic outcomes for patients with adverse prognostic features or T2 disease and is limited to those patients who are in a very well-defined low risk subset or who have prohibitive medical contraindications to major surgery (32). Certain guidelines have been established by the National Comprehensive Cancer Network (NCCN) to define which patients can be considered for transanal excision. These guidelines include tumor stage T1 only, involvement of less than 30% of the rectal circumference, less than 3 cm in size, surgical margins clear by greater than 3 mm, a lesion that is mobile and nonfixed within 8 cm of the anal verge, no lymphovascular or perineural invasion, well to moderately differentiated, and no evidence of lymphadenopathy on pretreatment imaging (33). These are highly selected patients who should be counseled regarding their options carefully and be informed of the intensive endoscopic surveillance required post transanal excision.

The role of radiation therapy in the setting of transanal excision of rectal cancer has been examined in two prospective phase II trials (34,35). RTOG 89–02 was a phase II study in which patients with distal rectal cancer were assigned to local excision using either a transanal or transsacral approach with anal sphincter preservation. The lesions had to be less than 4 cm in diameter, involve 40% or less of the rectal circumference, and be located below the peritoneal reflection (middle or lower rectum). Patients were then assigned to one of three arms based on tumor size, T classification, grade, and adequacy of surgical margins. Patients with negative margins and without adverse prognostic features were observed. Patients with negative margins and at least one adverse feature but at least 3-mm surgical margins were treated with concurrent continuous infusional 5-fluorouracil (5-FU) 1000 mg/m^2/24 hour × 96 hour week 1 and 5 and RT to a dose of 50 to 56 Gy. Those with positive margins were treated with concurrent 5-FU and RT to a dose of 59.4 to 65 Gy. At a median follow up of 6.1 years, the loco-regional failure rates were found to be unacceptably high in patients with T2 or greater tumors. Specifically, crude loco-regional failure rates for T1, T2, and T3 tumors were 4%, 16%, and 23%, respectively. It was also demonstrated that patients with circumferential involvement of less than or equal to 20% had a lower chance of recurrence versus those with greater than 20%. Not surprisingly, the rate of distant metastases also correlated with T stage (4% for T1, 12% for T2, and 31% for T3). The major conclusions of this early series were that sphincter-sparing local excision alone is a feasible alternative for highly selected low risk patients, but the rates of local recurrence after local excision escalate with increasing T stage, even with adjuvant chemoradiation (35).

Along with the phase II trial done by the RTOG, the CALBG conducted a similar study. In CALGB 8984, patients with tumors that were less than 10 cm from the dentate line, less than 4 cm in diameter, had involvement of less than 40% of the rectal circumference, and with negative surgical margins were assigned to local excision alone if T1 and local excision followed by adjuvant RT (54.0 Gy) and 5-FU (500 mg/m^2 days 1–3 and 29–31) if T2. With a median follow up of 7.1 years, local excision alone for T1 rectal cancer was associated with low recurrence and high OS that remain durable with long-term follow up. Ten-year actuarial OS and local recurrence rates (T1 vs T2) were 84% vs 66% and 8% vs 18%, respectively. This again demonstrated that the role of transanal excision is limited and patients that undergo this technique should be carefully selected and counseled regarding the alternatives. Chemotherapy and RT are not able to prevent high rates of local recurrence in patients with T2 or greater tumors that undergo transanal excision (34).

There are ongoing research efforts to use neoadjuvant chemoradiation for cT2N0 low rectal tumors in an attempt to downstage tumors before local excision. ACOSOG Z6041 was a phase II study of RT with concurrent capecitabine and oxaliplatin in cT2N0 patients prior to local excision. Early results have shown that 44% of patients achieved a pathologic complete response and that 64% of patients were downstaged to ypT0-T1 (36). The patients in this study are still being followed for recurrence and survival.

■ THE ROLE OF ADJUVANT RADIATION AND CHEMOTHERAPY IN RECTAL CANCER

The risk of loco-regional recurrence remains unacceptably high after radical surgery alone for patients with Stages II and III rectal cancer. As a consequence, numerous trials have examined the role of adjuvant radiation therapy and chemotherapy following up-front surgical resection. An overview of the role of adjuvant chemotherapy in conjunction with radiation therapy is presented.

The primary advantage of adjuvant therapy is the ability to selectively treat patients with a high risk of local recurrence based on pathologic results. Despite this advantage, there are several disadvantages that exist when giving RT in the adjuvant setting. These disadvantages include a larger amount of small bowel in the treatment field, larger treatment volumes, the possibility of decreased oxygenation of tissues and potential delays in adjuvant therapy if surgical complications occur. This decreased oxygenation of tissues in the postoperative setting could theoretically lead to increased radioresistance and a lower therapeutic gain from adjuvant therapy (37).

An early and important trial designed to examine the role of postoperative RT alone vs chemotherapy alone vs observation was NSABP R-01 (37). Patients with Stage II to III rectal cancer were treated with up-front surgery and then randomized to receive no further treatment versus adjuvant chemotherapy alone with 5-FU 325 mg/m^2 bolus on days 1 to 5 and 375 mg/m^2 on days 36 to 40, semustine 130 mg/m^2 orally on day 1, and vincristine 1 mg/m^2 to 2 mg maximum dose IV on days 1 and 36 (MOF) q10 weeks × 8 cycles, or postoperative RT alone (46–47 Gy in 26–27 fractions). If a perineal boost was given, the maximum dose to the perineum was 51–53 Gy. Major conclusions of this analysis were that there was an improvement in OS (53% vs 43%) and disease-free survival (DFS; 42% vs 30%) for postoperative chemotherapy, but that this benefit was restricted to males. The use of postoperative RT reduced the incidence of local regional recurrence from 26%–16% (P = .06), but failed to affect OS and DFS (37).

During the same time period the Gastrointestinal Tumor Study Group (GITSG) was performing a seminal study (GI-7175) examining the role of observation vs adjuvant RT vs chemotherapy vs concurrent chemoradiotherapy (38,39). This was a four-arm study that examined the benefit of chemoradiotherapy in patients with Stage II to III rectal cancer. Only patients with an R0 resection were eligible. Patients were treated with either surgery alone, postoperative chemotherapy (bolus 5-FU 325 mg/m^2 days 1–5 and 375 mg/m^2 days 36–40 and semustine 130 mg/m^2 day 1 q10 weeks for up to 18 months of therapy), postoperative RT (40–48 Gy), or postoperative chemo-RT (40–44 Gy) with bolus 5-FU (500mg/m^2 on the first and last 3 days of radiation), which was then followed by adjuvant 5-FU/semustine at the same doses as the chemotherapy alone arm except for the first 5 weeks, which was given with 5-FU 300 mg/m^2 and semustine 100 mg/m^2. This trial was terminated early due to a significant benefit of the chemoradiotherapy arm. The major conclusions of the analysis were that patients benefited most from a combination of adjuvant chemotherapy and RT, based on decreases in loco-regional (10% vs 25%), distant (25% vs 35%), and any recurrence rates (33% vs 55%), when compared to observation. The differences between chemoradiation and radiation alone or chemotherapy alone were nonsignificant. While the initial publication demonstrated a trend toward increased OS in patients undergoing postoperative chemoradiotherapy vs observation, further follow up demonstrated a significant OS benefit of approximately 25% (7 years OS 55% chemoradiation vs 30% observation). Again, the comparison of chemoradiation with chemotherapy alone or radiation alone was nonsignificant (38).

NSABP R-02 built upon the results of NSABP R-01 to examine whether the addition of RT to chemotherapy added to the benefit of adjuvant chemotherapy previously seen in NSABP R-01 (40). Male patients with Stages II to III rectal cancer were randomized to one of four postoperative treatment arms: adjuvant chemotherapy (5-FU 500 mg/m^2/leucovorin [LV] 500 mg/m^2 weekly × 6 weeks q 8 weeks × 6 cycles or MOF [5-FU 325 mg/m^2 days 1–5 and 375 mg/m^2 days 36–40; semustine 130 mg/m^2 day 1, vincristine 1 mg/m^2 to a maximum dose of 2 mg total dose on days 1 and 36] q10 weeks × 5 cycles) with or without the addition of RT (50.4 Gy) after the first cycle of chemotherapy. Female patients with Stages II to III rectal cancer were randomized to adjuvant 5-FU and LV with or without RT. For those patients assigned to radiation on either the 5-FU/LV or MOF arms, bolus 5-FU at 400 mg/m^2 was given during the first 3 and last 3 days of radiation. The main objective of this study was to determine if the addition of RT resulted in improved disease-free survival and OS. In male patients, treatment with 5-FU and LV resulted in a statistically significant benefit in relapse free survival (RFS) and DFS compared to treatment with MOF (5 years DFS 55% vs 47%, respectively, P = .009; 5 years RFS 61% vs 55% respectively, P = .046). With a median follow-up of 7.8 years, postoperative RT did not have a beneficial effect on DFS or OS, regardless of which chemotherapy regimen was used, although it reduced 5-year loco-regional relapse from 13% to 8% (P = .02; 41). More than two-thirds of relapses presented as a metastatic lesion outside the radiation field, which may explain why there was not an improvement in DFS or OS with the addition of RT despite an improvement in loco-regional control.

The Medical Research Council (MRC) conducted a study (MRC-3) examining the role of surgery alone vs surgery followed by radiation therapy for mobile cancer of the rectum (42). Patients with T3-T4 or node-positive cancer were randomized to either surgery alone vs surgery followed by RT (40 Gy in 20 fractions). Major conclusions of this analysis were that a trend existed toward a benefit of RT for OS, however, this did not reach statistical significance (46% surgery alone vs 52% surgery + RT). Again, an improvement in rates of local recurrence was demonstrated (34% surgery alone vs 21% surgery + RT).

After the GITSG study demonstrated a significant benefit of adjuvant concurrent chemoradiation (CRT) vs observation, a controversy still existed as to whether concurrent chemoradiation was superior to RT alone. A comparison of postoperative RT with postoperative chemoradiotherapy was the subject of a study by the North Central Cancer Treatment Group (NCCTG; 43). The Mayo-NCCTG study examined patients with T3-T4 or node-positive tumors who underwent surgery and were then randomized to either RT alone (50.4 Gy) or 1 cycle of 5-FU 300 mg/m^2 days 1 to 5 and 400 mg/m^2 on day 36/semustine 130 mg/m^2, followed by concurrent CRT (50.4 Gy) starting on day 64 with 5-FU 500 mg/m^2 days 1 to 3 in weeks 1 and 5 of radiation, followed 1 month later by semustine 100 mg/m^2 day 1 and 5-FU 300 mg/m^2 days 1 to 5 followed 1 month later by 5-FU 400 mg/m^2 days 1 to 5. The major conclusions of this analysis were that patients treated with combined modality therapy with postoperative CRT had reduced local recurrence (25%

vs 14%; P = .036) and distant metastases rates (46% vs 29%; P = .011), as well as a significantly increased OS rate (approximately 55% vs 45%; 43). Interestingly, there was treatment interaction observed for type of surgery, with no OS benefit seen with combined therapy in patients who underwent APR versus a striking benefit seen in those patients who underwent LAR.

Most of the studies up to this point had used 3 to 5 day infusions of 5-FU concurrent with RT, and adjuvant chemotherapy consisting of 5-FU and semustine. The NCCTG conducted a study looking at the role of semustine in adjuvant chemotherapy as well as bolus versus continuous infusion (CI) 5-FU concurrent with RT. Patients with Stage II and III rectal cancer underwent resection and were then randomized in a 2 × 2 fashion to bolus 5-FU 500 mg/m^2 days 1 to 3 during weeks 1 and 5 of radiation vs CI5-FU 225 mg/m^2 daily for the duration of radiation with RT and adjuvant 5-FU alone 500 mg/m^2 days 1 to 5 and days 36 to 40 and 450 mg/m^2 on days 134 to 138 and days 169 to 173 vs 5-FU 350 mg/m^2 days 1 to 5, 400 mg/m^2 days 36 to 40, 300 mg/m^2 days 134 to 138, and 350 mg/m^2 day 169 to 173 + semustine 130 mg/m^2 day 1 and 100 mg/m^2 day 134 (40). Patients must have had an R0 resection for trial inclusion. RT was to 50.4 Gy ± an additional 3.6 Gy boost if small bowel was out of the field. Patients were analyzed as two groups: (a) ± semustine and (b) bolus 5-FU versus CI 5-FU concurrent with RT. There was no difference in loco-regional control, 4-year DFS, or 4-year OS between the ± semustine arms. There was a significant benefit observed with CI 5-FU over bolus 5-FU in terms of 4-year OS (70% vs 60%, P = .005), 4-year DFS (63% vs 53%, P = .01), and distant metastases (31% vs 40%, P = .03). There was no difference in loco-regional control rates. The benefit of CI 5-FU may have been due to the protracted exposure of tumor cells to the drug, the significantly higher doses of 5-FU received with CI vs bolus therapy, or a combination of both factors.

THE ROLE OF NEOADJUVANT RT IN RECTAL CANCER

Starting in the early 1970s, the concept of treating patients with rectal cancer before surgery was introduced. The potential ability to downstage tumors, increase sphincter preservation rates, and improve resectability drove the transition from postoperative to preoperative RT with several studies showing increased local control with preoperative RT (45).

Preoperative RT Versus Surgery Alone

Several randomized trials have shown that preoperative RT decreases local recurrence; however, there has been no demonstrated benefit toward OS with preoperative RT in the setting of modern day surgical techniques.

Beginning in 1987, the Swedish Rectal Cancer Trial was initiated and randomized patients to preoperative RT vs surgery alone (46). The surgical intervention took place 1 week after the RT was completed. This trial included patients staged with Dukes A-C, which translates to AJCC Stages I to III rectal cancer. Important to note in this study was that the surgical intervention was not a TME. The RT was delivered 5 Gy × 5 using either AP/PA, 3-field, or 4-field technique given 1 week preoperatively. There are several issues that exist in interpreting the results due to the trial design. First, the surgical intervention is not considered the current standard of care (TME) and resulted in a high local failure rate of 27% with surgery alone. Additionally, the short course radiation schedule was considered to put patients at high risk for late toxicity, and the short time period between radiation and surgery may not have allowed for optimal downstaging. Nevertheless, the trial did demonstrate an impressive advantage to preoperative RT, with a 5-year local recurrence rate of 12% with RT vs 27% for surgery alone, as well as an absolute 10% 5-year OS benefit for preoperative RT (58% vs 48%, P = .004). This benefit was maintained for 13-year OS in an analysis that included R0 resection patients only (38% vs 30%, $P < .05$; 46). There was also an advantage in cancer-specific survival among patients in the preoperative RT arm (74% vs 65%, P = .002), which was also maintained in R0 patients at 13 years (72% vs 62%). Neoadjuvant RT was associated with increased toxicity, with significantly higher rates of any small bowel obstruction (14% vs 6%) and small bowel obstruction requiring surgery (7% vs 2%) in an analysis that included R0 resection patients only (47).

The question of the preoperative fractionation schedule and interval to surgery was examined with the French Lyon 90–01 trial (48). Patients with T2-T3 NX rectal cancer that was accessible to DRE were randomized to RT (39 Gy/13 fx) delivered with either a short interval to surgery, mandated as surgery within 2 weeks after completion of RT, vs a long interval, mandated as surgery within 6 to 8 weeks. A total of 201 patients were enrolled in the study. The clinical tumor response was significantly better in the long interval group (72%) as compared to the short interval group (53%, P = .007). Pathologic downstaging was also significantly higher in the long interval group (26% vs 10%, P = .005). There were no differences with respect to sphincter preservation rate, morbidity, local relapse, or short-term survival. Major conclusions of this analysis were that a long interval between preoperative irradiation and surgery provides increased tumor downstaging without any negative effects on toxicity. Furthermore, there was a nonstatistically significant trend toward a higher rate of sphincter-preserving surgery in the long interval group (48).

As the TME surgical technique gained popularity, the question was raised regarding the ability of TME alone to control rectal cancer with low recurrence rates. Consequently in 1996, the Dutch TME trial (CKVO 95–04) set out to examine the role of preoperative short-course RT in the treatment of patients with rectal cancer in combination with TME (49). Patients with Stages I to III rectal cancer were randomized to preop short course RT (5 Gy × 5) vs TME alone with the primary endpoint of local recurrence. Surgery occurred within 1 week of the completion of RT in the neoadjuvant arm. Long-term results have recently been published and have shown that the 10-year cumulative incidence of local recurrence was 5% in the group assigned to RT and TME and 11% in the surgery-alone group ($P < .0001$). Despite this impressive reduction in local recurrence, there was no demonstrated OS benefit with the addition of preoperative short course RT (49). In a subgroup analysis, patients with Stage III cancer and R0 resection did have significant 10-year OS benefit (50% vs 40%), but this was exploratory in nature with small patient numbers. There was increased long-term toxicity associated with radiation therapy, with significantly higher rates of fecal incontinence (62% vs 38%), anal blood loss (11% vs 3%), and anal mucus loss (27% vs 15%) compared to TME alone (50).

As previously mentioned, the involvement of a CRM is a negative prognostic factor for recurrence in rectal cancer and a logical question is whether or not the addition of RT can compensate for the presence of a positive resection margin. The Dutch TME trial mandated the use of postoperative RT for patients in the TME alone arm with a positive CRM (defined as a margin of less than or equal to 1 mm). Despite this mandate, only 47% of patients received postoperative RT when they had a positive CRM. This allowed for an analysis of the ability of adjuvant RT to enhance local control in patients with a positive CRM. It was shown that the local recurrence rate for patients with a positive CRM who received postoperative RT was 17.3% compared to 15.7% in the patients with a positive CRM who did not undergo postoperative RT. There was no difference between the two arms. Neoadjuvant RT significantly improved local control for patients with a narrow resection margin (1.1 to 2 mm) or a wide resection margin (greater than 2 mm) but could not compensate for a positive resection margin (16).

With an inconsistent benefit to RT with respect to OS, two large meta-analyses have been conducted in an attempt to determine the benefit of preoperative RT (51,52). The first of these analyses demonstrated that RT was associated with a significant improvement in local control, cause specific survival and OS, but with no effect on distant metastases rates. Therefore, prognostic factors were needed which could identify which patients would benefit most from preoperative RT (51). The second meta-analysis, performed by the CRC Collaborative Group, included a mixture of neoadjuvant RT and adjuvant RT studies. There was a significant reduction in local recurrence and death from rectal cancer with the addition of RT, but no difference in OS. Important to consider is that an improvement in the rate of R0 resection was not demonstrated, and that there was an increased rate of early deaths from other causes in the RT group. The increased risk of other deaths was a possible reason why an OS benefit was not demonstrated with the addition of preoperative RT (51).

Neoadjuvant Chemoradiation

EMILY CHAN

The addition of chemotherapy to neoadjuvant RT has been the subject of several clinical trials, and the precise role of chemotherapy in the neoadjuvant setting continues to evolve. The French FFCD 9203 study examined the role of chemoradiotherapy vs RT alone (53). With a primary endpoint of OS, patients with resectable T3–T4 NX adenocarcinoma of the rectum, accessible to digital rectal exam, were randomized to RT (45 Gy/25) with concurrent bolus 5-FU 350 mg/m^2/d and LV 20 mg/m^2/d days 1 to 5 and days 29 to 33 vs RT alone. Both arms were followed by surgery planned for 3 to 10 weeks after the end of RT, with an additional four cycles of postoperative 5-FU and LV chemotherapy q4 weeks using the same schedule as preoperatively. There was no difference in protocol compliance with adjuvant chemotherapy between arms (70% CRT vs 65% RT). Grades 3 and 4 acute toxicity was significantly more frequent in the chemoradiotherapy arm compared to RT alone (15% vs 3%). There was a significant decrease in local recurrence with chemoradiotherapy compared to RT alone (8.1% vs 16.5%, $P = .004$), as well as an increase in pathologic complete response (pCR) (11.4% vs 3.6%; $P < .0001$); however, this did not translate to a difference in 5-year OS between the two arms (67.9% CRT vs 67.4% RT, $P = .684$). There was also no difference in the rates of sphincter preservation (57.7% CRT vs 58.3% RT, $P = .837$). Given the significantly improved local control with only a moderate increase in toxicity, neoadjuvant chemoradiotherapy was recommended over RT alone for this patient population.

EORTC 22941 explored the role of adding chemotherapy to neoadjuvant radiation and adding adjuvant chemotherapy for locally advanced rectal cancer (54,55). Patients with T3–4 NX resectable rectal cancer were randomized in a 2 × 2 design to preoperative RT vs preoperative chemoradiotherapy vs preoperative RT and postoperative chemotherapy vs preoperative chemoradiotherapy and postoperative chemotherapy. TME was instituted during study accrual, hence only approximately 35% of patients underwent TME. The analysis was done using two groups: (a) neoadjuvant RT vs CRT and (b) ± adjuvant chemotherapy. The RT in this study was given as 45 Gy/25 fractions to the pelvis. Preoperative chemotherapy consisted of 5-FU 350 mg/m^2/d and LV 20 mg/m^2/d × 5 days given on weeks 1 and 5 of RT. Postoperative chemotherapy was given at the same doses every 3 weeks × 4 cycles. There was no difference in 5-year OS or DFS based on the addition of neoadjuvant therapy (OS: 64.8% preoperative RT vs 65.8% preoperative chemoradiation; $P = .84$. DFS: 54.4% preoperative RT vs 56.1% preoperative chemoradiation; $P = .52$) or adjuvant chemotherapy (OS: 63.2% no adjuvant chemotherapy vs 67.2% adjuvant chemotherapy; $P = .12$. 52.2% no adjuvant chemotherapy vs 58.2% adjuvant chemotherapy; $P = .13$), or both. Five-year loco-regional recurrence was significantly reduced with the addition of chemotherapy, regardless of timing, when compared to neoadjuvant RT alone (8.7% vs 17.1%). A later subset analysis found that patients who had a response to neoadjuvant therapy (ypT0–2 rectal cancers) derived a selective benefit in both DFS and OS from adjuvant chemotherapy ($P = .011$) vs none in those patients with ypT3-T4 tumors (54).

In the United States, the standard of care is long course neoadjuvant chemoradiation in order to maximize tumor downstaging, while in Europe, short course 5 Gy × 5 fractionation has a more established role. The question of neoadjuvant long course CRT versus short course RT was examined in a Polish study (56). Patients with cT3–4 resectable adenocarcinoma of the rectum, accessible by DRE, were randomized to preoperative short course RT (5 Gy × 5 fractions) and surgery performed within 7 days versus preoperative CRT with bolus 5-FU 325 mg/m^2/d and LV 20 mg/m^2/d × 5 days during weeks 1 and 5 of radiation and RT (50.4 Gy/28 fx) followed by surgery 4 to 6 weeks later. Postoperative chemotherapy was optional. If subjects received preoperative chemoradiation, they would get 4 months of 5-FU/LV. If subjects had short course radiation, they would get 6 months of 5-FU/LV. There was no difference observed between the short course and long course regimens in terms of 4-year actuarial loco-regional relapse (11% vs 16%), DFS (58% vs 56%; $P = .82$), or OS (67% vs 66%; $P = .96$). However, the chemo-RT arm did have a significantly higher pCR rate (16% vs 0.7%) and lower positive CRM rate (4% vs 13%; $P = .017$). Important to note was the significant difference in grade 3 or higher acute toxicity between arms, with the short course RT arm having 3% as compared to 18% in the chemo-RT arm ($P < .001$). However, at a median follow up of 48 months, there was no difference in late toxicity. Major criticisms of this study include the lack of quality assurance with any treatment modality, differences in the rates of adjuvant chemotherapy, and the primary endpoint of sphincter preservation, which most likely led to insufficient power to detect smaller differences in other endpoints (56).

In an attempt to again answer the question as to the role of short vs long course neoadjuvant RT, the

Trans-Tasman Radiation Oncology Group (TROG) conducted a similar trial to the Polish study examining the same preoperative fractionation schedules of 5 Gy × 5 fractions vs 50.4 Gy of conventionally fractionated RT with 5-FU-based chemotherapy (57). The primary reason this trial was undertaken was the suboptimal chemotherapy that was used in the Polish study, which consisted of bolus 5-FU and LV. Additionally, in the Polish study the use of adjuvant chemotherapy was optional, and EUS and MRI were not performed for all patients. The TROG study showed that for all patients there was not a statistically significant difference in the 3-year local recurrence rate for the short course versus long course RT. It did appear from the TROG study that for distal tumors (less than 5 cm) long course might be more effective in reducing local recurrence, which is consistent with the results of past series. Several critiques of the TROG study exist, namely that it was not designed as a noninferiority trial, and was powered to detect a difference and not equality between the treatment arms. Furthermore, the follow up in this series is relatively short, so late toxicity has not been completely accounted for. Ultimately, this trial was not viewed as changing the standard of care to short course RT given the lack of power to show the two schedules are equivalent, along with the relatively short follow up (57). However, if a particular patient has a compelling reason to shorten the course of preoperative RT, such as social or compliance challenges with prolonged RT delivery, a course of 5 Gy × 5 could potentially be considered with little evidence supporting a worse overall outcome. Trials are currently ongoing examining the sequencing of short course RT with chemotherapy; the results of these data are much anticipated.

Preoperative CRT Versus Postoperative CRT

The question regarding the optimal timing of RT in patients with rectal cancer has remained a point of controversy. Several major clinical trials have been conducted in an attempt to answer this important question; however, there is still a lack of consensus in the international community as to the ideal sequencing of RT in patients with rectal cancer.

A multicenter randomized study performed by the MRC (CR07) and NCIC (C016) examined the role of short course preoperative RT compared with selective postoperative CRT (58). Patients with operable carcinoma of the rectum, required to be less than 15 cm from the anal verge, were included. They were randomized to short course preoperative RT consisting of 25 Gy over five fractions followed by surgical resection vs surgery upfront with selective postoperative CRT restricted to those patients where the CRM was positive. The postoperative RT was 45 Gy delivered over 25 fractions to the pelvis with either concurrent bolus 5-FU 300 mg/m^2 and LV 20 mg/m^2 weekly chemotherapy or concurrent continuous infusional 5-FU 200 mg/m^2 daily during radiation. Adjuvant chemotherapy was given to 40% of patients in the preoperative arm and 45% in the postoperative arm (P = NS). The primary outcome was local recurrence. Patients in the preoperative RT arm had a significantly lower rate of local recurrence compared to selective adjuvant CRT (4.4% vs 10.6%, $P < .0001$). While there was a DFS benefit with preoperative RT (77.5% vs 71.5%, $P = .013$), OS did not differ between the two arms. This trial provided more evidence that preoperative short course RT is an effective treatment for patients with operable rectal cancer and that postoperative radiation therapy cannot compensate for a positive CRM.

A seminal trial was conducted by the German Rectal Cancer Study Group (CAO/ARO/AIO) to examine the role of preoperative CRT vs postoperative chemoradiotherapy (59). Patients with clinical stage II to III rectal cancer with the inferior margin of tumor within 16 cm from the anal verge were randomized to receive either surgical resection (TME) followed by CRT consisting of 50.4 Gy/28 fractions with an additional 5.4 Gy boost to the tumor bed with concurrent continuous infusional 5-FU 1000 mg/m^2/d × 120 hours during week 1 and 5 vs preoperative treatment with RT to a dose of 50.4 Gy/28 fractions and the same concurrent continuous infusional 5-FU dosing. Patients in the preoperative arm underwent surgery (TME) 6 weeks after chemoradiation. Both arms were to receive four cycles of adjuvant bolus 5-FU 500 mg/m^2/d × 5 days q4 weeks. The primary endpoint of OS was not different between the two arms (76% preop vs 74% postop, $P = .8$). There were several statistically significant benefits observed in the preoperative group including reduced local relapse (6% vs 13%; $P = .006$), reduced rates of pathologic nodal involvement (25% vs 40%), and increased rates of sphincter preservation in the patients originally planned to undergo APR (39% vs 19%; $P = .004$). Furthermore, the rates of both acute (27% vs 40%, $P = .001$) and late (14% vs 24%, $P = .01$) grade 3 to 4 toxicity were significantly better in the preoperative arm as compared with the postoperative arm. The German Rectal Cancer Study Group provided the foundation favoring preoperative treatment compared with postoperative treatment. Important to consider in this study is the relatively high percentage of patients (20%) who were considered clinical Stages II to III, but were found to be pathologic Stage I after upfront surgery and did not undergo adjuvant therapy. Preoperative therapy does have the risk of potentially overtreating patients who are not staged pathologically.

The NSABP R-03 study also attempted to answer the RT timing question (60). In this trial, which closed prematurely secondary to poor accrual, patients with clinically staged T3-T4 or node positive rectal cancer were randomized to preoperative chemotherapy with 5-FU

500 mg/m² and LV 500 mg/m² weekly × 6 weeks followed by CRT (50.4 Gy/28 fractions with concurrent bolus 5-FU 325 mg/m²/d and LV 20 mg/m²/d × 5 days weeks 1 and 5 of radiation) followed by four additional cycles of chemotherapy vs upfront surgery with the same regimen delivered adjuvantly. In the preoperative arm, surgery was performed within 8 weeks of completion of chemoradiation (TME was not mandated). This study demonstrated that 5-year DFS in patients with preoperative therapy was significantly improved vs postoperative therapy (64.7% vs 53.4%, *P* = .011). There was also a trend toward improved 5-year OS with preoperative therapy (74.5% vs 65.6%, *P* = .065). A pCR was demonstrated in 15% of preoperative patients, and it is important to note that no recurrences were seen in patients that achieved a complete response. There was no difference in the rates of sphincter preservation (47.8% preoperative vs 39.2% postoperative, *P* = .23). Therefore, preoperative CRT improved DFS and had a trend toward improved OS as compared to postoperative chemoradiation (60).

■ THE ROLE OF RT DOSE ESCALATION

The optimal dosing and fractionation of RT in rectal cancer have been subject to much investigation and are important factors to consider for the radiation oncologist. In a publication by Wiltshire et al from Princess Margaret Hospital, three consecutive phase II studies of preoperative RT and concurrent 5-FU were reported, with primary endpoints of acute toxicity and pCR (61). In addition, secondary endpoints of recurrence free survival, DFS, and OS were examined. Patients enrolled had clinical T3–4 or node positive adenocarcinoma of the rectum and three different fractionation schedules were examined. The fractionation schedules consisted of 40 Gy in 20 fractions vs 46 Gy in 23 fractions vs 50 Gy in 25 fractions. These were given with continuous infusion 5-FU (225 mg/m²/d). Treatment was generally well tolerated, with grade 3 or 4 acute toxicity observed in 13%, 4%, and 14% of patients in the 40 Gy, 46 Gy, and 50 Gy cohorts, respectively (*P* = .20). Pathologic complete response was documented in 15%, 23%, and 33% of patients, respectively (*P* = .07). The 2-year loco-regional control rate was 72%, 90%, and 89% (*P* = .02), DFS was 62%, 84%, and 78% (*P* = .02), and OS was 72%, 94%, and 92%, respectively (*P* = .03). Conclusions from this study were that doses of 46 Gy and higher were associated with improved outcomes, but there was no difference between 46 and 50 Gy.

The RTOG conducted an important trial to answer the question of the optimal RT fractionation schedule in the randomized phase II study RTOG 00–12 (62). Patients with T3–4 NX distal rectal tumors (up to 9 cm from the anal verge) were randomized between two arms. Arm 1 included continuous infusion (CI) 5-FU (225 mg/m²/d) with hyperfractionated RT (HF-RT) to a dose of 55.2 to 60 Gy given at 1.2 Gy BID. This was compared to CI 5-FU given 5 days per week and irinotecan 50 mg/m² weekly × 4 weeks with conventionally fractionated RT to doses of 50.4 to 54 Gy at 1.8 Gy per fraction. Surgery (not TME in most cases) was performed 4 to 10 weeks after the completion of the neoadjuvant therapy. The pCR rate for patients who underwent surgery was 28% in both arms. This study demonstrated that a high pCR rate is achievable through altered fractionation or the addition of chemotherapeutic agents.

In addition to the variety of RT doses and fractionation schedules, an important question regarding the role of higher doses was examined at in the Lyon R 96–02 trial. Patients with low rectal cancers (inferior tumor edge within 6 cm of the anal verge), stage T2 or T3 NX, and not involving more than two-thirds of the rectal circumference were randomly assigned to one of two groups. Arm 1 was preoperative RT to 39 Gy over 13 fractions vs the same EBRT dose with the addition of a boost of 85 Gy over three fractions using endocavitary contact x-ray therapy. The addition of the high dose boost resulted in significant improvement in complete clinical response (24% vs 2%, *P* < .05) and complete or near complete pathologic response (57% vs 34%, *P* = .027). There was also a significant increase in the rate of sphincter preservation in the boost arm as compared to the EBRT only arm (76% vs 44%, *P* = .004; 63). The 10-year follow up of this study shows no significant difference in local recurrence, disease-free survival, or OS between the two groups (64). The concept of higher dose boost irradiation in the treatment of rectal cancers in the modern day era warrants exploration in future clinical trials.

■ CHEMOTHERAPY OPTIMIZATION

Early trials suggested that continuous infusional 5-FU may be a more effective radiation sensitizer than bolus 5-FU. INT-0144 (65) studied three different adjuvant chemoradiation regimens to formally address this issue. Patients with resected Stage II or III rectal cancer were randomized to one of three adjuvant arms: Arm 1: Bolus 5-FU (500 mg/m²/d on D1–5 and 29–33) before and after RT plus 5-FU via protracted vein infusion (PVI; 225 mg/m²/d) during RT; Arm 2: PVI 5-FU (300 mg/m²/d) × 42 days before and 56 days after RT + 5-FU PVI (225 mg/m²/d); and Arm 3: Bolus 5-FU (425 mg/m²/d before RT and 380 mg/m²/d after RT) and LV (20 mg/m²/d) in two 5-day cycles before and after RT plus bolus 5-FU (400 mg/m²/d) and LV (20 mg/m²/d) days 1 to 4 q28 days. Levamisole (50 mg tid) × 3 days q14 days was given. All three arms had similar relapse-free survival and OS, but had different toxicity profiles.

With the advent of more effective systemic therapy for metastatic CRC, efforts were undertaken to explore these therapies in earlier stage disease.

NSABP R-04 explored the roles of capecitabine, an oral fluoropyrimidine, and oxaliplatin as radiation sensitizers (66). Patients with clinical Stage II or III rectal cancer were randomized to one of four chemotherapy regimens to be given with radiation: Continuous infusional 5-FU (225 mg/m^2/d 5 days/week) with or without oxaliplatin (50 mg/m^2/week × 5) or capecitabine (825 mg/m^2 BID 5 days/week) with or without oxaliplatin (50 mg/m^2/week × 5). The capecitabine arms resulted in similar rates of pCR, sphincter-saving surgery, and surgical downstaging as the 5-FU arms. The patients in the oxaliplatin containing arms had similar rates of pCR, sphincter-saving surgery, and surgical downstaging as the arms without oxaliplatin but did result in significantly more grade 3 to 4 diarrhea than the non-oxaliplatin containing arms.

The STAR-01 phase III trial explored the addition of oxaliplatin to chemoradiation with 5-FU (67). Seven hundred forty-seven patients with clinical Stage II or III rectal cancer were randomized to neoadjuvant chemoradiation with infusional 5-FU (225 mg/m^2/d) with or without oxaliplatin (60 mg/m^2 weekly × 6). There was no statistically significant difference in the pCR rate or the rate of APRs but there were significantly more grade 3 to 4 adverse events in the oxaliplatin containing arm (24% vs 8%; $P < .001$).

The phase III ACCORD 12/0405-Prodige 2 trial also explored the addition of oxaliplatin to 5-FU based chemoradiation (68). Five hundred ninety-eight patients with T3–4 M0 rectal cancer were randomized to neoadjuvant chemoradiation with capecitabine (800 mg/m^2 twice daily 5 days/week during radiation)and 45 Gy of radiation or capecitabine (800 mg/m^2 twice daily 5 days/week during radiation), oxaliplatin (50 mg/m^2 weekly × 5), and 50 Gy of radiation. Similar to the STAR-01 study, the rate of conservative surgery and pCR rate was not statistically different between the two groups, but there were significantly more grade 3 to 4 preoperative toxicity in the oxaliplatin containing arm (25% vs 1%; $P < .001$). Given the disappointing results of the STAR-01 and ACCORD 12/0405-Prodige 2 trials, there is currently no role for the addition of oxaliplatin to chemoradiation in Stage II to III rectal cancer.

■ The Evolving Role of Intraoperative RT (IORT) in the Management of Rectal Cancer

CHARLES STALEY

The role of IORT in the management of patients with rectal cancer is continuing to evolve. By definition IORT is radiation therapy given at the time of surgical resection, usually directly to the tumor bed. The most common treatment modality is with electrons; however, IORT has also been delivered with orthovoltage units. Working directly with the surgeon to deliver RT at the time of the operation, with good exposure and visualization of the tumor bed, enables radiation to be delivered with high precision. Furthermore, critical normal structures, such as the small bowel, can be moved from the treatment field and the risk of toxicity to these structures is reduced. Finally, the use of electrons in the intraoperative RT devices also has dosimetric advantages when compared to photons. Critical to any new technology is the validation of the theoretical benefits of that technology in prospective randomized trials. Devices to deliver IORT come at a significant cost and their future use in radiation oncology should be evidence based.

IORT has been used in rectal cancer for decades. An early and large retrospective series was published from Sadahiro et al (69). In this series 78 patients underwent IORT between 1982 and 1998 in combination with curative surgical resection for adenocarcinoma of the middle to lower third of the rectum. Of these patients 62 had previously received preoperative RT to a dose of 20 Gy. These patients were compared to 248 patients that had been treated with surgery alone during this same period. There were no statistically significant differences with regard to tumor stage or surgical procedures between the two groups. OS, DFS, and local recurrence-free survival in the intraoperative RT group was significantly better than in the nonintraoperative group. The differences in survival were seen in patients with Stage II rectal cancer, but not in patients with Stage I or III rectal cancer. The local failure rates were 2.6% in the intraoperative group and 11.3% in the nonintraoperative group ($P = .02$). There was a statistically significant difference in the rate of wound infections, with the intraoperative group having more wound infections that the nonintraoperative group. None of these infections were considered to be serious according to the authors. This series provided some early data as to the possible benefit of IORT in the management of patients with rectal cancer. Several other retrospective series have emerged that have shown a benefit to the use of IORT in the management of patients with rectal cancer. These series have shown a reduction in local recurrence with the use of IORT; however, the limitations of these series include their retrospective nature and the evolving role of rectal cancer chemotherapy in the management of rectal cancer (69–71).

IORT has been applied to patients with locally advanced rectal cancer deemed unresectable at the time of initial presentation. In a series by Kim et al, 40 patients with locally advanced unresectable adenocarcinoma of the rectum were treated with preoperative external beam RT to a median dose of 50.4 Gy. Of the 40 patients 30 received concurrent 5-FU based chemotherapy (72). Four to 6 weeks following the completion of the neoadjuvant therapy surgical resection was then undertaken and if microscopic disease was found, IORT was delivered to the tumor bed. The median dose of IORT was 12.5 Gy with a range of 8 to 20 Gy, using a 300 kVp orthovoltage unit. This dose was typically prescribed to a depth of 1 to 2 cm. With a median follow up of 33 months, 83% of the patients were able to undergo a curative resection. The crude local control rates in patients that underwent a complete resection with negative margins was 92% for those treated with IORT and 33% without IORT. The 5-year actuarial OS was 64% for those patients that underwent a gross total resection and IORT, and local control rates were 75% for this same group. Complications were higher in the IORT arm with 65% of the IORT patients experiencing some sort of pelvic complication as compared with two patients that did not receive IORT. Major conclusions of this early, small retrospective series were that in patients with minimal residual disease, IORT could have therapeutic merit in the treatment of rectal cancer. The role may be particularly important in the setting of minimal residual disease at the time of surgery (72).

An area that has been examined to potentially have advantages in IORT is that of functional preservation in patients with advanced lower rectal cancer, particularly with respect to the function of the pelvic autonomic nerves. This is secondary to the frequent necessity of these nerves to be sacrificed in advanced disease to ensure an adequate resection. In a study published in 2008 by Masaki et al, 41 patients with advanced lower rectal cancer were enrolled into a two-arm study that included a TME with bilateral lymph node dissection with limited pelvic autonomic nervous system preservation vs TME with bilateral lymph node dissection with complete pelvic autonomic lymph node preservation, along with IORT (73). There was no difference seen with regard to local recurrence, DFS, or OS. There was improved time to indwelling catheter and voiding function. This did provide encouraging data as to the benefit of IORT in preservation of the pelvic autonomic nerves.

More recent data have shown a lack of benefit to IORT. In a multicenter, comparative, prospective phase III study, 142 patients with locally advanced (T3, T4, or N+) disease underwent neoadjuvant chemo-RT (40 Gy) and were randomly assigned to either surgical resection alone or surgical resection combined with 18 Gy of IORT. There was no benefit seen with regard to OS, DFS, or probability of metastatic relapse in the group undergoing IORT. There was a lack of additional postoperative complications seen in the group undergoing IORT as compared with the group undergoing surgery alone. The technical feasibility of IORT was confirmed and the authors concluded that it should be the subject of future evaluation (74).

As the data for IORT continue to evolve, it remains to be seen if IORT can provide substantial advantages to conformal postop external beam RT. One of the most promising areas for further investigation of IORT appears to be in those patients with limited surgical resectability. Additionally, the ability for functional preservation of pelvic autonomic nerves has shown great promise.

■ FUTURE DIRECTIONS

As progress is made in the treatment of cancer and as patients live longer, there is an increasing recognition of the long-term effects of cancer therapy. While chemoradiation decreases the rate of local recurrence, radiation can result in long-term effects of proctitis, muscle damage, bone damage, and loss of sexual function. NCCTG N1048, also known as PROSPECT, is a randomized phase II/III trial of the selective use of radiation in intermediate risk rectal cancer. With the advent of more effective systemic chemotherapy regimens, the trial is seeking to address the issue of whether radiation is necessary in all cases. Patients with locally advanced rectal cancer will be randomized to neoadjuvant chemoradiation with infusional 5-FU or preoperative chemotherapy with FOLFOX with the selective use of chemoradiation therapy with 5-FU in patients who have an inadequate response (defined as less than 20% response) to FOLFOX. This trial is ongoing, and the results are eagerly anticipated.

■ REFERENCES

1. Jemal A, Siegel R, Xu J, Ward E. Cancer statistics, 2010. *CA Cancer J Clin.* 2010;60(5):277–300.
2. Edwards BK, Ward E, Kohler BA, et al. Annual report to the nation on the status of cancer, 1975–2006, featuring colorectal cancer trends and impact of interventions (risk factors, screening, and treatment) to reduce future rates. *Cancer.* 2010;116(3):544–573.
3. van Gijn W, Krijnen P, Lemmens VE, den Dulk M, Putter H, van de Velde CJ. Quality assurance in rectal cancer treatment in the Netherlands: a catch up compared to colon cancer treatment. *Eur J Surg Oncol.* 2010;36(4):340–344.
4. Augestad KM, Lindsetmo RO, Reynolds H, et al. International trends in surgical treatment of rectal cancer. *Am J Surg.* 2011;201(3):353–7; discussion 357.
5. Wils J, O'Dwyer P, Labianca R. Adjuvant treatment of colorectal cancer at the turn of the century: European and US perspectives. *Ann Oncol.* 2001;12(1):13–22.
6. Eglinton T, Luck A, Bartholomeusz D, Varghese R, Lawrence M. Positron-emission tomography/computed tomography (PET/CT) in the initial staging of primary rectal cancer. *Colorectal Dis.* 2010;12(7):667–673.
7. Gearhart SL, Frassica D, Rosen R, Choti M, Schulick R, Wahl R. Improved staging with pretreatment positron emission tomography/computed tomography in low rectal cancer. *Ann Surg Oncol.* 2006;13(3):397–404.
8. Davey K, Heriot AG, Mackay J, et al. The impact of 18-fluorodeoxyglucose positron emission tomography-computed tomography on the staging and management of primary rectal cancer. *Dis Colon Rectum.* 2008;51(7):997–1003.
9. Edge SB, Zwelling LA, Hohn DC. The anticipated and unintended consequences of the patient protection and affordable care act on cancer research. *Cancer J.* 2010;16(6):606–613.
10. Gunderson LL, Sargent DJ, Tepper JE, et al. Impact of T and N stage and treatment on survival and relapse in adjuvant rectal cancer: a pooled analysis. *J Clin Oncol.* 2004;22(10):1785–1796.
11. Gunderson LL, Sargent DJ, Tepper JE, et al. Impact of T and N substage on survival and disease relapse in adjuvant rectal cancer: a pooled analysis. *Int J Radiat Oncol Biol Phys.* 2002;54(2):386–396.
12. Adam IJ, Mohamdee MO, Martin IG, et al. Role of circumferential margin involvement in the local recurrence of rectal cancer. *Lancet.* 1994;344(8924):707–711.
13. Nagtegaal ID, Quirke P. What is the role for the circumferential margin in the modern treatment of rectal cancer? *J Clin Oncol.* 2008;26(2):303–312.
14. Birbeck KF, Macklin CP, Tiffin NJ, et al. Rates of circumferential resection margin involvement vary between surgeons and predict outcomes in rectal cancer surgery. *Ann Surg.* 2002;235(4): 449–457.
15. Wibe A, Rendedal PR, Svensson E, et al. Prognostic significance of the circumferential resection margin following total mesorectal excision for rectal cancer. *Br J Surg.* 2002;89(3):327–334.
16. Marijnen CA, Nagtegaal ID, Kapiteijn E, et al.; Cooperative investigators of the Dutch Colerectal Cancer Group. Radiotherapy does not compensate for positive resection margins in rectal cancer patients: report of a multicenter randomized trial. *Int J Radiat Oncol Biol Phys.* 2003;55(5):1311–1320.
17. Stocchi L, Nelson H, Sargent DJ, et al.; North Central Cancer Treatment Group. Impact of surgical and pathologic variables in rectal cancer: a United States community and cooperative group report. *J Clin Oncol.* 2001;19(18):3895–3902.
18. Hall NR, Finan PJ, al-Jaberi T, et al. Circumferential margin involvement after mesorectal excision of rectal cancer with curative intent. Predictor of survival but not local recurrence? *Dis Colon Rectum.* 1998;41(8):979–983.
19. Minsky BD, Mies C, Rich TA, Recht A. Lymphatic vessel invasion is an independent prognostic factor for survival in colorectal cancer. *Int J Radiat Oncol Biol Phys.* 1989;17(2): 311–318.
20. Minsky BD, Mies C, Recht A, Rich TA, Chaffey JT. Resectable adenocarcinoma of the rectosigmoid and rectum. II. The influence of blood vessel invasion. *Cancer.* 1988;61(7):1417–1424.
21. Matsumoto K, Nakayama Y, Inoue Y, et al. Lymphatic microvessel density is an independent prognostic factor in colorectal cancer. *Dis Colon Rectum.* 2007;50(3):308–314.

22. Liang P, Nakada I, Hong JW, et al. Prognostic significance of immunohistochemically detected blood and lymphatic vessel invasion in colorectal carcinoma: its impact on prognosis. *Ann Surg Oncol.* 2007;14(2):470–477.
23. Liebig C, Ayala G, Wilks J, et al. Perineural invasion is an independent predictor of outcome in colorectal cancer. *J Clin Oncol.* 2009;27(31):5131–5137.
24. Lo DS, Pollett A, Siu LL, Gallinger S, Burkes RL. Prognostic significance of mesenteric tumor nodules in patients with stage III colorectal cancer. *Cancer.* 2008;112(1):50–54.
25. Rödel C, Martus P, Papadoupolos T, et al. Prognostic significance of tumor regression after preoperative chemoradiotherapy for rectal cancer. *J Clin Oncol.* 2005;23(34):8688–8696.
26. Compton CC, Fielding LP, Burgart LJ, et al. Prognostic factors in colorectal cancer. College of American Pathologists Consensus Statement 1999. *Arch Pathol Lab Med.* 2000;124(7):979–994.
27. Samowitz WS, Curtin K, Wolff RK, Tripp SR, Caan BJ, Slattery ML. Microsatellite instability and survival in rectal cancer. *Cancer Causes Control.* 2009;20(9):1763–1768.
28. Enker WE. Sphincter-preserving operations for rectal cancer. *Oncology (Williston Park, NY).* 1996;10(11):1673–84, 1689; discussion 1690.
29. Kirklin JW, Dockerty MB, Waugh JM. The role of the peritoneal reflection in the prognosis of carcinoma of the rectum and sigmoid colon. *Surg Gynecol Obstet.* 1949;88(3):326–331.
30. Enker WE, Thaler HT, Cranor ML, Polyak T. Total mesorectal excision in the operative treatment of carcinoma of the rectum. *J Am Coll Surg.* 1995;181(4):335–346.
31. Buess G, Theiss R, Günther M, Hutterer F, Pichlmaier H. Endoscopic surgery in the rectum. *Endoscopy.* 1985;17(1):31–35.
32. Nash GM, Weiser MR, Guillem JG, et al. Long-term survival after transanal excision of T1 rectal cancer. *Dis Colon Rectum.* 2009;52(4):577–582.
33. National Comprehensive Cancer Network(NCCN), www.nccn.org/professionals/physician-gls/f-guidelines.asp#
34. Greenberg JA, Shibata D, Herndon JE 2nd, Steele GD Jr, Mayer R, Bleday R. Local excision of distal rectal cancer: an update of cancer and leukemia group B 8984. *Dis Colon Rectum.* 2008;51(8):1185–91; discussion 1191.
35. Russell AH, Harris J, Rosenberg PJ, et al. Anal sphincter conservation for patients with adenocarcinoma of the distal rectum: long-term results of radiation therapy oncology group protocol 89–02. *Int J Radiat Oncol Biol Phys.* 2000;46(2):313–322.
36. Garcia-Aguilar J, Shi Q, Thomas CR Jr, et al. A phase II trial of neoadjuvant chemoradiation and local excision for T2N0 rectal cancer: preliminary results of the ACOSOG Z6041 trial. *Ann Surg Oncol.* 2012;19(2):384–391.
37. Fisher B, Wolmark N, Rockette H, et al. Postoperative adjuvant chemotherapy or radiation therapy for rectal cancer: results from NSABP protocol R-01. *J Natl Cancer Inst.* 1988;80(1):21–29.
38. Douglass HO Jr, Moertel CG, Mayer RJ, et al. Survival after postoperative combination treatment of rectal cancer. *N Engl J Med.* 1986;315(20):1294–1295.
39. Prolongation of the disease-free interval in surgically treated rectal carcinoma. Gastrointestinal Tumor Study Group. *N Engl J Med.* 1985;312:1465–1472.
40. O'Connell MJ, Martenson JA, Wieand HS, et al. Improving adjuvant therapy for rectal cancer by combining protracted-infusion fluorouracil with radiation therapy after curative surgery. *N Engl J Med.* 1994;331(8):502–507.
41. Wolmark N, Wieand HS, Hyams DM, et al. Randomized trial of postoperative adjuvant chemotherapy with or without radiotherapy for carcinoma of the rectum: National Surgical Adjuvant Breast and Bowel Project Protocol R-02. *J Natl Cancer Inst.* 2000;92(5):388–396.
42. Randomised trial of surgery alone versus surgery followed by radiotherapy for mobile cancer of the rectum. Medical Research Council Rectal Cancer Working Party. *Lancet.* 1996;348:1610–1614.
43. Krook JE, Moertel CG, Gunderson LL, et al. Effective surgical adjuvant therapy for high-risk rectal carcinoma. *N Engl J Med.* 1991;324(11):709–715.
44. WHO Handbook for reporting results of cancer treatment. World Health Organization, Publication number 48, Geneva; 1979.
45. Frykholm GJ, Glimelius B, Påhlman L. Preoperative or postoperative irradiation in adenocarcinoma of the rectum: final treatment results of a randomized trial and an evaluation of late secondary effects. *Dis Colon Rectum.* 1993;36(6):564–572.
46. Folkesson J, Birgisson H, Pahlman L, Cedermark B, Glimelius B, Gunnarsson U. Swedish Rectal Cancer Trial: long lasting benefits from radiotherapy on survival and local recurrence rate. *J Clin Oncol.* 2005;23(24):5644–5650.
47. Birgisson H, Påhlman L, Gunnarsson U, Glimelius B. Late gastrointestinal disorders after rectal cancer surgery with and without preoperative radiation therapy. *Br J Surg.* 2008;95(2):206–213.
48. Francois Y, Nemoz CJ, Baulieux J, et al. Influence of the interval between preoperative radiation therapy and surgery on downstaging and on the rate of sphincter-sparing surgery for rectal cancer: the Lyon R90–01 randomized trial. *J Clin Oncol.* 1999;17(8):2396.
49. van Gijn W, Marijnen CA, Nagtegaal ID, et al.; Dutch Colorectal Cancer Group. Preoperative radiotherapy combined with total mesorectal excision for resectable rectal cancer: 12-year follow-up of the multicentre, randomised controlled TME trial. *Lancet Oncol.* 2011;12(6):575–582.
50. Peeters KC, van de Velde CJ, Leer JW, et al. Late side effects of short-course preoperative radiotherapy combined with total mesorectal excision for rectal cancer: increased bowel dysfunction in irradiated patients–a Dutch colorectal cancer group study. *J Clin Oncol.* 2005;23(25):6199–6206.
51. Adjuvant radiotherapy for rectal cancer: a systematic overview of 8,507 patients from 22 randomised trials. *Lancet.* 2001;358:1291–1304.
52. Cammà C, Giunta M, Fiorica F, Pagliaro L, Craxì A, Cottone M. Preoperative radiotherapy for resectable rectal cancer: A meta-analysis. *JAMA.* 2000;284(8):1008–1015.
53. Gérard JP, Conroy T, Bonnetain F, et al. Preoperative radiotherapy with or without concurrent fluorouracil and leucovorin in T3–4 rectal cancers: results of FFCD 9203. *J Clin Oncol.* 2006;24(28):4620–4625.
54. Collette L, Bosset JF, den Dulk M, et al. Patients with curative resection of cT3–4 rectal cancer after preoperative radiotherapy or radiochemotherapy: does anybody benefit from adjuvant fluorouracil-based chemotherapy? A trial of the European Organisation for Research and Treatment of Cancer Radiation Oncology Group. *J Clin Oncol.* 2007;25:4379–4386.
55. Bosset JF, Collette L, Calais G, et al.; EORTC Radiotherapy Group Trial 22921. Chemotherapy with preoperative radiotherapy in rectal cancer. *N Engl J Med.* 2006;355(11):1114–1123.
56. Bujko K, Nowacki MP, Nasierowska-Guttmejer A, Michalski W, Bebenek M, Kryj M. Long-term results of a randomized trial comparing preoperative short-course radiotherapy with preoperative conventionally fractionated chemoradiation for rectal cancer. *Br J Surg.* 2006;93(10):1215–1223.
57. Ngan SY, Burmeister B, Fisher RJ, et al. Randomized trial of short-course radiotherapy versus long-course chemoradiation comparing rates of local recurrence in patients with T3 rectal cancer: Trans-Tasman Radiation Oncology Group trial 01.04. *J Clin Oncol.* 2012;30(31):3827–3833.
58. Sebag-Montefiore D, Stephens RJ, Steele R, et al. Preoperative radiotherapy versus selective postoperative chemoradiotherapy in patients with rectal cancer (MRC CR07 and NCIC-CTG C016): a multicentre, randomised trial. *Lancet.* 2009;373(9666):811–820.
59. Sauer R, Becker H, Hohenberger W, et al.; German Rectal Cancer Study Group. Preoperative versus postoperative chemoradiotherapy for rectal cancer. *N Engl J Med.* 2004;351(17):1731–1740.

60. Roh MS, Colangelo LH, O'Connell MJ, et al. Preoperative multimodality therapy improves disease-free survival in patients with carcinoma of the rectum: NSABP R-03. *J Clin Oncol.* 2009;27(31):5124–5130.
61. Wiltshire KL, Ward IG, Swallow C, et al. Preoperative radiation with concurrent chemotherapy for resectable rectal cancer: effect of dose escalation on pathologic complete response, local recurrence-free survival, disease-free survival, and overall survival. *Int J Radiat Oncol Biol Phys.* 2006;64(3):709–716.
62. Mohiuddin M, Winter K, Mitchell E, et al.; Radiation Therapy Oncology Group Trial 0012. Randomized phase II study of neoadjuvant combined-modality chemoradiation for distal rectal cancer: Radiation Therapy Oncology Group Trial 0012. *J Clin Oncol.* 2006;24(4):650–655.
63. Gerard JP, Chapet O, Nemoz C, et al. Improved sphincter preservation in low rectal cancer with high-dose preoperative radiotherapy: the Lyon R96-02 randomized trial. *J Clin Oncol.* 2004;22(12):2404–2409.
64. Ortholan C, Romestaing P, Chapet O, Gerard JP. Correlation in rectal cancer between clinical tumor response after neoadjuvant radiotherapy and sphincter or organ preservation: 10-year results of the Lyon R 96–02 randomized trial. *Int J Radiat Oncol Biol Phys.* 2012;83(2):e165–e171.
65. Smalley SR, Benedetti JK, Williamson SK, et al. Phase III trial of fluorouracil-based chemotherapy regimens plus radiotherapy in postoperative adjuvant rectal cancer: GI INT 0144. *J Clin Oncol.* 2006;24(22):3542–3547.
66. Roh Gay MS, O'Connell MJ, Beart RW, et al. The impact of capecitabine and oxaliplatin in the preoperative multimodality treatment in patients with carcinoma of the rectum: NSABP R-04. *J Clin Oncol.* 2011;29.
67. Aschele C, Cionini L, Lonardi S, et al. Primary tumor response to preoperative chemoradiation with or without oxaliplatin in locally advanced rectal cancer: pathologic results of the STAR-01 randomized phase III trial. *J Clin Oncol.* 2011;29(20):2773–2780.
68. Gérard JP, Azria D, Gourgou-Bourgade S, et al. Comparison of two neoadjuvant chemoradiotherapy regimens for locally advanced rectal cancer: results of the phase III trial ACCORD 12/0405-Prodige 2. *J Clin Oncol.* 2010;28(10):1638–1644.
69. Sadahiro S, Suzuki T, Ishikawa K, et al. Intraoperative radiation therapy for curatively resected rectal cancer. *Dis Colon Rectum.* 2001;44(11):1689–1695.
70. Huber FT, Stepan R, Zimmermann F, Fink U, Molls M, Siewert JR. Locally advanced rectal cancer: resection and intraoperative radiotherapy using the flab method combined with preoperative or postoperative radiochemotherapy. *Dis Colon Rectum.* 1996; 39(7):774–779.
71. Calvo FA, Gómez-Espí M, Díaz-González JA, et al. Intraoperative presacral electron boost following preoperative chemoradiation in T3-4Nx rectal cancer: initial local effects and clinical outcome analysis. *Radiother Oncol.* 2002;62(2):201–206.
72. Kim HK, Jessup JM, Beard CJ, et al. Locally advanced rectal carcinoma: pelvic control and morbidity following preoperative radiation therapy, resection, and intraoperative radiation therapy. *Int J Radiat Oncol Biol Phys.* 1997;38(4):777–783.
73. Masaki T, Takayama M, Matsuoka H, et al. Intraoperative radiotherapy for oncological and function-preserving surgery in patients with advanced lower rectal cancer. *Langenbecks Arch Surg.* 2008;393(2):173–180.
74. Dubois JB, Bussieres E, Richaud P, et al. Intra-operative radiotherapy of rectal cancer: results of the French multi-institutional randomized study. *Radiother Oncol.* 2011;98(3):298–303.

9 Management of Synchronous Metastases

Surgical Considerations in the Treatment of Synchronous Stage IV Disease

JEFFREY M. FARMA
ELIN R. SIGURDSON

In 2012, there will be approximately 143,000 patients diagnosed with colorectal cancer (CRC) annually in the United States, with CRC being the third cause of cancer-related death in men and women (1). At presentation approximately 15%–25% of these patients will have metastatic disease (2–5), with the most common sites being the liver (15%–20%), lung (10%–15%), and less commonly, the peritoneum, ovary, adrenal, and bone (2,5,6). Management of patients with Stage IV CRC at presentation is complex and requires a multidisciplinary approach. This section will concentrate on the role of surgery in the care of these patients.

At initial presentation, the treating multidisciplinary team should classify the patient into 1 of 3 groups. The first are those who have resectable primary and metastatic disease; these patients are potentially curable. The second are those who are initially unresectable due to their metastatic disease, but have the potential of being converted to resectable following chemotherapy; these patients may become "curable" if they respond to chemotherapy. The third are unresectable; these patients should be treated with palliative intent. The treating team should also consider whether the primary tumor is symptomatic in terms of bleeding or obstruction and therefore requires resection. For these reasons, it is key to have the surgeon involved early in treatment planning.

Patients who are candidates for complete surgical resection of both their primary and metastatic disease have a 5-year survival approaching 24%–58% (7–13; Table 9.1). If untreated, median survival is 6 to 12 months (5). Without resection, the median survival of patients with liver metastases treated with aggressive systemic chemotherapy alone ranges from 11 to 24 months, and 5-year survival of patients with even solitary liver metastases is rare (4,14–16).

Resection of the Primary Tumor

Modern day chemotherapy including irinotecan and oxaliplatin has led to a trend toward lower rates of elective primary tumor resection (17). In 1999, Scoggins reported that contrary to traditional surgical teaching and belief, malignant obstruction occurred in only 8.7% of patients managed with an intact primary tumor in Stage IV CRC, with no cases of bleeding or perforation reported while on chemotherapy (18). Using the SEER database, Temple evaluated surgical practice in patients with Stage IV CRC over 65 years of age from 1991 to 1999 and found that 72% received primary cancer directed surgery, with a much lower rate of administration of chemotherapy (18). Using the SEER database, Cook et al evaluated treatment of 26,754 patients with Stage IV CRC from 1988 to 2000 and found that 66% initially underwent primary tumor resection (19). In a study from Memorial Sloan-Kettering, in patients who were initially managed with modern combination chemotherapy regimens, only 7% of patients treated with oxaliplatin- or irinotecan-based therapy required surgical palliation for their intact primary tumor (20). In 255 patients at Fox Chase Cancer Center there was a low rate (9.8%) of obstruction or perforation related to an intact primary tumor in patients with metastatic colorectal cancer (MCRC) who did not initially require surgical intervention (21). All of these series confirm a low rate of complications related to the primary tumor, and need for initial surgical management of the primary tumor in the setting of MCRC, unless the patient has acute obstructive symptoms or significant bleeding on presentation. Frequently patients can be bridged through chemotherapy and ultimately resection with serial endoscopic dilations or endoscopic stents for

Table 9.1 Survival After Hepatic Resection for Colorectal Metastases

Studies	Patient (N)	Operative Mortality (%)	5/10 Year Survival (%)
Kokudo (149)	736	0	51
Dexiang et al (137)	530	2.2	47
Rees et al (138)	929	1.5	36/23
Mutsaerts et al (13)	102	-	29
Abdalla et al (7)	190	-	58
Bramhall et al (8)	212	2.8	28
Liu et al (139)	72	4	32
Choti et al (9)	226	0.9	40/26
Fong et al (140)	1001	3	37/22
Bradley et al (141)	134	4	36/23

near obstructing lesions of the colon and rectum, rather than requiring up front resection or colostomy.

Radiation to the Primary Tumor

There is limited literature regarding the use of pelvic radiation to control the primary cancer and decrease the chance of local recurrence in Stage IV CRC. Kim et al recently reviewed their series in Korea (22) comparing all patients with rectal cancer and synchronous liver metastasis, and identified 27 patients who received adjuvant pelvic radiation, compared to 62 patients who did not receive radiation. Pelvic recurrence occurred in 15% with radiation vs 34% without radiation. Similarly, Crane reported on a cohort of patients with metastatic rectal cancer treated with pelvic chemoradiation on initial presentation, with 94% resolution of primary tumor symptoms and a pelvic control rate of 81%–91% (23). Platell evaluated 313 patients with Stage IV CRC and on univariate analysis use of radiation to the primary was an independent predictor of overall survival (HR, 0.543; 95% CI, 0.352–0.835, $P = .05$; 24). In their study, radiation was used to improve symptoms and control local disease; however, many of these patients also had their primary tumors removed and there are no local recurrence data on this specific subset of patients.

Potentially Resectable Stage IV Rectal Cancer

Modern series demonstrate 5-year survival rate of 22%–38% in patients initially deemed unresectable who respond to chemotherapy and proceed to surgery (25–30). Adam evaluated a highly selected group of patients initially deemed unresectable who were converted to resectable. Five- and 10-year overall survival were 33% and 27%, respectively, and of 148 patients with a follow up of greater than or equal to 5 years, 16% were considered cured of their disease. Multivariate analysis found size of metastases less than 3 cm at diagnosis, number of metastases less than three and complete pathologic response to predict cure (29). Results of the phase II CELIM trial were reported evaluating cetuximab with FOLFOX6 or FOLFIRI in patients with unresectable or greater than four colorectal liver metastases (29). There were higher response rates of 68% in the cetuximab/FOLFOX6 group, with an overall rate of 34% of patients who were able to go on to achieve R0 resections.

There may be a role for hepatic resection in select patients with limited extrahepatic metastases (31,32). Elias reported results of 75 patients who underwent R0 resection of extrahepatic disease in combination with hepatic resection. Extrahepatic sites of disease included peritoneal, ovarian, hilar lymph nodes, local recurrence, retroperitoneal lymph nodes, lung, and abdominal wall metastases. Operative mortality was 2.7% with a morbidity of 25%. At a median follow up of 4.9 years, the overall 3- and 5-year survival was 45% and 28%, respectively. R0 resection could not be accomplished in 50% of patients who underwent surgical exploration, and negative prognostic factors included greater than five liver lesions and multiple sites of extrahepatic disease.

Chemotherapy-Induced Hepatotoxicity

Due to the risk of hepatotoxicity related to newer chemotherapeutic agents we emphasize the importance of limited preoperative treatment (33–35). Chemotherapy-induced steatohepatitis has been associated with the use of 5-fluorouracil (5-FU) and irinotecan as well as increased postoperative mortality (36–39). Oxaliplatin has been associated with vascular sinusoidal injury in the liver, occurs in 19%–52% of patients and can lead to increased intraoperative bleeding (40–43). Nakano evaluated the relationship of sinusoidal injury and outcomes in patients after hepatectomy for colorectal liver metastases after receiving oxaliplatin. It correlated with female gender, greater than or equal to 6 cycles, preoperative AST value greater than 36 IU/L, and abnormal preoperative indocyanine green retention greater than 10% with sinusoidal injury (41). Patients with steatohepatitis demonstrated an increased 90-day mortality compared to those who did not have steatohepatitis

(14.7% vs 1.6%; P = .01). In general, we recommend initially treating patients with 6 cycles of chemotherapy followed by restaging imaging to plan resection prior to the development of induced hepatotoxicity.

Simultaneous or Staged Resections

Timing and coordination of surgery has been studied in retrospective series, evaluating the ability to perform simultaneous resections of the primary and metastatic disease (Table 9.2; 44–50). Martin et al reviewed their experience with 70 patients with simultaneous resection of the primary colorectal tumor and hepatectomy for liver metastases and compared this to 160 patients who underwent staged resections (47) and found no difference in size of metastases, number of lesions, or percentage of major liver resections. Patients with simultaneous resection required shorter hospitalization with no difference in morbidity or mortality rates. Reddy et al performed a multi-institutional study evaluating simultaneous resection of synchronous CRC and liver metastases, comparing 135 patients who had simultaneous resection to 475 patients with staged resections (44). In this study, patients with simultaneous resections had fewer and smaller metastases and were less likely to undergo major hepatectomy (greater than three segments).

Resection of Lung Metastases

The international registry of lung metastases demonstrated a 5- and 10-year overall survival rate of 37% and 22%, respectively (51). A summary of recent studies on lung metastasectomy for CRC is listed in Table 9.3. Negri et al reviewed their series of patients undergoing pulmonary metastasectomy for CRC and identified 31 patients; 35% received preoperative chemotherapy and 65% proceeded directly to surgery (52). In their series, the majority of patients had either a wedge resection or segmentectomy and there was no operative mortality, less than 20% had postoperative complications, with an overall 3- and 5-year survival rate of 65.2% and 26.1%, respectively. Suemitsu identified 57 patients treated between 1996 and 2008 who underwent pulmonary metastasectomy for CRC; 32 of these patients also had a previous liver resection for metastases (53). The majority of patients had resection of a single metastatic lesion, 91% had less than a lobectomy, with a 5-year survival after first pulmonary metastasectomy of 53.9%. In select patients with resectable pulmonary metastases from CRC metastasectomy can be performed with low morbidity and can potentially lead to prolonged survival.

Conclusions

With modern day chemotherapy regimens and newer agents on the horizon, patients with Stage IV rectal cancer are living longer and more patients are being considered for surgical resection of all sites of their disease, both the primary and metastatic, in hopes of prolonging survival. There are still many unanswered questions related to timing and sequencing of therapies and future clinical trials need to address these questions in these complex patients.

Table 9.2 Staged or Synchronous Resection of Colorectal Liver Metastases and Primary Tumor

Studies	Patient (N) (Staged/ Synchronous)	Mortality (%) (Staged/ Synchronous)	Morbidity (%) (Staged/ Synchronous)	
Luo et al (142)	276/129	2%/1.5%	54.3%/47.3%	
deHaas et al (143)	173/55	0.6%/0%	25.4%/11%	
Martin et al (47)	160/70	1%/0%	55%/56%	
Reddy (44)	475/135	0.5 %/1 %	13%/14%	Minor hepatectomy
		1.4%/8.3%	15.1%/36.1%	Major hepatectomy
Martin et al (144)	106/134	2%/2%	67%/49%	
Lyass et al (48)	86/26	2.3%/0%	35%/27%	

Table 9.3 Outcomes After Resection of Colorectal Lung Metastases

Studies	Patient (N)	Operative Mortality (%)	5/10 Year Survival (%)
Suemitsu et al (53)	57	nr	54
Hornbech et al (145)	53	1.9	50
Kanzaki et al (146)	156	0	56/44
Lin et al (147)	63	nr	44
Lee et al (148)	59	0	50
Negri et al (52)	31	0	26

nr, not reported.

Chemotherapy for the Treatment of Synchronous Stage IV Disease

LAURA GOFF

The improvement in MCRC median survival can be attributed in large part to advances in the multidisciplinary care of these patients. Systemic therapy may provide a palliative benefit in terms of symptom control as well as improve the median survival of patients from a few months without treatment to several years in the era of modern chemotherapy. Moreover, systemic therapy may ultimately lead to a potential cure if a patient's cancer is rendered resectable. The possibility of resection must be considered in order to plan therapy for patients with synchronous metastatic disease.

Patients Unlikely to Come to Resection

For patients with widespread metastatic disease unlikely to come to resection, systemic chemotherapy is generally the only modality of therapy that is appropriate, especially if the primary tumor is minimally symptomatic. The focus for these patients is on improving survival with appropriate quality of life. The rate of tumor shrinkage as evaluated by response rates is less important.

Early Versus Delayed Chemotherapy

In asymptomatic patients, the question arises regarding when to initiate chemotherapy. Although all recommendations must be tailored to an individual, there are some data to suggest that early initiation of chemotherapy leads to symptomatic and survival benefits. The Nordic Gastrointestinal Tumor Adjuvant Therapy Group randomized asymptomatic patients to receive either initial combination chemotherapy or to holding chemotherapy until symptoms appeared. Early treatment led to both an improvement in median survival by approximately 5 months as well as a prolonged "asymptomatic period" (54). Therefore, for patients who are physiologically fit for chemotherapy, prompt initiation of treatment should be considered.

Combination Versus Sequential Chemotherapy

Many different drugs and combination regimens have demonstrated activity in MCRC. Early data suggested that the response rate to first-line chemotherapy translated into an increase in overall survival for patients with CRC, thereby validating the use of combination regimens with higher response rates early in the course of a patient's disease (55). In a later analysis of the role of 5-FU, leucovorin, irinotecan, and oxaliplatin in CRC, the use of combination therapy first-line did result in improved survival (56). However, the median overall survival was more closely related to the administration of all 3 drugs during the course of the disease, rather than the sequence or combination used. Two later studies subsequently challenged this dogma that combination chemotherapy was the best initial approach for patients with MCRC. In the CAIRO study, Dutch investigators randomized 820 patients to either sequential or combination treatment (57). Sequential treatment consisted of capecitabine, followed by single-agent irinotecan, followed by capecitabine with oxaliplatin while combination treatment consisted of first-line capecitabine plus irinotecan followed by second-line capecitabine with oxaliplatin. In this analysis, combination therapy did not improve overall survival (median survival of 17.4 months). In the MRC FOCUS study, several potential treatment strategies were explored including sequential single agent therapy, combination therapy from the outset of treatment, or single-agent therapy followed by combination therapy (58). This study found that initial single-agent therapy escalating to combination therapy when required was not inferior to initial combination therapy. Median survival times were in the range of 14 to 16 months. No biologic therapy such as bevacizumab or epidermal growth factor receptor (EGFR) inhibitors was included, limiting the ability to compare these survival times across trials. In summary, although initial combination chemotherapy for MCRC is generally well-tolerated, for patients in whom the treatment goal is palliation, front-line single-agent chemotherapy is a reasonable choice, saving combination therapy for when it is needed.

Patients With Potentially Resectable Disease

While patients with extensive metastatic disease are unlikely to ever benefit from surgical intervention, some patients with initially unresectable disease can undergo sufficient tumor shrinkage to undergo resection, which may lead to long-term disease control and probable cure. Therefore, choosing a regimen that has a high response rate and consequently, improved tumor shrinkage, can have significant clinical implications.

Combination Chemotherapy

Combination chemotherapy in MCRC generally leads to higher response rates. Exactly which combination is best is unclear. When irinotecan is combined with 5-FU/LV in the front-line treatment of MCRC, response rates are generally around 50% and median survival times range from 15 to 23 months (59–62). Oxaliplatin as a single agent in MCRC demonstrates response rates of 10% or less (16,63–65). However, it is very active in MCRC when given in combination with either 5-FU or capecitabine, even in 5-FU-refractory disease (16,66–68). Response rates to oxaliplatin and fluoropyrimidine combinations are also around 50% and median survival times around 20 months. Early suggestion from the large North Central Cancer Treatment Group study that FOLFOX was the superior regimen in terms of response rate was likely due to the lack of infusional 5-FU used in the comparator arms of IROX or IFL (69). Subsequent comparisons of FOLFOX and the infusional regimen FOLFIRI demonstrate similar response rates as well as overall survival times, and both regimens represent reasonable chemotherapy options upon which to build (70,71). The FOLFOX regimen is preferred in the setting of initially resectable metastatic disease as there is a progression-free survival advantage for the perioperative administration of FOLFOX in patients with resectable liver metastases (72). Conversely, FOLFIRI was no more effective after liver metastasectomy than infusional 5-FU in terms of disease-free survival (73).

Tritherapy

Because both FOLFOX and FOLFIRI lead to high response rates, attempts have been made to combine these regimens in the hopes of increasing the likelihood of conversion to resectability. Two closely related regimens, FOLFOXIRI and FOLFIRINOX, have been investigated in patients with initially unresectable MCRC (74,75). Response rates for both regimens was 70%. Of 34 patients treated with FOLFIRINOX, 26.5% were eventually able to undergo an R0 resection. One hundred ninety-six patients were treated with FOLFOXIRI, which uses a slightly lower dose of irinotecan and a slightly higher dose of infusional 5FU. In this study, 19% of patients were able to undergo an R0 resection. Not unexpectedly, the toxicity of these "tritherapy" regimens is increased with high rates of neutropenia, diarrhea, and fatigue. Appropriate patient selection is important, but some patients may benefit from this aggressive approach.

Bevacizumab

In addition to escalating cytotoxic chemotherapy, the addition of biologic agents to chemotherapy can lead to improved outcomes. Bevacizumab is used in conjunction with chemotherapy in both first- and second-line regimens due to improvements in survival (14,76–80). In addition to improved survival, in general, response rates are improved as well, nearing 60%–70% depending on the series. While it is unclear if the addition of bevacizumab to chemotherapy will add to the conversion rate, there is ample evidence that the use of bevacizumab prior to liver resection does not increase postoperative morbidity (81–84). Although the optimal timing of liver resection after bevacizumab is unclear, most published series demonstrate safety in the range of 6 to 8 weeks following the last bevacizumab dose.

Epidermal Growth Factor Receptor (EGFR) Inhibitors

The drugs cetuximab and panitumumab are monoclonal antibodies to the EGFR and were originally developed in advanced MCRC (85–88). These agents are not effective in colorectal tumors, which harbor activating mutations in the *K-ras* gene that encodes the downstream effector of EGFR (89). As efficacy was demonstrated in the refractory setting, cetuximab and panitumumab were added to cytotoxic chemotherapy in the first-line setting in the hopes of improving response rates and survival. In the front-line setting, EGFR inhibition with either panitumumab or cetuximab improves the response rates of irinotecan or oxaliplatin-based chemotherapy for *K-ras* wild-type tumors to about 60% (90–93). The percentage of completed R0 resections for metastatic disease appears to be improved as well, but the numbers are small and the true effect on improved rate of cure for patients is unclear.

Dual Antibody Therapy

It is clear, however, that unlike cytotoxic chemotherapy, combining biologic therapy does not result in additive response. When bevacizumab, chemotherapy, and either cetuximab or panitumumab are given in combination, the outcomes are inferior (94,95). Response rates are not improved and toxicity, quality of life, and progression-free survival are worse. Dual antibody therapy should not be used.

Summary

In order to appropriately care for patients with synchronous metastatic disease, a multidisciplinary approach is essential. The goals of therapy must be outlined in the context of whether a patient has potentially resectable disease or widespread metastases unlikely to come to resection. For patients with potentially resectable disease, combination regimens of doublet chemotherapy given with biologic agents or possibly even tritherapy may yield the highest response rates, providing a potential opportunity for curative surgery. On the other hand, less toxic doublets or even single-agent therapy may be optimal for patients with widespread metastases for whom palliation is the goal.

The Role of Radiotherapy for Liver Metastases

MONIQUE J. YOUL
LAURA A. DAWSON

As discussed earlier in this chapter, surgical resection of liver metastases is potentially curative in appropriately selected patients. However, a substantial proportion of patients with liver-confined metastases have disease unsuitable for surgery, even after chemotherapy. This is due to anatomical location or medical contraindications. These patients may be candidates for local ablative treatment modalities.

Radiofrequency ablation (RFA) is the most common nonsurgical local therapy for unresectable liver metastases (7,96–99). There is a wide range of reported local recurrence rates (3.6%–60%; 100). However, in studies where the median tumor size is 3 cm or smaller and the median number of tumors per patient is less than or equal to 3, lower local recurrence rates of 1.6%–24% (101–108) are reported. Five-year overall survival rates range between 14% and 55% (100). A suggestion of overall benefit to patients from obtaining local control was shown in an EORTC intergroup phase II study (109). This study randomized 119 patients with unresectable CRC liver metastases to systemic therapy alone vs systemic therapy with RFA. While only reported in abstract form, improved progression-free survival was seen in the patients treated with local therapy in addition to systemic therapy. Other local therapies that are currently under investigation include microwave ablation, cryotherapy, and high-intensity focused ultrasound (HIFU; 110,111).

The first use of external beam radiation therapy for liver metastases was by the University of Michigan (112). Twenty-two patients with liver metastases from CRC were treated with conformal radiation therapy delivered with concurrent hepatic intra-arterial (HAI) fluoro-deoxyuridine. The doses ranged from 48–73 Gy in 1.5–1.65 Gy fractions given twice daily. The response rate was 50%; only 25% of the patients were free of hepatic progression at 1 year. It was hypothesized that a higher dose of conformal radiation would be required to achieve a durable response. A subsequent dose-escalation study of conformal radiation therapy (median dose 60.75 Gy, range, 40–90 Gy, 1.5 Gy twice daily) and concurrent HAI fluoro-deoxyuridine, found that the total dose was the only significant predictor of survival. The median survival of patients with liver metastases secondary to CRC was 17.2 months, significantly longer than historical controls (113).

In the last decade there have been significant technological advances in radiation planning, organ motion management, radiation delivery, and image guided radiotherapy (IGRT). This has facilitated the development of stereotactic body radiotherapy (SBRT). SBRT is a noninvasive, radiotherapy technique that allows an ablative dose of radiotherapy to be safely delivered to extracranial metastases, with rapid fall off of dose to adjacent normal tissues. SBRT is different from conventional radiotherapy, which typically delivers 1.8–2 Gy per fraction over a 5 to 7 week course. SBRT, in comparison, uses only 1–10 fractions over a 1–2 week course. The short overall treatment time of SBRT makes it more attractive to patients and caregivers due to increased efficiency. The SBRT dose per fraction is much higher than conventional fraction size, ranging from 5–30 Gy per fraction. This high dose per fraction necessitates a steep dose gradient outside of the target to avoid the delivery of high dose to surrounding normal tissues. This is achieved by the use of multiple nonopposing beams (typically 5–9), which enter the patient at different angles, possibly noncoplanar or delivered in a rotation or arc to produce doses with high conformality around the target volume and sparing of normal tissues (Figure 9.1).

This steep dose gradient outside the target is designed to spare normal tissues and relies on additional technology to ensure the accurate delivery of the planned treatment. This includes IGRT, which refers to the use of frequent (daily in the case of SBRT) imaging prior to treatment to ensure the appropriate set up of the patient. This reduces the risk of a marginal miss," which refers to the delivery

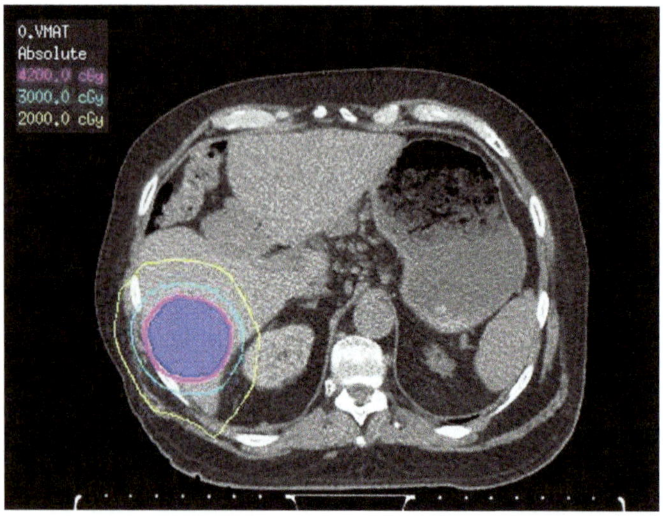

FIGURE 9.1 SBRT treatment for CRC liver metastasis. The planned target volume (treated volume) is in blue color wash. The prescription isodose (42 Gy in 6 fractions) is highly conformal around the planned target volume. There is a sharp drop off of dose within the normal liver.

of the high dose of radiation to normal tissues and underdosage of the tumor. Other technologies are designed to account for, or lessen, intrafractional tumor movement (ie, respiratory movement of the liver, up to 3 cm, occurring as the radiation is delivered). Examples of techniques to reduce the amplitude of respiration include respiratory gating, breath-holding techniques, and abdominal compression. Combining motion management technologies with IGRT leads to improved treatment precision and accuracy.

Patient Selection for SBRT

The criteria to determine appropriate candidates for SBRT are not well defined. The following criteria, from SBRT series and surgical data, may be helpful in the selection of patients with liver metastases from CRC who are most likely to benefit from SBRT:

- Good performance status (ECOG 0–1).
- Adequate liver function (Child Pugh A).
- Greater than 700 cc of uninvolved liver.
- Number of liver metastases less than or equal to 5.
- Size of the largest lesion less than or equal to 6 cm.
- No extrahepatic disease.
- Greater than 1.5 cm away from luminal GI tissues.
- CEA less than or equal to 200 ng/mL.

In practice, however, the candidates for SBRT depend to a large degree on local expertise and referral patterns in addition to the patient and tumor characteristics. Given the undisputable survival advantage of surgical resection, patients referred for SBRT are either unresectable, medically inoperable, or have declined surgery. They are, therefore, at an inherently greater risk of recurrence compared with surgical patients with CRC metastases. Very often, the liver metastases referred for SBRT exceed 6 cm, where despite initial responses to SBRT, long-term control may be reduced, especially as the burden of metastases increases.

The criteria for selecting the most appropriate patients for local therapy are being continuously challenged. Improved chemotherapy regimens can substantially "downstage" patients who would previously not have been considered for radical therapy for extensive liver metastases. Larger tumors have been documented to have a reduced chance of sustained local control in some SBRT series (114,115). A confounding factor, however, is that larger tumors often receive a lower dose of radiation in order to keep normal tissues within tolerance. Despite this probable reduced chance of sustained local control, larger tumors may have local control for many months (or years), which may benefit the patient by delaying the need for chemotherapy and/or reducing symptoms from growing liver metastases. Also, today, the absolute number of metastases is not a contraindication to surgery or SBRT; rather, adequate liver reserve is the final determinant of feasibility (116). Chang et al showed that a single metastasis vs 2 to 4 metastases did not correlate with survival (117). Five metastases is included in the above selection list as an arbitrary limit beyond which the risk of micrometastases increases and the ability to deliver ablative SBRT doses safely is reduced.

Active extrahepatic disease has been consistently shown to correlate with poorer survival outcomes in both surgical (6,118–120) and SBRT series (117). However, studies on SBRT for liver metastases often include patients with extrahepatic disease. It is thought that these patients may still gain benefit from local control, especially if the hepatic disease is the largest burden of disease or if the extrahepatic disease is controlled or potentially treatable.

If surgery has been ruled out but local treatment is still felt to be beneficial, then it is often challenging to determine which local treatment should be offered. Once again, referral patterns and local expertise may influence this decision, but discussion in a multidisciplinary setting is essential. RFA and SBRT have the most data regarding local control and results appear comparable for similarly selected patients (121). Local control outcomes following RFA for metastases less than 3 cm are excellent, whereas relapse rates increase for larger lesions or those adjacent to vasculature due to a heat sink effect (100,122). For example, the portahepatic region, with its large vessels and the main bile tracts, is generally considered an inappropriate region for RFA (123,124) but may be suitable for SBRT. Other tumor positions may also make one modality more favorable over another. For example, tumors close to the diaphragm may risk diaphragmatic injury with RFA but may be suitable for SBRT. Metastases close to bowel or stomach may be at risk of intestinal perforation with RFA and likewise have an increased risk of bleeding, ulceration, and/or perforation with SBRT. There is currently one accruing randomized trial comparing RFA vs SBRT for CRC liver metastases that should provide useful data (www.clinicaltrials.gov; Radiofrequency ablation vs stereotactic radiotherapy in colorectal liver metastases; NCT01233544).

Regarding patient workup, all patients should have recent imaging (CT or whole body PET) of the chest, abdomen, and pelvis. A liver MRI may be valuable, especially in the setting of hepatic steatosis, to determine the number of metastases and further characterize the lesions. Baseline blood work to confirm adequate liver function (Child-Pugh score A) and a CEA should be performed. A CEA of greater than 200 ng/mL is predictive of more widespread metastatic disease and a patient may be more suitable for upfront palliative chemotherapy rather than local therapies (106).

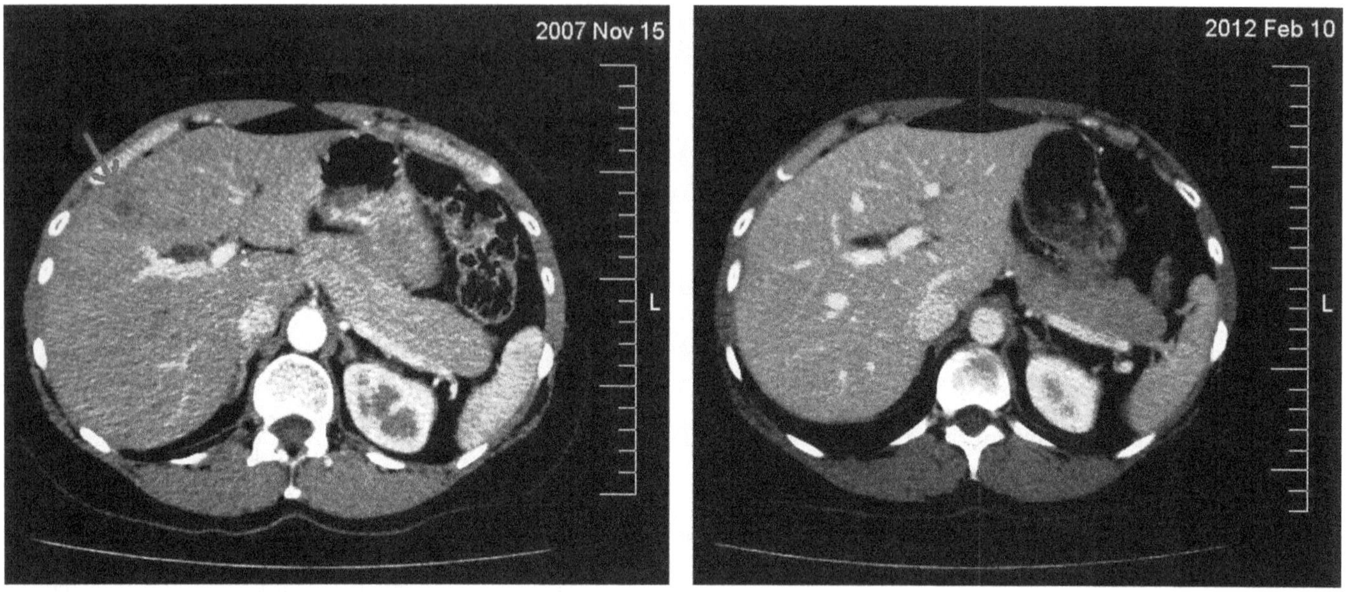

FIGURE 9.2 Pre-SBRT (45 Gy in 10 fractions) CT scan (left) illustrating the liver metastasis (arrow) and more than 4 years after treatment, a follow-up CT scan (right) continues to show no evidence of disease within the liver and the patient has also remained free of distance relapse.

Outcomes of SBRT

Local control at 2 years ranges from 55%–92% and the 2-year overall survival rates range from 32%–83% (115,117,125–127). An excellent response is shown in Figure 9.2. Sustained local control has been shown to correlate with overall survival (117). Although there is an increasing number of prospective studies being published, there are no completed randomized trials of conformal radiation therapy or SBRT for CRC metastases. Table 9.4 summarizes the available studies and retrospective series on SBRT for liver metastases that included at least 15 patients with CRC liver metastases. There are other prospective series of liver SBRT for metastases that demonstrate similar or improved sustained local control; however, they included smaller numbers of patients with CRC liver metastases (128–131). The first three studies in Table 9.1 (117,126,127) only included patients with colorectal metastases. The other studies (114,115,123,125,132,133), in comparison, incorporated multiple histologies, although colorectal metastases were still the most common histology. Colorectal liver metastases have a worse local control rate compared to the results of SBRT for liver metastases from other primary sites, particularly breast cancer (114,125,134,135). Høyer et al (127) hypothesized this may be due to the fact that patients with colorectal liver metastases are often heavily pretreated with both systemic and local treatments prior to being referred for SBRT (Table 9.4).

Patient heterogeneity including different histologies, prior systemic chemotherapy, the presence of extrahepatic disease, and volume of disease treated does make comparison of the trials difficult, and leads to the relatively large ranges in local control and survival rates quoted above. However, despite these limitations, SBRT appears to be an effective local treatment for colorectal liver metastases, and it should be considered, especially if surgery or RFA are not feasible.

Appropriate Dose/Fractionation Schedules

Studies have demonstrated that there is a dose-response for local control following SBRT (117,125,134). Chang et al (117) demonstrated that 18-month local control was 84% for total doses greater than or equal to 42 Gy compared with only 43% for total doses less than 42 Gy. In practice, liver tolerance or close proximity of the metastasis to small bowel, stomach, or right kidney may limit the maximal dose that is able to be safely delivered.

Potential Toxicity of SBRT

SBRT is generally well tolerated with the most common acute side effects being fatigue. Nausea may also occur, especially if the metastases are adjacent to the stomach. Late toxicity is infrequent but may include:

- Hepatotoxicity (usually transient increase in liver enzymes). Liver failure is rare as long as greater than 700 to 800 cc of liver is spared from radiation therapy.
- Gastric and small or large bowel ulceration, hemorrhage, perforation, or obstruction.
- Chest wall pain and rib fracture.
- Renal toxicity.

Table 9.4 SBRT Studies and Series in Liver Metastases

Study and Design*	No. Patients	No. Metastases Treated	No. Metastases/ Patient	% CRC LM	Median Volume or Size of Metastases (Range)	Dose/Fractionation (Range)	Outcomes
Chang et al (117) (pooled patients (114,115,130)) Retrospective	65	102	1 to 4	100%	30.1 cc (0.6–3088 cc)	Median 42 Gy in 6# Median 42 Gy in 6#	1-yr LC: 67% 2-yr LC: 55% 1-yr OS: 72% 2-yr OS: 38%
van der Pool et al (126) Retrospective	20	31	1 to 3	100%	2.3 cm (0.7–6.2 cm)	37.5 to 45 Gy in 3#	2-yr LC: 74% 2-yr OS: 83%
Hoyer et al (127) Phase II	64[a] 44 LM	141 69% LM	1 to 6	100%	3.5 cm (1.0–8.8 cm)	45 Gy in 3#	2-yr LC: 79% 1-yr OS: 67% 2-yr OS: 38%
Vautravers-Dewas et al (133) Retrospective	42	62	1 to 4	67%	3.4 cm (Mean) (0.7–10 cm)	40 Gy in 4# 45 Gy in 3#	1-yr LC: 90% 2-yr LC: 86% 1-yr OS: 94% 2-yr OS: 48%
Lee et al (114) Phase I	68	~143	1 to 8	59%	75.2 cc 134.8 cc (CRC)	Median 41.8 Gy in 6# (27.7–60 Gy in 6#)	1-yr LC: 71% 1-yr OS: 60%
Herfarth et al (132) Phase I–II	35[b]	60	1 to 3	49%	10 cc (1–132 cc)	Escalated dose: 14–26 Gy in 1#[c]	18-m LC: 68% (overall) 18-m LC: 81% (dose esc group) Median OS: 25 m
Wulf et al (125) Retrospective	39[d]	51	Not stated	45%	53 cc (CTV) (9–355 cc CTV)	30 to 37.5 Gy in 3#[e] 26 Gy in 1#[c]	1-yr LC: 92% 2-yr LC: 66% 1-yr OS: 72% 2-yr OS: 32%
Rusthoven et al (115) Phase I–II	47	63	1 to 3	32%	2.7 cm (0.4–6.8 cm) 14.93 cc (0.75–97.98 cc)	Escalated dose: 36 to 60 Gy in 3#	1-yr: LC: 95% 2-yr LC: 92% Median RFS: 20.5 m
Katz et al (123) Retrospective	69	174	1 to 6	29%	2.7 cm (0.6–12.2 cm)	Median 48 Gy (30–55 Gy) 7 to 20# (mean 11)	10-m LC: 76% 20-m LC: 57% Median OS: 14.5 months

[a]Included patients with CRC metastases to lung, lymph nodes, and adrenal gland in addition to liver metastases.

[b]Included 4 patients with primary liver cancer.

[c]Prescribed to the 80% isodose.

[d]Included 5 patients with primary liver cancer.

[e]Prescribed to the 65% isodose.

CRC, colorectal cancer; LM, liver metastases; #, fraction; LC, local control; OS, OS; RFS, recurrence free survival; esc, escalated; m, month; yr, year.

*In Vautravers-Dewas et al, Chang et al, and Herfarth et al, the majority of patients (~2/3) had either no EH disease or no active EH disease. In van der Pool et al, Rusthoven et al, and Wulf et al, EH disease was permitted as long as it was potentially treatable or controlled. In Lee et al, and Katz et al, EH disease was permitted as long as the largest burden of disease was hepatic or the hepatic disease was considered the most life limiting component of their disease respectively.

While the tolerance of normal tissues to conventional fractionation is well documented, their tolerance in the setting of SBRT is less well understood and further investigation regarding the most appropriate normal tissue SBRT dose limits is being undertaken.

Follow Up After SBRT

Clinical history, examination, and blood work are required to monitor for late effects of SBRT. Surveillance imaging is also warranted, as new sites of disease within the liver may be salvageable via either surgery, other localized treatments such as RFA or possibly re-irradiation (although this may not be possible due to normal tissue limits). A well-demarcated hypodense region around the treated metastasis may be seen on follow-up CT imaging at a median time interval of 1.8 months (range, 1.2–4.6 months) posttreatment (136). This may be incorrectly interpreted as recurrent tumor. The treated tumor, however, is usually of lower density than the radiation reaction, which can be helpful in distinguishing between radiation-induced reaction and viable tumor. If the imaging is still challenging to interpret then a repeat follow-up CT should show a reduction of the hypodense region if it is truly a radiation reaction (136). The volume of liver which has been irradiated to a very high dose may show evidence of fibrosis.

■ FUTURE DIRECTIONS

Determining the role of systemic therapy in combination with SBRT is an important question that is just starting to be explored. Most SBRT experience is in patients who have exhausted their systemic options. If disease is confined to the liver, and surgery has been ruled out as an option, SBRT should, perhaps, be considered earlier in a patient's natural history. Discussion in a multidisciplinary setting is recommended for patients with CRC liver metastases who are possibly suitable for SBRT. Local control has been shown to correlate with total dose delivered and a dose schedule of at least 48 Gy in 3 fractions (respecting normal tissue tolerances) or equivalent biologic dose has been recommended (117). Further studies will help confirm the ideal dose/fractionation schedule and provide further information on normal tissue tolerances in the setting of hypo-fractionation.

■ REFERENCES

1. Siegel R, Naishadham D, Jemal A. Cancer statistics, 2012. *CA Cancer J Clin.* 2012;62(1):10–29.
2. Labianca R, Beretta GD, Kildani B, et al. Colon cancer. *Crit Rev Oncol Hematol.* 2010;74(2):106–133.
3. Ridge JA, Daly JM. Treatment of colorectal hepatic metastases. *Surg Gynecol Obstet.* 1985;161(6):597–607.
4. Ballantyne GH, Quin J. Surgical treatment of liver metastases in patients with colorectal cancer. *Cancer.* 1993;71 (12 Suppl):4252–4266.
5. Bengmark S, Hafström L. The natural history of primary and secondary malignant tumors of the liver. I. The prognosis for patients with hepatic metastases from colonic and rectal carcinoma by laparotomy. *Cancer.* 1969;23(1):198–202.
6. Fong Y, Cohen AM, Fortner JG, et al. Liver resection for colorectal metastases. *J Clin Oncol.* 1997;15(3):938–946.
7. Abdalla EK, Vauthey JN, Ellis LM, et al. Recurrence and outcomes following hepatic resection, radiofrequency ablation, and combined resection/ablation for colorectal liver metastases. *Ann Surg.* 2004;239(6):818–25; discussion 825.
8. Bramhall SR, Gur U, Coldham C, et al. Liver resection for colorectal metastases. *Ann R Coll Surg Engl.* 2003;85(5):334–339.
9. Choti MA, Sitzmann JV, Tiburi MF, et al. Trends in long-term survival following liver resection for hepatic colorectal metastases. *Ann Surg.* 2002;235(6):759–766.
10. Fong Y. Surgical therapy of hepatic colorectal metastasis. *CA Cancer J Clin.* 1999;49(4):231–255.
11. Gayowski TJ, Iwatsuki S, Madariaga JR, et al. Experience in hepatic resection for metastatic colorectal cancer: analysis of clinical and pathologic risk factors. *Surgery.* 1994;116(4):703–10; discussion 710.
12. Jamison RL, Donohue JH, Nagorney DM, Rosen CB, Harmsen WS, Ilstrup DM. Hepatic resection for metastatic colorectal cancer results in cure for some patients. *Arch Surg.* 1997;132(5):505–10; discussion 511.
13. Mutsaerts EL, van Ruth S, Zoetmulder FA, Rutgers EJ, Hart AA, van Coevorden F. Prognostic factors and evaluation of surgical management of hepatic metastases from colorectal origin: a 10-year single-institute experience. *J Gastrointest Surg.* 2005;9(2):178–186.
14. Hurwitz H, Fehrenbacher L, Novotny W, et al. Bevacizumab plus irinotecan, fluorouracil, and leucovorin for metastatic colorectal cancer. *N Engl J Med.* 2004;350(23):2335–2342.
15. Bilchik AJ, Poston G, Curley SA, et al. Neoadjuvant chemotherapy for metastatic colon cancer: a cautionary note. *J Clin Oncol.* 2005;23(36):9073–9078.
16. Rothenberg ML, Oza AM, Bigelow RH, et al. Superiority of oxaliplatin and fluorouracil-leucovorin compared with either therapy alone in patients with progressive colorectal cancer after irinotecan and fluorouracil-leucovorin: interim results of a phase III trial. *J Clin Oncol.* 2003;21(11):2059–2069.
17. Kleespies A, Füessl KE, Seeliger H, et al. Determinants of morbidity and survival after elective non-curative resection of stage IV colon and rectal cancer. *Int J Colorectal Dis.* 2009;24(9):1097–1109.
18. Scoggins CR, Meszoely IM, Blanke CD, Beauchamp RD, Leach SD. Nonoperative management of primary colorectal cancer in patients with stage IV disease. *Ann Surg Oncol.* 1999;6(7):651–657.
19. Cook AD, Single R, McCahill LE. Surgical resection of primary tumors in patients who present with stage IV colorectal cancer: an analysis of surveillance, epidemiology, and end results data, 1988 to 2000. *Ann Surg Oncol.* 2005;12(8):637–645.
20. Poultsides GA, Servais EL, Saltz LB, et al. Outcome of primary tumor in patients with synchronous stage IV colorectal cancer receiving combination chemotherapy without surgery as initial treatment. *J Clin Oncol.* 2009;27(20):3379–3384.
21. Nitzkorski JR, Farma JM, Watson JC, et al. Outcome and natural history of patients with stage IV colorectal cancer receiving chemotherapy without primary tumor resection. *Ann Surg Oncol.* 2012;19(2):379–383.
22. Kim JW, Kim YB, Kim NK, et al. The role of adjuvant pelvic radiotherapy in rectal cancer with synchronous liver metastasis: a retrospective study. *Radiat Oncol.* 2010;5:75.
23. Crane CH, Janjan NA, Abbruzzese JL, et al. Effective pelvic symptom control using initial chemoradiation without colostomy in metastatic rectal cancer. *Int J Radiat Oncol Biol Phys.* 2001; 49(1):107–116.

24. Platell C, Ng S, O'bichere A, Tebbutt N. Changing management and survival in patients with stage IV colorectal cancer. *Dis Colon Rectum*. 2011;54(2):214–219.
25. Giacchetti S, Itzhaki M, Gruia G, et al. Long-term survival of patients with unresectable colorectal cancer liver metastases following infusional chemotherapy with 5-fluorouracil, leucovorin, oxaliplatin and surgery. *Ann Oncol*. 1999;10(6):663–669.
26. Meric F, Patt YZ, Curley SA, et al. Surgery after downstaging of unresectable hepatic tumors with intra-arterial chemotherapy. *Ann Surg Oncol*. 2000;7(7):490–495.
27. Adam R, Pascal G, Castaing D, et al. Tumor progression while on chemotherapy: a contraindication to liver resection for multiple colorectal metastases? *Ann Surg*. 2004;240(6):1052–61; discussion 1061.
28. Rivoire M, De Cian F, Meeus P, Négrier S, Sebban H, Kaemmerlen P. Combination of neoadjuvant chemotherapy with cryotherapy and surgical resection for the treatment of unresectable liver metastases from colorectal carcinoma. *Cancer*. 2002;95(11):2283–2292.
29. Adam R, Wicherts DA, de Haas RJ, et al. Patients with initially unresectable colorectal liver metastases: is there a possibility of cure? *J Clin Oncol*. 2009;27(11):1829–1835.
30. Brouquet A, Nordlinger B. Neoadjuvant therapy of colorectal liver metastases: lessons learned from clinical trials. *J Surg Oncol*. 2010;102(8):932–936.
31. Elias D, Lasser P, Ducreux M, et al. Liver resection (and associated extrahepatic resections) for metastatic well-differentiated endocrine tumors: a 15-year single center prospective study. *Surgery*. 2003;133(4):375–382.
32. Elias D, Sideris L, Pocard M, et al. Results of R0 resection for colorectal liver metastases associated with extrahepatic disease. *Ann Surg Oncol*. 2004;11(3):274–280.
33. Nordlinger B, Benoist S. Benefits and risks of neoadjuvant therapy for liver metastases. *J Clin Oncol*. 2006;24(31):4954–4955.
34. Nordlinger B, Van Cutsem E, Rougier P, et al.; European Colorectal Metastases Treatment Group. Does chemotherapy prior to liver resection increase the potential for cure in patients with metastatic colorectal cancer? A report from the European Colorectal Metastases Treatment Group. *Eur J Cancer*. 2007;43(14):2037–2045.
35. Chun YS, Laurent A, Maru D, Vauthey JN. Management of chemotherapy-associated hepatotoxicity in colorectal liver metastases. *Lancet Oncol*. 2009;10(3):278–286.
36. Kooby DA, Fong Y, Suriawinata A, et al. Impact of steatosis on perioperative outcome following hepatic resection. *J Gastrointest Surg*. 2003;7(8):1034–1044.
37. Vauthey JN, Pawlik TM, Ribero D, et al. Chemotherapy regimen predicts steatohepatitis and an increase in 90-day mortality after surgery for hepatic colorectal metastases. *J Clin Oncol*. 2006;24(13):2065–2072.
38. Fernandez FG, Ritter J, Goodwin JW, Linehan DC, Hawkins WG, Strasberg SM. Effect of steatohepatitis associated with irinotecan or oxaliplatin pretreatment on resectability of hepatic colorectal metastases. *J Am Coll Surg*. 2005;200(6):845–853.
39. Donadon M, Vauthey JN, Loyer EM, Charnsangavej C, Abdalla EK. Portal thrombosis and steatosis after preoperative chemotherapy with FOLFIRI-bevacizumab for colorectal liver metastases. *World J Gastroenterol*. 2006;12(40):6556–6558.
40. Soubrane O, Brouquet A, Zalinski S, et al. Predicting high grade lesions of sinusoidal obstruction syndrome related to oxaliplatin-based chemotherapy for colorectal liver metastases: correlation with post-hepatectomy outcome. *Ann Surg*. 2010;251(3):454–460.
41. Nakano H, Oussoultzoglou E, Rosso E, et al. Sinusoidal injury increases morbidity after major hepatectomy in patients with colorectal liver metastases receiving preoperative chemotherapy. *Ann Surg*. 2008;247(1):118–124.
42. Aloia T, Sebagh M, Plasse M, et al. Liver histology and surgical outcomes after preoperative chemotherapy with fluorouracil plus oxaliplatin in colorectal cancer liver metastases. *J Clin Oncol*. 2006;24(31):4983–4990.
43. Rubbia-Brandt L, Audard V, Sartoretti P, et al. Severe hepatic sinusoidal obstruction associated with oxaliplatin-based chemotherapy in patients with metastatic colorectal cancer. *Ann Oncol*. 2004;15(3):460–466.
44. Reddy SK, Pawlik TM, Zorzi D, et al. Simultaneous resections of colorectal cancer and synchronous liver metastases: a multi-institutional analysis. *Ann Surg Oncol*. 2007;14(12): 3481–3491.
45. Weber JC, Bachellier P, Oussoultzoglou E, Jaeck D. Simultaneous resection of colorectal primary tumour and synchronous liver metastases. *Br J Surg*. 2003;90(8):956–962.
46. Tanaka K, Shimada H, Matsuo K, et al. Outcome after simultaneous colorectal and hepatic resection for colorectal cancer with synchronous metastases. *Surgery*. 2004;136(3):650–659.
47. Martin RC 2nd, Augenstein V, Reuter NP, Scoggins CR, McMasters KM. Simultaneous versus staged resection for synchronous colorectal cancer liver metastases. *J Am Coll Surg*. 2009;208(5):842–50; discussion 850.
48. Lyass S, Zamir G, Matot I, Goitein D, Eid A, Jurim O. Combined colon and hepatic resection for synchronous colorectal liver metastases. *J Surg Oncol*. 2001;78(1):17–21.
49. Nordlinger B, Guiguet M, Vaillant JC, et al. Surgical resection of colorectal carcinoma metastases to the liver. A prognostic scoring system to improve case selection, based on 1568 patients. Association Française de Chirurgie. *Cancer*. 1996;77(7): 1254–1262.
50. Bolton JS, Fuhrman GM. Survival after resection of multiple bilobar hepatic metastases from colorectal carcinoma. *Ann Surg*. 2000;231(5):743–751.
51. Pastorino U. Lung metastasectomy for colorectal cancer. *Tumori*. 1997;83(1 Suppl):S28–S30.
52. Negri F, Musolino A, Cunningham D, Pastorino U, Ladas G, Norman AR. Retrospective study of resection of pulmonary metastases in patients with advanced colorectal cancer: the development of a preoperative chemotherapy strategy. *Clin Colorectal Cancer*. 2004;4(2):101–106.
53. Suemitsu R, Takeo S, Kusumoto E, Hamatake M, Ikejiri K, Saitsu H. Results of a pulmonary metastasectomy in patients with colorectal cancer. *Surg Today*. 2011;41(1):54–59.
54. Nordic Gastrointestinal Tumor Adjuvant Therapy Group. Expectancy or primary chemotherapy in patients with advanced asymptomatic colorectal cancer: a randomized trial. *J Clin Oncol*. 1992;10:904–911.
55. Buyse M, Thirion P, Carlson RW, Burzykowski T, Molenberghs G, Piedbois P. Relation between tumour response to first-line chemotherapy and survival in advanced colorectal cancer: a meta-analysis. Meta-Analysis Group in Cancer. *Lancet*. 2000;356(9227):373–378.
56. Grothey A, Sargent D, Goldberg RM, Schmoll HJ. Survival of patients with advanced colorectal cancer improves with the availability of fluorouracil-leucovorin, irinotecan, and oxaliplatin in the course of treatment. *J Clin Oncol*. 2004;22(7): 1209–1214.
57. Koopman M, Antonini NF, Douma J, et al. Sequential versus combination chemotherapy with capecitabine, irinotecan, and oxaliplatin in advanced colorectal cancer (CAIRO): a phase III randomised controlled trial. *Lancet*. 2007;370(9582): 135–142.
58. Seymour MT, Maughan TS, Ledermann JA, et al.; FOCUS Trial Investigators; National Cancer Research Institute Colorectal Clinical Studies Group. Different strategies of sequential and combination chemotherapy for patients with poor prognosis advanced colorectal cancer (MRC FOCUS): a randomised controlled trial. *Lancet*. 2007;370(9582):143–152.
59. Douillard JY, Cunningham D, Roth AD, et al. Irinotecan combined with fluorouracil compared with fluorouracil alone as first-line treatment for metastatic colorectal cancer: a multicentre randomised trial. *Lancet*. 2000;355(9209): 1041–1047.

60. Saltz LB, Cox JV, Blanke C, et al. Irinotecan plus fluorouracil and leucovorin for metastatic colorectal cancer. Irinotecan Study Group. *N Engl J Med.* 2000;343(13):905–914.
61. Köhne CH, van Cutsem E, Wils J, et al.; European Organisation for Research and Treatment of Cancer Gastrointestinal Group. Phase III study of weekly high-dose infusional fluorouracil plus folinic acid with or without irinotecan in patients with metastatic colorectal cancer: European Organisation for Research and Treatment of Cancer Gastrointestinal Group Study 40986. *J Clin Oncol.* 2005;23(22):4856–4865.
62. Fuchs CS, Marshall J, Mitchell E, et al. Randomized, controlled trial of irinotecan plus infusional, bolus, or oral fluoropyrimidines in first-line treatment of metastatic colorectal cancer: results from the BICC-C Study. *J Clin Oncol.* 2007;25(30):4779–4786.
63. Bécouarn Y, Ychou M, Ducreux M, et al. Phase II trial of oxaliplatin as first-line chemotherapy in metastatic colorectal cancer patients. Digestive Group of French Federation of Cancer Centers. *J Clin Oncol.* 1998;16(8):2739–2744.
64. Díaz-Rubio E, Sastre J, Zaniboni A, et al. Oxaliplatin as single agent in previously untreated colorectal carcinoma patients: a phase II multicentric study. *Ann Oncol.* 1998;9(1):105–108.
65. Machover D, Diaz-Rubio E, de Gramont A, et al. Two consecutive phase II studies of oxaliplatin (L-OHP) for treatment of patients with advanced colorectal carcinoma who were resistant to previous treatment with fluoropyrimidines. *Ann Oncol.* 1996;7(1):95–98.
66. Cassidy J, Tabernero J, Twelves C, et al. XELOX (capecitabine plus oxaliplatin): active first-line therapy for patients with metastatic colorectal cancer. *J Clin Oncol.* 2004;22(11):2084–2091.
67. Giacchetti S, Perpoint B, Zidani R, et al. Phase III multicenter randomized trial of oxaliplatin added to chronomodulated fluorouracil-leucovorin as first-line treatment of metastatic colorectal cancer. *J Clin Oncol.* 2000;18(1):136–147.
68. de Gramont A, Figer A, Seymour M, et al. Leucovorin and fluorouracil with or without oxaliplatin as first-line treatment in advanced colorectal cancer. *J Clin Oncol.* 2000;18(16):2938–2947.
69. Goldberg RM, Sargent DJ, Morton RF, et al. A randomized controlled trial of fluorouracil plus leucovorin, irinotecan, and oxaliplatin combinations in patients with previously untreated metastatic colorectal cancer. *J Clin Oncol.* 2004;22(1):23–30.
70. Colucci G, Gebbia V, Paoletti G, et al.; Gruppo Oncologico Dell'Italia Meridionale. Phase III randomized trial of FOLFIRI versus FOLFOX4 in the treatment of advanced colorectal cancer: a multicenter study of the Gruppo Oncologico Dell'Italia Meridionale. *J Clin Oncol.* 2005;23(22):4866–4875.
71. Tournigand C, André T, Achille E, et al. FOLFIRI followed by FOLFOX6 or the reverse sequence in advanced colorectal cancer: a randomized GERCOR study. *J Clin Oncol.* 2004;22(2):229–237.
72. Nordlinger B, Sorbye H, Glimelius B, et al.; EORTC Gastro-Intestinal Tract Cancer Group; Cancer Research UK; Arbeitsgruppe Lebermetastasen und-tumoren in der Chirurgischen Arbeitsgemeinschaft Onkologie (ALM-CAO); Australasian Gastro-Intestinal Trials Group (AGITG); Fédération Francophone de Cancérologie Digestive (FFCD). Perioperative chemotherapy with FOLFOX4 and surgery versus surgery alone for resectable liver metastases from colorectal cancer (EORTC Intergroup trial 40983): a randomised controlled trial. *Lancet.* 2008;371(9617):1007–1016.
73. Ychou M, Hohenberger W, Thezenas S, et al. A randomized phase III study comparing adjuvant 5-fluorouracil/folinic acid with FOLFIRI in patients following complete resection of liver metastases from colorectal cancer. *Ann Oncol.* 2009;20(12):1964–1970.
74. Masi G, Loupakis F, Pollina L, et al. Long-term outcome of initially unresectable metastatic colorectal cancer patients treated with 5-fluorouracil/leucovorin, oxaliplatin, and irinotecan (FOLFOXIRI) followed by radical surgery of metastases. *Ann Surg.* 2009;249(3):420–425.
75. Ychou M, Viret F, Kramar A, et al. Tritherapy with fluorouracil/leucovorin, irinotecan and oxaliplatin (FOLFIRINOX): a phase II study in colorectal cancer patients with non-resectable liver metastases. *Cancer Chemother Pharmacol.* 2008;62(2):195–201.
76. Giantonio BJ, Catalano PJ, Meropol NJ, et al.; Eastern Cooperative Oncology Group Study E3200. Bevacizumab in combination with oxaliplatin, fluorouracil, and leucovorin (FOLFOX4) for previously treated metastatic colorectal cancer: results from the Eastern Cooperative Oncology Group Study E3200. *J Clin Oncol.* 2007;25(12):1539–1544.
77. Hochster HS, Hart LL, Ramanathan RK, et al. Safety and efficacy of oxaliplatin and fluoropyrimidine regimens with or without bevacizumab as first-line treatment of metastatic colorectal cancer: results of the TREE Study. *J Clin Oncol.* 2008;26(21):3523–3529.
78. Kabbinavar FF, Schulz J, McCleod M, et al. Addition of bevacizumab to bolus fluorouracil and leucovorin in first-line metastatic colorectal cancer: results of a randomized phase II trial. *J Clin Oncol.* 2005;23(16):3697–3705.
79. Kozloff M, Yood MU, Berlin J, et al.; Investigators of the BRiTE study. Clinical outcomes associated with bevacizumab-containing treatment of metastatic colorectal cancer: the BRiTE observational cohort study. *Oncologist.* 2009;14(9):862–870.
80. Van Cutsem E, Rivera F, Berry S, et al.; First BEAT investigators. Safety and efficacy of first-line bevacizumab with FOLFOX, XELOX, FOLFIRI and fluoropyrimidines in metastatic colorectal cancer: the BEAT study. *Ann Oncol.* 2009;20(11):1842–1847.
81. D'Angelica M, Kornprat P, Gonen M, et al. Lack of evidence for increased operative morbidity after hepatectomy with perioperative use of bevacizumab: a matched case-control study. *Ann Surg Oncol.* 2007;14(2):759–765.
82. Gruenberger B, Tamandl D, Schueller J, et al. Bevacizumab, capecitabine, and oxaliplatin as neoadjuvant therapy for patients with potentially curable metastatic colorectal cancer. *J Clin Oncol.* 2008;26(11):1830–1835.
83. Kesmodel SB, Ellis LM, Lin E, et al. Preoperative bevacizumab does not significantly increase postoperative complication rates in patients undergoing hepatic surgery for colorectal cancer liver metastases. *J Clin Oncol.* 2008;26(32):5254–5260.
84. Reddy SK, Morse MA, Hurwitz HI, et al. Addition of bevacizumab to irinotecan- and oxaliplatin-based preoperative chemotherapy regimens does not increase morbidity after resection of colorectal liver metastases. *J Am Coll Surg.* 2008;206(1):96–106.
85. Cunningham D, Humblet Y, Siena S, et al. Cetuximab monotherapy and cetuximab plus irinotecan in irinotecan-refractory metastatic colorectal cancer. *N Engl J Med.* 2004;351(4):337–345.
86. Van Cutsem E, Peeters M, Siena S, et al. Open-label phase III trial of panitumumab plus best supportive care compared with best supportive care alone in patients with chemotherapy-refractory metastatic colorectal cancer. *J Clin Oncol.* 2007;25(13):1658–1664.
87. Hecht JR, Patnaik A, Berlin J, et al. Panitumumab monotherapy in patients with previously treated metastatic colorectal cancer. *Cancer.* 2007;110(5):980–988.
88. Peeters M, Price TJ, Cervantes A, et al. Randomized phase III study of panitumumab with fluorouracil, leucovorin, and irinotecan (FOLFIRI) compared with FOLFIRI alone as second-line treatment in patients with metastatic colorectal cancer. *J Clin Oncol.* 2010;28(31):4706–4713.
89. Amado RG, Wolf M, Peeters M, et al. Wild-type K-ras is required for panitumumab efficacy in patients with metastatic colorectal cancer. *J Clin Oncol.* 2008;26(10):1626–1634.
90. Bokemeyer C, Bondarenko I, Makhson A, et al. Fluorouracil, leucovorin, and oxaliplatin with and without cetuximab in the first-line treatment of metastatic colorectal cancer. *J Clin Oncol.* 2009;27(5):663–671.
91. Douillard JY, Siena S, Cassidy J, et al. Randomized, phase III trial of panitumumab with infusional fluorouracil, leucovorin, and oxaliplatin (FOLFOX4) versus FOLFOX4 alone as first-line treatment in patients with previously untreated metastatic colorectal cancer: the PRIME study. *J Clin Oncol.* 2010;28(31):4697–4705.

92. Maughan TS, Adams RA, Smith CG, et al.; MRC COIN Trial Investigators. Addition of cetuximab to oxaliplatin-based first-line combination chemotherapy for treatment of advanced colorectal cancer: results of the randomised phase 3 MRC COIN trial. *Lancet.* 2011;377(9783):2103–2114.
93. Van Cutsem E, Köhne CH, Hitre E, et al. Cetuximab and chemotherapy as initial treatment for metastatic colorectal cancer. *N Engl J Med.* 2009;360(14):1408–1417.
94. Hecht JR, Mitchell E, Chidiac T, et al. A randomized phase IIIB trial of chemotherapy, bevacizumab, and panitumumab compared with chemotherapy and bevacizumab alone for metastatic colorectal cancer. *J Clin Oncol.* 2009;27(5):672–680.
95. Tol J, Koopman M, Cats A, et al. Chemotherapy, bevacizumab, and cetuximab in metastatic colorectal cancer. *N Engl J Med.* 2009;360(6):563–572.
96. Otto G, Düber C, Hoppe-Lotichius M, König J, Heise M, Pitton MB. Radiofrequency ablation as first-line treatment in patients with early colorectal liver metastases amenable to surgery. *Ann Surg.* 2010;251(5):796–803.
97. Lencioni R, Crocetti L, Cioni D, Della Pina C, Bartolozzi C. Percutaneous radiofrequency ablation of hepatic colorectal metastases: technique, indications, results, and new promises. *Invest Radiol.* 2004;39(11):689–697.
98. Berber E, Pelley R, Siperstein AE. Predictors of survival after radiofrequency thermal ablation of colorectal cancer metastases to the liver: a prospective study. *J Clin Oncol.* 2005;23(7):1358–1364.
99. Gillams AR, Lees WR. Five-year survival in 309 patients with colorectal liver metastases treated with radiofrequency ablation. *Eur Radiol.* 2009;19(5):1206–1213.
100. Wong SL, Mangu PB, Choti MA, et al. American Society of Clinical Oncology 2009 clinical evidence review on radiofrequency ablation of hepatic metastases from colorectal cancer. *J Clin Oncol.* 2010;28(3):493–508.
101. Abitabile P, Hartl U, Lange J, Maurer CA. Radiofrequency ablation permits an effective treatment for colorectal liver metastasis. *Eur J Surg Oncol.* 2007;33(1):67–71.
102. Chow DH, Sinn LH, Ng KK, et al. Radiofrequency ablation for hepatocellular carcinoma and metastatic liver tumors: a comparative study. *J Surg Oncol.* 2006;94(7):565–571.
103. Geyik S, Akhan O, Abbasoglu O, et al. Radiofrequency ablation of unresectable hepatic tumors. *Diagn Interv Radiol.* 2006;12(4):195–200.
104. Joosten J, Jager G, Oyen W, Wobbes T, Ruers T. Cryosurgery and radiofrequency ablation for unresectable colorectal liver metastases. *Eur J Surg Oncol.* 2005;31(10):1152–1159.
105. Kosari K, Gomes M, Hunter D, Hess DJ, Greeno E, Sielaff TD. Local, intrahepatic, and systemic recurrence patterns after radiofrequency ablation of hepatic malignancies. *J Gastrointest Surg.* 2002;6(2):255–263.
106. Machi J, Oishi AJ, Sumida K, et al. Long-term outcome of radiofrequency ablation for unresectable liver metastases from colorectal cancer: evaluation of prognostic factors and effectiveness in first- and second-line management. *Cancer J.* 2006;12(4):318–326.
107. Martin RC 2nd, McGuffin SA, Roetzer LM, Abell TD, Studts JL. Method of presenting oncology treatment outcomes influences patient treatment decision-making in metastatic colorectal cancer. *Ann Surg Oncol.* 2006;13(1):86–95.
108. White TJ, Roy-Choudhury SH, Breen DJ, et al. Percutaneous radiofrequency ablation of colorectal hepatic metastases—initial experience. An adjunct technique to systemic chemotherapy for those with inoperable colorectal hepatic metastases. *Dig Surg.* 2004;21(4):314–320.
109. Ruers T, Punt CJ, Van Coevorden F, Borel Rinkes I, Ledermann JA, Poston JG. Final results of the EORTC intergroup randomized study 40004 (CLOCC) evaluating the benefit of radiofrequency ablation (RFA) combined with chemotherapy for unresectable colorectal liver metastases (CRC LM). *J Clin Oncol.* 2010;28:3526.
110. Illing RO, Kennedy JE, Wu F, et al. The safety and feasibility of extracorporeal high-intensity focused ultrasound (HIFU) for the treatment of liver and kidney tumours in a Western population. *Br J Cancer.* 2005;93(8):890–895.
111. Garcea G, Lloyd TD, Aylott C, Maddern G, Berry DP. The emergent role of focal liver ablation techniques in the treatment of primary and secondary liver tumours. *Eur J Cancer.* 2003;39(15):2150–2164.
112. Robertson JM, Lawrence TS, Walker S, Kessler ML, Andrews JC, Ensminger WD. The treatment of colorectal liver metastases with conformal radiation therapy and regional chemotherapy. *Int J Radiat Oncol Biol Phys.* 1995;32(2):445–450.
113. Ben-Josef E, Normolle D, Ensminger WD, et al. Phase II trial of high-dose conformal radiation therapy with concurrent hepatic artery floxuridine for unresectable intrahepatic malignancies. *J Clin Oncol.* 2005;23(34):8739–8747.
114. Lee MT, Kim JJ, Dinniwell R, et al. Phase I study of individualized stereotactic body radiotherapy of liver metastases. *J Clin Oncol.* 2009;27(10):1585–1591.
115. Rusthoven KE, Kavanagh BD, Cardenes H, et al. Multi-institutional phase I/II trial of stereotactic body radiation therapy for liver metastases. *J Clin Oncol.* 2009;27(10):1572–1578.
116. Charnsangavej C, Clary B, Fong Y, Grothey A, Pawlik TM, Choti MA. Selection of patients for resection of hepatic colorectal metastases: expert consensus statement. *Ann Surg Oncol.* 2006;13(10):1261–1268.
117. Chang DT, Swaminath A, Kozak M, et al. Stereotactic body radiotherapy for colorectal liver metastases: a pooled analysis. *Cancer.* 2011;117(17):4060–4069.
118. Hotokezaka M, Jimi S, Hidaka H, et al. Factors influencing outcome after surgery for stage IV colorectal cancer. *Surg Today.* 2008;38(9):784–789.
119. Hotta T, Takifuji K, Arii K, et al. Potential predictors of long-term survival after surgery for patients with stage IV colorectal cancer. *Anticancer Res.* 2006;26(2B):1377–1383.
120. Carpizo DR, D'Angelica M. Liver resection for metastatic colorectal cancer in the presence of extrahepatic disease. *Lancet Oncol.* 2009;10(8):801–809.
121. Høyer M, Swaminath A, Bydder S, et al. Radiotherapy for liver metastases: a review of evidence. *Int J Radiat Oncol Biol Phys.* 2012;82(3):1047–1057.
122. de Meijer VE, Verhoef C, Kuiper JW, Alwayn IP, Kazemier G, Ijzermans JN. Radiofrequency ablation in patients with primary and secondary hepatic malignancies. *J Gastrointest Surg.* 2006;10(7):960–973.
123. Katz AW, Carey-Sampson M, Muhs AG, Milano MT, Schell MC, Okunieff P. Hypofractionated stereotactic body radiation therapy (SBRT) for limited hepatic metastases. *Int J Radiat Oncol Biol Phys.* 2007;67(3):793–798.
124. Wood TF, Rose DM, Chung M, Allegra DP, Foshag LJ, Bilchik AJ. Radiofrequency ablation of 231 unresectable hepatic tumors: indications, limitations, and complications. *Ann Surg Oncol.* 2000;7(8):593–600.
125. Wulf J, Guckenberger M, Haedinger U, et al. Stereotactic radiotherapy of primary liver cancer and hepatic metastases. *Acta Oncol.* 2006;45(7):838–847.
126. van der Pool AE, Méndez Romero A, Wunderink W, et al. Stereotactic body radiation therapy for colorectal liver metastases. *Br J Surg.* 2010;97(3):377–382.
127. Hoyer M, Roed H, Traberg Hansen A, et al. Phase II study on stereotactic body radiotherapy of colorectal metastases. *Acta Oncol.* 2006;45(7):823–830.
128. Méndez Romero A, Wunderink W, Hussain SM, et al. Stereotactic body radiation therapy for primary and metastatic liver tumors: A single institution phase I–II study. *Acta Oncol.* 2006;45(7):831–837.
129. Rule W, Timmerman R, Tong L, et al. Phase I dose-escalation study of stereotactic body radiotherapy in patients with hepatic metastases. *Ann Surg Oncol.* 2011;18(4):1081–1087.

130. Goodman KA, Wiegner EA, Maturen KE, et al. Dose-escalation study of single-fraction stereotactic body radiotherapy for liver malignancies. *Int J Radiat Oncol Biol Phys.* 2010;78(2):486–493.
131. Ambrosino G, Polistina F, Costantin G, et al. Image-guided robotic stereotactic radiosurgery for unresectable liver metastases: preliminary results. *Anticancer Res.* 2009;29(8):3381–3384.
132. Herfarth KK, Debus J, Wannenmacher M. Stereotactic radiation therapy of liver metastases: update of the initial phase-I/II trial. *Front Radiat Ther Oncol.* 2004;38:100–105.
133. Vautravers-Dewas C, Dewas S, Bonodeau F, et al. Image-guided robotic stereotactic body radiation therapy for liver metastases: is there a dose response relationship? *Int J Radiat Oncol Biol Phys.* 2011;81(3):e39–e47.
134. Swaminath A, Jacks L, Massey C, et al. Accumulated delivered dose-response of stereotactic body radiotherapy (SBRT) for liver metastases. *Int J Radiat Oncol Biol Phys.* 2011;81:S347.
135. Milano MT, Katz AW, Schell MC, Philip A, Okunieff P. Descriptive analysis of oligometastatic lesions treated with curative-intent stereotactic body radiotherapy. *Int J Radiat Oncol Biol Phys.* 2008;72(5):1516–1522.
136. Herfarth KK, Hof H, Bahner ML, et al. Assessment of focal liver reaction by multiphasic CT after stereotactic single-dose radiotherapy of liver tumors. *Int J Radiat Oncol Biol Phys.* 2003;57(2):444–451.
137. Dexiang Z, Li R, Ye W, et al. Outcome of patients with colorectal liver metastasis: analysis of 1,613 consecutive cases. *Ann Surg Oncol.* 2012;19(9):2860–2868.
138. Rees M, Tekkis PP, Welsh FK, O'Rourke T, John TG. Evaluation of long-term survival after hepatic resection for metastatic colorectal cancer: a multifactorial model of 929 patients. *Ann Surg.* 2008;247(1):125–135.
139. Liu CL, Fan ST, Lo CM, Law WL, Ng IO, Wong J. Hepatic resection for colorectal liver metastases: prospective study. *Hong Kong Med J.* 2002;8(5):329–333.
140. Fong Y, Fortner J, Sun RL, Brennan MF, Blumgart LH. Clinical score for predicting recurrence after hepatic resection for metastatic colorectal cancer: analysis of 1001 consecutive cases. *Ann Surg.* 1999;230(3):309–18; discussion 318.
141. Bradley AL, Chapman WC, Wright JK, et al. Surgical experience with hepatic colorectal metastasis. *Am Surg.* 1999;65(6):560–6; discussion 566.
142. Luo Y, Wang L, Chen C, et al. Simultaneous liver and colorectal resections are safe for synchronous colorectal liver metastases. *J Gastrointest Surg.* 2010;14(12):1974–1980.
143. de Haas RJ, Adam R, Wicherts DA, et al. Comparison of simultaneous or delayed liver surgery for limited synchronous colorectal metastases. *Br J Surg.* 2010;97(8):1279–1289.
144. Martin R, Paty P, Fong Y, et al. Simultaneous liver and colorectal resections are safe for synchronous colorectal liver metastasis. *J Am Coll Surg.* 2003;197(2):233–41; discussion 241.
145. Hornbech K, Ravn J, Steinbrüchel DA. Outcome after pulmonary metastasectomy: analysis of 5 years consecutive surgical resections 2002–2006. *J Thorac Oncol.* 2011;6(10):1733–1740.
146. Kanzaki R, Higashiyama M, Oda K, et al. Outcome of surgical resection for recurrent pulmonary metastasis from colorectal carcinoma. *Am J Surg.* 2011;202(4):419–426.
147. Lin BR, Chang TC, Lee YC, Lee PH, Chang KJ, Liang JT. Pulmonary resection for colorectal cancer metastases: duration between cancer onset and lung metastasis as an important prognostic factor. *Ann Surg Oncol.* 2009;16(4):1026–1032.
148. Lee WS, Yun SH, Chun HK, et al. Pulmonary resection for metastases from colorectal cancer: prognostic factors and survival. *Int J Colorectal Dis.* 2007;22(6):699–704.
149. World J Surg. 2012 Sep;36(9):2171-8. doi: 10.1007/s00268-012-1616-y. Authors are Saiura A, Yamamamot J, Hasegawa K, Koga R, Sakamoto Y, Hata S, Makuuchi M and Kokudo N PMID 22547015

10 Management of Potentially Resectable Recurrent Disease

■ Systemic Therapy Considerations

E. GABRIELA CHIOREAN
PATRICK J. LOEHRER

Of the 141,210 patients diagnosed annually with colorectal cancer (CRC), almost 25% will also have synchronous metastatic disease. An additional 35%–40% of patients with resected Stage II and III tumors will develop distant disease sometime during the course of their disease (1). Due to venous drainage through the portal venous system the liver is the most prevalent site of metastasis (69%–87%), followed by lung (24%–31%) and peritoneum (10%). Unfortunately, most patients with metastatic CRC have unresectable disease, but 15%–20% of patients with isolated recurrence or spread are potential candidates for resection, with the opportunity for long-term survival.

Patients who undergo liver metastasectomy generally have 5-year survival rates of 30%–50% depending on prognostic scores, with negative markers including tumor size (greater than 5 cm), disease-free interval after primary colorectal surgery (less than 12 months), number of tumors (greater than 1), lymph node–positive primary, and preoperative carcinoembryonic antigen (CEA; greater than 200 ng/mL; 2,3). Almost 75% of patients will eventually relapse, half the time within the liver (4–6). Lung metastasectomy from CRC can also be accomplished with curative intent either for isolated lesions (survival rates 37% at 5 years and 22% at 10 years; 7,8), or in conjunction by either synchronous or staged resection of liver metastases, with 5-year survival rates around 50% (9–12). These data are important when considering methods of improving the odds of recurrence for potentially resectable/curable metastatic CRC.

The primary goal of administering neoadjuvant chemotherapy prior to surgical resection of metastatic disease is to achieve sufficient downsizing to allow metastasectomy. Using contemporary chemotherapeutic regimens with or without molecularly targeted agents against the vascular endothelial growth factor (VEGF) or the epidermal growth factor receptor (EGFR) confers response rates of 30%–60% and 12.5%–47.5% rates of conversion to resectability for patients with initially unresectable disease (13–17). There are no universally accepted criteria for what represents "resectability" (18). The optimal sequence of treatment administration (preoperative [neoadjuvant] chemotherapy, chemotherapy both before and after surgery [perioperative] or postoperative [adjuvant] for resectable disease), as well as the mode of delivery (systemic versus local), have been debated, but few randomized studies with adequate patient numbers were completed to reach meaningful conclusions.

■ ADJUVANT HEPATIC ARTERIAL INFUSION (HAI) OF CHEMOTHERAPY

Due to the preponderance of liver metastases in the course of CRC progression and spread, locoregional chemotherapy via hepatic arterial infusion (HAI) has been studied to diminish the incidence of intrahepatic recurrence after initial resection, as well as for patients with initially unresectable but limited to the liver disease. Anatomically, established liver metastases receive blood supply from the hepatic arteries, while the normal hepatocytes and newly developing metastases are nourished by the portal venous system (19). While HAI has been performed for selected patients in specialized centers for the last 3 decades, more recently its role has been emphasized in combination with systemic therapies after surgery, to aid in the prevention of systemic relapse.

Initial studies of HAI used 5-fluorouracil (5-FU) with modest results compounded by toxicity and poor bioavailability (20). Subsequent trials used floxuridine (FUDR), a 5-FU prodrug with higher selectivity in the hepatic rather than the general circulation, thus reducing systemic toxicities. FUDR has a high hepatic to systemic ratio (400) and a high hepatic extraction rate (95%), compared to a hepatic-systemic ratio of 10 to 100 and hepatic extraction of 20%–55% for 5-FU (21). Concerns regarding the use of locally delivered FUDR are that fluoropyrimidine alone is suboptimal treatment, and that toxicity associated with this treatment can be considerable, particularly chemical hepatitis, biliary sclerosis, and gastroduodenal ulcers (22,23).

Results with HAI alone after surgery, even with the use of FUDR (Table 10.1) were tempered by no benefit in overall or disease-free survival (DFS), clearly justifying the addition of systemic chemotherapy to improve the odds of preventing extrahepatic recurrence.

■ ADJUVANT HAI WITH SYSTEMIC CHEMOTHERAPY

Over the past 2 decades several post-liver metastasectomy trials compared adjuvant HAI using FUDR with or without the addition of systemic chemotherapy to surgery alone, or to surgery plus systemic therapy (Table 10.2). The need for systemic chemotherapy became obvious when extrahepatic progression offset the locoregional control with HAI alone (24). In a landmark MSKCC study, HAI with FUDR plus systemic 5-FU increased 5-year survival rates vs systemic 5-FU from 50%–60% (24), and after 10 years of follow-up survival rates increased from 28%–41% (P = .11). The rate of 2-year hepatic relapse-free survival was 90% in the combined therapy arm, vs 60% in the systemic therapy arm (P < .001), but the rates of extrahepatic recurrence were similar. An Eastern Oncology Cooperative Group trial assessed postoperative HAI with FUDR plus systemic 5-FU vs surgery alone, and noted an improvement in 4-year DFS from 25%–46% (P = .04) and for median survival from 49 to 63.7 months (P = .6; 25). Similarly, Lygidakis et al (26) reported significantly improved 4-year DFS (58% vs 34%, P = .002) and 4-year survival (73% vs 60%, P = .05) with HAI plus systemic chemoimmunotherapy versus systemic therapy alone.

In recent years combination multidrug regimens such as 5-FU/leucovorin or capecitabine with oxaliplatin (FOLFOX, XELOX) or irinotecan (FOLFIRI), as well as molecularly targeted therapies against the VEGF or the EGFR antibody have led to improved responses and survival in metastatic CRC, thus these agents have been incorporated in systemic regimens, both in addition to HAI, and as control arms in randomized trials. Phase I/II studies tested systemic irinotecan or oxaliplatin-based chemotherapy with FUDR HAI with encouraging results, particularly with the use of FOLFOX: 2-year survival of 89% with systemic irinotecan (27), and 4-year survival rates of 88% with FOLFOX (28). To capitalize on the potential benefit of adding oxaliplatin to a systemic fluoropyrimidine, an NCCTG/NSABP phase II single-arm trial used systemic XELOX (capecitabine and oxaliplatin) with FUDR HAI (29). With a median follow-up of 4.8 years, the 2-year hepatic relapse-free survival was 75.5%, the median OS has not been reached, and the 2-year survival was 89%. These outcomes were not superior to prior results with HAI plus systemic 5-FU (24). Kemeny et al added bevacizumab to systemic FOLFOX or FOLFIRI and HAI, with disappointing results (4-year relapse-free survival [RFS] and OS were 37% and 81% with bevacizumab, versus 46% and 85% in the control arm, respectively; P = .5; 30).

The use of modern systemic chemotherapy with or without HAI has been evaluated in a retrospective review of 250 patients treated at MSKCC between 2001 and 2005. Five-year liver recurrence-free survival rates were 75% with systemic therapy plus HAI vs 55% with systemic therapy alone (P < .01), overall RFS was 48% vs 25% (P < .01), and 5-year survival rates were 79% vs 55% (HR, 0.39, P < .01; 31).

Some of the best long-term outcomes with combination HAI plus systemic chemotherapy have been 4- to 5-year disease/relapse-free survival rates of 40%–50%, and 4 to 5 years overall survival of 60%–80%,

■ Table 10.1 Clinical Trials of Adjuvant HAI Therapy

Authors	No. Pts.	Treatment	mOS (Months) HAI	mOS (Months) Control	5-Year OS HAI	5-Year OS Control	DFS/RFS (Months) HAI	DFS/RFS (Months) Control
Lorenz et al (20)	226	HAI 5-FU /LV vs surgery	34.5	40.8			13.7	14.2
Ambiru et al* (174)	174	HAI 5-FU, aclarubicin, mitomycin vs surgery	NR	NR	40%	20%	35% 5-yr	9% 5-yr
Lygidakis et al (175)	40	HAI 5-FU /LV, mitomycin, IL-2 (FMI) vs surgery	20	11	–	–		
Rudroff et al (176)	42	HAI mitomycin, 5-FU vs surgery	–	–	25%	31%	15% 5-yr	23% 5-yr
Tono et al (177)	19	HAI 5-FU vs surgery	–	–	78%	50%	62.6	13.8
Wagman et al (178)	21	HAI FUDR vs surgery	28.5	28.3	35%	50%	23.1	8.7

*Retrospective study.
NR, not reached.

Table 10.2 Clinical Trials of Adjuvant HAI and Systemic Chemotherapy

			mOS (Months)		Overall Survival		DFS/RFS (Months)	
Authors	No. Pts.	Treatment	HAI	Control	HAI	Control	HAI	Control
Kemeny et al (179) and Kemeny and Gonen (180)	156	HAI FUDR + 5-FU/LV vs 5-FU/LV	72.2	59.3	61% 5-yr 41% 10-yr	49% 5-yr 27% 10 yr	31.3 48% 4-yr	17.2 33% 4-yr
Kemeny et al (181)	75	HAI FUDR + 5-FU/LV vs none	63.7	49	62% 4-yr 58% 5-yr	53% 4-yr 40% 5-yr	46% 4-yr 40% 5-yr	25% 4-yr 20% 5-yr
Lygidakis et al (182)	122	HAI 5-FU /LV, mitomycin, IL-2 (FMI) + FMI vs FMI	N/A	N/A	73% 5-yr	60% 5-yr	58% 4-yr	33% 4-yr
Kemeny et al (183)	96	HAI FUDR + irinotecan	N/A		89% 2-yr		57% 18-mo	
Kemeny et al (184)	35	HAI FUDR + FOLFOX	N/A		88%		50%	
Alberts et al (185)	55	HAI FUDR + XELOX	NR		88% 2yr		32.7	
Kemeny et al (186)	73	HAI + FOLFOX/ FOLFIRI ± Bevacizumab	NR		81% versus 85% 4-yr		37% versus 46% 4-yr	
House* et al (187)	250	HAI + FOLFOX/ FOLFIRI vs FOLFOX/FOLFIRI	NR	NR	79% 5-yr	55% 5-yr	48% 5-yr	25% 5-yr

*, Retrospective study; FUDR, fluoxuridine; HAI, hepatic arterial infusion; N/A, not applicable; NR, not reached.

numerically higher than the historical 30%–40% 5-year survival seen with surgery alone. Nevertheless, the results with HAI plus systemic chemotherapy are not uniformly superior to systemic chemotherapy alone, even with the use of oxaliplatin-based chemotherapy or the addition of anti-VEGF targeted agents. Randomized trials of modern chemo-/biotherapy with or without HAI are clearly needed. NSABP-C09 attempted to address the role of adding HAI with FUDR in a randomized manner to XELOX, but unfortunately closed early due to poor accrual. The low rates of HAI use and its successful implementation in only select academic centers will most likely make such a trial very difficult to accrue.

NEOADJUVANT HAI

High response rates of 50% observed with HAI are the rationale for using HAI prior to metastasectomy primarily for patients with unresectable disease. In the setting of potentially curable metastases neoadjuvant HAI treatment is hampered by biliary toxicity thus decreasing the hepatic reserve prior to surgery. Given that similar high response rates can be obtained with systemic chemotherapy, HAI does not have a major role prior to metastasectomy for primarily resectable disease.

SYSTEMIC CHEMOTHERAPY

Preoperative Chemotherapy

Multiple clinical trials in the last decade using chemotherapy combined with molecularly targeted agents, both anti-EGFR and anti-VEGF, or three-drug chemotherapy regimens (ie, FOLFOXIRI) reported response rates of greater than 50% and survival rates averaging 24 months, making these regimens attractive for first-line use in metastatic CRC (14,15,32–34).

While these studies report resectability outcomes, patients' recruitment criteria most commonly did not require formal evaluation of resectability before study enrollment, therefore not enabling assessment of selective benefit for initially resectable vs unresectable patients. In the CRYSTAL (Cetuximab Combined with Irinotecan in First-Line Therapy for Metastatic CRC) study, among patients with *K-ras* wild type disease, the addition of cetuximab to FOLFIRI conferred responses of 57% vs 40% with FOLFIRI alone, and R0 metastasectomy rates were 5.1% vs 2.0% ($P = .0265$; 15). The OPUS (Oxaliplatin and Cetuximab in First-Line Treatment of MCRC trial) tested FOLFOX with or without cetuximab and showed responses of 61% vs 37% in the *K-ras* wild-type population and the R0 metastases resection rate was 9.8% vs 4.1% (34). The CELIM study used FOLFOX or FOLFIRI and cetuximab for initially "considered" unresectable disease (technically unresectable or greater than or equal to 5 metastases) and demonstrated 70% responses in *K-ras* wild-type patients and 34% of patients underwent R0 resections. Upon study's conclusion a retrospective review panel showed that resectability rates increased from 32% (at baseline) to 60% (after treatment; $P < .0001$), further questioning the interpretation of "resectability" at study entry 16. Bevacizumab with oxaliplatin-based chemotherapy regimens did not yield superior resection rates in the randomized phase III study NO16966, as 6.3% of patients treated with bevacizumab and 4.9% in the control arm underwent R0 metastasectomy (17,35).

Naturally, resection rates are higher for patients who present with potentially curable or limited disease. Very few studies were designed to address the role of neoadjuvant therapy alone on long-term outcomes, as most investigators have used pre- and postoperative approaches instead. Wein et al reported 100% responses and 80% resectability with two 8-week cycles of oxaliplatin (biweekly × 4/cycle) and weekly 5-FU-based chemotherapy (weekly × 6 for every 8-week cycle). The 2-year DFS was 52% and the 2-year survival was 80% (36). A large review of randomized and nonrandomized trials encompassing 3278 patients treated with neoadjuvant chemotherapy, yielded radiological responses in 64% of patients, median DFS of 21 months and median OS of 46 months (37).

The rationale of using preoperative systemic chemotherapy for resectable metastatic disease stems from a few considerations: (a) facilitates surgery; (b) obtaining predictive and prognostic information; and (c) delivering early systemic therapy for poor prognosis patients. It is clear that the pathological response to preoperative therapy correlates with survival outcomes postresection (38). Achieving a pathologic response to preoperative chemotherapy (oxaliplatin or irinotecan-based) in a large series of 305 patients treated at the MD Anderson Cancer Center correlated with improved survival, with 5-year survival rates of 75% in complete responders (no residual cancer cells), 56% in major responders (1%–49% residual cancer cells) and 33% in minor responders (greater than or equal to 50% residual cancer cells; $P = .034$; 38). In addition, progression of disease during neoadjuvant chemotherapy may preclude benefit from surgical resection (39), but data are still controversial (40).

The duration of preoperative chemotherapy is subject to debate, as long-term treatment has been associated with steatosis and steatohepatitis ("yellow liver") from 5-FU and irinotecan (up to 20% incidence), and capillary injury and sinusoidal obstruction syndrome ("blue liver") from oxaliplatin (incidence ranges between 20% and 50%; 41–44). Steatohepatitis has been associated with increased 90-day mortality after surgical resection in some series (14.7% vs 1.6%; 42), and steatosis significantly impairs wound healing (23% incidence in patients with severe steatosis vs 1% in those with no steatosis), and causes more biliary complications and infections (45) raising concerns regarding prolonged irinotecan-based therapy in neoadjuvant setting. Recent data suggest a beneficial role for neoadjuvant bevacizumab when combined with oxaliplatin-based regimens due to a reduction in sinusoidal dilatation (46) or obstruction (47), but its effects on liver regeneration have been debatable (48–51). In general, there has been no evidence that bevacizumab increases perioperative morbidity (52–54).

Another potential deleterious aspect associated with preoperative chemotherapy could be the radiological or gross disappearance of metastases, which therefore will not be visible intraoperatively and not resected. In one large series of treated colorectal metastases who obtained complete radiological response, one-third was visible during laparoscopy; among the remaining lesions which "disappeared," one-third was resected and still revealed pathologically visible tumor in 80% of the samples, and among those not seen and left behind, 74% recurred (55).

No trial to date had demonstrated an unequivocal benefit from preoperative chemotherapy alone for resectable colorectal metastases. Most studies adopted perioperative approaches, by combining neoadjuvant with adjuvant chemotherapy, thus limiting the preoperative component to try to preserve the liver functional capacity.

Perioperative Systemic Chemotherapy (Tables 10.3 and 10.4)

The European Organization for Research and Treatment of Cancer (EORTC) Intergroup 40983 study randomized 364 patients with resectable metastatic CRC to surgery alone vs 3 months of pre- and postoperative 5-FU and oxaliplatin (FOLFOX4; 56). Patients had to have up to four potentially resectable liver metastases and underwent surgery in highly skilled institutions. Eighty percent of patients in the chemotherapy arm completed the preoperative treatment and 76% received postoperative therapy. Toxicities were mild and while there were slightly more postoperative complications in the chemotherapy arm (25% vs 16%; $P = .04$), including biliary fistulae (8% vs 4%), hepatic failure (bilirubin greater than 10 mg/d for longer than 3 days: 6% vs 3%), and wound infections (3% vs 2%), they were reversible and the postoperative mortality was not affected (1% in both arms). With a median follow-up of 3.9 years, the 3-year DFS in the intent-to-treat population was 28% with surgery alone, and 35% with perioperative chemotherapy (HR, 0.79; $P = .058$), with statistical significance in the group of patients who underwent resection: 33% with surgery alone, and 42.4% with chemotherapy (HR, 0.73; $P = .025$). Survival data are not yet mature. In a retrospective analysis of EORTC 40983, the investigators observed that elevated CEA levels (greater than 5 ng/mL), good performance status (ECOG PS0) and body mass index (BMI) lower than 30, but not the number of metastatic lesions (1 vs 2–4), were predictive of benefit from perioperative therapy (57).

Table 10.3 Perioperative/Neoadjuvant Chemotherapy Trials

Authors	No. Pts.	Treatment	Resection Rate %	mOS (Months)	5-Year OS	DFS/RFS (Months)
Nordlinger et al (56)	364	FOLFOX + surgery + FOLFOX vs surgery	83% vs 84%	n/a	n/a	18.7 vs 11.7*
Gruenberger et al (48)	56	XELOX + bevacizumab + surgery + XELOX + bevacizumab	93%	n/a	n/a	n/a
Bathe et al (59)	35	IFL/FOLFIRI + surgery + IFL/ FOLFIRI	86%	51.6	Greater than 50%	23
Chiappa et al (58)	25	FOLFOX/FOLFIRI + surgery + FOLFOX/FOLFIRI	100%		71% responders 15% non-responders	
Taïeb et al (70)	22	FOLFOX + surgery + FOLFIRI	91%	NR	89% 2-yr 61% 3-yr	21 47% 2-yr 33% 3-yr
Wein et al (36)	20	5-FU/oxaliplatin + surgery	80%	n/a	80% 2-yr	52% 2-yr

*3-year DFS survivals: 35% vs 28%, respectively.

n/a, not available; NR, not reached.

Table 10.4 Adjuvant Chemotherapy Trials

Authors	No. Pts.	Treatment	Median OS (Months)		DFS/PFS (Months)	
			Chemo	Control	Chemo	Control
Portier et al (61)	173	surgery + 5-FU/LV vs surgery	62.1	46.4	24.4	17.6
Mitry et al (63)	278	surgery + 5-FU/LV vs surgery	62.2	47.3	27.9	18.8
Ychou et al (67)	306	surgery + FOLFIRI vs surgery + 5-FU/LV	n/a	n/a	24.7	21.6

n/a, not available.

Chiappa et al tested perioperative oxaliplatin or irinotecan-based chemotherapy for resectable CRC patients and demonstrated differentially higher 5-year survival rates of 71% for patients who responded to preoperative treatment, vs 15% for nonresponders (58). In this study, most patients continued to receive adjuvant chemotherapy after resection, the same one to which they responded for the responding patients, or alternative chemotherapy for the initial nonresponders. Similarly, good outcomes were reported with perioperative IFL/FOLFIRI with 86% resection rates and 51.6 months median survival (59). A small 56-patient study tested the safety, response, and resectability rates with bevacizumab plus six 2-week cycles of capecitabine/oxaliplatin (XELOX) and showed 73% responses, and 93% of patients successfully underwent liver resection. After surgery patients resumed six more cycles of XELOX and bevacizumab (48). The rates of postoperative bleeding (0% vs 3%) and wound healing (0% vs 0%) complications in this trial versus historical data with chemotherapy alone (such as in EORTC 40983) showed no increased morbidity with the addition of bevacizumab. Unfortunately, this study did not assess long-term outcomes.

Preoperative chemotherapy is not considered standard for all resectable metastatic CRC patients, but it is an accepted conversion strategy for borderline or unresectable patients, and it can be used successfully for disease downstaging. The duration of perioperative treatment is also a matter of debate. Due to reported toxicities from chemotherapy, the duration of treatment should be restricted to 3 months or less, and surgery should be performed as soon as metastases are resectable by skilled surgeons. The general agreement is to discontinue chemotherapy ± cetuximab 4 weeks prior to, and bevacizumab treatment 5 to 8 weeks prior to surgery (60).

The question of whether resectable patients could benefit as much or more from peri- or postoperative treatment, and the effects of chemotherapy on postoperative morbidity was to be addressed in a randomized phase III trial NSABP C-11, where patients would receive FOLFOX with or without bevacizumab in six 2-week cycles prior to and postoperatively, vs 12 cycles postoperatively. This study recently closed due to low patient enrollment, leaving this important question of peri- vs postoperative therapy unanswered. Building upon EORTC 40983, an ongoing phase II study in Europe, EORTC 40051-BOS (Biologics, Oxaliplatin, and Surgery) will test two FOLFOX-based perioperative regimens: FOLFOX and cetuximab with or without bevacizumab.

Postoperative Systemic Therapy

Randomized phase III trials described below support the use of postoperative adjuvant chemotherapy with 5-FU after resection of metastatic disease, due to a trend in improved survival, albeit lack of sufficient patient accrual hinder definitive conclusions.

Portier et al (61) showed benefit from 6 months of adjuvant bolus 5-FU in the Fédéracion Francophone de Cancérologie Digestive (FFCD) 9002 trial, after a median follow-up of 87.4 months. The 5-year RFS rates were 33.5% vs 26.7% with surgery alone (*P* = .028). The median and 5-year survival rates were not significantly better (62 vs 46 months, and 51% vs 41%, respectively, *P* = .13). An additional randomized EORTC/NCI-CTG/GIVIO (ENG) study with adjuvant bolus 5-FU after liver or lung metastasectomy demonstrated a benefit in RFS (median, 39 vs; 20 months, *P* = .35) and survival (median, 53 vs; 43 months, *P* = .39), in favor of the chemotherapy arm, but neither were statistically significant (62).

A meta-analysis of these similarly designed trials (173 patients in the FFCD trial and 129 patients in the ENG trial) was conducted in order to increase statistical power, but only showed a trend toward benefit in both RFS (median, 27.9 vs 18.8 months; *P* = .058; HR, 1.32; 95% confidence interval [CI], 1.00–1.76) and overall survival (62.2 vs 47.3 months, *P* = .095; HR, 1.32; 95% CI, 0.95–1.82) with postoperative 5-FU (63). Multivariate analysis found that adjuvant chemotherapy was independently associated with PFS (*P* = .036) and OS (*P* = .046), and the number of metastases (greater than or equal to 2) was associated with OS (*P* = .023).

Supporting these data, a retrospective analysis of a SEER-Medicare database of 923 patients had shown survival benefit from adjuvant chemotherapy with a hazard ratio of 0.62 (95% CI, 0.5–0.78; 64). Other large retrospective reports demonstrated that adjuvant chemotherapy after resection is a positive independent predictor for outcome (65,66).

More recently investigators have been trying to intensify the postoperative chemotherapy regimens with the addition of irinotecan (FOLFIRI) or oxaliplatin (FOLFOX). FOLFIRI did not demonstrate superior results when compared to 5-FU alone (DFS 24.7 vs 21.6 months; *P* = .44), mimicking the lack of benefit with adjuvant FOLFIRI in the PETACC-3 trial for resected primary CRC (67).

Given the results of the Multicenter International Study of Oxaliplatin/5-Fluorouracil/Leucovorin in the Adjuvant Treatment of Colon Cancer (MOSAIC) study for patients with resected Stage III colon cancer, with improved disease-free and overall survival with FOLFOX vs 5-FU, as well as the NO16968 study with XELOX vs 5-FU (68), trials using FOLFOX or XELOX postmetastasectomy are awaited. A retrospective Korean study assessed adjuvant therapy with either fluoropyrimidines alone (5-FU or capecitabine), FOLFOX or FOLFIRI. While flawed by small patient numbers (28–58 per group), after a median follow-up of 3.7 years there was a trend toward a benefit in DFS with FOLFOX (3-year DFS 35% vs 25% with FOLFIRI or 5-FU/capecitabine; *P* = .068; 69). With a different approach, Taïeb et al studied irinotecan plus oxaliplatin strategy (MIROX) by using adjuvant chemotherapy with six cycles of FOLFOX-7 followed by six cycles of FOLFIRI (*N* = 25 patients) or perioperative chemotherapy (six cycles of neoadjuvant FOLFOX-7 followed by surgery and six additional cycles of adjuvant FOLFIRI, *N* = 22 patients; 70). The median overall survival has not been reached for the overall group of patients, and the median DFS was 21 months.

From existing data with average DFS rates of 19 to 23 months for perioperative chemotherapy and 24 to 28 months for adjuvant systemic therapies, it is unclear what the best approach is for resectable colorectal metastases. Results of adjuvant and perioperative studies incorporating biological therapies (bevacizumab or cetuximab), are eagerly awaited.

■ CONCLUSIONS

Metastatic CRC poses a significant burden worldwide, and efforts for increasing the odds of cure involve multiple international cooperative groups as well as small novel institutional trials. A meta-analysis of eight trials including 1174 patients since 1990 concluded that perioperative chemotherapy, with or without the addition of intraarterial chemotherapy is effective to improve outcomes in addition to metastasectomy. In general, HAI improved recurrence-free survival with a HR of 0.78 (95% CI, 0.65–0.95, *P* = .01) and systemic therapy conferred a HR of 0.75 (95% CI, 0.62–0.91, *P* = .003; 71). While HAI alone does not affect survival, HAI in combination with systemic chemotherapy has produced some of the highest survival rates to date, justifying its use in centers of excellence. Perhaps, influenced by patient selection and center expertise, HAI plus chemotherapy trials conferred seemingly higher DFS rates, generally over 30 months and median survival rates of 64 to 70 months (Table 10.2). Unfortunately, given the difficulty in accruing to these studies it is unlikely that future attempts comparing systemic therapy with or without HAI chemotherapy will be possible. The expertise of surgeons and interventional radiologists, as well as modern systemic regimens thoughtfully planned and conducted by the oncology community, are critical for obtaining the best possible outcomes for this disease. In addition, using risk stratification strategies may aid in determining the best strategy for individual patients (2,72). At this time, "curable" CRC metastases should be treated with a combined regimen of 6 months of perioperative or postoperative chemotherapy, with no more than 3 months of neoadjuvant therapy if possible. Best clinical practices will hopefully be established with the completion of ongoing randomized clinical trials.

■ *Liver Metastases: Surgical Considerations*

YUN SHIN CHUN

The liver is the most common site of distant metastases from CRC, with approximately 25% of patients presenting with synchronous liver metastases at diagnosis and another 30% developing metachronous disease, usually within the first 2 years following primary tumor resection (73). Complete surgical resection is the only potentially curative treatment for colorectal liver metastases, with 5-year overall survival rates up to 58% after liver resection (Table 10.5; 74–76). Using traditional criteria for resectability, such as tumor size and number, only 10% of patients were considered candidates for hepatectomy. Recent advances in high-resolution imaging, systemic therapy, and innovative perioperative strategies have increased the number of patients eligible for surgical resection (77). The current definition of resectability is the ability to achieve a margin-negative resection while preserving adequate functional liver remnant volume, sparing two contiguous hepatic segments, and maintaining adequate vascular inflow and outflow and biliary drainage (78).

Preoperative planning requires high-resolution imaging to assess the relationship of tumors to vascular and biliary structures, plan extent of hepatectomy, and identify extrahepatic disease. Unless the diagnosis is in doubt, percutaneous or open liver biopsy should be avoided, since biopsy of resectable colorectal liver metastases is associated with needle-track deposits and inferior survival after hepatectomy (79). Triple-phase, helical CT is the preferred imaging modality, with attention to the portal venous phase, because it provides the anatomic detail necessary for surgical planning. In patients with hepatic steatosis, MRI is more sensitive than CT. [18F] 2-fluoro-2-deoxyglucose (FDG)–positron emission tomography (PET) may detect CT-occult intra- and extrahepatic disease, particularly in high-risk patients with poor prognostic factors. However, the sensitivity of FDG-PET is diminished in patients receiving neoadjuvant chemotherapy and in tumors that lack sufficient cellular density to accumulate FDG (80,81). In addition, subcentimeter metastases below the spatial resolution of FDG-PET may not be detected.

The definition of resectability for colorectal liver metastases has evolved from traditional morphologic criteria to the current definition, which is the ability to achieve a margin-negative resection while ensuring a sufficient functional liver remnant volume (78). An absolute contraindication to liver resection is an inadequate volume of liver remaining, leading to hepatic failure. The volume of the functional liver remnant can be precisely measured with CT scan and normalized to patients' body surface area (82). In patients with a normal liver, a standardized functional liver remnant volume of 20% is recommended for safe hepatic resection, and in patients who have received extensive chemotherapy, 30% is recommended.

When the volume of the functional liver remnant is insufficient for safe liver resection, portal vein embolization is employed to induce hypertrophy of the remnant liver (Figure 10.1; 83). Portal vein embolization is performed by interventional radiologists who percutaneously access a branch of the portal vein and embolize the entire portal territory to be resected with microcoils and microparticles. The nonembolized remnant liver hypertrophies during the first 2 months after portal vein embolization, with the greatest increase in remnant liver volume during the initial 3 weeks. Thus, a period of 3 to 4 weeks is recommended after portal vein embolization to assess adequate liver hypertrophy in patients with a normal liver (84). A longer time interval may be necessary in patients with underlying chronic liver disease.

Bilateral metastases represent a relative contraindication to portal vein embolization because of the risk of tumor progression in the nonembolized liver segments

■ Table 10.5 Outcomes After Resection of Colorectal Liver Metastases

Author	Year	No. Pts.	Perioperative Mortality (%)	Preoperative Chemotherapy (%)	Postoperative Chemotherapy (%)	5-Year DFS (%)	5-Year OS (%)
Adson et al (188)	1984	141	2	0	0	n/a	25
Scheele et al (189)	1991	207	5.6	0	6	22	39
Nordlinger et al (190)	1996	1568	2.3	0	35	15	28
Minagawa et al (191)	2000	235	0	0	0	26	38
Choti et al (192)	2002	226	0.9	52	n/a	20	40
Pawlik et al (193)	2005	557	0.9	n/a	60	n/a	58
House et al (194)	2010	563	1	66	65	33	51

DFS, disease-free survival; OS, overall survival; n/a, not available.

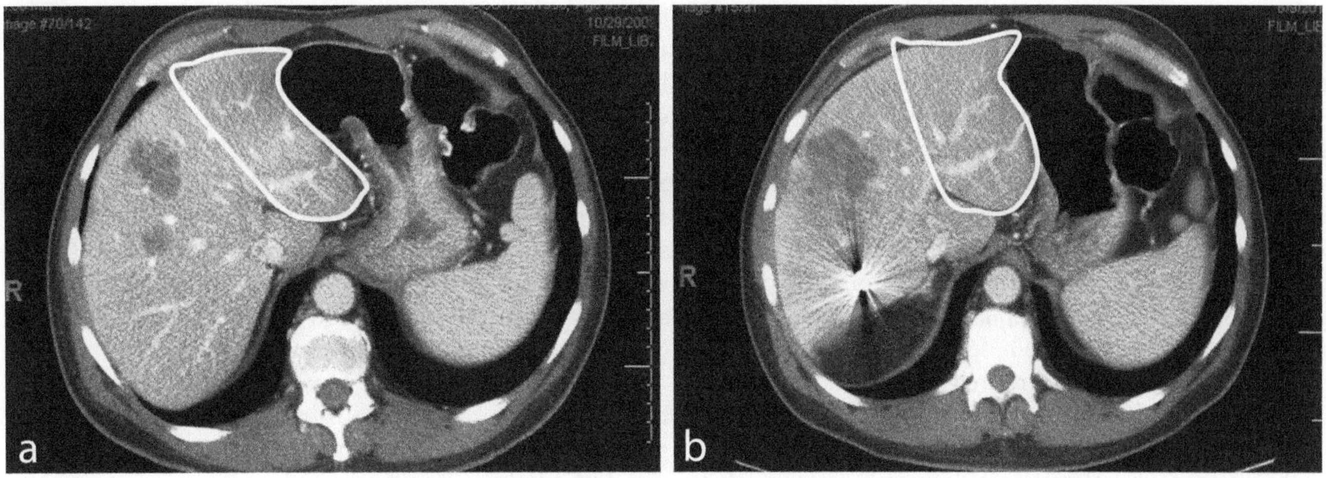

FIGURE 10.1 CT scans showing hypertrophy of future liver remnant volume before (a) and after (b) portal vein embolization.

while undergoing hypertrophy. For these patients, resection of metastases in the future liver remnant is recommended before portal vein embolization as a two-stage procedure. Two-stage hepatectomy is a novel strategy that enables resection of multiple, bilateral metastases that cannot be resected in a single procedure (85). The first stage involves a minor hepatectomy for lesions in the future liver remnant, usually the left liver, followed by a period of liver regeneration and portal vein embolization if the remnant liver volume is insufficient. Approximately 2 months later, a second-stage major liver resection is performed, typically a right or extended right hepatectomy. Chemotherapy is given before the first-stage and after the second-stage hepatectomy. Investigators at the University of Texas M. D. Anderson Cancer Center reported their results in 65 patients who underwent first-stage liver resection (86). Eighteen patients (28%) were unable to undergo second-stage hepatectomy because of disease progression or poor performance status. The 5-year overall survival of the 47 patients who completed 2-stage hepatectomy was 64%. This high survival rate in patients with advanced disease was attributed to selection of patients with favorable tumor biology who responded to preoperative chemotherapy and to complete surgical resection of all metastatic disease.

As noted above, modern chemotherapy and biologic agents have enabled more patients to undergo potentially curative resection of colorectal liver metastases (77). The benefits of preoperative chemotherapy include downsizing of liver metastases, treatment of occult micrometastases, and identification of patients with tumor progression on chemotherapy who would not benefit from surgery. The EORTC Intergroup trial 40983 randomized patients with resectable colorectal liver metastases to surgery alone or six cycles of oxaliplatin-based chemotherapy before and after surgery (56). Among 171 eligible patients randomized to the perioperative chemotherapy arm, 12 patients (7%)

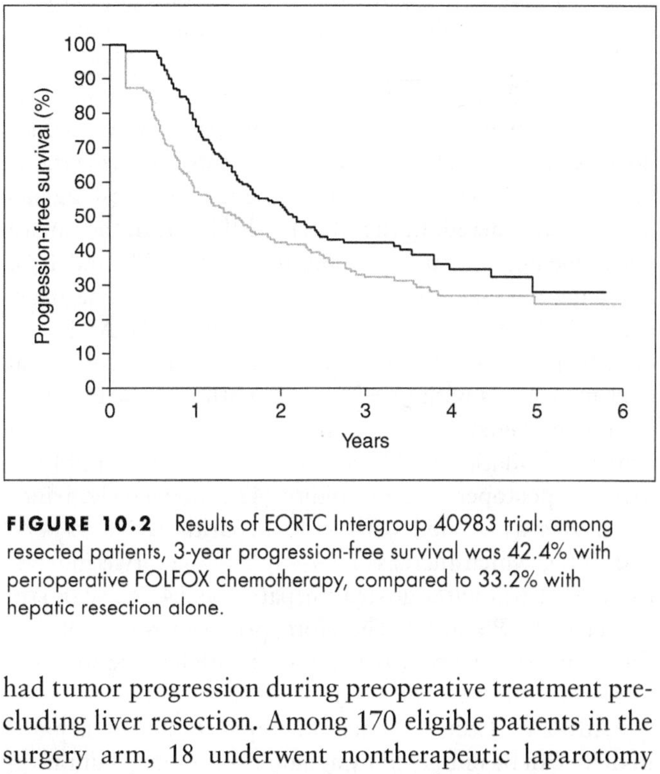

FIGURE 10.2 Results of EORTC Intergroup 40983 trial: among resected patients, 3-year progression-free survival was 42.4% with perioperative FOLFOX chemotherapy, compared to 33.2% with hepatic resection alone.

had tumor progression during preoperative treatment precluding liver resection. Among 170 eligible patients in the surgery arm, 18 underwent nontherapeutic laparotomy because of unexpected, extensive disease. Three-year progression-free survival rates in resected patients were 42.4% and 33.2% in the perioperative chemotherapy and surgery alone arms, respectively (P = .025; Figure 10.2). Based on data from this trial, patients with resectable colorectal liver metastases and high risk features, such as multiple metastases, synchronous presentation, and bilateral disease, are recommended to receive preoperative chemotherapy. Conversely, patients with small (less than 2 cm), solitary metastases should undergo liver resection first to avoid the risk of disappearing metastases with chemotherapy.

Response to preoperative chemotherapy is emerging as an important outcome end point after resection of colorectal liver metastases. Blazer et al evaluated pathologic response in 305 patients undergoing liver resection after chemotherapy (38). Pathologic response was stratified as complete, major, or minor, based on the percent residual tumor cells. On multivariate analysis, pathologic response and surgical margin status were the sole predictors of overall survival. Complete pathologic response occurred in a minority of patients (9%), similar to a study by Adam and coworkers, who reported a complete pathologic response rate of 4% (87). Radiographic response using the conventional, size-based Response Evaluation Criteria in Solid Tumors correlated poorly with complete pathologic response (88). In patients receiving preoperative chemotherapy with bevacizumab, novel CT-based morphologic criteria of response assessment were found to correlate with pathologic response and overall survival after liver resection (89). Patients treated with bevacizumab, which is thought to have a cytostatic mechanism of action, may exhibit cystic changes in tumors, indicating pathologic response, without change in tumor size.

Although modern chemotherapy can convert unresectable metastases to resectable in select patients and reduce postoperative recurrence rates in patients with resectable disease, the potential liver injury caused by these agents must be considered. In the EORTC 40983 trial, the rate of reversible postoperative complications was 25% and 16% in the perioperative chemotherapy and surgery alone arms, respectively ($P = .04$; 56). In a study from M. D. Anderson of 406 patients who underwent resection of colorectal liver metastases with (n = 248) and without (n = 158) preoperative chemotherapy, oxaliplatin was associated with sinusoidal dilation (19% vs 2%; $P < .001$), which did not increase postoperative morbidity (42). Conversely, irinotecan was associated with steatohepatitis (20% vs 4%; $P < .001$), which increased 90-day postoperative mortality rates (1.6% without steatohepatitis vs 14.7% with steatohepatitis, $P = .001$). Therefore, preoperative irinotecan should be used cautiously in patients with hepatic steatosis and other chronic liver diseases.

Adverse effects of chemotherapy-associated hepatotoxicity can be mitigated by avoiding a prolonged duration of preoperative chemotherapy and by ensuring a sufficient time interval between date of last chemotherapy and hepatectomy. Karoui et al reported higher postoperative morbidity rates in patients who received six or more cycles of preoperative chemotherapy compared with those who received less than six cycles (54% vs 19%; $P = .047$; 90). Similarly, Nakano et al showed that patients who received six or more cycles of oxaliplatin were at increased risk of sinusoidal dilatation (91). The optimal duration of preoperative chemotherapy to minimize hepatotoxicity while attaining tumor response is 2 to 3 months in most patients (92,93).

A longer time interval between date of last chemotherapy and hepatectomy is associated with reduced postoperative complications; however, this interval should be balanced with the risk of tumor progression off chemotherapy. Welsh et al demonstrated a surgical complication rate of 11% in patients undergoing hepatectomy less than or equal to 4 weeks after stopping chemotherapy, compared with 5.5% in those undergoing surgery after 5 to 8 weeks (94). Thus, an interval of 5 weeks is recommended between date of last chemotherapy and hepatectomy. In a phase II trial of neoadjuvant therapy in patients with colorectal liver metastases, bevacizumab administered 5 weeks before liver resection was not associated with an increased rate of surgical or wound complications (48).

The role of laparoscopic hepatectomy for colorectal liver metastases is expanding in specialized centers. Benefits of the laparoscopic approach include smaller incisions, less pain, and shorter length of hospital stay. Challenges of laparoscopic liver resection are the inability to perform bimanual palpation, potential for bleeding, and technical demands of liver mobilization and obtaining vascular control. Retrospective data suggest that oncologic outcomes, including 5-year overall survival rates and resection margins, are not compromised by laparoscopic liver resection (95). Small, peripheral tumors, particularly in the left lateral section, are most amenable to the laparoscopic approach. The learning curve for laparoscopic hepatectomy is significant, and laparoscopic major hepatectomy requires advanced laparoscopy and ultrasound skills.

■ *Pulmonary Metastases: Surgical Considerations*

PRASHANT SHAH

It has long been recognized that the lung is a frequent site for colorectal metastases, second only to the liver. With respect to incidence, approximately 10%–20% of patients with colorectal carcinoma will develop metastatic pulmonary involvement at some point during the course of their disease process (96). Historically, the presence of extrahepatic disease was regarded as a poor prognostic factor, irrespective of metastatic tumor burden. However, over the past 2 decades, numerous studies have demonstrated that select patients with lung colorectal metastases will have a survival advantage with complete pulmonary metastasectomy, similar to select patients undergoing hepatic metastasectomy (97,98). It is now standard practice to consider surgery in the multidisciplinary treatment of the Stage IV CRC patient with isolated metastatic disease to lung and liver.

Recent survival data from large series indicate an improving overall survival trend postmetastasectomy for this patient subgroup. Resection of colorectal liver metastases is associated with a 5-year survival as high as 58% (74), whereas resection of colorectal pulmonary metastases is associated with a 5-year survival as high as 68% (99). Brouquet et al have similarly evaluated CRC patients who underwent both hepatic and pulmonary metastasectomies and noted a 5-year survival as high as 50% (11). These survival rates for these subgroups of oligometastatic CRC patients far exceeds that of Stage IV CRC patients with unresectable or widespread disease, where 5-year survival is close to 0%.

When evaluating a patient undergoing treatment for CRC, it is important to provide close surveillance to help facilitate early detection of recurrences or metastatic disease. Radiographic imaging and periodic serum CEA levels are both implemented in most CRC surveillance protocols. CEA levels when elevated are more indicative of metastatic disease compared to locoregional recurrence and should prompt the clinician to pursue CT scan imaging of the chest, abdomen, and pelvis (100).

When an incidental solitary pulmonary nodule is identified in a CRC patient, there is a near equal probability of the nodule being a primary lung cancer versus a colorectal metastasis. In these patients, the clinician should obtain a CEA level to help elaborate on the possible histology of the nodule. While a positive CEA level (in the setting of a pulmonary nodule) has good predictive value, a negative or normal CEA level does not exclude the possibility of a colorectal metastasis. A preoperative biopsy (transthoracic needle biopsy or transbronchial needle biopsy) is often, but not always, helpful in distinguishing between these two histologies. In particular, thyroid transcription factor-1 (TTF-1) is a highly specific immunohistochemical tumor marker expressed only by primary lung adenocarcinomas, but a negative result is not diagnostic of an extrapulmonary adenocarcinoma (101).

The utility of obtaining a preoperative biopsy for a pulmonary nodule in a CRC patient has been debated. In either scenario (early lung primary cancer vs solitary colorectal pulmonary metastasis), complete resection is still warranted. However, a preoperative or intraoperative diagnosis of nonsmall cell lung carcinoma will prompt the thoracic surgeon to perform an anatomical resection (eg, lobectomy, segmentectomy). In the other instances, a diagnosis of a colorectal metastasis will not necessitate a lobar resection; instead, a "lesser" resection that is lung sparing will suffice (eg, wedge resection or segmentectomy). Often, when the preoperative workup is inconclusive, the surgeon can utilize a diagnostic wedge resection (at the time of lung resection) and submit the nodule for intraoperative "frozen-section" analysis to help determine the actual histological diagnosis. This intraoperative analysis will then help to determine the extent of further lung resection in the same operative setting. In the instance when the preoperative CEA level and intraoperative frozen-section analysis are both inconclusive in differentiating the histology and site of origin, it seems more reasonable to pursue an anatomical resection, as this serves as a complete resection in either histological scenario. In the instance when confronted with a CRC patient with either multiple pulmonary nodules or a moderately-elevated CEA level, it is very reasonable to assume metastatic disease and to proceed with a lung-sparing approach without a preoperative biopsy (102,103). Here, however, metastatic colorectal histology should still be confirmed by intraoperative "frozen-section" analysis, in an effort to avoid missing a possible primary lung cancer diagnosis.

A number of studies have evaluated different prognostic factors that directly influence survival after pulmonary metastectomy for CRC patients. Saito et al evaluated 165 patients with colorectal carcinoma who underwent pulmonary metastectomy (104). Overall survivals at 5 and 10 years postmetastasectomy were 39.6% and 37.2%, respectively. Differences in age, gender, location, grade, and stage of the primary CRC were not found to have influence on survival postmetastasectomy. The factors found to have a statistically significant increase in long-term survival included absence of hilar or mediastinal lymph node metastasis, normal preoperative CEA level (less than 10 ng/mL), and completeness of resection. Twenty-one patients underwent a second or third metastasectomy for recurrent colorectal carcinoma. Overall

5-year survival from the date of the second metastasectomy was 52.1%, suggesting that repeat resection is associated with acceptable long-term survival. The 34.1% 10-year survival for the 26 patients with hepatic metastases resected before pulmonary resection did not differ significantly from that of patients without hepatic metastases ($P = .38$), suggesting that concomitant (hepatic and pulmonary) metastatic disease should be treated with aggressive sequential metastasectomies when possible. McAfee et al at the Mayo Clinic evaluated 139 patients who similarly underwent pulmonary resection for metastatic CRC (105). They identified longer 5-year survival for patients with a solitary pulmonary metastasis and for patients with a near-normal preoperative CEA level (less than 4 ng/mL), as opposed to patients with multiple nodules or patients with an abnormal CEA level. The size of the metastasis (less than 3 cm) was not found to be associated with improved survival, however. Lin et al evaluated 63 patients who underwent curative pulmonary resection for colorectal metastases, and found that the time interval from CRC resection to detection of lung metastasis had prognostic significance (106). The 5-year overall survival rate was significantly higher for those with a time interval greater than 1 year (53% vs 13%; $P = .004$); similarly, the 5-year DFS (postmetastasectomy) was also higher for those with a time interval greater than 1 year (27% vs 0%, $P = .001$). Size and number of pulmonary metastases did not have prognostic significance in this study. Brouquet et al evaluated 112 colorectal patients who underwent both liver and lung metastasectomies (11). In their study, the location of the primary tumor (rectal vs colonic) and preoperative CEA level were the only factors that were independently associated with survival. Patients with a rectal primary had a 5-year survival of 28%, whereas those with a colon primary had a 5-year survival of 58% ($P = .01$). As in other studies, higher preoperative CEA levels (greater than 5 ng/mL) were associated with shorter survival (HR, 2.1; 95% CI 1.1 to 4.4; $P = .04$). Interestingly, this study also demonstrated that the following factors did not have prognostic significance on survival: synchronous liver metastases, preoperative chemotherapy before liver metastasectomy, multiple liver metastases, liver metastasis size greater than 5 cm, postoperative chemotherapy after liver metastasectomy, disease-free interval less than 12 months between resection of first and last metastatic site, synchronous lung metastases, preoperative chemotherapy before lung metastasectomy, bilateral lung metastases, lung metastasis size greater than 2 cm, and postoperative chemotherapy after lung metastasectomy.

In many CRC patients, pulmonary metastases will be detected either synchronously or metachronously with hepatic metastases. In either scenario, studies have indicated that aggressive attempts at complete resection of pulmonary and hepatic metastases will improve survival, provided that all metastatic lesions are confined to the liver and lung, that these metastatic lesions are all resectable, and that the patient is low operative risk for all of the entailed surgical resections. Labow et al evaluated 21 patients with colorectal pulmonary metastases, identified after hepatic metastasectomy, of which only 12 underwent pulmonary metastasectomy (107). There was a significant survival benefit noted at 3 years for the group that underwent pulmonary metastasectomy vs the group with unresected pulmonary metastases (60% vs 31%). In another study, Robinson et al at the Cleveland Clinic investigated the influence of the sequence and timing of hepatic and pulmonary colorectal metastases with respect to long-term survival (98). They evaluated 48 CRC patients with metastatic disease confined to both liver and lung, of which 25 had undergone metastasectomies, and 23 did not. Median survival was longer after resection of the last metastasis (lung or liver) in the resection group than in the nonresection group (16 months vs 6 months; $P < .001$). Interestingly, patients who underwent metachronous resections had a median survival after colorectal resection that was longer than that of patients who underwent synchronous resections (70 months vs; 22 months; $P < .001$). The authors concluded that those most likely to benefit long term from dual (liver and lung) metastasectomies included younger patients (less than 50 years of age), patients with a metachronous metastatic pattern (first liver, then lung), patients with only a solitary liver metastasis, and patients with a long (greater than 4 year) disease-free interval between colorectal resection and the development of the first pulmonary metastasis. Interestingly, however, patients who had risk factors for shorter survival (eg, greater than 70 years of age, multiple liver metastases, synchronous metastatic pattern, and a short disease-free interval) still had better survival with metastasectomies than without metastasectomies.

While more recent studies are identifying other potential predictors of survival for CRC patients with pulmonary metastases, it is important to note that "completeness of resection" has the most influence on prognosis and overall survival in this cohort. Unfortunately, there has been only little progress with improving the potential for survival with the use of chemotherapy or other nonsurgical options in this group. Given these circumstances, the clinician should pursue aggressive attempts at "complete" resection of pulmonary and hepatic colorectal metastases in the majority of these patients whenever possible, in an effort to improve overall survival. When patients cannot be completely resected, or are unresectable, survival is anticipated to be poor. In this setting, palliative options should be considered, including palliative chemotherapy. On the other hand, when a patient is a potential candidate for "complete" resection, the clinician should still evaluate each patient individually using the prognostic factors described above, to help determine the actual survival benefit that resection offers for that particular patient. But the clinician should still place an overwhelming emphasis on the potential for "completeness" of resection of both hepatic and pulmonary metastases, which is the most important factor for enhancing survival in this group.

■ *Pelvic Recurrences: Surgical Considerations*

JULIO GARCIA-AGUILAR
JULIAN SANCHEZ
LISA A. KACHNIC

■ INTRODUCTION

The surgical field is the third most common site of tumor relapse, after the liver and lung, following a curative-intent resection for CRC (108,109). The surgical field is defined as the site of the primary tumor, the regional and retroperitoneal lymph nodes, the surgical anastomosis, the drain tracts, and any surgical scars. Recurrences involving the omentum, or peritoneal surfaces not adjacent to the tumor bed, require special consideration and a different treatment approach because they probably have a different pathogenesis. Local recurrence is particularly morbid and debilitating, often causing chronic pain and obstruction of the digestive and urinary systems. Without treatment, most patients die within a year of diagnosis. Radiation and/or chemotherapy can provide palliation. However, surgery is the only curative option for patients with locally recurrent colon and rectal cancer. It is the treatment most likely to provide sustained pain control and improvement in quality of life (110). Although many patients with local recurrence are potentially resectable, few have curative-intent surgery. Additionally, patients with local recurrence are less likely to have salvage surgery than patients with distant metastasis. This nihilistic approach toward locally recurrent CRC is related to the magnitude and morbidity associated with the procedures required to control the disease. Improvements in surgical techniques and perioperative care, better imaging studies to help select patients who are more likely to benefit from an aggressive resection, and a multidisciplinary approach involving multiple specialists have increased the proportion of patients undergoing salvage surgery who are potentially curable, or who may be palliated from this devastating condition (111).

Risk Factors

Similar to distant metastasis, the risk of local recurrence is related to the biology of the tumor, and is greater in patients with higher grade and more advanced stage tumors (112). Local recurrence is also related to the completeness of resection of the primary tumor, being more common after surgical resection with close or positive margins (113). Additionally, local recurrence is more common after surgery for rectal cancer compared to colon cancer (114); this is probably related to the anatomical location of the rectum within the smaller pelvic cavity and the dual lymphatic drainage of the rectum, cephalad along the inferior mesenteric vessels, and laterally toward the internal iliac vessels. However, the risk of local recurrence in patients treated for rectal cancer has decreased significantly in the last 2 decades. This is largely due to advances in preoperative tumor staging and patient selection, improved surgical techniques, and the use of neoadjuvant therapies (115,116).

Diagnosis

Most local recurrences are identified within 2 years after treatment of the primary tumor, but some may be diagnosed many years after the initial operation, particularly in patients with rectal cancer who received preoperative radiation (117). Some local recurrences are diagnosed during surveillance visits, which aim to identify recurrences before they become symptomatic, and are still potentially resectable (118). Several meta-analyses of six prospective randomized trials suggest that intensive surveillance may provide a small survival advantage; however, there is no consensus on the frequency of clinic visits or type of diagnostic tests (119,120). The guidelines put forth by most professional societies recommend CEA testing every 3 months and annual CT scan of the chest and abdomen (as well as the pelvis in rectal cancer) for the first 3 years in patients with Stage II or III disease (121). However, in most series, only one-third of local recurrences are diagnosed at a scheduled surveillance visit; the remainder of patients are symptomatic at the time of diagnosis (122,123).

The symptoms of local recurrence depend on the location of the tumor, the initial operation, and the structures affected. The most common symptoms are pain, bowel obstruction, rectal or vaginal bleeding, and urinary symptoms. A nonhealing perineal wound is a common manifestation of local recurrence in rectal cancer patients treated with abdominoperineal resection. Patients with symptoms suggestive of locally recurrent colon and rectal cancer should be evaluated to confirm the diagnosis, exclude distant metastasis, assess resectability, and evaluate the risks of major surgery. A detailed history should include inquiry about the nature of the pain and symptoms suggesting involvement of other organs. A complete physical examination is mandatory. Digital rectal examination in patients who have had a sphincter-saving procedure, and pelvic exam in female patients, are particularly important in evaluating a suspected pelvic recurrence because they provide an idea of the extent of recurrence and the potential involvement of adjacent organs. Most intraluminal recurrences are easily diagnosed by endoscopy and biopsy; therefore, patients with potential local recurrence should have a colonoscopy. Symptoms and signs related to the urogenital tract are predictors of pathologic invasion of the ureter and bladder by recurrent tumor. A cystoscopy should be performed in patients with urinary symptoms (124).

CEA elevation in patients under surveillance is often the first indication of a potential tumor recurrence (125). In patients whose CEA levels were elevated prior to their initial surgery but normalized after treatment of the primary tumor, rising CEA is very specific for the development of recurrence; however, its sensitivity is low because serum CEA is only elevated in approximately half of CRC patients. Patients with rising CEA should undergo additional evaluation with endoscopy and imaging studies (100).

The imaging modalities used in diagnosing local recurrence and distant metastasis include CT scan, MRI, and PET (126,127). High-resolution CT scan has been the preferred test for diagnosing tumor recurrence because it provides good anatomical resolution of the thoracic, abdominal, and pelvic structures. However, CT imaging cannot distinguish between scar and tumor. MRI has excellent tissue resolution, and differences in signal intensity can help differentiate scar from tumor more accurately than CT. MRI is particularly useful in assessing the proximal extension along the presacral fascia in patients with locally recurrent rectal cancer. PET-CT combines the anatomical resolution of the CT scan (albeit limited by lack of intravenous contrast) with PET-detected elevated fluorodeoxyglucose-18 uptake characteristic of neoplastic tissue. PET-CT is useful in confirming or excluding a diagnosis of recurrence when the results of conventional imaging are equivocal; in excluding distant metastasis in patients with seemingly localized resectable recurrence; and in investigating unexplained elevation in CEA when CT or MRI are normal (128). However, PET-CT has some limitations. PET positivity depends on the size of the lesion and the FDG uptake. Lesions less than 1 cm in diameter are difficult to detect, and mucinous tumors have poor FDG uptake. Furthermore, PET may not be useful in the setting of residual inflammation in the tumor bed, which is found in patients with chronic-leak anastomosis. Endorectal ultrasound (ERUS) may help diagnose pelvic recurrences after local excision or sphincter-sparing surgery for rectal cancer (129). Nevertheless, whichever imaging modality is used to potentially diagnose local recurrence, it is important to confirm the diagnosis by performing a biopsy of the lesion. This is done either through the bowel (in the case of an anastomotic recurrence) or percutaneously under radiological guidance to identify an extraluminal recurrence.

Surgical Considerations

A complete surgical resection with negative margins is the only curative option for patients with recurrent CRC (108,130,131). A noncurative resection exposes the patient to the risk of significant postoperative morbidity, but does not offer any advantage over nonsurgical palliation in terms of survival or quality of life (130,132). A significant proportion of patients with locoregional recurrence are potentially resectable with negative margins at the time of diagnosis, but are not offered surgery due to the technical complexity and morbidity associated with these procedures. Often, patients who are resectable at the time of diagnosis are referred to surgeons later in the course of their disease, when the tumor has progressed and become unresectable. This is why, in some population-based series, only half of the patients with locoregional recurrences undergo surgery, and less than 20% have a complete resection with curative intent (133).

The precise location of a local recurrence is important when assessing whether the tumor is amenable to surgical resection with curative intent, particularly in patients with rectal cancer. Most pelvic recurrences start in the perirectal tissue and are located posteriorly (134). The sacrum and coccyx are involved more often than the lateral pelvic sidewall. Recurrences involving the lumen are usually located within 1 cm of the anastomosis. There are a number of classifications of rectal cancer recurrence based on location within the pelvis (135–137), but all essentially distinguish between centrally and posteriorly located recurrences and those involving the pelvic sidewalls, because these locations are associated with different resectability and outcomes (130). Locoregional recurrences after curative resection for colon cancer are usually located around the anastomosis, in the mesentery, in the retroperitoneal lymph nodes, or in the peritoneum (138). In many patients, adjacent organs and structures are involved.

Curative resection should be considered for patients with locoregional recurrences that are potentially resectable with negative margins; for patients who have no distant metastasis; and for patients who otherwise have a reasonable life expectancy. Similar to primary tumors, some locally recurrent colon and rectal cancers respond to chemotherapy and/or radiation. Patients with local recurrence who did not have chemotherapy or radiation therapy during treatment of their primary tumor should receive preoperative combined-modality therapy to increase the possibility of achieving negative surgical margins (139). In many centers, patients with locally recurrent rectal cancer who initially received neoadjuvant radiation or chemoradiation are now treated with re-irradiation (doses up to 30.6 to 45 Gy in patients previously treated with 50.4 Gy), with or without sensitizing chemotherapy (140,141).

The first important step in assessing a patient for locoregional recurrence is to exclude peritoneal disease, which is often missed on imaging studies. Patients with peritoneal carcinomatosis are considered to have metastatic disease and require a different treatment approach, including cytoreductive surgery and intraperitoneal chemotherapy. When planning the operation it is important to remember that, in these patients, the anatomic planes are distorted as a result of their initial surgery; it is almost impossible to distinguish between scar and tissue; and the planes opened at the time of the previous resection may be affected by tumor. Consequently, the surgeon must prepare to perform a wide resection through uninvolved planes, even if this requires resecting adjacent organs or anatomic structures. Most patients undergoing resection for locally recurrent colon cancer require an extended resection with en bloc removal of adjacent organs or structures, including the abdominal wall, small bowel, uterus and ovaries, ureter and bladder, pancreas, and duodenum (142).

Centrally located pelvic recurrences are often resectable, although recurrent tumor attached to the internal genitalia or the urologic system often requires a complete pelvic exenteration (143,144). Posterior recurrences adjacent to the sacrum at or below the level of S3 can often be treated with a partial sacrectomy (145). Lateral recurrences involving the lateral pelvic sidewall or the sciatic notch are more difficult to resect with negative margins. As a simple guideline, if the fat plane medial to the internal obturator internus is obliterated, the tumor is rarely resectable. The main contraindications to surgery in patients with recurrent rectal cancer are invasion of the sacrum above S2, or invasion of the pelvic sidewall, both of which preclude a complete resection.

Surgical treatment of locally recurrent colon or rectal cancer often requires multivisceral resection (131,142). The urinary system is frequently involved, necessitating resection of the prostate, seminal vesicles, ureters and/or bladder (124,146). Resection of some abdominal recurrences involving the bowel wall, and rectal recurrences warranting a perineal resection, also require complex reconstruction with prosthetic material or tissue transfers (147). Posterior pelvic recurrences involving the sacrum often necessitate major sacral resection with control of the dural sac and resection of sacral nerves. Therefore, the treatment of patients with local recurrence usually requires a multidisciplinary team comprising medical and radiation oncologists, a surgical oncologist or colorectal surgeon, urologist, plastic surgeon, and orthopedic surgeon or neurosurgeon (148). Given the length and extent of these procedures and the potential for significant bleeding and large fluid shifts, even apparently fit patients must undergo exhaustive preoperative evaluation by the anesthesia team.

Patient Outcomes

According to a report on salvage surgery for recurrence in patients with Stage II and III colon cancer who were treated with curative intent and followed according to an established protocol, only 24 of 44 patients undergoing salvage surgery for local recurrence had a curative-intent resection; only 7 (29%) of those undergoing curative-intent surgery were alive and free of disease at the end of follow up (122). Interestingly, median survival after salvage surgery for local recurrence (26 months) did not differ from the median survival of patients who had salvage surgery for liver (22 months) or lung (22 months) metastasis (122). More recent series have reported better results, probably due to patient selection and improvements in surgical technique and perioperative care. In the Memorial Sloan-Kettering Cancer Center (MSKCC) series, only 56% of patients undergoing surgical exploration had an R0 resection; 57% were alive at 5 years, compared to 5% of patients with an R1/2 resection (138). Akiyoshi et al recently reported their experience of salvage surgery in 45 patients with locoregional recurrence of colon cancer. Forty patients (89%) had an R0 resection. The 5-year cancer-specific survival for the entire group was 46%; 50% for patients with an R0 resection. None of the 10 patients with an R2 resection were alive at 5 years (142). Both series reported that patients with peri-anastomotic recurrences had a better prognosis compared to patients with retroperitoneal and mesenteric recurrences. Mortality was less than 2%, and the rates of perioperative complications were 21% and 38%, respectively.

Tepper et al reported the results of salvage surgery for rectal cancer patients enrolled in Intergroup Study 0114, which investigated the effects of adjuvant therapy in patients undergoing curative surgery for Stages II and III disease (123). A total of 715 patients were diagnosed with recurrent disease at almost 9 years of follow up: 171; (34% of those recurring) recurred at a single organ or site. Only 37% of the 47 patients with isolated local recurrences underwent surgical resection, compared to 32% of patients with isolated liver metastasis and 38% with pulmonary metastasis. Patients with disease limited to a single organ or site who underwent surgical resection had improved survival compared to those who had no surgery. The 5-year DFS in patients who had surgery for local recurrence was 20%, compared to 30% in patients who had surgery for recurrences limited to the liver or lungs. Resection with negative margins (R0) was the main predictor of survival in all three groups.

A number of series published over the last decade have reported 5-year overall survival rates ranging from 37%–60% in patients who had R0 resections for locally recurrent rectal cancer (111,131,136,143,144,149–154). According to a recent report from the Swedish Rectal Cancer Registry, a total of 57 (10.1%) of 562 rectal cancer patients treated with curative intent developed local recurrence, alone or combined with distant metastasis. Only 10 (18%) patients had surgery, with an R0 resection accomplished in eight. Only two patients were alive 5 years after the initial operation (133). A second population-based registry from the Amsterdam metropolitan area found 10% local recurrence among 632 patients treated with curative intent. Of the 32 patients with isolated local recurrence, only 10 had an R0 resection, and half were alive at 5 years. Patients with an R0 resection did better than patients who had noncurative surgery (24 months), radiation and/or chemotherapy (7 months), or supportive care (5 months; 116,155). These data suggest that surgical salvage is possible in as many as one-third of patients with resectable locally recurrent rectal cancer.

Surgical treatment of recurrent rectal cancer often requires extensive resections with complex reconstruction, creation of stomas, and plastic procedures to cover large pelvic and perineal defects. These operations are associated with some perioperative mortality (0%–9%), postoperative complications (24%–44%), and prolonged recovery (111,131,136,143,144,148,150–154). The oncologic outcomes of posterior pelvic exenteration with sacral resection, for posterior recurrences attached to or involving the sacrum, are not very different from the outcomes of operations performed for pelvic recurrences in other locations. The reported operative mortality ranges from 0%–5%. In all series, greater than 50% of patients had postoperative complications—especially dehiscence of the perineal wound, or pelvic sepsis. Five-year survival ranged from 20%–42%, being higher for patients with R0 resections (145,156–161).

Intraoperative Radiation

In spite of adequate planning and strict selection criteria, a resection with negative microscopic margins cannot be achieved in every patient. Because of the risk of local relapse, patients with a close or microscopically positive resection margin who have already received the maximal doses of external beam radiation are considered candidates for intraoperative radiotherapy (IORT). IORT has the advantage of directing treatment to the specific area of residual tumor, sparing vital adjacent structures. Radiation can be delivered directly to the tumor bed after resection by electron beam radiotherapy (EB-IORT; 111) or intraoperative brachytherapy (HDR-IORT), or placement of radioactive seeds in the areas of highest risk eved in every patient. The use of direct IORT has the advantage of directing treatment to the specific area of residual tumor, sparing vital adjacent structures. Radiation therapy can be delivered directly to the tumor bed after resection by EB-IORT or by intraoperative brachytherapy (HDR-IORT) or placement of radioactive seeds in the areas of highest risk (162). Intraoperative electron beam radiation has a deeper penetration; however, it can be difficult to aim the beam at certain areas of the pelvis. In addition, EB-IORT requires a dedicated operating room and a radiation accelerator available at only a small number of institutions. The HDR-IORT applicator is flexible and adjusts better to the concavity of the pelvis than the fixed cones used for electron beam therapy, but this technology is not widely available either. Local radiation can also be delivered with the placement of I-125 seeds or after-loading catheters using I-192. The brachytherapy catheters are easy to adapt to the area requiring treatment; however, the catheters can migrate after surgery, can be difficult to load, and may be uncomfortable for patients (163–165).

The literature on the efficacy of IORT in patients undergoing resection for locally recurrent CRC is difficult to interpret because it is based on relatively small institutional case series, with heterogeneous patient selection criteria, and differences in presurgical treatment. The lack of a control group of patients treated by surgery alone also makes interpretation difficult. However, most authors suggest a 30% survival advantage in patients with microscopically positive or close resection margins who undergo IORT, compared to those undergoing surgery alone (140,166–170). Patients with an R0 resection or macroscopic residual disease (R2 resection) do not seem to benefit from IORT as much as patients with R1 resections.

Patients with recurrent CRC who are not candidates for surgical resection are often given chemotherapy and radiation with palliative intent. Pain control is possible with radiotherapy but the relief is temporary; averaging 4 months in patients treated with radiation alone and 7.8 months in patients treated with combined chemoradiation (171). Patients who have exhausted all surgical, chemotherapy, and radiotherapy options still need supportive care to control their symptoms. Pain is particularly devastating in recurrent CRC—the most important factor affecting quality of life (172,173). Other common complications such as bowel obstruction and bleeding can be treated with stomas, stents, fulguration, laser or radiofrequency ablation, or image-guided interstitial radiation implants. Ureteral obstruction often requires stents, or even percutaneous nephrostomy.

REFERENCES

1. Siegel R, Naishadham D, Jemal A. Cancer statistics, 2012. *CA Cancer J Clin.* 2012;62:10–29.
2. Fong Y, Fortner J, Sun RL, Brennan MF, Blumgart LH. Clinical score for predicting recurrence after hepatic resection for metastatic colorectal cancer: analysis of 1001 consecutive cases. *Ann Surg.* 1999;230:309–318; discussion 18–21.
3. Merkel S, Bialecki D, Meyer T, Muller V, Papadopoulos T, Hohenberger W. Comparison of clinical risk scores predicting prognosis after resection of colorectal liver metastases. *J Surg Oncol.* 2009;100:349–357.

4. Nordlinger B, Guiguet M, Vaillant JC, et al. Surgical resection of colorectal carcinoma metastases to the liver. A prognostic scoring system to improve case selection, based on 1568 patients. Association Francaise de Chirurgie. *Cancer.* 1996;77:1254–1262.
5. Fong Y, Cohen AM, Fortner JG, et al. Liver resection for colorectal metastases. *J Clin Oncol.* 1997;15:938–946.
6. Petrelli NJ. Perioperative or adjuvant therapy for resectable colorectal hepatic metastases. *J Clin Oncol.* 2008;26:4862–4863.
7. Borasio P, Gisabella M, Bille A, et al. Role of surgical resection in colorectal lung metastases: analysis of 137 patients. *Int J Colorectal Dis.* 2011;26:183–190.
8. Chao YK, Chang HC, Wu YC, et al. Management of lung metastases from colorectal cancer: video-assisted thoracoscopic surgery versus thoracotomy: a case-matched study. *Thorac Cardiovasc Surg.* 2012;60:398–404.
9. Headrick JR, Miller DL, Nagorney DM, et al. Surgical treatment of hepatic and pulmonary metastases from colon cancer. *Ann Thorac Surg.* 2001;71:975–979; discussion 9–80.
10. Mineo TC, Ambrogi V, Tonini G, et al. Long-term results after resection of simultaneous and sequential lung and liver metastases from colorectal carcinoma. *J Am Coll Surg.* 2003;197:386–391.
11. Brouquet A, Vauthey JN, Contreras CM, et al. Improved survival after resection of liver and lung colorectal metastases compared with liver-only metastases: a study of 112 patients with limited lung metastatic disease. *J Am Coll Surg.* 2011;213:62–69; discussion 9–71.
12. Nojiri K, Tanaka K, Nagano Y, et al. Efficacy of surgery for lung metastases from colorectal cancer synchronous to or following that for liver metastases. *Anticancer Res.* 2011;31:1049–1054.
13. Carpenter S, Fong Y. Management of disappearing colorectal hepatic metastases. *Adv Surg.* 2010;44:269–279.
14. Falcone A, Ricci S, Brunetti I, et al. Phase III trial of infusional fluorouracil, leucovorin, oxaliplatin, and irinotecan (FOLFOXIRI) compared with infusional fluorouracil, leucovorin, and irinotecan (FOLFIRI) as first-line treatment for metastatic colorectal cancer: the Gruppo Oncologico Nord Ovest. *J Clin Oncol.* 2007;25:1670–1676.
15. Van Cutsem E, Kohne CH, Lang I, et al. Cetuximab plus irinotecan, fluorouracil, and leucovorin as first-line treatment for metastatic colorectal cancer: updated analysis of overall survival according to tumor K-ras and BRAF mutation status. *J Clin Oncol.* 2011;29:2011–2019.
16. Folprecht G, Gruenberger T, Bechstein WO, et al. Tumour response and secondary resectability of colorectal liver metastases following neoadjuvant chemotherapy with cetuximab: the CELIM randomised phase 2 trial. *Lancet Oncol.* 2010;11:38–47.
17. Okines A, Puerto OD, Cunningham D, et al. Surgery with curative-intent in patients treated with first-line chemotherapy plus bevacizumab for metastatic colorectal cancer First BEAT and the randomised phase-III NO16966 trial. *Br J Cancer.* 2009;101:1033–1038.
18. Poston GJ, Figueras J, Giuliante F, et al. Urgent need for a new staging system in advanced colorectal cancer. *J Clin Oncol.* 2008;26:4828–4833.
19. Ridge JA, Bading JR, Gelbard AS, Benua RS, Daly JM. Perfusion of colorectal hepatic metastases. Relative distribution of flow from the hepatic artery and portal vein. *Cancer.* 1987;59:1547–1553.
20. Lorenz M, Muller HH, Schramm H, et al. Randomized trial of surgery versus surgery followed by adjuvant hepatic arterial infusion with 5-fluorouracil and folinic acid for liver metastases of colorectal cancer. German Cooperative on Liver Metastases (Arbeitsgruppe Lebermetastasen). *Ann Surg.* 1998;228:756–762.
21. Ensminger WD, Rosowsky A, Raso V, et al. A clinical-pharmacological evaluation of hepatic arterial infusions of 5-fluoro-2'-deoxyuridine and 5-fluorouracil. *Cancer Res.* 1978;38:3784–3792.
22. Kemeny MM, Battifora H, Blayney DW, et al. Sclerosing cholangitis after continuous hepatic artery infusion of FUDR. *Ann Surg.* 1985;202:176–181.
23. Barnett KT, Malafa MP. Complications of hepatic artery infusion: a review of 4580 reported cases. *Int J Gastrointest Cancer.* 2001;30:147–160.
24. Kemeny N, Huang Y, Cohen AM, et al. Hepatic arterial infusion of chemotherapy after resection of hepatic metastases from colorectal cancer. *N Engl J Med.* 1999;341:2039–2048.
25. Kemeny MM, Adak S, Gray B, et al. Combined-modality treatment for resectable metastatic colorectal carcinoma to the liver: surgical resection of hepatic metastases in combination with continuous infusion of chemotherapy--an intergroup study. *J Clin Oncol.* 2002;20:1499–1505.
26. Lygidakis NJ, Sgourakis G, Vlachos L, et al. Metastatic liver disease of colorectal origin: the value of locoregional immunochemotherapy combined with systemic chemotherapy following liver resection. Results of a prospective randomized study. *Hepatogastroenterology.* 2001;48:1685–1691.
27. Kemeny N, Jarnagin W, Gonen M, et al. Phase I/II study of hepatic arterial therapy with floxuridine and dexamethasone in combination with intravenous irinotecan as adjuvant treatment after resection of hepatic metastases from colorectal cancer. *J Clin Oncol.* 2003;21:3303–3309.
28. Kemeny N, Capanu M, D'Angelica M, et al. Phase I trial of adjuvant hepatic arterial infusion (HAI) with floxuridine (FUDR) and dexamethasone plus systemic oxaliplatin, 5-fluorouracil and leucovorin in patients with resected liver metastases from colorectal cancer. *Ann Oncol.* 2009;20:1236–1241.
29. Alberts SR, Roh MS, Mahoney MR, et al. Alternating systemic and hepatic artery infusion therapy for resected liver metastases from colorectal cancer: a North Central Cancer Treatment Group (NCCTG)/ National Surgical Adjuvant Breast and Bowel Project (NSABP) phase II intergroup trial, N9945/CI-66. *J Clin Oncol.* 2010;28:853–858.
30. Kemeny NE, Jarnagin WR, Capanu M, et al. Randomized phase II trial of adjuvant hepatic arterial infusion and systemic chemotherapy with or without bevacizumab in patients with resected hepatic metastases from colorectal cancer. *J Clin Oncol.* 2011;29:884–889.
31. House MG, Kemeny NE, Gonen M, et al. Comparison of adjuvant systemic chemotherapy with or without hepatic arterial infusional chemotherapy after hepatic resection for metastatic colorectal cancer. *Ann Surg.* 2011;254:851–856.
32. Hurwitz H, Fehrenbacher L, Novotny W, et al. Bevacizumab plus irinotecan, fluorouracil, and leucovorin for metastatic colorectal cancer. *N Engl J Med.* 2004;350:2335–2342.
33. Tournigand C, Andre T, Achille E, et al. FOLFIRI followed by FOLFOX6 or the reverse sequence in advanced colorectal cancer: a randomized GERCOR study. *J Clin Oncol.* 2004; 22:229–237.
34. Bokemeyer C, Bondarenko I, Makhson A, et al. Fluorouracil, leucovorin, and oxaliplatin with and without cetuximab in the first-line treatment of metastatic colorectal cancer. *J Clin Oncol.* 2009;27:663–671.
35. Saltz LB, Clarke S, Diaz-Rubio E, et al. Bevacizumab in combination with oxaliplatin-based chemotherapy as first-line therapy in metastatic colorectal cancer: a randomized phase III study. *J Clin Oncol.* 2008;26:2013–2019.
36. Wein A, Riedel C, Bruckl W, et al. Neoadjuvant treatment with weekly high-dose 5-Fluorouracil as 24-hour infusion, folinic acid and oxaliplatin in patients with primary resectable liver metastases of colorectal cancer. *Oncology.* 2003;64:131–138.
37. Chua TC, Saxena A, Liauw W, Kokandi A, Morris DL. Systematic review of randomized and nonrandomized trials of the clinical response and outcomes of neoadjuvant systemic chemotherapy for resectable colorectal liver metastases. *Ann Surg Oncol.* 2010;17:492–501.
38. Blazer DG, III, Kishi Y, Maru DM, et al. Pathologic response to preoperative chemotherapy: a new outcome end point after resection of hepatic colorectal metastases. *J Clin Oncol.* 2008;26:5344–5351.

39. Adam R, Pascal G, Castaing D, et al. Tumor progression while on chemotherapy: a contraindication to liver resection for multiple colorectal metastases? *Ann Surg.* 2004;240:1052–1061; discussion 61–64.
40. Neumann UP, Thelen A, Rocken C, et al. Nonresponse to preoperative chemotherapy does not preclude long-term survival after liver resection in patients with colorectal liver metastases. *Surgery.* 2009;146:52–59.
41. Benoist S, Nordlinger B. The role of preoperative chemotherapy in patients with resectable colorectal liver metastases. *Ann Surg Oncol.* 2009;16:2385–2390.
42. Vauthey JN, Pawlik TM, Ribero D, et al. Chemotherapy regimen predicts steatohepatitis and an increase in 90-day mortality after surgery for hepatic colorectal metastases. *J Clin Oncol.* 2006;24:2065–2072.
43. Rubbia-Brandt L, Audard V, Sartoretti P, et al. Severe hepatic sinusoidal obstruction associated with oxaliplatin-based chemotherapy in patients with metastatic colorectal cancer. *Ann Oncol.* 2004;15:460–466.
44. Chun YS, Laurent A, Maru D, Vauthey JN. Management of chemotherapy-associated hepatotoxicity in colorectal liver metastases. *Lancet Oncol.* 2009;10:278–286.
45. Kooby DA, Fong Y, Suriawinata A, et al. Impact of steatosis on perioperative outcome following hepatic resection. *J Gastrointest Surg.* 2003;7:1034–1044.
46. Ribero D, Wang H, Donadon M, et al. Bevacizumab improves pathologic response and protects against hepatic injury in patients treated with oxaliplatin-based chemotherapy for colorectal liver metastases. *Cancer.* 2007;110:2761–2767.
47. Klinger M, Eipeldauer S, Hacker S, et al. Bevacizumab protects against sinusoidal obstruction syndrome and does not increase response rate in neoadjuvant XELOX/FOLFOX therapy of colorectal cancer liver metastases. *Eur J Surg Oncol.* 2009;35:515–520.
48. Gruenberger B, Tamandl D, Schueller J, et al. Bevacizumab, capecitabine, and oxaliplatin as neoadjuvant therapy for patients with potentially curable metastatic colorectal cancer. *J Clin Oncol.* 2008;26:1830–1835.
49. Ellis LM, Curley SA, Grothey A. Surgical resection after downsizing of colorectal liver metastasis in the era of bevacizumab. J Clin Oncol. 2005;23:4853–4855.
50. Aussilhou B, Dokmak S, Faivre S, Paradis V, Vilgrain V, Belghiti J. Preoperative liver hypertrophy induced by portal flow occlusion before major hepatic resection for colorectal metastases can be impaired by bevacizumab. *Ann Surg Oncol.* 2009;16:1553–1559.
51. Wicherts DA, de Haas RJ, Sebagh M, et al. Impact of bevacizumab on functional recovery and histology of the liver after resection of colorectal metastases. *Br J Surg.* 2011;98:399–407.
52. D'Angelica M, Kornprat P, Gonen M, et al. Lack of evidence for increased operative morbidity after hepatectomy with perioperative use of bevacizumab: a matched case-control study. *Ann Surg Oncol.* 2007;14:759–765.
53. Reddy SK, Morse MA, Hurwitz HI, et al. Addition of bevacizumab to irinotecan- and oxaliplatin-based preoperative chemotherapy regimens does not increase morbidity after resection of colorectal liver metastases. *J Am Coll Surg.* 2008;206:96–106.
54. Kesmodel SB, Ellis LM, Lin E, et al. Preoperative bevacizumab does not significantly increase postoperative complication rates in patients undergoing hepatic surgery for colorectal cancer liver metastases. *J Clin Oncol.* 2008;26:5254–5260.
55. Benoist S, Brouquet A, Penna C, et al. Complete response of colorectal liver metastases after chemotherapy: does it mean cure? *J Clin Oncol.* 2006;24:3939–3945.
56. Nordlinger B, Sorbye H, Glimelius B, et al. Perioperative chemotherapy with FOLFOX4 and surgery versus surgery alone for resectable liver metastases from colorectal cancer (EORTC Intergroup Trial 40983): a randomised controlled trial. *Lancet.* 2008;371:1007–1016.
57. Sorbye H, Mauer M, Gruenberger T, et al. Predictive factors for the benefit of perioperative FOLFOX for resectable liver metastasis in colorectal cancer patients (EORTC Intergroup Trial 40983). *Ann Surg.* 2012;255:534–539.
58. Chiappa A, Bertani E, Makuuchi M, et al. Neoadjuvant chemotherapy followed by hepatectomy for primarily resectable colorectal cancer liver metastases. *Hepatogastroenterology.* 2009;56:829–834.
59. Bathe OF, Ernst S, Sutherland FR, et al. A phase II experience with neoadjuvant irinotecan (CPT-11), 5-fluorouracil (5-FU) and leucovorin (LV) for colorectal liver metastases. *BMC cancer.* 2009;9:156.
60. Nordlinger B, Vauthey JN, Poston G, Benoist S, Rougier P, Van Cutsem E. The timing of chemotherapy and surgery for the treatment of colorectal liver metastases. *Clin Colorectal Cancer.* 2010;9:212–218.
61. Portier G, Elias D, Bouche O, et al. Multicenter randomized trial of adjuvant fluorouracil and folinic acid compared with surgery alone after resection of colorectal liver metastases: FFCD ACHBTH AURC 9002 trial. *J Clin Oncol.* 2006;24:4976–4982.
62. Bernard Langer HB, Labianca R, Shepherd L, Nitti D, Marsoni S, Tu D, et al. Fluorouracil (FU) plus l-leucovorin (l-LV) versus observation after potentially curative resection of liver or lung metastases from colorectal cancer (CRC): results of the ENG (EORTC/NCIC CTG/GIVIO) randomized trial. *Proc Am Soc Clin Oncol.* 2002;21.
63. Mitry E, Fields AL, Bleiberg H, et al. Adjuvant chemotherapy after potentially curative resection of metastases from colorectal cancer: a pooled analysis of two randomized trials. *J Clin Oncol.* 2008;26:4906–4911.
64. Wang X, Hershman DL, Abrams JA, et al. Predictors of survival after hepatic resection among patients with colorectal liver metastasis. *Br J Cancer.* 2007;97:1606–1612.
65. Parks R, Gonen M, Kemeny N, et al. Adjuvant chemotherapy improves survival after resection of hepatic colorectal metastases: analysis of data from two continents. *J Am Coll Surg.* 2007;204:753–61; discussion 61–63.
66. Figueras J, Torras J, Valls C, et al. Surgical resection of colorectal liver metastases in patients with expanded indications: a single-center experience with 501 patients. *Dis Colon Rectum.* 2007;50:478–488.
67. Ychou M, Hohenberger W, Thezenas S, et al. A randomized phase III study comparing adjuvant 5-fluorouracil/folinic acid with FOLFIRI in patients following complete resection of liver metastases from colorectal cancer. *Ann Oncol.* 2009;20:1964–1970.
68. Haller DG, Tabernero J, Maroun J, et al. Capecitabine plus oxaliplatin compared with fluorouracil and folinic acid as adjuvant therapy for stage III colon cancer. *J Clin Oncol.* 2011;29:1465–1471.
69. Kim SY, Kim HJ, Hong YS, et al. Resected colorectal liver metastases: does the survival differ according to postoperative chemotherapy regimen? *J Surg Oncol.* 2009;100:713–718.
70. Taieb J, Artru P, Paye F, et al. Intensive systemic chemotherapy combined with surgery for metastatic colorectal cancer: results of a phase II study. *J Clin Oncol.* 2005;23:502–509.
71. Wieser M, Sauerland S, Arnold D, Schmiegel W, Reinacher-Schick A. Peri-operative chemotherapy for the treatment of resectable liver metastases from colorectal cancer: A systematic review and meta-analysis of randomized trials. *BMC cancer.* 2010;10:309.
72. Kattan MW, Gonen M, Jarnagin WR, et al. A nomogram for predicting disease-specific survival after hepatic resection for metastatic colorectal cancer. Ann Surg. 2008;247:282–287.
73. Scheele J, Stang R, Altendorf-Hofmann A, Paul M. Resection of colorectal liver metastases. *World J Surg.* 1995;19:59–71.
74. Abdalla EK, Vauthey JN, Ellis LM, et al. Recurrence and outcomes following hepatic resection, radiofrequency ablation, and combined resection/ablation for colorectal liver metastases. *Ann Surg.* 2004;239:818–25; discussion 25–27.
75. Choti MA, Sitzmann JV, Tiburi MF, et al. Trends in long-term survival following liver resection for hepatic colorectal metastases. *Ann Surg.* 2002;235:759–766.

76. Fernandez FG, Drebin JA, Linehan DC, Dehdashti F, Siegel BA, Strasberg SM. Five-year survival after resection of hepatic metastases from colorectal cancer in patients screened by positron emission tomography with F-18 fluorodeoxyglucose (FDG-PET). *Ann Surg.* 2004;240:438–47; discussion 47–50.
77. Chun YS, Vauthey JN. Extending the frontiers of resectability in advanced colorectal cancer. *Eur J Surg Oncol.* 2007;33 Suppl 2:S52-S58.
78. Charnsangavej C, Clary B, Fong Y, Grothey A, Pawlik TM, Choti MA. Selection of patients for resection of hepatic colorectal metastases: expert consensus statement. *Ann Surg Oncol.* 2006;13:1261–1268.
79. Jones OM, Rees M, John TG, Bygrave S, Plant G. Biopsy of resectable colorectal liver metastases causes tumour dissemination and adversely affects survival after liver resection. *Br J Surg.* 2005;92:1165–1168.
80. Ramos E, Valls C, Martinez L, et al. Preoperative staging of patients with liver metastases of colorectal carcinoma. Does PET/CT really add something to multidetector CT? *Ann Surg Oncol.* 2011;18:2654–2661.
81. Akhurst T, Kates TJ, Mazumdar M, et al. Recent chemotherapy reduces the sensitivity of [18F]fluorodeoxyglucose positron emission tomography in the detection of colorectal metastases. *J Clin Oncol.* 2005;23:8713–8716.
82. Vauthey JN, Abdalla EK, Doherty DA, et al. Body surface area and body weight predict total liver volume in Western adults. Liver transplantation: official publication of the American Association for the Study of Liver Diseases and the International Liver Transplantation Society 2002;8:233–240.
83. Abdalla EK, Hicks ME, Vauthey JN. Portal vein embolization: rationale, technique and future prospects. *Br J Surg.* 2001;88:165–175.
84. Ribero D, Abdalla EK, Madoff DC, Donadon M, Loyer EM, Vauthey JN. Portal vein embolization before major hepatectomy and its effects on regeneration, resectability and outcome. *Br J Surg.* 2007;94:1386–1394.
85. Chun YS, Vauthey JN, Ribero D, et al. Systemic chemotherapy and two-stage hepatectomy for extensive bilateral colorectal liver metastases: perioperative safety and survival. *J Gastrointest Surg.* 2007;11:1498–1504; discussion 504–505.
86. Brouquet A, Abdalla EK, Kopetz S, et al. High survival rate after two-stage resection of advanced colorectal liver metastases: response-based selection and complete resection define outcome. *J Clin Oncol.* 2011;29:1083–1090.
87. Adam R, Wicherts DA, de Haas RJ, et al. Patients with initially unresectable colorectal liver metastases: is there a possibility of cure? *J Clin Oncol.* 2009;27:1829–1835.
88. Therasse P, Arbuck SG, Eisenhauer EA, et al. New guidelines to evaluate the response to treatment in solid tumors. European Organization for Research and Treatment of Cancer, National Cancer Institute of the United States, National Cancer Institute of Canada. *J Natl Cancer Inst.* 2000;92:205–216.
89. Chun YS, Vauthey JN, Boonsirikamchai P, et al. Association of computed tomography morphologic criteria with pathologic response and survival in patients treated with bevacizumab for colorectal liver metastases. *JAMA.* 2009;302:2338–2344.
90. Karoui M, Penna C, Amin-Hashem M, et al. Influence of preoperative chemotherapy on the risk of major hepatectomy for colorectal liver metastases. *Ann Surg.* 2006;243:1–7.
91. Nakano H, Oussoultzoglou E, Rosso E, et al. Sinusoidal injury increases morbidity after major hepatectomy in patients with colorectal liver metastases receiving preoperative chemotherapy. *Ann Surg.* 2008;247:118–124.
92. White TJ, Roy-Choudhury SH, Breen DJ, et al. Percutaneous radiofrequency ablation of colorectal hepatic metastases - initial experience. An adjunct technique to systemic chemotherapy for those with inoperable colorectal hepatic metastases. *Dig Surg.* 2004;21:314–320.
93. Vauthey JN, Nordlinger B, Kopetz S, Poston G. Sequenced chemotherapy and surgery for potentially resectable colorectal liver metastases: a debate over goals of research and an approach while the jury remains out. *Ann Surg Oncol.* 2010;17:1983–1986.
94. Welsh FK, Tilney HS, Tekkis PP, John TG, Rees M. Safe liver resection following chemotherapy for colorectal metastases is a matter of timing. *Br J Cancer.* 2007;96:1037–1042.
95. Nguyen KT, Geller DA. Outcomes of laparoscopic hepatic resection for colorectal cancer metastases. *J Surg Oncol.* 2010;102:975–977.
96. McCormack PM, Burt ME, Bains MS, Martini N, Rusch VW, Ginsberg RJ. Lung resection for colorectal metastases. 10-year results. *Arch Surg.* 1992;127:1403–1406.
97. Murata S, Moriya Y, Akasu T, Fujita S, Sugihara K. Resection of both hepatic and pulmonary metastases in patients with colorectal carcinoma. *Cancer.* 1998;83:1086–1093.
98. Robinson BJ, Rice TW, Strong SA, Rybicki LA, Blackstone EH. Is resection of pulmonary and hepatic metastases warranted in patients with colorectal cancer? J *Thorac Cardiovasc Surg.* 1999;117:66–75; discussion 6.
99. Watanabe K, Nagai K, Kobayashi A, Sugito M, Saito N. Factors influencing survival after complete resection of pulmonary metastases from colorectal cancer. *Br J Surg.* 2009;96:1058–1065.
100. Abir F, Alva S, Longo WE, Audiso R, Virgo KS, Johnson FE. The postoperative surveillance of patients with colon cancer and rectal cancer. *Am J Surg.* 2006;192:100–108.
101. Reis-Filho JS, Carrilho C, Valenti C, et al. Is TTF1 a good immunohistochemical marker to distinguish primary from metastatic lung adenocarcinomas? *Pathol Res Pract.* 2000;196:835–840.
102. Vogelsang H, Haas S, Hierholzer C, Berger U, Siewert JR, Prauer H. Factors influencing survival after resection of pulmonary metastases from colorectal cancer. *Br J Surg.* 2004;91:1066–1071.
103. Pfannschmidt J, Dienemann H, Hoffmann H. Surgical resection of pulmonary metastases from colorectal cancer: a systematic review of published series. *Ann Thorac Surg.* 2007;84:324–338.
104. Saito Y, Omiya H, Kohno K, et al. Pulmonary metastasectomy for 165 patients with colorectal carcinoma: A prognostic assessment. *J Thorac Cardiovasc Surg.* 2002;124:1007–1013.
105. McAfee MK, Allen MS, Trastek VF, Ilstrup DM, Deschamps C, Pairolero PC. Colorectal lung metastases: results of surgical excision. *Ann Thorac Surg.* 1992;53:780–785; discussion 5–6.
106. Lin BR, Chang TC, Lee YC, Lee PH, Chang KJ, Liang JT. Pulmonary resection for colorectal cancer metastases: duration between cancer onset and lung metastasis as an important prognostic factor. *Ann Surg Oncol.* 2009;16:1026–1032.
107. Labow DM, Buell JE, Yoshida A, Rosen S, Posner MC. Isolated pulmonary recurrence after resection of colorectal hepatic metastases—is resection indicated? *Cancer J.* 2002; 8:342–347.
108. Abulafi AM, Williams NS. Local recurrence of colorectal cancer: the problem, mechanisms, management and adjuvant therapy. *Br J Surg.* 1994;81:7–19.
109. Bouchard P, Efron J. Management of recurrent rectal cancer. *Ann Surg Oncol.* 2010;17:1343–1356.
110. Chen J, Zhao G. Multimodality therapy for patients with locally recurrent rectal cancer. *Colorectal disease: the official journal of the Association of Coloproctology of Great Britain and Ireland.* 2011;13:944–945; author reply 5–6.
111. Hahnloser D, Nelson H, Gunderson LL, et al. Curative potential of multimodality therapy for locally recurrent rectal cancer. *Ann Surg.* 2003;237:502–508.
112. de Chaisemartin C, Penna C, Goere D, et al. Presentation and prognosis of local recurrence after total mesorectal excision. *Colorectal disease: the official journal of the Association of Coloproctology of Great Britain and Ireland.* 2009;11:60–66.
113. Adam IJ, Mohamdee MO, Martin IG, et al. Role of circumferential margin involvement in the local recurrence of rectal cancer. *Lancet.* 1994;344:707–711.
114. Andre T, Boni C, Mounedji-Boudiaf L, et al. Oxaliplatin, fluorouracil, and leucovorin as adjuvant treatment for colon cancer. *N Engl J Med.* 2004;350:2343–2351.

115. Palmer G, Martling A, Cedermark B, Holm T. A population-based study on the management and outcome in patients with locally recurrent rectal cancer. *Ann Surg Oncol.* 2007;14:447–454.
116. Visser O, Bakx R, Zoetmulder FA, et al. The influence of total mesorectal excision on local recurrence and survival in rectal cancer patients: a population-based study in Greater Amsterdam. *J Surg Oncol.* 2007;95:447–454.
117. Kusters M, Marijnen CA, van de Velde CJ, et al. Patterns of local recurrence in rectal cancer; a study of the Dutch TME trial. *Eur J Surg Oncol.* 2010;36:470–476.
118. Baca B, Beart RW, Jr., Etzioni DA. Surveillance after colorectal cancer resection: a systematic review. *Dis Colon Rectum.* 2011;54:1036–1048.
119. Figueredo A, Rumble RB, Maroun J, et al. Follow-up of patients with curatively resected colorectal cancer: a practice guideline. *BMC cancer.* 2003;3:26.
120. Renehan AG, Egger M, Saunders MP, O'Dwyer ST. Impact on survival of intensive follow-up after curative resection for colorectal cancer: systematic review and meta-analysis of randomised trials. *BMJ.* 2002;324:813.
121. Desch CE, Benson AB, 3rd, Somerfield MR, et al. Colorectal cancer surveillance: 2005 update of an American Society of Clinical Oncology practice guideline. *J Clin Oncol.* 2005;23:8512–8519.
122. Goldberg RM, Fleming TR, Tangen CM, et al. Surgery for recurrent colon cancer: strategies for identifying resectable recurrence and success rates after resection. Eastern Cooperative Oncology Group, the North Central Cancer Treatment Group, and the Southwest Oncology Group. *Ann Intern Med.* 1998;129: 27–35.
123. Tepper JE, O'Connell M, Hollis D, et al. Analysis of surgical salvage after failure of primary therapy in rectal cancer: results from Intergroup Study 0114. *J Clin Oncol.* 2003;21:3623–3628.
124. Balbay MD, Slaton JW, Trane N, Skibber J, Dinney CP. Rationale for bladder-sparing surgery in patients with locally advanced colorectal carcinoma. *Cancer.* 1999;86:2212–2216.
125. Tan E, Gouvas N, Nicholls RJ, Ziprin P, Xynos E, Tekkis PP. Diagnostic precision of carcinoembryonic antigen in the detection of recurrence of colorectal cancer. *Surg Oncol.* 2009;18:15–24.
126. Schaefer O, Langer M. Detection of recurrent rectal cancer with CT, MRI and PET/CT. *Eur Radiol.* 2007;17:2044–2054.
127. Potter KC, Husband JE, Houghton SL, Thomas K, Brown G. Diagnostic accuracy of serial CT/magnetic resonance imaging review vs. positron emission tomography/CT in colorectal cancer patients with suspected and known recurrence. *Dis Colon Rectum.* 2009;52:253–259.
128. Maas M, Rutten IJ, Nelemans PJ, et al. What is the most accurate whole-body imaging modality for assessment of local and distant recurrent disease in colorectal cancer? A meta-analysis: imaging for recurrent colorectal cancer. *Eur J Nucl Med Mol Imaging.* 2011;38:1560–1571.
129. de Anda EH, Lee SH, Finne CO, Rothenberger DA, Madoff RD, Garcia-Aguilar J. Endorectal ultrasound in the follow-up of rectal cancer patients treated by local excision or radical surgery. *Dis Colon Rectum.* 2004;47:818–824.
130. Garcia-Aguilar J, Cromwell JW, Marra C, Lee SH, Madoff RD, Rothenberger DA. Treatment of locally recurrent rectal cancer. *Dis Colon Rectum.* 2001;44:1743–1748.
131. Heriot AG, Byrne CM, Lee P, et al. Extended radical resection: the choice for locally recurrent rectal cancer. *Dis Colon Rectum.* 2008;51:284–291.
132. You YN, Habiba H, Chang GJ, Rodriguez-bigas MA, Skibber JM. Prognostic value of quality of life and pain in patients with locally recurrent rectal cancer. *Ann Surg Oncol.* 2011;18:989–996.
133. Kodeda K, Derwinger K, Gustavsson B, Nordgren S. Local recurrence of rectal cancer: a population-based cohort study of diagnosis, treatment and outcome. *Colorectal disease: the official journal of the Association of Coloproctology of Great Britain and Ireland.* 2012;14:e230–237.
134. Enriquez-Navascues JM, Borda N, Lizerazu A, et al. Patterns of local recurrence in rectal cancer after a multidisciplinary approach. World journal of gastroenterology: *WJG.* 2011;17:1674–1684.
135. Suzuki K, Dozois RR, Devine RM, et al. Curative reoperations for locally recurrent rectal cancer. *Dis Colon Rectum.* 1996;39:730–736.
136. Moore HG, Shoup M, Riedel E, et al. Colorectal cancer pelvic recurrences: determinants of resectability. *Dis Colon Rectum.* 2004;47:1599–1606.
137. Boyle KM, Sagar PM, Chalmers AG, Sebag-Montefiore D, Cairns A, Eardley I. Surgery for locally recurrent rectal cancer. *Dis Colon Rectum.* 2005;48:929–937.
138. Bowne WB, Lee B, Wong WD, et al. Operative salvage for locoregional recurrent colon cancer after curative resection: an analysis of 100 cases. *Dis Colon Rectum.* 2005;48:897–909.
139. Lee JH, Kim DY, Kim SY, et al. Clinical outcomes of chemoradiotherapy for locally recurrent rectal cancer. *Radiation oncology.* 2011;6:51.
140. Vermaas M, Nuyttens JJ, Ferenschild FT, Verhoef C, Eggermont AM, de Wilt JH. Reirradiation, surgery and IORT for recurrent rectal cancer in previously irradiated patients. *Radiother Oncol.* 2008;87:357–360.
141. Mohiuddin M, Marks G, Marks J. Long-term results of reirradiation for patients with recurrent rectal carcinoma. *Cancer.* 2002;95:1144–1150.
142. Akiyoshi T, Fujimoto Y, Konishi T, et al. Prognostic factors for survival after salvage surgery for locoregional recurrence of colon cancer. *Am J Surg.* 2011;201:726–733.
143. Park JK, Kim YW, Hur H, et al. Prognostic factors affecting oncologic outcomes in patients with locally recurrent rectal cancer: impact of patterns of pelvic recurrence on curative resection. *Langenbecks Arch Surg.* 2009;394:71–77.
144. Kusters M, Dresen RC, Martijn H, et al. Radicality of resection and survival after multimodality treatment is influenced by subsite of locally recurrent rectal cancer. *Int J Radiat Oncol Biol Phys.* 2009;75:1444–1449.
145. Wanebo HJ, Antoniuk P, Koness RJ, et al. Pelvic resection of recurrent rectal cancer: technical considerations and outcomes. *Dis Colon Rectum.* 1999;42:1438–1448.
146. Saito N, Suzuki T, Sugito M, et al. Bladder-sparing extended resection of locally advanced rectal cancer involving the prostate and seminal vesicles. *Surg Today.* 2007;37:845–852.
147. Nisar PJ, Scott HJ. Myocutaneous flap reconstruction of the pelvis after abdominoperineal excision. *Colorectal disease: the official journal of the Association of Coloproctology of Great Britain and Ireland.* 2009;11:806–816.
148. Mirnezami AH, Sagar PM, Kavanagh D, Witherspoon P, Lee P, Winter D. Clinical algorithms for the surgical management of locally recurrent rectal cancer. *Dis Colon Rectum.* 2010;53:1248–1257.
149. Saito N, Koda K, Takiguchi N, et al. Curative surgery for local pelvic recurrence of rectal cancer. *Dig Surg.* 2003;20:192–199; discussion 200.
150. Valentini V, Morganti AG, Gambacorta MA, et al. Preoperative hyperfractionated chemoradiation for locally recurrent rectal cancer in patients previously irradiated to the pelvis: A multicentric phase II study. *Int J Radiat Oncol Biol Phys.* 2006;64:1129–1139.
151. Bedrosian I, Giacco G, Pederson L, et al. Outcome after curative resection for locally recurrent rectal cancer. *Dis Colon Rectum.* 2006;49:175–182.
152. Asoglu O, Karanlik H, Muslumanoglu M, et al. Prognostic and predictive factors after surgical treatment for locally recurrent rectal cancer: a single institute experience. *Eur J Surg Oncol.* 2007;33:1199–1206.

153. Schurr P, Lentz E, Block S, et al. Radical redo surgery for local rectal cancer recurrence improves overall survival: a single center experience. *J Gastrointest Surg.* 2008;12:1232–1238.
154. Pacelli F, Tortorelli AP, Rosa F, et al. Locally recurrent rectal cancer: prognostic factors and long-term outcomes of multimodal therapy. *Ann Surg Oncol.* 2010;17:152–162.
155. Bakx R, Visser O, Josso J, Meijer S, Slors JF, van Lanschot JJ. Management of recurrent rectal cancer: a population based study in greater Amsterdam. *World J Gastroenterol.* 2008;14:6018–6023.
156. Yamada K, Ishizawa T, Niwa K, Chuman Y, Aikou T. Pelvic exenteration and sacral resection for locally advanced primary and recurrent rectal cancer. *Dis Colon Rectum.* 2002;45:1078–1084.
157. Moriya Y, Akasu T, Fujita S, Yamamoto S. Total pelvic exenteration with distal sacrectomy for fixed recurrent rectal cancer. *Surg Oncol Clin N Am.* 2005;14:225–238.
158. Melton GB, Paty PB, Boland PJ, et al. Sacral resection for recurrent rectal cancer: analysis of morbidity and treatment results. *Dis Colon Rectum.* 2006;49:1099–1107.
159. Akasu T, Yamaguchi T, Fujimoto Y, et al. Abdominal sacral resection for posterior pelvic recurrence of rectal carcinoma: analyses of prognostic factors and recurrence patterns. *Ann Surg Oncol.* 2007;14:74–83.
160. Sagar PM, Gonsalves S, Heath RM, Phillips N, Chalmers AG. Composite abdominosacral resection for recurrent rectal cancer. *Br J Surg.* 2009;96:191–196.
161. Dozois EJ, Privitera A, Holubar SD, et al. High sacrectomy for locally recurrent rectal cancer: Can long-term survival be achieved? J Surg Oncol. 2011;103:105–109.
162. Harrison LB, Minsky BD, Enker WE, et al. High dose rate intraoperative radiation therapy (HDR-IORT) as part of the management strategy for locally advanced primary and recurrent rectal cancer. *Int J Radiat Oncol Biol Phys.* 1998;42:325–330.
163. Kumar PP, Good RR, Conlan MG, Edney JA, Hodgson PE, McCaul GF. Postoperative adjuvant irradiation of rectal and rectosigmoid cancer. *Radiat Med.* 1988;6:289–296.
164. Yamazaki H, Inoue T, Ikeda H, et al. High-dose-rate remote afterloading intestinal radiotherapy employing the template technique for recurrent cancer in the pelvic area. *Strahlenther Onkol.* 1993;169:481–485.
165. Tanderup K, Hellebust TP, Honore HB, et al. Dose optimisation in single plane interstitial brachytherapy. *Radiother Oncol.* 2006;81:105–111.
166. Wiig JN, Tveit KM, Poulsen JP, Olsen DR, Giercksky KE. Preoperative irradiation and surgery for recurrent rectal cancer. Will intraoperative radiotherapy (IORT) be of additional benefit? A prospective study. *Radiother Oncol.* 2002;62:207–213.
167. Pezner RD, Chu DZ, Ellenhorn JD. Intraoperative radiation therapy for patients with recurrent rectal and sigmoid colon cancer in previously irradiated fields. *Radiother Oncol.* 2002;64:47–52.
168. Alektiar KM, Zelefsky MJ, Paty PB, et al. High-dose-rate intraoperative brachytherapy for recurrent colorectal cancer. *Int J Radiat Oncol Biol Phys.* 2000;48:219–226.
169. Dresen RC, Gosens MJ, Martijn H, et al. Radical resection after IORT-containing multimodality treatment is the most important determinant for outcome in patients treated for locally recurrent rectal cancer. *Ann Surg Oncol.* 2008;15:1937–1947.
170. Idrees K, Minsky B, Alektiar K, et al. Surgical resection and high dose rate intraoperative radiation therapy for locally recurrent rectal cancer. *Acta Chir Iugosl.* 2004;51:11–18.
171. Ito Y, Ohtsu A, Ishikura S, et al. Efficacy of chemoradiotherapy on pain relief in patients with intrapelvic recurrence of rectal cancer. *Jpn J Clin Oncol.* 2003;33:180–185.
172. Esnaola NF, Cantor SB, Johnson ML, et al. Pain and quality of life after treatment in patients with locally recurrent rectal cancer. *J Clin Oncol.* 2002;20:4361–4367.
173. Swarm R, Abernethy AP, Anghelescu DL, et al. Adult cancer pain. *J Natl Compr Canc Netw.* 2010;8:1046–1086.
174. Ambiru S, Miyazaki M, Ito H, Nakagawa K, Shimizu H, Nakajima N. Adjuvant regional chemotherapy after hepatic resection for colorectal metastases. *Br J Surg.* 1999;86:1025–1031.
175. Lygidakis NJ, Ziras N, Parissis J. Resection versus resection combined with adjuvant pre- and post-operative chemotherapy—immunotherapy for metastatic colorectal liver cancer. A new look at an old problem. *Hepatogastroenterology.* 1995;42:155–161.
176. Rudroff C, Altendorf-Hoffmann A, Stangl R, Scheele J. Prospective randomised trial on adjuvant hepatic-artery infusion chemotherapy after R0 resection of colorectal liver metastases. *Langenbecks Arch Surg.* 1999;384:243–249.
177. Tono T, Hasuike Y, Ohzato H, Takatsuka Y, Kikkawa N. Limited but definite efficacy of prophylactic hepatic arterial infusion chemotherapy after curative resection of colorectal liver metastases: a randomized study. *Cancer.* 2000;88:1549–1556.
178. Wagman LD, Kemeny MM, Leong L, et al. A prospective, randomized evaluation of the treatment of colorectal cancer metastatic to the liver. *J Clin Oncol.* 1990;8:1885–1893.
179. Kemeny N, Huang Y, Cohen AM, et al. Hepatic arterial infusion of chemotherapy after resection of hepatic metastases from colorectal cancer. *N Engl J Med.* 1999;341:2039–2048.
180. Kemeny NE, Gonen M. Hepatic arterial infusion after liver resection. *N Engl J Med.* 2005;352:734–735.
181. Kemeny MM, Adak S, Gray B, et al. Combined-modality treatment for resectable metastatic colorectal carcinoma to the liver: surgical resection of hepatic metastases in combination with continuous infusion of chemotherapy—an intergroup study. *J Clin Oncol.* 2002;20:1499–1505.
182. Lygidakis NJ, Sgourakis G, Vlachos L, et al. Metastatic liver disease of colorectal origin: the value of locoregional immunochemotherapy combined with systemic chemotherapy following liver resection. Results of a prospective randomized study. *Hepatogastroenterology.* 2001;48:1685–1691.
183. Kemeny N, Jarnagin W, Gonen M, et al. Phase I/II study of hepatic arterial therapy with floxuridine and dexamethasone in combination with intravenous irinotecan as adjuvant treatment after resection of hepatic metastases from colorectal cancer. *J Clin Oncol.* 2003;21:3303–3309.
184. Kemeny N, Capanu M, D'Angelica M, et al. Phase I trial of adjuvant hepatic arterial infusion (HAI) with floxuridine (FUDR) and dexamethasone plus systemic oxaliplatin, 5-fluorouracil and leucovorin in patients with resected liver metastases from colorectal cancer. *Ann Oncol.* 2009;20:1236–1241.
185. Alberts SR, Roh MS, Mahoney MR, et al. Alternating systemic and hepatic artery infusion therapy for resected liver metastases from colorectal cancer: a North Central Cancer Treatment Group (NCCTG)/ National Surgical Adjuvant Breast and Bowel Project (NSABP) phase II intergroup trial, N9945/CI-66. *J Clin Oncol.* 2010;28:853–858.
186. Kemeny NE, Jarnagin WR, Capanu M, et al. Randomized phase II trial of adjuvant hepatic arterial infusion and systemic chemotherapy with or without bevacizumab in patients with resected hepatic metastases from colorectal cancer. *J Clin Oncol.* 2011;29:884–889.
187. House MG, Kemeny NE, Gonen M, et al. Comparison of adjuvant systemic chemotherapy with or without hepatic arterial infusional chemotherapy after hepatic resection for metastatic colorectal cancer. *Ann Surg.* 2011;254:851–856.
188. Adson MA, van Heerden JA, Adson MH, Wagner JS, Ilstrup DM. Resection of hepatic metastases from colorectal cancer. *Arch Surg.* 1984;119:647–651.
189. Scheele J, Stangl R, Altendorf-Hofmann A, Gall FP. Indicators of prognosis after hepatic resection for colorectal secondaries. *Surgery.* 1991;110:13–29.
190. Nordlinger B, Guiguet M, Vaillant JC, et al. Surgical resection of colorectal carcinoma metastases to the liver. A prognostic scoring system to improve case selection, based on 1568 patients. Association Francaise de Chirurgie. *Cancer.* 1996;77:1254–1262.

191. Minagawa M, Makuuchi M, Torzilli G, et al. Extension of the frontiers of surgical indications in the treatment of liver metastases from colorectal cancer: long-term results. *Ann Surg.* 2000;231:487–499.
192. Choti MA, Sitzmann JV, Tiburi MF, et al. Trends in long-term survival following liver resection for hepatic colorectal metastases. *Ann Surg.* 2002;235:759–766.
193. Pawlik TM, Scoggins CR, Zorzi D, et al. Effect of surgical margin status on survival and site of recurrence after hepatic resection for colorectal metastases. *Ann Surg.* 2005;241:715–22, discussion 22–24.
194. House MG, Ito H, Gonen M, et al. Survival after hepatic resection for metastatic colorectal cancer: trends in outcomes for 1,600 patients during two decades at a single institution. *J Am Coll Surg.* 2010;210:744–52, 52–55.

II Systemic Therapy

First-Line Chemotherapy

JAYKUMAR THUMAR
HOWARD S. HOCHSTER

Approximately 20% of patients with colorectal cancers (CRC) will present with distant metastasis at time of presentation. Although a subset of these patients will have oligometastatic disease to lung or liver that can be cured with aggressive multimodality approaches, for the majority of patients treatment remains palliative. Although the goals of systemic therapy differ with each clinical scenario, prolongation of overall survival and improving quality of life (QOL) are the main objectives for the majority of patients.

In the last decade, the development of combination regimens and the addition of multiple biological agents has revolutionized the treatment of CRC. The overall survival, which was estimated to be around 12 months in the era of single-agent 5-fluorouracil (5-FU), has more than doubled (1).

AGENTS APPROVED FOR FIRST-LINE THERAPY FOR METASTATIC COLON CANCER

Fluropyrimidines

5-FU and Leucovorin

5-FU, a key member of the pyrimidine antimetabolite family, remains the backbone of treatment regimens for metastatic CRC (MCRC). It inhibits thymidylate synthetase (TS) by its metabolite fluorodeoxyuridine monophosphate (FdUMP), which leads to inhibition of methylation of deoxyuridylic acid and thus impairs DNA synthesis (2).

Leucovorin (LV, folinic acid), a reduced form of folic acid and biochemical modulator, enhances the cytotoxic effects of 5-FU. It stabilizes the binding of FdUMP and TS, forming a stable ternary complex and thus prolonging inhibition of the TS by 5-FU. Systematic analysis of 19 randomized trials concluded that combining LV with FU provided a higher response rate (RR) compared to bolus 5-FU alone and translated into a small but statistically significant improvement in 1-year survival (3). Between 1980 and 2000, several clinical trials were conducted to study the efficacy and toxicity of various dosing schedules of 5-FU/LV. A meta-analysis of six randomized trials with 1219 patients concluded that infusional 5-FU was superior to 5-FU bolus in terms of RR and achieved a slight increase in the overall survival (3).

Since 2000, a regimen of a bolus followed by a 24 to 48 hours infusion of 5-FU/LV (de Gramont regimen; 4) has become the standard of care, especially when combining this with newer agents (irinotecan and oxaliplatin). This has led to the development of first-line regimens that use the de Gramont regimen as its backbone 5-FU plus LV plus oxaliplatin (FOLFOX [FOLinic acid, 5-FU and OXaliplatin]) and 5-FU plus LV plus irinotecan (FOLFIRI [same with IRInotecan]; Table 11.1). In elderly patients with poor performance status, 5-FU/LV alone is the preferred first-line regimen. A short infusional protocol (de Gramont type) is preferred to the bolus regimen (Mayo regimen) due to its favorable toxicity profile and better tumor response.

Capecitabine

Capecitabine (Xeloda) is an orally active fluoropyrimidine analogue. It is absorbed through the intestinal tract and is converted to 5-FU, via a three-step enzymatic process. The liver is the primary site of its metabolism, where it is converted initially to 5-deoxy-5-fluorocytidine and then to 5′-deoxy-5-fluorouridine (5′DFUR). The daily administration of capecitabine results in the antitumor and toxicity profile of infusional 5-FU, thus eliminating the need for central venous line and infusion pump (5).

Two randomized trials have shown similar efficacy for capecitabine monotherapy (1250 mg/m^2 twice daily

Table 11.1 Select Chemotherapy Regimens for Metastatic Colon Cancer

Regimen	Fluorouracil/Capecitabine	Leucovorin	Oxaliplatin	Irinotecan	Cycle Schedule
Mayo regimen	Bolus 5-FU: 425 mg/m^2 days 1 to 5	20 mg/m^2 days 1 to 5			Every 4 to 6 weeks
deGramont regimen (LV5FU2)	Bolus 5-FU: 400 mg/m^2 Infusion 5-FU: 600 mg/m^2 × 22 hr both on Days 1 and 2	200 mg/m^2 Over 2 hr before on days 1 and 2			Every 2 weeks
FOLFOX-4	Bolus 5-FU: 400 mg/m^2 Infusion 5-FU: 600 mg/m^2 for 22 hr both on days 1 and 2	400 mg/m^2 Over 2 hr days 1 and 2	85 mg/m^2 Day 1		Every 2 weeks
FOLFOX-6	Bolus 5-FU: 400 mg/m^2 Infusion 5-FU: 2400 mg/m^2 for 46 hr	400 mg/m^2 Over 2 hr day 1	100 mg/m^2 Day 1		Every 2 weeks
mFOLFOX-6	Bolus 5-FU: 400 mg/m^2 Infusion 5-FU: 2400 mg/m^2 for 46 hr	400 mg/m^2 Over 2 hr before 5-FU	85 mg/m^2 day 1		Every 2 weeks
(m)FOLFOX-7 Optimox and CONcePT	Infusion: 5-FU 2400-3000 mg/m^2 over 46 hr	400 mg/m^2 Over 2 hr day 1	85–130 mg/m^2 Day 1		Every 2 weeks
CapeOX TREE-1 and TREE-2	Capecitabine 850–1000 mg/m^2 orally twice daily days 1 to 14		130 mg/m^2 Day 1		Every 3 weeks
Douillard regimen	Bolus 5-FU: 400 mg/m^2 Infusion 5-FU: 600 mg/m^2 for 22 hr both on days 1 and 2	200 mg/m^2 Over 2 hrs days 1 and 2 before 5-FU 5-FU		180 mg/m^2 day 1	Every 2 weeks
FOLFIRI GERCORstudy	Bolus 5-FU: 400 mg/m^2 Infusion 5-FU: 2400–3000 mg/m^2 for 46 hr	400 mg/m^2 Over 2 hr day 1		180 mg/m^2 day 1	Every 2 weeks

for 14 of every 21 days) as compared to 5-FU/LV (the Mayo regimen) for the first-line treatment of MCRC (6,7). Capecitabine was associated with a lower incidence of mucositis, neutropenia, and alopecia, but a higher incidence of hand and foot syndrome (HFS) and hyperbilirubinemia. Capecitabine is approved as monotherapy when single-agent fluoropyrimidine is indicated. It should be noted that capecitabine is cleared by the kidneys and requires dose reduction patients with reduced growth factor receptor (GFR).

Multiple phase III trials have compared the efficacy of capecitabine plus oxaliplatin (CapeOX) to various combinations of 5-FU and oxaliplatin. CapeOX was shown to be noninferior compared to FOLFOX. A systematic review of six randomized phase II and III trials concluded that CapeOX was associated with a lower RR when compared with infusional 5-FU regimens, but that this did not translate into significant differences in progression-free survival (PFS) and overall survival (OS). CapeOX regimens were associated with more grade 3 to 4 thrombocytopenia and grade 2 to 3 HFS (8).

In summary, CapeOX is probably as effective as FOLFOX in the treatment of MCRC. Substituting capecitabine for infusional 5-FU may add the convenience of oral administration. However, the cost of therapy (variations in reimbursement policies) and toxicities (higher in certain population) are the key issues to be considered in decision making. The safety and efficacy data for the capecitabine-based regimes were established in European trials, where 1000 mg/m^2 twice daily is the standard dose. In the United States, this dosing schedule as part of the CapeOX regimen, when studied in the TREE-1 trial, was associated with significant toxicities including grade 3/4 diarrhea (31%) and dehydration (27%). A reduced dose of 850 mg/m^2 twice daily in the subsequent amendment in the TREE-2 arm showed improved tolerability as well as clinical efficacy. Based on the TREE-2 trial results, for the U.S. patient population, 850 mg/m^2 twice daily dose is preferable (9).

The bolus and infusional protocols differ in their toxicity profiles. Hematologic toxicities are more common with bolus 5-FU (31% vs 4%), while hand-foot syndrome (HFS) is more common in infusional 5-FU (34% vs 13%; 3). Dihydropyrimidine dehydrogenase (DPD) is a rate-limiting enzyme in 5-FU catabolism, which converts 5-FU to inactive dihydrofluorouracil (DHFU). Patients with partial or total deficiency of DPD develop severe life-threatening toxicities, including severe diarrhea, mucositis, and pancytopenia. Certain genetic polymorphisms in the promoter region of TS gene (TYMS) are also associated with higher toxicities. Commercially available molecular testing (TheraGuide 5-FU, Myriad Laboratories) is indicated in patients who experience severe adverse reactions after receiving a fluoropyrimidine-containing regimen, but upfront testing to diagnose DPD deficiency for all patients undergoing treatment with 5-FU is not cost effective and not routinely performed (10).

Camptothecins

Irinotecan

Irinotecan, a topoisomerase I inhibitor, is a pro-drug and semi-synthetic analog of the parent compound camptothecin. It is active as monotherapy in advanced CRC and is converted to its active metabolite SN-38 (7-ethyl-10-hydroxy-camptothecin) in the liver by carboxylesterase enzymes. SN-38 reversibly binds to the topoisomerase I-DNA complex and prevents the re-ligation of the cleaved DNA strands, resulting in "replication fork collision," which leads to cell death in the S-phase of the replication cycle. The combinations of irinotecan with 5-FU and biological agents (bevacizumab and cetuximab) have synergistic cytotoxicity and translate into higher clinical efficacy.

Three pivotal trials showed a survival benefit of combining irinotecan with 5-FU/LV (FOLFIRI type regimen in two European trials and bolus IFL regimen in one USA trial) compared to 5-FU/LV alone in the first-line setting (11–13). The FOLFIRI regimen was associated with a significantly higher RR (35% vs 22%; $P < .005$), median PFS (6.7 vs 4.4 months; $P < .001$) and median OS (17.4 vs 14.1 months; $P = .031$). Higher rates of toxicities were seen in FOLFIRI arm, mainly grade 3/4 diarrhea (24% vs 11%; $P = .05$) and grade 3/4 neutropenia (15% vs 1%; $P < .001$) but they were manageable and noncumulative (12).

The IFL regimen in a US study showed similar benefits when compared to bolus 5-FU/LV given by the Mayo schedule but was associated with significantly higher toxicities (13). A retrospective review of two clinical trials (Cancer and Leukemia Group B protocol C89803 and North Center Cancer Treatment Group protocol N9741) showed that the IFL regimen was associated with increased toxicities and 30-day mortality (14). This was confirmed in the BICC-C randomized phase III trial, which showed higher toxicity and lower efficacy for even a modified IFL regimen as compared with FOLFIRI. In the bevacizumab-containing arms, the reported median OS was higher than any other reported trial (15). The IFL regimen has therefore fallen out of favor in clinical practice.

The adverse reactions commonly associated with irinotecan are early and late phase diarrhea, dehydration, and neutropenia. SN-38, the active metabolic of irinotecan, is conjugated by UDP-glucuronosyl transferase 1A1 (UGT1A1) to form a glucuronide metabolite. Patients with genetic polymorphism of UGT1A1 (the UGT1A1*28 allele, 10% of North Americans are homozygous for this allele) may have more severe toxicities, mainly neutropenia. FDA-approved genetic testing is available (Invader UGT1A1 Molecular Assay) but data regarding the benefits and role of testing are controversial. In clinical practice, irinotecan should be used with caution in patients with Gilbert disease and elevated bilirubin.

In summary, FOLFIRI is considered a standard first-line treatment regimen for MCRC. However, in clinical practice in the United States, oncologists generally use this regimen as second-line therapy after failure of first-line FOLFOX regimen. FOLFIRI is the preferred first-line regimen in patients with preexisting neuropathy.

Platinum Compounds

Oxaliplatin

Oxaliplatin, a third-generation platinum compound and an alkylating agent, does not have significant activity as a single-agent but has significant synergism with 5-FU in MCRC (16). The cytotoxic action is cell-cycle nonspecific and mediated by formation of DNA cross-links leading to inhibition of DNA transcription and replication.

The benefit of adding oxaliplatin to 5-FU/LV (FOLFOX-4) was reported in the first-line setting in a phase III trial in which 420 patients were randomly assigned to 5-FU with LV (de Gramont regimen), either alone or with oxaliplatin (85 mg/m^2 on day 1). The FOLFOX4 regimen had a significantly higher objective RR and median PFS but similar median OS (16.2 vs 14.7 months; $P = .12$). Higher rates of grade 3/4 neutropenia, grade 3/4 diarrhea, and grade 3 neurotoxicity were noted in the FOLFOX arm (17).

The FOLFOX regimen (oxaliplatin, short-term infusional 5-FU and LV) is considered a standard first-line treatment option for MCRC. Over the last 10 years, several variations of FOLFOX were studied in clinical trials (Table 11.1) and modified FOLFOX6 (mFOLFOX6) is the most commonly used regimen in the United States.

Neurotoxicity is the major dose limiting toxicity of oxaliplatin. There are two distinct clinical entities: (a) chronic cumulative sensory neuropathy with distal sensory loss, and (b) acute and short-lived neurotoxicity, which includes paresthesia and dysesthesia involving extremities, face, jaw, laryngo-pharynx (pharyngo-laryngodysesthesias), and cold-induced pseudolaryngospasm. Acute hypersensitivity reactions are also commonly reported and the main symptoms are varying degree of skin rash, fever, and respiratory distress. Premedications with steroids and antihistamines are usually given for prevention of these infusion reactions.

Empirical use of Ca/Mg administration was associated with significant decrease in the incidence and intensity of acute oxaliplatin-induced symptoms when compared to controls (16). The CONcePT (Combined Oxaliplatin Neurotoxicity Prevention Trial) trial was as a 2 × 2 factorial study with two study interventions: (a) intermittent use of oxaliplatin in eight cycle blocks in the setting of FOLFOX-bevacizumab treatment (OPTIMOX concept); and (b) use of IV Ca/Mg pre- and postoxaliplatin infusion (18). An unplanned interim analysis by the independent data monitoring committee in the first 174 patients found that those patients who received Ca/Mg salts had significantly lower RR than the control group and the study was terminated (19). Subsequently, a blinded independent radiology review committee reviewed the actual scans of the randomized patients and found no differences in response rates. TTF was significantly longer in patients with the intermittent oxaliplatin strategy.

In a retrospective analysis of data collected in the phase III CAIRO II clinical trial, prophylactic use of Ca/Mg infusions was found to decrease oxaliplatin-related sensory neurotoxicity and have no effect on RR, PFS, or OS (20). In summary, the available literature suggests that the supplemental use of Ca/Mg reduces oxaliplatin associated neurotoxicity, though the benefit on the cumulative dose delivery remains uncertain. Despite the concerns that were raised by an interim analysis in the CONcePT trial, the use of Ca/Mg does not have a detrimental effect on response rate. In the metastatic setting, supplemental Ca/Mg infusions (1 g calcium gluconate plus 1 g magnesium sulfate 30 minutes pre- and postoxaliplatin) are recommended to decrease the severity of oxaliplatin-induced peripheral neurotoxicity.

Biological Agents

Anti-VEGF Targeted Therapy: Bevacizumab (Avastin)

Bevacizumab (Avastin, Genentech), is a humanized monoclonal antibody directed against all isoforms of the vascular endothelial growth factor-A (VEGF-A), a member of the family of VEGF-receptor activating ligands. In a pivotal trial, the combination of IFL with bevacizumab resulted in significant improvement in RR, PFS, and OS (20). Based on these data, bevacizumab was approved by the FDA for the treatment of MCRC in combination with fluoropyrimidine based regimens.

Subsequently, multiple trials have investigated combining bevacizumab with both irinotecan and oxaliplatin-based regimens. The addition of bevacizumab to bolus 5-FU/LV when compared to bolus 5-FU/LV alone resulted in a higher median PFS and RR (21). Studies combining bevacizumab to cytotoxic chemotherapy did not demonstrate as large a benefit for the combination as was seen in the initial trial (Table 11.3).

In the TREE-2 trial, patients were assigned to bevacizumab (5 mg/kg every 2 weeks) and one of three different oxaliplatin and 5-FU-containing regimens (mFOLFOX6, bFOL, CapeOx). The addition of bevacizumab showed an increase in median OS when compared to the historical control of the TREE-1 trial (9).

In the N016966 trial, patients were randomly assigned to CapeOX vs FOLFOX4 in a 2 × 2 factorial design, and then to bevacizumab vs placebo (22). Median PFS was significantly better in the two bevacizumab-containing groups (9.4 vs 8.0 months; $P < .0023$); however, the magnitude of benefit was smaller compared to the other trials.

Combining bevacizumab with first-line FOLFIRI has not been tested in a large randomized trial. The Bevacizumab Expanded Access Trial (BEAT) was an open-label, noncomparative study where 1927 previously untreated patients received bevacizumab plus a chemotherapy regimen chosen by the individual clinician. This study found that the median PFS and OS for patients treated with FOLFIRI/bevacizumab was 11.6 and 23.7 months, respectively (23).

Bevacizumab is associated with rare, but potentially life-threatening side effects. Commonly encountered side effects are proteinuria, hypertension, bleeding, bowel perforation, impaired wound healing, arterial (but not venous) thromboembolic events (such as transient ischemic attack, stroke, angina, myocardial infarction), and reversible posterior multifocal leucoencephalopathy.

About one-third of the patients report epistaxis. Fatal hemoptysis has been reported in squamous cell lung cancer patients and, therefore, a recent history of hemoptysis is an absolute contraindication to the use of this drug. Lung metastasis from colon primary is not a contraindication for the treatment with bevacizumab.

Patients receiving bevacizumab have an increased risk of arterial thromboembolic events (ATEs). A recent meta-analysis of data in Genentech-supported trials demonstrated an overall risk ratio of 1.46 for bevacizumab compared with chemotherapy alone. Age over 65 years (hazard ratio [HR], 2.1) and prior history of ATEs (HR, 4.18) were independent risk factor for ATEs (24). The role of aspirin in prevention of ATEs is not established but is recommended for high-risk patients.

Table 11.2 Select Clinical Trials of Capecitabine

Clinical Trials	Trial Arms	5-FU	Leucovorin	Capecitabine	Oxaliplatin	Response Rate (%)	Median Overall Survival (Months)	Time to Progression (Months)
Monotherapy								
Van Cutsem (7) 2001 $N = 602$	A: Capecitabine vs B:5-FU/LV	bolus 425 mg/m² 1–5/every 4 weeks	20 mg/m² day 1 to 5/every 4 weeks	1250 mg/m² BID days 1 to 14 every 21 days		A: 18.9 vs B: 15	A: 13.2 vs B: 12.1 $P = 0.33$	A: 5.2 vs B: 4.7 $P = .65$ HR 0.92
Hoff (6) $N = 605$	A: Capecitabine vs B: 5-FU/LV	bolus 425 mg/m² 1–5/every 4 weeks.	20 mg/m² days 1 to 5/every 4 weeks	C: 1250 mg/m² BID days 1 to 14 every 21 days		A: 24.8 vs B: 15.5 $P = .005$	A: 12.5 vs B: 13.3 $P = .974$ HR 1.00	A: 4.3 vs B: 4.7 $P = .72$ HR 1.03
Combination Regimen								
Porschen AIO Trial $N = 474$	A: CapeOX vs B: FUFOX	5-FU 2000 mg/m², 22 hr infusion days 1, 8, 15,22 every 36 days	500 mg/m² days 1,8, 15,22 every 36 days	1000 mg/m² bid days 1 to 14 every 21 days	CAPOX: 70 mg/m² days 1 and 8 FUFOX: 50 mg/m² days 1,8,15, and 22, repeated every 36 days	A: 48 vs B: 54 $P = .7$	A: 16.8 vs B: 18.8 $P = .26$ HR 1.12	A: 7.1 vs B: 8.0 $P = .117$ HR 1.17
Díaz-Rubio 2007 Spanish Cooperative Group Trial 9 $N = 348$	A: CapeOX vs B: FUOX	FU 2250 mg/m² 48 hrs infusion on days 1, 8, 15, 22, 29, and 36		1000 mg/m² bid days 1 to 14 every 21 days	85 mg/m² on days 1, 15, and 29 every 6 weeks	A: 37 vs B: 46 P = .539	A: 18.1 vs B: 20.8 $P = .145$	A: 8.9 vs B: 9.5 $P = .153$
Cassidy, 2007 NO16966A $N = 2034$	2×2 design A: CapeOX with or without bevacizumab vs B: FOLFOX-4 with or without bevacizumab	Bolus 400 mg/m² then 600 mg/m² over 22 hr, days 1 and 2	400 mg/m² days 1 and 2	1000 mg/m² bid days 1 to 14 every 21 days	A: 130 mg/m² day 1 B: 85 mg/m² day 1	A: 37 vs B: 37	A: 19.8 vs B: 19.6 HR 0.99	A: 8.0 vs B: 8.5 HR 1.04
Ducreux 2011 ML16987 $N = 306$	A: CapeOX vs B: FOLFOX-6	Bolus 400 mg/m² than 2400–3000 mg/m² over 46 hr every 2 weeks	400 mg/m² day 1	1000 mg/m² bid days 1 to 14 every 21 days	A: 130 mg/m² day 1 B: 100 mg/m² on day 1	A: 42 vs B: 46	A: 19.9 vs B: 20.5 HR 1.02	A: 8.8 vs B:9.3 HR 1.0

Table 11.3 Select Clinical Trials of Biologics

Selected Clinical Trials	Arms	Response Rate (%)	Overall Survival (Months)	Progression-Free Survival (Months)
Bevacizumab				
Hurwitz (25) phase III *N* = 813	A: IFL with bevacizumab B: IFL	A: 44.8 vs B: 34.8 *P* = .004	A: 20.3 vs B: 15.6 *P* < .001 HR 0.66	A: 10.6 vs B: 6.2 *P* < .001 HR 0.54
Kabbinavar (21) phase II *N* = 209	A: 5-FU/LV bolus with bevacizumab B: 5-FU/LV	A:2 6.0 vs B: 15.2 *P* = .05	A: 16.6 vs B: 12.9 *P* = .16 HR 0.79	A: 9.2 vs B: 5.5 *P* = .002 HR 0.50
Saltz (22) N016966 (2×2 design) phase III *N* =1401	A: FOLFOX vs CapeOx with bevacizumab B: FOLFOX vs CapeOx	A: 47 vs B: 49 *P* = .31	A: 21.3 vs B: 19.9 *P* = .07 HR 0.89	A: 9.4 vs B: 8.0 *P* = .0023 HR 0.83
Hochster (9) TREE-1 and TREE-2 phase II N:TREE-1 = 150 N:TREE-2 = 223	TREE-1 A: mFOLFOX6 C: bFOL E: CapeOx TREE-2 B: mFOLFOX6 with bevacizumab D:bFOL with bevacizumab F:CapeOx with bevacizumab	B: 52 vs A: 41 D: 39 vs C: 20 F: 46 vs E: 27	B: 26.1 vs A: 19.2 D: 20.4 vs C: 17.9 F: 24.6 vs E: 17.2	B: 9.9 vs A: 8.7 D: 8.3 vs C: 6.9 F: 10.3 vs E: 5.9
Cetuximab				
Cunningham (27) BOND trial, phase III *N* =329 third or fourth line	A: Irinotecan with cetuximab B: Cetuximab	A: 22.9 vs B: 10.8 *P* = .007	A: 8.6 vs B: 6.9 *P* = .48	A: 4.1 vs B: 1.5 *P* < .001
Van Cutsem (29) CRYSTAL trial, Phase III *N* =1198	A: FOLFIRI with cetuximab B: FOLFIRI	A: 46.9 vs B: 38.7 *P* = .004 A: 59.3 vs B: 43.2* OR = 1.91 95% CI: 1.24–2.93	A: 19.9 vs B: 18.6 A: 24.9 vs B: 21.0* HR 0.84 95% CI 0.64–1.11	A: 8.9 vs B: 8.0 *P* = .48 A: 9.9 vs B: 8.4* *P* = .02 HR 0.68
Bokemeyer 2009 (30) OPUS trial, phase II *N* =337	A: FOLFOX4 with cetuximab B: FOLFOX4	A: 45.6 vs B: 35.7 *P* = 0 .064 A: 61 vs B: 37* *P* = .01	NR	A: 7.7 vs B: 7.2* *P* = .02 HR 0.57
Maughan, 2011 (31) Medical Research Council-COIN, phase III *N* = 1630	A: FOLFOX or CapeOX B: Combination plus cetuximab C: Intermittent chemotherapy	A: 57 vs B: 64* *P* = 0·049	A: 17·9 vs B: 17·0* *P* = 0·67	A: 8.6 vs B: 8·6* *P* = 0·60
Panitumumab				
Van Cutsem, 2007 (32) phase III *N* =463 previously treated	A: Panitumumab B: BSC	A: 10 vs B: 0 *P* < .0001 A: 17 vs B: 0*	NR	A: 8 vs B: 7.3 *P* < .0001 HR 0.54 A: 12.3 vs B: 7.3* *P* < .0001 HR 0.45

(Continued)

Table 11.3 *(Continued)*

Peeters, 2010 (73) phase III N = 1186 (second line)	A: Panitumumab with FOLFIRI B: FOLFIRI	A: 35 vs B: 10* P < .001	A: 14.5 vs B: 12.5* P = .12 HR 0.85	A: 5.9 vs B: 3.9* P = .004 HR 0.73
Douillard, 2010 (33) PRIME trial phase III N = 1183 first line	A: FOLFOX4 with panitumumab B: FOLFOX4	A: 55 vs B: 48 P = .068	A: 29.3 vs B: 19.7 P = .072 HR 0.83	A: 9.6 vs B: 8.0 P = .02

The risk of a wound healing complication in patients undergoing surgery was reported to be 13% (25). Due to its long half-life of 20 days, it is generally recommended to avoid major elective surgeries for 6 to 8 weeks of the last dose.

In summary, to date, many randomized phase III trials have been conducted to study the benefit of bevacizumab in first-line treatment when added to bIFL-, FOLFIRI-, or FOLFOX- based regimens. These studies have shown variable benefit for adding bevacizumab to combination chemotherapy in the first-line therapy of CRC.

Anti-Epidermal Growth Factor Receptor Targeted Therapy

The over expression or upregulation of epidermal growth factor receptor (EGFR), a member of the ErbB family of receptors, is reported in 60%–80% patients with CRC and is associated with a poor survival. Two FDA approved monoclonal antibodies, cetuximab (Erbitux, chimeric human-mouse, IgG1) and panitumumab (Vectibix, recombinant fully human IgG2), block the ligand-binding site of the EGFR and inhibit the ligand-induced phosphorylation and intracellular signal transduction. Both antibodies have single-agent activity as well as synergistic cytotoxicity with chemotherapy agents in MCRC.

Approximately 40% of patients with MCRC harbor an activating mutation in the *K-ras* gene (mainly found in codons 12, 13, and 61), which isolates the downstream pathway from the effect of the EGFR signaling. The benefit of EGFR-based therapy is limited to patients with *K-ras* wild-type tumors. Neither of these agents should be used in patients with *K-ras* mutations in codons 12 or 13 (26).

Cetuximab (Erbitux)

Numerous studies have shown that cetuximab can be used both as a single-agent as well as combined with chemotherapy in the first-line setting. In the BOND trial, combining cetuximab with irinotecan partially circumvented irinotecan resistance translating into higher RR and median PFS as well as a trend toward better OS (27). EGFR expression in tumor samples by immunohistochemistry did not correlate significantly with the clinical RR (Table 11.3).

In the CRYSTAL trial, previously untreated patients were randomly assigned to FOLFIRI with or without cetuximab. In the initial results of unselected patients, the addition of cetuximab to FOLFIRI showed a modest impact on median PFS and no effect on OS (28). In the retrospective follow up of this trial, when *K-ras* mutation status was available for 89% of tumors, in patient with *K-ras* wild-type MCRC, the addition of cetuximab to FOLFIRI significantly improved median OS, median PFS, and RR compared with FOLFIRI alone (29). The rate of surgery for metastases was higher in the cetuximab–FOLFIRI group, as was the rate of R0 resection with curative intent (Table 11.3).

The role of cetuximab in combination with FOLFOX has been studied in multiple trials as first-line therapy. In the multicenter European OPUS trial (FOLFOX4 with or without cetuximab), the addition of cetuximab was associated with a higher RR and median PFS (30) (Table 11.3).

The UK-based phase III trial, Medical Research Council COIN, combined cetuximab with FOLFOX or CapeOx regimen and also addressed the role of intermittent therapy. The addition of cetuximab resulted in an increase in RR but overall survival did not improve (31). However, it should be noted that this survival is quite short when compared with recent comparable studies (Table 11.3).

Panitumumab (Vectibix)

Panitumumab has shown single-agent antitumor activity in refractory MCRC (32). Unlike cetuximab, adding panitumumab to an oxaliplatin-based regimen clearly improved clinical efficacy. The results of the PRIME trial showed that panitumumab improved the RR, PFS, and median OS when compared to FOLFOX4 (33). Panitumumab alone has not been studied in combination with the FOLFIRI in the first-line setting in a randomized trial.

The common adverse effects of the anti-EGFR therapies include acneiform rash, fatigue, malaise, nausea, diarrhea, and infusion reactions. Diffuse papulpo-pustular eruption is a common class specific side effect that occurs in more than 70% of unselected patients and can be severe in 5%–10% cases. This is a dose-dependent side effect and usually involves the face, trunk, and extremities. In patients with moderate to severe rash, dose modifications are required. The severity of rash generally correlates with better outcomes.

Infusion reaction occurs in 3% of the patients treated with cetuximab and most occur with the first dose. Premedication with an H1 blocker and steroids are usually administered for prevention. Panitumumab, being a fully human antibody, is associated with lower rates of infusion reactions and has an advantage over cetuximab in Midwest and Southern regions of the United States where a higher incidence of infusion reactions has been reported. These reactions are due to natural background immunity to cross-reacting antigens on cetuximab (34).

Magnesium wasting syndrome is seen in approximately 10%–20% of patients receiving anti-EFGR antibodies. Secondary hypokalemia and hypocalcaemia are also frequently reported side effects. Close monitoring and replacement of magnesium, calcium, and potassium is recommended.

In summary, EGFR-directed therapies are clinically beneficial. In patients with *K-ras* wild-type tumors (especially patients with contraindications to bevacizumab), adding EGFR-targeted therapy (cetuximab or panitumumab) to FOLFIRI or FOLFOX may provide higher RR and could be beneficial in patients with symptomatic disease. While the addition of cetuximab to FOLFOX improved the response rate and PFS in the OPUS and CAIRO trials, a survival advantage has not been reported in any of the phase III trials. In particular, the MRC COIN and NORDIC VII studies have shown divergent results.

GENERAL PRINCIPLES OF THE THERAPY FOR MCRC

Is Chemotherapy Beneficial in MCRC?

The estimated median survival of patients who receive only best supportive care is approximately 6 months. The 5YS of patients treated with 5-FU/LV alone is approximately 1% and is 9.8% with FOLFOX.

When to Initiate the Treatment?

Most patients with Stage IV colon cancer are asymptomatic at time of diagnosis. The benefit of initiating systemic treatment early (when the patient is asymptomatic) vs late phase (when the patient develops symptoms) has not been studied. In the era of single-agent 5-FU, clinical trials showed benefit to initiating early treatment and the results have been extrapolated to current regimens.

Single Versus Combination Chemotherapy as an Initial Treatment?

Based on the results of many phase III trials, median survival of patients correlates with exposure to all active agents (1). Hence it is conceivable that treatment with sequential single agents may provide a better outcome over combination chemotherapy, postulating that more options might be available to patients when they develop disease progression while on monotherapy.

This question of initial combination vs sequential single-agent therapy was directly studied in two randomized clinical trials (FOCUS and CAIRO; 36–38). In the United Kingdom Medical Research Council's FOCUS (Fluorouracil, Oxaliplatin, CPT-11: Use and Sequencing) trial, patients were randomized to one of three arms. Control arm A received 5-FU/LV followed by irinotecan monotherapy at the time of progression; experimental arm B received 5-FU/LV followed by FOLFOX or FOLFIRI; experimental arm C received initial combination FOLFOX or FOLFIRI. The CAIRO trial (CApecitabine, IRinotecan, Oxaliplatin trial) randomized patients in to sequential arm (capecitabine followed by irinotecan monotherapy and then CapeOx) vs combination arm (initial CapIRI followed by CapeOx). Both trials showed no difference in median survival among patients treated with first-line single-agents vs combination therapy. Multiple concerns were raised in both trials including the low median survival for all groups in both trials.

A pooled analysis of five phase III clinical trials have predicted 3.5 months improvement in median survival in patients receiving first-line combination chemotherapy compared to monotherapy in MCRC (1). Patients treated with first-line combination therapy are more likely to receive all three active agents in the course of their therapy than those who start with monotherapy.

In summary, the current data support combination regimens as frontline treatment for most patients. Such upfront treatment will maximize the RR, duration of response, and potentially improve chances of resection for patients with oligometastatic disease.

Sequence of Regimens: Does It Matter?

Based on a meta-analysis of several phase III clinical trials, overall survival of patients with advanced CRC is strongly correlated with administration of all active agents (1). The superiority of any particular first-line regimen has not been established. The GERCOR study was the largest, yet still underpowered, randomized phase III trial designed to investigate two sequences of first-line treatment: FOLFIRI followed by FOLFOX6 vs FOLFOX6 followed by FOLFIRI. RR, median survival, and PFS were similar in both arms but the toxicity profiles were different (35). Therefore the actual sequence of administration (ie, irinotecan- or oxaliplatin-based regimen as first-line therapy) appears to be less critical and, therefore, the specific regimen is based on the goals of therapy and toxicity profile.

Duration of the First-Line Therapy: Continuous Versus Intermittent?

Oxaliplatin causes cumulative neurotoxicity and the incidence of grade 3 to 4 neuropathy rapidly rises after a total dose of 640 mg/m^2 (usually after 4 months of biweekly regimen). Thus, intermittent rather than continuous treatment seems a logical approach to minimize the cumulative toxicity. Another option is to discontinue chemotherapy all together (chemotherapy "holiday") or to omit only a particular agent like oxaliplatin and continue maintenance regimen of 5-FU and bevacizumab or other antibody. The results of many randomized clinical trials investigating these questions have been inconsistent.

In the OPTIMOX1 trial, a "stop-and-go" approach for oxaliplatin was compared with the standard first-line therapy. A total of 620 previously untreated patients were randomly assigned to either control arm A of FOLFOX4 (administered every 2 weeks until disease progression) or experimental arm B of FOLFOX7 (with higher doses of oxaliplatin) given for six cycles only, followed by reintroduction of oxaliplatin after up to 12 cycles of a nonoxaliplatin-containing FU/LV maintenance regimen. The outcomes did not differ significantly among the groups in terms of RR (58.5% in arm A vs 59.2% in arm B), median progression-free survival (9.0 months in arm A vs 8.7 months in arm B), and overall survival (19.3 months in arm A vs 21.2 months in arm B). In follow-up analysis, authors concluded that oxaliplatin reintroduction had an independent and significant impact on the OS (HR, 0.56; $P = .009$), but the survival benefit for maintenance nonoxaliplatin chemotherapy could have been masked as only 40% patient received the planned oxaliplatin reintroduction (35).

A phase III Italian trial randomized patients to receive first-line FOLFIRI regimen in group A (intermittent 2 months on and 2 months off) and group B (continuous). The outcomes among the two arms were similar in terms of PFS and overall survival. Grades 3 to 4 toxicities (myelosuppression, fever, and diarrhea) were similar among the two groups and median chemotherapy free interval was 3.5 month in group A. The trial was, however, substantially underpowered to detect clinically relevant differences. Additional studies are needed to clarify the role of intermittent irinotecan-based regimen (36).

In NO16966 trial, the addition of bevacizumab to XELOX or FOLFOX4 regimens had significantly improved PFS. However, the extent of benefit was strikingly lower than seen in prior phase III trials and there was no impact on RR or OS. The authors have suggested that early discontinuation of both bevacizumab and fluoropyrimidine prior to disease progression may have weakened the influence of bevacizumab, thereby limiting its impact on OS and PFS (22,25,37).

In summary, patients receiving first-line FOLFOX regimen with or without bevacizumab, complete discontinuation of chemotherapy (no maintenance therapy) appears to be detrimental. Patients should be followed closely to detect early signs of progression and treatment can be reinitiated. Continuous therapy is preferred for patients with a good response, minimal toxicities, and aggressive and/or bulky disease. Intermittent oxaliplatin treatment (as in the CONcePT trial with 4 month blocks of therapy) can be helpful in extending TTF. It is reasonable to withhold oxaliplatin at the earliest onset of neuropathy to avoid developing severe neuropathy. 5-FU and bevacizumab could be continued and oxaliplatin can be reintroduced early at the first signs of disease progression. For patient who achieves CR after first-line FOLFOX, continuation of the therapy beyond two additional cycles was not associated with improved outcome and discontinuation of the therapy with close follow up can be considered.

Response Assessment

Radiographic evaluation (mainly CT scans) should be performed at 2 to 3 month intervals and RECIST (Response Evaluation Criteria In Solid Tumors) should be utilized for objective response measurements (38). Carcinoembryonic antigen (CEA) is an important biomarker in management of metastatic colon cancer. However, kinetics of CEA is clinically more relevant than variation in serum levels between 2 points (39). Persistent and more importantly a rapid rise in CEA level correlates with disease progression, but confirmation with imaging modalities is recommended prior to switching therapy (40). It is important to exercise caution in interpreting CEA levels in the first few weeks after starting first-line chemotherapy since a rapid surge in levels can occur in 10% of patients (41).

First Line FOLFOX Versus FOLFIRI?

FOLFOX is a commonly used first-line regimen in the United States. The North Central Cancer Treatment Group (NCCTG)/U.S. Intergroup trial N9741 randomly assigned patients to IFL, FOLFOX4, or Irinotecan plus oxaliplatin (IROX; oxaliplatin 85 mg/m^2, irinotecan 200 mg/m^2, both on days 1, 3 weekly cycle). In the final analysis FOLFOX4 emerged superior to both IFL and IROX with regard to response rate as well as toxicity profile (42,43). Since then, IFL and IROX have fallen out of favor and are not routinely used in clinical practice. Subsequently two clinical trials have confirmed the equal efficacy of adding oxaliplatin or irinotecan to 5-FU/LV (FOLFOX and FOLFIRI regimens; 44). In the GERCOR study when FOLFOX6 vs FOLFIRI were compared in the first-line treatment of MCRC where both groups were allowed to crossover at progression, overall survival was approximately 21 months in both groups (45).

A phase III Italian study randomized 336 patients to FOLFOX4 versus FOLFIRI and confirmed the findings reported in GERCOR (44). Both groups were similar in terms of RR, time to progression (TTP) and OS. Toxicity profiles of each regimen were different but the incidence of grade 3 to 4 toxicities were uncommon and similar in both arms.

Thus, FOLFOX and FOLFIRI are both considered acceptable choices for first-line therapy and the selection of regimens is generally based on the expected toxicity. FOLFOX is commonly used as first-line in the United States, but in patients with pre-existing neuropathy FOLFIRI is preferable. The original FOLFOX regimen described by deGramont (FOLFOX-4, bolus LV and 5-FU on days 1 and 2 and relatively low-dose 5-FU) has now been replaced in clinical practice by mFOLFOX6 (omits day 2 bolus) or modified FOLFOX7 (omits day 1 and 2 bolus).

■ CONCLUSIONS

Even though its goal is mainly palliative, the use of systemic therapy (with or without biologics) substantially prolongs survival in patients with MCRC. In the era of single-agent 5-FU, median survival was 12 to 13 months, which was increased to 16 to 17 months with the use of combination regimens (FOLFOX or FOLFIRI). The addition of biologics to chemotherapy has resulted in median survival of 24 months with many patients surviving longer than 3 years. A subset of patients with oligometastatic liver metastasis, an aggressive multimodality approach could be potentially curative. For patients with good performance status, doublet combinations (FOLFOX, FOLFIRI, or CapeOx) are considered the standard. These regimens have similar clinical efficacy and the choice of which first-line regimen to use is based on the toxicity profile. Bevacizumab should generally be added to the first-line chemotherapy regimen but the clinical benefit should be carefully balanced against the rare but potentially life-threatening side effects. For patients with *K-ras* wild-type tumors and/or contraindications to bevacizumab, anti-EGFR, based therapy (cetuximab or panitumumab) can be added to first-line combination chemotherapy.

A key concept in the treatment of metastatic colorectal cancer is that exposure to all available agents (fluoropyrimidines, irinotecan, oxaliplatin, bevacizumab, and anti-EGFR antibodies) will lead to the longest overall survival and best quality of life. Intermittent use of oxaliplatin or reintroduction of oxaliplatin plus treatment-free intervals should be used as clinically appropriate. Judicial use of these agents in combination and sequentially can yield the best outcomes.

■ Second- and Third-Line Therapy for MCRC

NEETA K. VENEPALLI
JORDAN BERLIN

■ THERAPY AFTER PROGRESSION

General Principles

In the past decade, the treatment paradigm for MCRC has shifted from separate "lines" of treatment to a continuum of care that emphasizes optimizing patient benefit through exposure to all active agents throughout therapy (46). A combined analysis of 11 phase III trials published in 2004, showed a positive correlation between survival and exposure to all cytotoxic drugs regardless of sequence of therapy (1,47). The five classes of active agents include fluoropyrimidines (5-fluorouracil [5-FU] and capecitabine), irinotecan, oxaliplatin, epidermal growth factor inhibitors (cetuximab and panitumumab), and vascular endothelial growth factor (VEGF) inhibitors (bevacizumab, aflibercept, and regorafenib). The optimal combination and sequencing of these agents is not yet established, but treatment strategies should be directed toward specific treatment goals (such as disease stability vs tumor shrinkage for resection), patient comorbidities, and disease characteristics (such as *K-ras* mutation status). The choice of subsequent lines of therapy is most dependent on the first-line regimen.

■ SECOND-LINE CHEMOTHERAPY AFTER FIRST-LINE PROGRESSION

Based on three large phase III trials, it is estimated that 50%–70% of patients progressing on first-line therapy will receive second-line therapy, and only 49% of patients progressing on second-line therapy will receive third-line therapy (48,49). These data highlight that only 25% to 33% of patients who fail first-line therapy ultimately receive third-line therapy (50).The highest response rates (RR) in the first-line setting are associated with doublet cytotoxic regimens in combination with bevacizumab. Regardless of the initial chemotherapy regimen, second-line therapy with active agents is associated with an OS benefit in comparison to best supportive care (BSC; Table 11.4). Exposure to all active agents and utilization of synergistic doublet combinations are more important than any particular sequencing. As in the first-line setting, active single-agents in further lines of treatment include 5-FU, irinotecan, cetuximab, and panitumumab; active agents with little single-agent activity include oxaliplatin and bevacizumab. Tournigand et al's crossover study was the first to report median OS in excess of 20 mos with exposure to all three cytotoxic agents, regardless of the sequence of doublet therapy (45; Table 11.4).

Postfailure of Single-Agent 5-FU

First-line 5-FU plus leucovorin (LV) is generally reserved for patients unable to tolerate chemotherapy doublets, and is associated with median OS of 13 to 14.6 months, progression-free survival (PFS) of 5.6 months, and RR of 24.5%. Phase III studies in 5-FU- resistant disease have demonstrated OS benefit for second-line irinotecan (single-agent and in combination with 5-FU) and oxaliplatin (in combination with 5-FU/LV (FOLFOX), and in combination with irinotecan; 51). Oxaliplatin monotherapy is not recommended because of poor single-agent activity (52). Table 11.4 summarizes phase III and selected phase II data for second-line treatment with irinotecan and oxaliplatin-based regimens after failure of 5-FU based chemotherapy in bevacizumab naïve patients.

After first-line 5-FU failure, second-line irinotecan yields superior OS and improved QOL in comparison to BSC (53), and superior OS with comparable toxicities in comparison to infusional 5-FU (54). Second-line irinotecan is associated with comparable efficacy whether given weekly or every 3 weeks (55). However, the addition of oxaliplatin (IROX) improves efficacy in comparison to irinotecan alone (56). IROX is associated with significant improvement in median OS, TTP, RR, tumor-related symptoms, as well as comparable grade 3 to 4 toxicities except for granulocytopenia, diarrhea, and sensory disturbances. The phase III Intergroup N9841 trial demonstrated noninferiority in terms of OS with second-line FOLFOX4 compared to irinotecan through randomization of 491 patients after first-line 5-FU failure and mandated crossover after second-line disease progression (50). Median OS was similar for both second-line arms although RR and TTP were significantly higher for the FOLFOX4 arm in comparison to irinotecan. For patients initiating third line therapy (46% of the initial population), median OS was similar in both arms despite higher RR and longer TTP in the third line FOLFOX arm.

Postfailure of Irinotecan

After progression of first-line irinotecan, second-line options with documented benefit include oxaliplatin in combination with 5-FU/LV or capecitabine (Table 11.4), FOLFOX plus bevacizumab (Table 11.5), and cetuximab

Table 11.4 Phase III Trials of Second-Line Treatment After Failure of First-Line 5-FU-Based Chemotherapy

Author	Phase	First-Line Treatment	Second-Line Treatment	N	RR (%) Second Line	PFS (Mos)	Median OS (Mos)
Cunningham et al (53)	III	5-FU	BSC	90	NR	NR	**6.5**
			IRI q 3 wk + BSC	189			**9.2 *P* = . 0001**
Rougier et al (54)	III	5-FU	CI 5-FU	134	NR	**2.9 *P* = .030**	**8.5 *P* = .035**
			IRI q 3 wk	133		**4.2**	**10.8**
Fuchs et al (55)	III	5-FU	IRI 125 mg/m² q 1 wk	95	NR	4.0 *P* = .54	9.9 *P* = .43
			IRI 300–350 mg/m² q 3 wk	196		3.0	9.9
Haller et al (56)	III	5-FU or	IROX	318	**22 *P* < 0.0001**	**5.3 *P* < 0.0001**	**13.8 *P* = 0.0069**
		Xeloda	IRI q 3 wk	310	**7**	**2.8**	**11.1**
Kim et al (50)	III	5-FU	FOLFOX4 → IRI	246 → 97	**13.6 *P* = .039**	**5.8 *P* = .0022**	15.9 *P* = .7691
			IRI q 3 wk → FOLFOX4	245 →130	**5.2****	**3.3****	14.9**
Rothenberg et al (52)	III	IFL	FOLFOX4	270	**9.6 *P* < .0001**	**5.6 *P* < .0001**	9.8 *P* = .07
			Infusional 5-FU/LV	272	**0.7**	**2.6**	8.7 HR = 0.84
			Oxaliplatin	274	1.1*	1.9*	8.1
Rothenberg et al (82)	III	IRI regimen	FOLFOX4	314	18	4.8	12.5
			CAPEOX	313	20	4.7 HR = 0.97	11.9 HR = 1.02
Tournigand et al (45)	III	FOLFIRI	FOLFOX6	82	15 *P* = 0.05	4.2 14.2**	21.5** *P* = 0.99
		FOLFOX6	FOLFIRI	68	4*	2.5* 10.9**	20.6**
Cunningham et al (53)	III	IRI + 5-FU	C	111	**22.9 *P* = .007**	**4.1 *P* < .001**	8.6 *P* = .48
		62% prior OX	C+IRI	218	**10.8**	**1.5 HR = 0.54**	6.9 HR = .91
Giantonio et al (37)	III	5-FU and IRI	FOLFOX4 + B	286	**22.7 *P* < .0001**	**7.3 *P* < .0001**	**12.9 *P* = .0011**
			FOLFOX4	291	**8.6**	**4.7** HR = 0.61	**10.8** HR = 0.75
			B	243	3.3	2.7	10.2
Bidard et al (57)	III	FOLFOX4	FOLFIRI-1	112	8	**3.0 *P* = .001**	NR
		FOLFOX 7	FOLFIRI-3	109	17	**3.7**	In total: 9.3
		(OX break)	Other: Irinotecan based	121	6	2.3	
Fornaro et al (59)	III	FOLFOXIRI	FOLFOXIRI	32	**38 *P* = .003**	**8.2 *P* = .001**	**19.3 *P* < .001**
			Doublets + B or + C	52	**28**	**6.3**	**14.0**

Bold: significant improvement with addition of agent.

*By independent review.

**OS of all lines (first plus second plus third).

5-FU, 5-fluorouracil; CI, continuous infusion; IRI, irinotecan; OX, oxaliplatin; IFL, bolus 5-FU plus irinotecan; FOLFOX, biweekly 5-FU (infusional and bolus) plus leucovorin plus oxaliplatin; FOLFIRI, biweekly 5-FU (infusional and bolus) plus leucovorin plus irinotecan; CAPEIRI, capecitabine plus irinotecan; CAPEOX, capecitabine plus oxaliplatin; FOLFOXIRI, biweekly 5-FU (infusional) plus leucovorin plus oxaliplatin plus irinotecan; S FOLFOXIRI: simplified FOLFOXIRI; C, cetuximab; B, bevacizumab; BSC, best supportive care; TX, treatment; N, number of patients; RR, response rates; PFS, median progression free survival; OS, overall survival; mos, months; NR, not reported; HR, hazard ratio for death (or progression, with PFS).

Table 11.5 Nonfirst-Line Treatment with Bevacizumab, Aflibercept, Regorafenib; Results of Phase III and Select Phase II Trials

Author	Phase	Agent	Prior TX	Study Arms	N	RR (%)	PFS (Mos)	Median OS (Mos)
Grothey et al (60)	PCS	B	First line chemo + B	Post progression TX + B Post progression TX no B No TX postprogression	642 531 253	NR	Total: 10.0	**31.8** ***P* < .001** **19.9** HR = 0.48 12.6
Giantonio et al (37)	III	B	First line 5-FU + IRI	FOLFOX4 + B FOLFOX4 B	286 291 243	**22.7** ***P* < .0001** **8.6** 3.3	**7.3** ***P* < .0001** **4.7** HR = 0.61 2.7	**12.9** ***P* = .0011** **10.8** HR = 0.75 10.2
Moriwaki et al (63)	PCS	B	First line 5-FU + IRI First line 5-FU + OX	FOLFOX + B FOLFIRI + B	45 115	29 25	7.8 8.3	16.5 21.6
Bennouna et al (61)	II	B	First line OX or IRI regimens	FOLFOX + B FOLFIRI, XELIRI, IRI + B	14 39	29 33	5.3 7.8 (total: 6.5)	13.9 22.4 (total: 19.3)
Chen et al (64)	II	B	Both OX and IRI regimens	Roswell Park 5-FU + B de Gramont 5-FU + B	73 27	4 (1*)	3.5	9.0
Vincenzi et al (65)	II	B	First line OX Second line IRI Third line C + IRI	de Gramont 5-FU + B	48	6.5	3.5	7.7
Van Cutsem et al (83)	III	A	First line OX Prior B 30.4%	FOLFIRI + aflibercept FOLFIRI + placebo	614 612	**19.8** ***P* = .0001** **11.1**	**6.9** ***P* = .0007** **4.67**	**13.5** ***P* = .0032** **12.06**
Grothey et al (78)	III*	R	Heavily pretreated	Regorafenib + BSC placebo + BSC	505 255	**1.6** ***P* < .000001** **0.4**	**1.9** ***P* < .000001** **1.7 HR = 0.493**	**6.4** ***P* = .0051** **5.0 HR = 0.773**

Bold: significant improvement with addition of agent.

*By independent review.

PCS, prospective cohort study; B, bevacizumab; A, aflibercept; R, regorafenib; 5FU, 5-fluorouracil; IRI, irinotecan; OX, oxaliplatin; FOLFOX, biweekly 5-FU (infusional and bolus) plus leucovorin plus oxaliplatin; FOLFIRI, biweekly 5-FU (infusional and bolus) plus leucovorin plus irinotecan; CAPEIRI, capecitabine + irinotecan; BSC, best supportive care; TX, treatment; N, number of patients; RR, response rates; PFS, median progression free survival; OS, overall survival; mos, months; NR, not reported; HR, hazard ratio for death (or progression, with PFS).

Table 11.6 Nonfirst-Line Treatment with Cetuximab and Panitumumab: Results of Phase III and Select Phase II Trials

Author	Phase	Agent	Prior Treatment	Study Arms	N	RR (%)	Median PFS (Mos)	Median OS (Mos)	*K-ras* avlb?
Sobrero et al (72)	III	C	First-line 5-FU + OX 12.8% prior B	IRI + C IRI	648 650	**16.4 *P* < .0001**	**4.0 *P* < .0001** **2.6 HR = 0.69**	10.7 *P* = .71 10 HR = 0.97	No
Peeters et al (73)	III	Pan	First line 5-FU 60% prior OX 17% prior B	FOLFIRI + Pan FOLFIRI	303** 294	**35 *P* < .001** 10	**5.9 *P* = .004** **3.9** HR = 0.73	14.5 *P* = .12 12.5 HR = 0.85	Yes
Cunningham et al (27)	III	C	IRI + 5-FU 62% with prior OX	IRI + C C	218 111	**22.9 *P* = .007** **10.8**	**4.1 *P* < .001** **1.5 HR = 0.54**	8.6 *P* = .48 6.9 HR = .91	No
Vincenzi et al (65)	II	C	First-line OX and second-line IRI	IRI + C	55	25.4	4.7	9.8	No
Jonker et al (75)	III	C	>96% with prior OX and IRI	C + BSC BSC	117* 113	12.8 0	**3.7 *P* < .001** **1.9 HR = 0.40**	**9.5 *P* < .001** **4.8 HR = 0.55**	Yes
Van Cutsem et al (84)	III	Pan	At least two lines prior treatment	Pan + BSC BSC (76% crossover)	231 232	**10 *P* < .0001** 0	**8w *P* < .0001** **7.3w** HR = 0.54	NR HR = 1	No

Bold: significant improvement with addition of agent.

*Only *K-ras* WT patients included in this table.

C, cetuximab; Pan = panitumumab; B, bevacizumab; 5FU, 5-fluorouracil; IRI, irinotecan; OX, oxaliplatin; FOLFOX, biweekly; 5-FU (infusional and bolus) plus leucovorin plus oxaliplatin; FOLFIRI, biweekly 5-FU (infusional and bolus) plus leucovorin plus irinotecan; BSC, best supportive care; TX, treatment; N, number of patients; RR, response rates; PFS, median progression free survival; OS, overall survival; mos, months; NR, not reported; HR, hazard ratio for death (or progression, with PFS); avlb, available.

plus irinotecan (Table 11.6). The phase III EFC4584 trial confirmed superiority of second-line FOLFOX to single-agent infusional 5-FU and single-agent oxaliplatin after first-line failure of IFL (bolus 5-FU, LV, and irinotecan; 51). Second-line FOLFOX was associated with a significantly higher RR, TTP, and improvement in tumor-related symptoms without an increase in treatment discontinuation or 60-day mortality. Following first-line bolus 5-FU, infusional 5-FU demonstrated minimal yet significant improvement in TTP, and improved RR and OS in comparison to oxaliplatin monotherapy. Second-line capecitabine plus oxaliplatin (XELOX) demonstrated similar PFS to FOLFOX4 in a phase III noninferiority trial (55). Sequencing trials (phase III study of FOLFOX6 → FOLFIRI, vs. FOLFIRI → FOLFOX6 (45) have determined that the sequence of cytotoxics does not influence outcomes; both studies reported noninferiority of either sequencing with similar OS. The addition of biologics to second-line cytotoxic therapy after irinotecan failure improves efficacy (27,37).

Postfailure Oxaliplatin

Second-line irinotecan (in combination with 5-FU/LV or capecitabine) is efficacious after first-line oxaliplatin plus fluoropyrimidine failure (Table 11.4). Both the GERCOR study (45) as well as the OPTIMOX 1 phase III study (56). Interestingly, despite comparable OS in the Tournigand study with both doublet sequences of FOLFOX ï FOLFIRI and FOLFIRI ïFOLFOX, the FOLFIRI ï FOLFOX arm had longer PFS (4.2 vs 2.5 months) and higher RR (15% vs 4%). It is unclear whether irinotecan is less active following oxaliplatin failure, as OS between both arms was similar. Bidard et al evaluated second-line irinotecan regimens in patients on the OPTIMOX 1 phase III study with all patients receiving first-line FOLFOX; while second-line regimen was not specified on protocol, second-line data were prospectively registered. Of the 342 patients receiving second line irinotecan treatment, 109 received FOLFIRI-3, 112 received FOLFIRI-1, and 121 received other irinotecan regimens. PFS was highest for the FOLFIRI-3 arm (respectively: 3.7 vs 3.0 vs 2.3 months; 56).

Postfailure of FOLFOXIRI

First-line 5-FU plus leucovorin plus oxaliplatin plus irinotecan (FOLFOXIRI) has demonstrated superior OS, RR, and PFS in comparison to FOLFIRI in a phase III trial (58). Optimal second-line therapy after FOLFOXIRI failure is uncertain. Fornaro et al evaluated patients progressing on the phase III trial above, and reported high RR and OS with a variety of second-line treatment (59; Table 11.4). Interestingly, rechallenge with FOLFOXIRI was associated with longer PFS and OS in comparison to second-line doublet therapy. More mature data are needed prior to establishing second-line regimens post FOLFOXIRI failure.

■ BEVACIZUMAB IN THE NONFIRST-LINE SETTING

Since FDA approval of bevacizumab as first-line treatment for MCRC (in combination with IV 5-FU based therapy) in 2004, the most common first-line treatment for patients with MCRC in the United States is bevacizumab in combination with FOLFOX. When other chemotherapy backbones such as FOLFIRI, 5-FU/LV, or capecitabine are utilized, bevacizumab is frequently included (60).

In the second-line setting, phase III data are available for FOLFOX plus bevacizumab in bevacizumab-naïve patients (37) while smaller phase II and observational data are available for FOLFIRI plus bevacizumab. Table 11.5 summarizes phase III and selected phase II data for non-first-line treatment with bevacizumab.

Continuation of Bevacizumab After First-Line Progression

Data are limited as to the efficacy of continuing bevacizumab after disease progression with prior bevacizumab. A survival advantage for ongoing bevacizumab exposure was suggested in a multivariate analysis of the BRiTE observational cohort study which followed 1953 MCRC patients receiving first-line chemotherapy and bevacizumab (Table 11.5). Of the 1445 patients with disease progression, 642 patients continued bevacizumab while 531 patients received second-line treatment without bevacizumab. Median OS and PFS for the entire group were high (25.1 mos; 10.0 mos), and in multivariate analysis, ongoing bevacizumab was significantly and independently associated with improved survival (HR, 0.48; $P < .001$) as well as more frequent hypertension (60). The TML randomized phase III intergroup study assigned 820 patients with progressive MCRC on prior bevacizumab to second-line chemotherapy (choice of oxaliplatin or irinotecan, depending on first first-line progression) with or without ongoing bevacizumab 2.5 mg/kg/week (2012). Continuation of bevacizumab after first progression resulted in improved median overall survival (11.2 vs 9.8 mos, $P = .0062$; 61). Until prospective data are available and have been evaluated for clinical significance and cost–benefit ratios are analyzed, continuation of bevacizumab after progression cannot yet routinely be recommended.

Addition of Bevacizumab to Second-Line Therapy (Bevacizumab Naïve)

Addition of bevacizumab to second-line 5-FU-based therapy is associated with improved OS, PFS, and high RR (Table 11.5). In 2006, the FDA approved bevacizumab as second-line treatment for MCRC (in combination with IV 5-FU-based therapy) on the basis of the phase III ECOG 3200 trial. E3200 randomized 829 MCRC patients (bevacizumab naïve) with progression on prior 5-FU and irinotecan treatment to FOLFOX4, FOLFOX4 plus bevacizumab, or bevacizumab alone. The bevacizumab arm was closed early after interim analysis suggested inferior survival in comparison to the FOLFOX4 control arm. Besides establishing a significant survival benefit for the addition of bevacizumab to FOLFOX4 in the second-line setting (in comparison to FOLFOX4 alone), E3200 also demonstrated a lack of efficacy for single-agent bevacizumab with reported RR of 3.3% and inferior survival in comparison to chemotherapy alone (37).

While phase III data are lacking for bevacizumab plus second-line irinotecan, a number of smaller studies report OS benefit (62). A Japanese observational cohort study found that the addition of bevacizumab to FOLFIRI for 115 patients with prior oxaliplatin progression yielded comparable improvements in OS and PFS to the E3200 study. Interestingly, median OS and PFS reported for second-line FOLFOX plus bevacizumab were notably lower than the E3200 study, likely confounded by differences in patient population and nonprotocol therapeutic management (63). The AVASIRI phase II trial evaluated 25 patients receiving FOLFIRI plus bevacizumab after progression on first-line chemotherapy without irinotecan or bevacizumab. The primary endpoint of RR was 32%, with median PFS 11.6 months, and median OS of 21.4 months (62).

Addition of Bevacizumab in Heavily Pretreated Patients

Addition of bevacizumab to third or fourth line 5-FU/LV yields poor RR with rare reports of efficacy in patients with progression after both oxaliplatin and irinotecan-based regimens (Table 11.5). A multicenter phase II trial of 5-FU/LV (de Gramont and Roswell Park regimens) plus bevacizumab after prior oxaliplatin and irinotecan failure reported low RR of 1%, and modest PFS and OS (respectively, 3.5 mos, 9 mos; 64). Safety profile was comparable to first-line settings with similar regimens with a 5% rate of grade 3 or 4 hemorrhage. A smaller phase II study of fourth line 5-FU/LV (de Gramont) plus bevacizumab in 48 heavily pretreated patients noted slightly higher RR but similar PFS and OS (respectively, 6.5%, 3.5 mos, 7.7 mos; 65). These data are in sharp contrast to phase II data for first-line bevacizumab plus 5-FU/LV (respectively, as above, 26%, 9.2 mos, 16.6 mos; 66), suggesting that bevacizumab efficacy is highest in the first- or second-line setting.

■ CETUXIMAB AND PANITUMUMAB IN THE NONFIRST-LINE SETTING

Cetuximab and panitumumab only benefit patients with *K-ras* wild-type (*K-ras* WT) tumors; the presence of mutations in codon 12 or 13 of the *K-ras* gene is a negative predictive marker for benefit from EGFR antibody therapy. Mutations in other codons exist and are rare but their significance is not yet known. The following section relates only to those patients with *K-ras* WT tumors. Of note, the subset of *K-ras* WT tumors with mutations in *BRAF*, *NRAS*, and PI3K appear to show little or no response to EGFR antibody treatment (67).

Continuation/Switching of Cetuximab and Panitumumab After First-Line Progression

Data are limited as to the efficacy of continuing EGFR antibody therapy after disease progression with prior EGFR therapy. Data are limited to small studies of cetuximab-irinotecan rechallenge after prior failure (68), or cetuximab rechallenge with dual antibody therapy (69). The safety and efficacy of panitumumab after progression on cetuximab, or vice versa, has not been well established. Two small retrospective series reported mild clinical benefit and tolerability of panitumumab in patients previously treated with cetuximab (70,71) but prospective data are lacking. At this time, neither continuation nor switching of EGFR antibodies is recommended after progression on prior EGFR therapy.

Addition of Cetuximab and Panitumumab to Second-Line Therapy (Irinotecan Naïve)

In the second-line irinotecan naive *K-ras* WT setting, the addition of cetuximab or panitumumab to FOLFIRI or single-agent irinotecan is associated with significant improvement in PFS and RR without OS benefit (Table 11.6). At present, there are no prospective trials evaluating second-line oxaliplatin regimens in combination with cetuximab or panitumumab.

The phase III EPIC trial randomized 1298 patients (*K-ras* mutation status not checked) with disease progression on first-line 5-FU plus oxaliplatin to irinotecan with or without weekly cetuximab (72). Despite significant improvement in PFS, RR, disease control, and QOL with the addition of cetuximab to irinotecan, median OS was comparable in the cetuximab-irinotecan and irinotecan arms. This lack of difference was partially attributed to crossover of 46.4% of the irinotecan patients to third-line cetuximab (87% in combination with irinotecan). Rates of treatment discontinuation were comparable in both arms, despite a higher frequency of rash, diarrhea, and electrolyte imbalances with cetuximab.

A phase III trial randomized 1186 patients to FOLFIRI with or without panitumumab after failure of first-line 5-FU based treatment (approximately 65% with prior oxaliplatin, 20% with prior bevacizumab; 73). In the *K-ras* WT subgroup (*K-ras* mutation status available for 91% of patients), the addition of panitumumab to FOLFIRI significantly improved PFS and RR in comparison to FOLFIRI, and was associated with comparable adverse events (except for more rash and electrolyte abnormalities). *K-ras* mutant patients did not benefit from panitumumab addition.

Addition to Second- or Third-Line Irinotecan (Irinotecan Refractory Setting)

Combined irinotecan and cetuximab salvage therapy in the setting of prior irinotecan failure is associated with a significant improvement in RR and PFS without OS benefit (Table 11.6). Cunningham et al randomized 329 patients with EGFR positive tumors and prior progression on irinotecan (62% with prior oxaliplatin as well) to cetuximab monotherapy or cetuximab plus irinotecan therapy (27); combination therapy was associated with significantly higher RR of 23% and TTP of 4.1 mos in irinotecan refractory patients, establishing the role of cetuximab in reversing irinotecan resistance. Comparable third-line efficacy for cetuximab plus irinotecan was also demonstrated in a phase II study of 55 patients with prior oxaliplatin and irinotecan failure (65), with RR of 25.4% and TTP of 4.7 mos.

Addition of Cetuximab and Panitumumab in Heavily Pretreated Patients

In the salvage setting of heavily pretreated patients, both cetuximab (74,75) and panitumumab monotherapy (76) have demonstrated improved RR and PFS in comparison to BSC. Cetuximab monotherapy was also shown to improve median OS in comparison to BSC in the *K-ras* WT setting (Table 11.6). A phase II study evaluating cetuximab monotherapy in 57 patients (EGFR + via IHC) with documented irinotecan failure reported a modest benefit with partial responses seen in six patients (RR 9%; 74).

The NCI CTG phase III study compared cetuximab monotherapy to BSC in 572 heavily pretreated patients (greater than 80% had progressed through three or more regimens including irinotecan, oxaliplatin, and 5-FU) and found cetuximab monotherapy to be associated with significant improvements in median OS, PFS, RR, and QOL, despite a higher incidence of grade 3 to 4 toxicities (75). This study did not allow crossover. A subsequent analysis evaluating *K-ras* mutation status (available for 69% of patients) reported that cetuximab benefit was limited to patients with *K-ras* WT tumors (26). Panitumumab's efficacy as monotherapy was demonstrated in a large phase III study in which 463 heavily pretreated patients were randomized to BSC or panitumumab. The study met its primary endpoint of PFS; panitumumab significantly improved PFS and RR without grade 3 or 4 toxicities. However, panitumumab monotherapy did not prolong OS; this was attributed to crossover of 76% BSC arm to subsequent panitumumab (76).

■ DUAL ANTIBODY THERAPY IN THE NONFIRST-LINE SETTING

The PACCE and CAIRO-2 trials both showed detrimental effects from combining dual VEGF and EGFR inhibition with chemotherapy in the first-line MCRC setting. Addition of panitumumab to bevacizumab and chemotherapy resulted in higher toxicity and death rates, and lower PFS, regardless of *K-ras* mutation status (77), while addition of cetuximab to CAPOX plus bevacizumab resulted in lower PFS for the entire study group (later found to be restricted to the *K-ras* mutant group; 30). In contrast, the BOND-2 study demonstrated high RR and a tolerable toxicity profile similar to that of each agent separately (22; Table 11.6). The phase II trial randomized 83 heavily pretreated patients who were irinotecan refractory and bevacizumab-cetuximab naïve to either cetuximab-bevacizumab (CB) or cetuximab-bevacizumab-irinotecan (CBI). RR, TTP, and median OS were all higher than historical controls (of cetuximab alone, or cetuximab plus irinotecan).

It is unclear if dual antibody therapy may be a promising therapeutic option in the salvage setting for heavily pretreated patients, possibly with fewer chemotherapy agents than were tested in the first-line setting, but without further carefully controlled studies, dual antibody therapy is not recommended in any setting at this time.

■ NOVEL AGENTS WITH RECENT FDA APPROVAL

Until the approval of regorafenib and aflibercept in late 2012, no new agents had been FDA approved for the second- or third-line treatment of MCRC since panitumumab approval in 2006 (Table 11.5). Aflibercept, a humanized recombinant protein comprised of extracellular VEGFR-1 and VEGFR-2 domains, in combination with FOLFIRI, was approved in August 2012 for the treatment of patients with MCRC progression on prior oxaliplatin regimens (2012). Regorafenib, an oral multikinase and VEGF inhibitor, was approved in September 2012 for the treatment of patients with MCRC progression on prior 5-FU, oxaliplatin, irinotecan, anti-VEGF, and anti-EGFR therapy (78). The VELOUR trial randomized 1226 patients (28% with prior bevacizumab exposure) with ECOG PS 0 to 2 after first-line oxaliplatin progression to FOLFORI plus placebo or FOLFIRI plus aflibercept 4 mg/kg (79). Results presented at ESMO 2011 reported significant improvement in median OS, PFS, and RR with aflibercept (respectively, 13.5 vs 12.06 mos; 6.9 vs 4.7 mos; 19.8% vs 11%). Adverse effects such as grade 3 or 4 diarrhea, fatigue, hypertension, proteinuria, and neutropenia led to discontinuation in 26.6% and 12.1 of patients in the aflibercept vs placebo arm, with a median of 9 vs 8 cycles. Planned subset analyses for OS yielded an HR of 0.86 (95% CI, 0.68–1.1) in patients with prior bevacizumab exposure, and an HR of 0.79 (95% CI, 0.67–0.93) in bevacizumab naïve patients (80).

The CORRECT trial assigned 760 patients with ECOG PS 0 to 1 in a 2:1 randomization to either regorafenib 160 mg daily plus BSC, or placebo plus BSC for 21 days of a 28-day cycle. Median number of prior lines of therapy was 3, and all patients had received prior treatment with 5-FU, oxaliplatin, irinotecan, bevacizumab; all but one *K-ras* WT patient received anti-EGFR therapy. Preliminary results presented at ASCO reported a statistically significant improvement in median OS and PFS in patients treated with regorafenib vs placebo. Adverse effects reported in at least 30% of patients included asthenia, hand-food skin reactions, diarrhea, mucositis, infection, hypertension; grade 3 to 4 toxicities also included hemorrhage, hepatotoxicity, and GI perforation. These led to discontinuation in 8.2% and 1.2% of patients in the regorafenib vs placebo arm, with a mean duration of treatment 12 vs 8 weeks (81).

CONCLUSIONS

The optimal combination and sequencing of cytotoxic and biologic agents for MCRC is not yet established. Patients benefit from exposure to all active agents over a continuum of care, rechallenge with previously utilized therapies may be beneficial in select cases. Selection of first- and second-line regimens should be individualized with respect to treatment goals and patient comorbidities. Bevacizumab is associated with lower response rates in third and fourth lines of therapy, and should ideally be utilized in the first or second-line setting in combination with 5-FU based chemotherapy. Cetuximab and panitumumab are beneficial only in the setting of *K-ras* WT tumors, require specific chemotherapy backbones for efficacy, and yield similar response rates in multiple lines of therapy. At present, continuation of bevacizumab after progression cannot yet be routinely recommended until mature data clarifying cost-benefit and survival analysis become available. Other pathways under investigation are PI3K-ATK, RAF/MEK/ERK, and VEGF pathways. Ongoing areas of research include optimal sequencing for biologics, novel drug development, patient toxicity and risk stratification, and further characterization of mutations and tumor biology.

REFERENCES

1. Grothey A, Sargent D, Goldberg RM, Schmoll HJ. Survival of patients with advanced colorectal cancer improves with the availability of fluorouracil-leucovorin, irinotecan, and oxaliplatin in the course of treatment. *J Clin Oncol.* 2004;22:1209–1214.
2. Longley DB, Harkin DP, Johnston PG. 5-fluorouracil: mechanisms of action and clinical strategies. *Nat Rev Cancer.* 2003;3:330–338.
3. Efficacy of intravenous continuous infusion of fluorouracil compared with bolus administration in advanced colorectal cancer. Meta-analysis Group In Cancer. *J Clin Oncol.* 1998;16:301–308.
4. de Gramont A, Bosset JF, Milan C, et al. Randomized trial comparing monthly low-dose leucovorin and fluorouracil bolus with bimonthly high-dose leucovorin and fluorouracil bolus plus continuous infusion for advanced colorectal cancer: a French intergroup study. *J Clin Oncol.* 1997;15:808–815.
5. Silvestris N, Maiello E, De Vita F, et al. Update on capecitabine alone and in combination regimens in colorectal cancer patients. *Cancer Treat Rev.* 2010;36 Suppl 3:S46–55.
6. Hoff PM, Ansari R, Batist G, et al. Comparison of oral capecitabine versus intravenous fluorouracil plus leucovorin as first-line treatment in 605 patients with metastatic colorectal cancer: results of a randomized phase III study. *J Clin Oncol.* 2001;19:2282–2292.
7. Van Cutsem E, Twelves C, Cassidy J, et al. Oral capecitabine compared with intravenous fluorouracil plus leucovorin in patients with metastatic colorectal cancer: results of a large phase III study. *J Clin Oncol.* 2001;19:4097–4106.
8. Arkenau HT, Arnold D, Cassidy J, et al. Efficacy of oxaliplatin plus capecitabine or infusional fluorouracil/leucovorin in patients with metastatic colorectal cancer: a pooled analysis of randomized trials. *J Clin Oncol.* 2008;26:5910–5917.
9. Hochster HS, Hart LL, Ramanathan RK, et al. Safety and efficacy of oxaliplatin and fluoropyrimidine regimens with or without bevacizumab as first-line treatment of metastatic colorectal cancer: results of the TREE Study. *J Clin Oncol.* 2008;26:3523–3529.
10. van Kuilenburg AB, Haasjes J, Richel DJ, et al. Clinical implications of dihydropyrimidine dehydrogenase (DPD) deficiency in patients with severe 5-fluorouracil-associated toxicity: identification of new mutations in the DPD gene. *Clin Cancer Res.* 2000;6:4705–4712.
11. Kohne CH, van Cutsem E, Wils J, et al. Phase III study of weekly high-dose infusional fluorouracil plus folinic acid with or without irinotecan in patients with metastatic colorectal cancer: European Organisation for Research and Treatment of Cancer Gastrointestinal Group Study 40986. *J Clin Oncol.* 2005;23:4856–4865.
12. Douillard JY, Cunningham D, Roth AD, et al. Irinotecan combined with fluorouracil compared with fluorouracil alone as first-line treatment for metastatic colorectal cancer: a multicentre randomised trial. *Lancet.* 2000;355:1041–1047.
13. Saltz LB, Cox JV, Blanke C, et al. Irinotecan plus fluorouracil and leucovorin for metastatic colorectal cancer. Irinotecan Study Group. *N Engl J Med.* 2000;343:905–14.
14. Rothenberg ML, Meropol NJ, Poplin EA, Van Cutsem E, Wadler S. Mortality associated with irinotecan plus bolus fluorouracil/leucovorin: summary findings of an independent panel. *J Clin Oncol.* 2001;19:3801–3807.

15. Fuchs CS, Marshall J, Mitchell E, et al. Randomized, controlled trial of irinotecan plus infusional, bolus, or oral fluoropyrimidines in first-line treatment of metastatic colorectal cancer: results from the BICC-C Study. *J Clin Oncol.* 2007;25:4779–4786.
16. Gamelin L, Boisdron-Celle M, Delva R, et al. Prevention of oxaliplatin-related neurotoxicity by calcium and magnesium infusions: a retrospective study of 161 patients receiving oxaliplatin combined with 5-Fluorouracil and leucovorin for advanced colorectal cancer. *Clin Cancer Res.* 2004;10:4055–4061.
17. de Gramont A, Figer A, Seymour M, et al. Leucovorin and fluorouracil with or without oxaliplatin as first-line treatment in advanced colorectal cancer. *J Clin Oncol.* 2000;18:2938–2947.
18. Grothey A, Nikcevich DA, Sloan JA, et al. Intravenous calcium and magnesium for oxaliplatin-induced sensory neurotoxicity in adjuvant colon cancer: NCCTG N04C7. *J Clin Oncol.* 2011;29:421–427.
19. Hochster HS, Grothey A, Childs BH. Use of calcium and magnesium salts to reduce oxaliplatin-related neurotoxicity. *J Clin Oncol.* 2007;25:4028–4029.
20. Knijn N, Tol J, Koopman M, et al. The effect of prophylactic calcium and magnesium infusions on the incidence of neurotoxicity and clinical outcome of oxaliplatin-based systemic treatment in advanced colorectal cancer patients. *Eur J Cancer.* 2011;47:369–374.
21. Kabbinavar FF, Hambleton J, Mass RD, Hurwitz HI, Bergsland E, Sarkar S. Combined analysis of efficacy: the addition of bevacizumab to fluorouracil/leucovorin improves survival for patients with metastatic colorectal cancer. *J Clin Oncol.* 2005;23:3706–3712.
22. Saltz LB, Clarke S, Diaz-Rubio E, et al. Bevacizumab in combination with oxaliplatin-based chemotherapy as first-line therapy in metastatic colorectal cancer: a randomized phase III study. *J Clin Oncol.* 2008;26:2013–2019.
23. Van Cutsem E, Rivera F, Berry S, et al. Safety and efficacy of first-line bevacizumab with FOLFOX, XELOX, FOLFIRI and fluoropyrimidines in metastatic colorectal cancer: the BEAT study. *Ann Oncol.* 2009;20:1842–1847.
24. Schutz FA, Je Y, Azzi GR, Nguyen PL, Choueiri TK. Bevacizumab increases the risk of arterial ischemia: a large study in cancer patients with a focus on different subgroup outcomes. *Ann Oncol.* 2011;22:1404–1412.
25. Hurwitz H, Fehrenbacher L, Novotny W, et al. Bevacizumab plus irinotecan, fluorouracil, and leucovorin for metastatic colorectal cancer. *N Engl J Med.* 2004;350:2335–2342.
26. Karapetis CS, Khambata-Ford S, Jonker DJ, et al. K-ras mutations and benefit from cetuximab in advanced colorectal cancer. *N Engl J Med.* 2008;359:1757–1765.
27. Cunningham D, Humblet Y, Siena S, et al. Cetuximab monotherapy and cetuximab plus irinotecan in irinotecan-refractory metastatic colorectal cancer. *N Engl J Med.* 2004;351:337–345.
28. Van Cutsem E, Kohne CH, Hitre E, et al. Cetuximab and chemotherapy as initial treatment for metastatic colorectal cancer. *N Engl J Med.* 2009;360:1408–1417.
29. Van Cutsem E, Kohne CH, Lang I, et al. Cetuximab plus irinotecan, fluorouracil, and leucovorin as first-line treatment for metastatic colorectal cancer: updated analysis of overall survival according to tumor K-ras and BRAF mutation status. *J Clin Oncol.* 2011;29:2011–2019.
30. Bokemeyer C, Bondarenko I, Makhson A, et al. Fluorouracil, leucovorin, and oxaliplatin with and without cetuximab in the first-line treatment of metastatic colorectal cancer. *J Clin Oncol.* 2009;27:663–671.
31. Maughan TS, Adams RA, Smith CG, et al. Addition of cetuximab to oxaliplatin-based first-line combination chemotherapy for treatment of advanced colorectal cancer: results of the randomised phase 3 MRC COIN trial. *Lancet.* 2011;377:2103–2114.
32. Van Cutsem E, Siena S, Humblet Y, et al. An open-label, single-arm study assessing safety and efficacy of panitumumab in patients with metastatic colorectal cancer refractory to standard chemotherapy. *Ann Oncol.* 2008;19:92–98.
33. Douillard JY, Siena S, Cassidy J, et al. Randomized, phase III trial of panitumumab with infusional fluorouracil, leucovorin, and oxaliplatin (FOLFOX4) versus FOLFOX4 alone as first-line treatment in patients with previously untreated metastatic colorectal cancer: the PRIME study. *J Clin Oncol.* 2010;28:4697–4705.
34. Chung CH, Mirakhur B, Chan E, et al. Cetuximab-induced anaphylaxis and IgE specific for galactose-alpha-1,3-galactose. *N Engl J Med.* 2008;358:1109–1117.
35. Tournigand C, Cervantes A, Figer A, et al. OPTIMOX1: a randomized study of FOLFOX4 or FOLFOX7 with oxaliplatin in a stop-and-go fashion in advanced colorectal cancer—a GERCOR study. *J Clin Oncol.* 2006;24:394–400.
36. Labianca R, Sobrero A, Isa L, et al. Intermittent versus continuous chemotherapy in advanced colorectal cancer: a randomised 'GISCAD' trial. *Ann Oncol.* 2011;22:1236–1242.
37. Giantonio BJ, Catalano PJ, Meropol NJ, et al. Bevacizumab in combination with oxaliplatin, fluorouracil, and leucovorin (FOLFOX4) for previously treated metastatic colorectal cancer: results from the Eastern Cooperative Oncology Group Study E3200. *J Clin Oncol.* 2007;25:1539–1544.
38. Therasse P, Arbuck SG, Eisenhauer EA, et al. New guidelines to evaluate the response to treatment in solid tumors. European Organization for Research and Treatment of Cancer, National Cancer Institute of the United States, National Cancer Institute of Canada. *J Natl Cancer Inst.* 2000;92:205–216.
39. Iwanicki-Caron I, Di Fiore F, Roque I, et al. Usefulness of the serum carcinoembryonic antigen kinetic for chemotherapy monitoring in patients with unresectable metastasis of colorectal cancer. *J Clin Oncol.* 2008;26:3681–3686.
40. Locker GY, Hamilton S, Harris J, et al. ASCO 2006 update of recommendations for the use of tumor markers in gastrointestinal cancer. *J Clin Oncol.* 2006;24:5313–5327.
41. Strimpakos AS, Cunningham D, Mikropoulos C, Petkar I, Barbachano Y, Chau I. The impact of carcinoembryonic antigen flare in patients with advanced colorectal cancer receiving first-line chemotherapy. *Ann Oncol.* 2010;21:1013–1019.
42. Goldberg RM, Sargent DJ, Morton RF, et al. A randomized controlled trial of fluorouracil plus leucovorin, irinotecan, and oxaliplatin combinations in patients with previously untreated metastatic colorectal cancer. *J Clin Oncol.* 2004;22:23–30.
43. Ashley AC, Sargent DJ, Alberts SR, et al. Updated efficacy and toxicity analysis of irinotecan and oxaliplatin (IROX): intergroup trial N9741 in first-line treatment of metastatic colorectal cancer. *Cancer.* 2007;110:670–677.
44. Colucci G, Gebbia V, Paoletti G, et al. Phase III randomized trial of FOLFIRI versus FOLFOX4 in the treatment of advanced colorectal cancer: a multicenter study of the Gruppo Oncologico Dell'Italia Meridionale. *J Clin Oncol.* 2005;23:4866–4875.
45. Tournigand C, Andre T, Achille E, et al. FOLFIRI followed by FOLFOX6 or the reverse sequence in advanced colorectal cancer: a randomized GERCOR study. *J Clin Oncol.* 2004;22:229–237.
46. Goldberg RM, Rothenberg ML, Van Cutsem E, et al. The continuum of care: a paradigm for the management of metastatic colorectal cancer. *Oncologist.* 2007;12:38–50.
47. Grothey A, Sargent D. Overall survival of patients with advanced colorectal cancer correlates with availability of fluorouracil, irinotecan, and oxaliplatin regardless of whether doublet or single-agent therapy is used first line. *J Clin Oncol.* December 20, 2005;23(36):9441 –9442. PMID: 16361649
48. Koopman M, Antonini NF, Douma J, et al. Sequential versus combination chemotherapy with capecitabine, irinotecan, and oxaliplatin in advanced colorectal cancer (CAIRO): a phase III randomised controlled trial. *Lancet.* 2007;370:135–142.
49. Seymour MT, Maughan TS, Ledermann JA, et al. Different strategies of sequential and combination chemotherapy for patients with poor prognosis advanced colorectal cancer (MRC FOCUS): a randomised controlled trial. *Lancet.* 2007;370:143–152.
50. Kim GP, Sargent DJ, Mahoney MR, et al. Phase III noninferiority trial comparing irinotecan with oxaliplatin, fluorouracil,

and leucovorin in patients with advanced colorectal carcinoma previously treated with fluorouracil: N9841. *J Clin Oncol.* 2009;27:2848–2854.
51. Guglielmi AP, Sobrero AF. Second-line therapy for advanced colorectal cancer. *Gastrointestinal cancer research: GCR.* 2007;1:57–63.
52. Rothenberg ML, Oza AM, Bigelow RH, et al. Superiority of oxaliplatin and fluorouracil-leucovorin compared with either therapy alone in patients with progressive colorectal cancer after irinotecan and fluorouracil-leucovorin: interim results of a phase III trial. *J Clin Oncol.* 2003;21:2059–2069.
53. Cunningham D, Pyrhonen S, James RD, et al. Randomised trial of irinotecan plus supportive care versus supportive care alone after fluorouracil failure for patients with metastatic colorectal cancer. *Lancet.* 1998;352:1413–1418.
54. Rougier P, Van Cutsem E, Bajetta E, et al. Randomised trial of irinotecan versus fluorouracil by continuous infusion after fluorouracil failure in patients with metastatic colorectal cancer. *Lancet.* 1998;352:1407–1412.
55. Fuchs CS, Moore MR, Harker G, Villa L, Rinaldi D, Hecht JR. Phase III comparison of two irinotecan dosing regimens in second-line therapy of metastatic colorectal cancer. *J Clin Oncol.* 2003;21:807–814.
56. Haller DG, Rothenberg ML, Wong AO, et al. Oxaliplatin plus irinotecan compared with irinotecan alone as second-line treatment after single-agent fluoropyrimidine therapy for metastatic colorectal carcinoma. *J Clin Oncol.* 2008;26:4544–4550.
57. Bidard FC, Tournigand C, Andre T, et al. Efficacy of FOLFIRI-3 (irinotecan D1, D3 combined with LV5-FU) or other irinotecan-based regimens in oxaliplatin-pretreated metastatic colorectal cancer in the GERCOR OPTIMOX1 study. *Ann Oncol.* 2009;20:1042–1047.
58. Falcone A, Ricci S, Brunetti I, et al. Phase III trial of infusional fluorouracil, leucovorin, oxaliplatin, and irinotecan (FOLFOXIRI) compared with infusional fluorouracil, leucovorin, and irinotecan (FOLFIRI) as first-line treatment for metastatic colorectal cancer: the Gruppo Oncologico Nord Ovest. J Clin Oncol. May 1, 2007;25(13):1670–1976. PMID: 17470860
59. Fornaro L, Vasile E, Masi G, et al. Outcome of second-line treatment after first-line chemotherapy with the GONO FOLFOXIRI regimen. *Clin Colorectal Cancer.* 2012;11:71–76.
60. Grothey A, Sugrue MM, Purdie DM, et al. Bevacizumab beyond first progression is associated with prolonged overall survival in metastatic colorectal cancer: results from a large observational cohort study (BRiTE). *J Clin Oncol.* 2008;26:5326–5334.
61. Bennouna J, Sastre J, Arnold D, et al. Continuation of bevacizumab after first progression in metastatic colorectal cancer (ML18147): a randomised phase 3 trial. *Lancet Oncol.* 2012.
62. Horita Y, Yamada Y, Kato K, et al. Phase II clinical trial of second-line FOLFIRI plus bevacizumab for patients with metastatic colorectal cancer: AVASIRI trial. *Int J Clin Oncol.* 2011.
63. Moriwaki T, Bando H, Takashima A, et al. Bevacizumab in combination with irinotecan, 5-fluorouracil, and leucovorin (FOLFIRI) in patients with metastatic colorectal cancer who were previously treated with oxaliplatin-containing regimens: a multicenter observational cohort study (TCTG 2nd-BV study). *Med Oncol.* 2012;29:2842–2848.
64. Chen HX, Mooney M, Boron M, et al. Phase II multicenter trial of bevacizumab plus fluorouracil and leucovorin in patients with advanced refractory colorectal cancer: an NCI Treatment Referral Center Trial TRC-0301. *J Clin Oncol.* 2006;24:3354–3360.
65. Vincenzi B, Santini D, Russo A, et al. Bevacizumab in association with de Gramont 5-fluorouracil/folinic acid in patients with oxaliplatin-, irinotecan-, and cetuximab-refractory colorectal cancer: a single-center phase 2 trial. *Cancer.* 2009;115:4849–4856.
66. Hurwitz H, Kabbinavar F. Bevacizumab combined with standard fluoropyrimidine-based chemotherapy regimens to treat colorectal cancer. *Oncology.* 2005;69 Suppl 3:17–24.
67. De Roock W, Claes B, Bernasconi D, et al. Effects of K-ras, BRAF, NRAS, and PIK3CA mutations on the efficacy of cetuximab plus chemotherapy in chemotherapy-refractory metastatic colorectal cancer: a retrospective consortium analysis. *Lancet Oncol.* 2010;11:753–762.
68. Santini D, Vincenzi B, Addeo R, et al. Cetuximab rechallenge in metastatic colorectal cancer patients: how to come away from acquired resistance? *Ann Oncol.* 2012;23:2313–2318.
69. Larsen FO, Pfeiffer P, Nielsen D, et al. Bevacizumab in combination with cetuximab and irinotecan after failure of cetuximab and irinotecan in patients with metastatic colorectal cancer. *Acta Oncol.* 2011;50:574–577.
70. Power DG, Shah MA, Asmis TR, Garcia JJ, Kemeny NE. Safety and efficacy of panitumumab following cetuximab: retrospective review of the Memorial Sloan-Kettering experience. *Invest New Drugs.* 2010;28:353–360.
71. Saif MW, Kaley K, Chu E, Copur MS. Safety and efficacy of panitumumab therapy after progression with cetuximab: experience at two institutions. *Clinical Colorectal Cancer.* 2010;9:315–318.
72. Sobrero AF, Maurel J, Fehrenbacher L, et al. EPIC: phase III trial of cetuximab plus irinotecan after fluoropyrimidine and oxaliplatin failure in patients with metastatic colorectal cancer. *J Clin Oncol.* 2008;26:2311–2319.
73. Peeters M, Price TJ, Cervantes A, et al. Randomized phase III study of panitumumab with fluorouracil, leucovorin, and irinotecan (FOLFIRI) compared with FOLFIRI alone as second-line treatment in patients with metastatic colorectal cancer. *J Clin Oncol.* 2010;28:4706–4713.
74. Saltz LB, Meropol NJ, Loehrer PJ, Sr., Needle MN, Kopit J, Mayer RJ. Phase II trial of cetuximab in patients with refractory colorectal cancer that expresses the epidermal growth factor receptor. *J Clin Oncol.* 2004;22:1201–1208.
75. Jonker DJ, O'Callaghan CJ, Karapetis CS, et al. Cetuximab for the treatment of colorectal cancer. *N Engl J Med.* 2007;357:2040–2048.
76. Amado RG, Wolf M, Peeters M, et al. Wild-type K-ras is required for panitumumab efficacy in patients with metastatic colorectal cancer. *J Clin Oncol.* 2008;26:1626–1634.
77. Hecht JR, Mitchell E, Chidiac T, et al. A randomized phase IIIB trial of chemotherapy, bevacizumab, and panitumumab compared with chemotherapy and bevacizumab alone for metastatic colorectal cancer. *J Clin Oncol.* 2009;27:672–680.
78. Grothey A, Cutsem EV, Sobrero A, et al. Regorafenib monotherapy for previously treated metastatic colorectal cancer (CORRECT): an international, multicentre, randomised, placebo-controlled, phase 3 trial. *Lancet.* 2012.
79. Van Cutsem E, Tabernero J, Lakomy R, et al. Intravenous (IV) aflibercept versus placebo in combination with irinotecan/5-FU (FOLFIRI) for second-line treatment of metastatic colorectal cancer (MCRC): results of a multinational phase III trial (EFC10262-VELOUR). *Ann Oncol.* 2011;22:v18.
80. Allegra CJ, Lakomy R, Tabernero J, et al. Effects of prior bevacizumab (B) use on outcomes from the VELOUR study: A phase III study of aflibercept (Afl) and FOLFIRI in patients (pts) with metastatic colorectal cancer (mCRC) after failure of an oxaliplatin regimen. *J Clin Oncol.* (Meeting Abstracts) 2012;30:3505.
81. Van Cutsem E, Sobrero A, Siena A, Siena S. Phase III CORRECT trial of regorafenib in metastatic colorectal cancer. In: *ASCO Annual Meeting*; 2012.
82. Rothenberg ML, Cox JV, Butts C, et al. Capecitabine plus oxaliplatin (XELOX) versus 5-fluorouracil/folinic acid plus oxaliplatin (FOLFOX-4) as second-line therapy in metastatic colorectal cancer: a randomized phase III noninferiority study. *Ann Oncol* 2008;19:1720-6.
83. Van Cutsem E, Josep Tabernero, Radek Lakomy, Jana Prausova, Paul Ruff, Guy Van Hazel, Vladimir Moiseyenko et al. Intravenous (IV) aflibercept versus placebo in combination with irinotecan/5-FU (FOLFIRI) for second-line treatment of metastatic colorectal cancer (MCRC): results of a multinational phase III trial (EFC10262-VELOUR). *Annals of Oncology* 2011;22:v18.
84. Van Cutsem E, Peeters M, Siena S, et al. Open-label phase III trial of panitumumab plus best supportive care compared with best supportive care alone in patients with chemotherapy-refractory metastatic colorectal cancer. *J Clin Oncol* 2007;25:1658-64.

12 Phase I/II Clinical Trials in Metastatic Colorectal Cancer

DAVENDRA P. S. SOHAL
RODOLFO F. PERINI
PETER J. O'DWYER

INTRODUCTION

Early-phase clinical trials bridge the transition of novel molecules from promising compounds in preclinical models to viable drugs ready for testing in large-scale clinical trials. Viable clinical candidates have substantial preclinical weight to support a rationale that they might be therapeutically useful in cancer patients. Key attributes include optimization for their chemical interaction with the target, structural modifications, formulation to ensure that the agent is bioavailable for its purpose, pharmacological evidence to support ability to achieve relevant exposure, as well as demonstration of pharmacodynamic (PD) effects. As a final step before clinical development, toxicology studies in animal models establish the safety of the initial doses to be used in human trials, and where possible, establish that the desired pharmacological effect can be achieved at tolerable doses. These molecules are developed in various laboratories—research universities, large pharmaceutical companies, and newer biotechnology firms are major suppliers of such drugs. Extensive research, involving considerable time, manpower and resources, is usually needed to generate a molecule ready to be tested on humans.

Phase I trials are the initial studies of new molecules in the clinic. The goals of phase I trials are to determine an appropriate and safe dose for clinical use, to understand the clinical pharmacokinetics (PKs; the effect of the body on the drug) and PDs (the effect of the drug on the body), to guide future studies. The results of these studies lend confidence that in trials intended to show activity, the new drug is being used at doses that will achieve the desired biological effect, and so prove or disprove the hypothesis that the study has been embarked upon. Randomized trials are expensive, and the success rate in oncology has not been as good as in other therapeutic areas. But in addition to the cost imperative, there is an ethical dimension that motivates us to choose regimens that have a high likelihood of success and have the scientific rigor to merit a patient consenting to risk, discomfort, and inconvenience.

Advances in the approach to drug development have modified the role of phase I trials, though the designs have not changed greatly. Upon introduction to the clinic, the dose of a new drug is chosen to have a low likelihood of side effects (based upon toxicity studies), then escalated in successive groups of patients to a level sufficient to undergo further efficacy testing. New drugs for cancer now almost always have a defined mechanism at their introduction, and often represent a refinement of previous attacks on a target. Monoclonal antibodies are being tested increasingly, and being large molecules, they have special PK properties. At the earliest stages this finding impacts patient selection and PD endpoints, and doses selected for further studies are often well tolerated, and not limited by toxicity. It is critical that insofar as it is possible, proof that the drug is achieving the desired effect on the target in tumor tissue be obtained. This goal extends from phase I through early phase II, often requires serial tumor biopsies, and in most companies is a requirement that must be met before further development can be supported.

Eligibility criteria based on the target maximize the potential for patient benefit. For this reason, it is now appropriate to say that in early phase studies in colon cancer and even in subsets of the disease (eg, *BRAF* mutant tumors), patients with extensive pretreatment are expected to be responsive to selected interventions. At the same time, more is asked of each participant, often including biopsies at the highest or target doses to ensure that the desired effects are indeed being achieved in the tumor.

Formally, the goal of a phase II trial is directed to identifying activity of a compound, with the assumption that the phase I trial has identified a safe and potentially effective dose. Selection of the phase II dose may be based on PK or PD or both. Commonly the lines between phase I and II objectives are blurred today, since a simple continuation of the phase I trial can provide vital information regarding the activity of a targeted agent. Expansion phases in specific diseases or subtypes of a disease are incorporated early in drug development. It is in this arena that phase I studies (in reality more phase I/Ib/II studies) have immediate relevance to the options available for colorectal cancer (CRC) patients. In the next sections, we will illustrate concepts through data from selected clinical trials.

■ OVERALL DESIGN OF PHASE I TRIALS

The first aspect of drug evaluation is to demonstrate that the drug may be safely administered to humans. By testing a new agent in a small number of patients treated at ever-higher doses, a description of toxicity is obtained. Treatment is started at a low dose, usually extrapolated from animal toxicology data, and the dose selected is often an order of magnitude lower than that associated with severe effects in murine models. Principles of allometry are used for such interspecies scaling (1). One must be careful with interspecies scaling of interspecies drugs such as chimeric antibodies, however, since varying receptor expression and drug affinity across species, along with altered intratumoral clearance may lead to erroneous PK estimates via interspecies scaling (2). The selection of initial doses has received much attention in recent years, since the consequence of a margin of safety is the likelihood that the initial dose levels of many drugs will be ineffective. Considerable thought has been given to alternative designs for "first-in-human" studies, with attention both to starting dose selection, and dose escalation (3,4). The dose is increased in prespecified increments and all toxicities are carefully monitored. At any dose level, a toxicity that is severe enough to necessitate treatment cessation or considerable dose reduction is usually deemed to be a dose-limiting toxicity (DLT). The definition of DLT depends on both drug and disease, but usually defines unacceptable toxicity such as prolonged/profound marrow suppression, severe nonmyeloid toxicity (usually grade 3 or worse), or the inability to deliver therapeutic schedules of the investigational drug. Severity is usually graded by the Common Terminology Criteria for Adverse Events (CTCAE) that are widely available (ctep.cancer.gov/protocolDevelopment/electronic_applications/ctc.htm).

By increasing the dose in a stepwise fashion, until DLT is observed, a dose level for testing efficacy in a phase II setting is reached. Escalation of dose can be done in various ways—the commonest method is a "3+3" design where three patients are treated at each dose level, with doses escalated done in a modified Fibonacci sequence (dose increased by 100%, 67%, 50%, 40%, 33%). Various alternative methods have been developed, including accelerated titration and model-based methods, where continuous assessment of PK is done to adjust dose in each subsequent patient (5). A recent innovation in trial design has been the phase 0 trial, designed to assess the pharmacologic behavior of a new agent in humans by giving ultra-low doses (6). As with PK-based escalation procedures, these trials have the potential to increase both safety and efficiency of phase I studies. In the current regulatory environment, a negative impact on speed of development is often viewed as a liability of this approach.

Phase I Combinations

Combination trials are a special form of phase I trial (often denoted as phase Ib) in which considerations of both dose and mechanism enter into the study design. Such trials can employ dose escalation of one or both drugs, to evaluate toxicities of the combination. The design of the combination regimen, including selection of schedules of administration, starting doses, and modifications for toxicity, may be informed by preclinical combination studies in vivo (optimal), or by PK and PD studies from previous human single-agent trials. For example, drugs that are commonly administered continuously as single agents may be given less frequently in combination, provided there is PK/PD justification. As is well known, cetuximab, which like most antibodies has a long half-life, though given weekly as a single agent, is now more commonly administered biweekly in combination. With sunitinib, which causes significant bone marrow and adrenal toxicities, an interrupted schedule was chosen early during its development (7), and has recently been proven superior (8). In other cases, schedules may be modified as the phase I is in progress—ipilimumab, the anti-CTLA4 antibody, was developed by evaluating immune-related adverse events closely. Based on appearance of these toxicities, their association with therapeutic response, and ability to manage these toxicities, effective but safe doses and schedules were chosen (9). These examples indicate that design flexibility and continuous monitoring of results is required to optimize regimens in advance of formal phase II studies.

There is no single optimal design of a phase I combination trial. In some combinations, the dose of one drug may be fixed, and the second escalated—this is a strategy often used in antibody trials, as was the design in a phase I trial of rad001 and cetuximab (Table 12.1). In others, there is a desire to define varying dose ratios, and to analyze PK/PD interactions. Such was the case in a phase I trial of sorafenib and irinotecan (Table 12.1). Here, the doses of each drug were escalated separately in a simultaneous accrual after the combination of equivalent doses (eg, 50% standard doses) was found to be tolerable. Interim dose levels were accrued together, and if both were tolerable the next level would comprise both escalations (see levels 3 and 5).

Early introduction of combination regimens is an attractive avenue when the phase I trial indicates a good toxicity profile and early evidence of target inhibition, and when preclinical data suggest that the novel compound may be most effective as a part of a combination regimen. For example, the Smac-mimetic IAP antagonist, TL32711, was studied initially as a single agent, but even while that approach was in progress, a 5-arm phase Ib combination trial (NCT01188499) was activated when biologically

Table 12.1 Designs for Combination Phase I Trials

Level	Drug A (Cetuximab)	Drug B (RAD001)	n
1	100%	50%	3
2	100%	75%	6
3	100%	100%	6

Level	Drug A (Irinotecan)	Drug B (Sorafenib)	n
1	120 mg/m^2 q2w	100 mg bid	3
2A	150 mg/m^2 q2w	100 mg bid	3
2B	120 mg/m^2 q2w	200 mg bid	6
3	150 mg/m^2 q2w	200 mg bid	6
4A	180 mg/m^2 q2w	200 mg bid	3
4B	150 mg/m^2 q2w	400 mg bid	6
5	180 mg/m^2 q2w	400 mg bid	6

active concentrations in plasma were shown to be achievable and well tolerated (10). Such an approach permits accelerated development to a setting in which the activity of the drug will be optimally assessed.

EARLY EVIDENCE OF ACTIVITY

Pharmacodynamics and Biomarker Identification

A sine qua non of targeted therapy development is the demonstration that the drug does what it is supposed to, preferably in tumor tissue. This PD objective is not easily accomplished. For various signaling inhibitors, Baselga, Tabernero, and the Barcelona group have led the way in demonstrating, through validated analyses of tumor and surrogate tissues, which investigational pathway inhibitors have the desired PD effects at tolerable doses (recent review [11]). Initially, for gefitinib and erlotinib, and subsequently for several inhibitors of the epidermal growth factor receptor (EGFR) pathway, they have shown evidence to link PD effects to therapeutic value (12–14). These studies have led most recently to advances with signaling inhibitors in breast cancer (15,16), as well as a better understanding of the role of novel targeted therapies in CRC (17).

With other targeted therapies, it may be even more difficult to demonstrate effects in tumor tissue histologically, and alternative approaches are required. Cell cycle inhibitors provide a case in point: Many colon tumors have relatively low fractions of cycling cells, and the assays for their quantification are nonspecific (eg, Ki67). In this setting, imaging may provide proof of concept. We studied the cell cycle inhibitor PD0332991, a potent inhibitor of cyclin-dependent kinases 4 and 6 (18). In our initial phase I trials an excellent relationship of dose to neutropenia, the main side-effect, was demonstrated (19). An even closer relationship with drug exposure was evident from the Hill plot (Figure 12.1A), which shows the expected relationship of higher exposure (AUC) and greater myelotoxicity (expressed as % change in neutrophils). This relationship is similar to that shown for carboplatin, a drug now commonly dosed based on projected PK exposure. In practical terms, the data demonstrate that a decrease in neutrophils should be sought as evidence of potentially therapeutic drug levels. Imaging methods can serve as PD markers as well. In a clinical trial of Rad001 and cetuximab, FDG-PET showed clearly that the uptake of the label in the tumor was decreased markedly after treatment (Figure 12.1B), verifying that the PD endpoint had been met in tumor tissue. FLT-PET uses fluoro-L-thymidine, the uptake of which is increased in cycling cells, and is another marker being studied in phase I/II settings. Similarly, MRI imaging has refined the development of sorafenib, and may provide early PD evidence for anti-angiogenic drugs directed to several targets.

Pharmacodynamic Refinement

In the early phase I setting, there is noise in the data principally from small numbers of patients, interpatient variability, and different dose levels. A more consistent relationship between drug dosing and PD response may therefore be obtained in the phase Ib/II setting. This is a key justification for expansion cohorts at the highest doses of phase I trials—in a more uniform population, the degree of target interaction and its variability can be quantified with greater accuracy. Further advantages include treating more patients, with perhaps more uniform disease characteristics, in a narrower dose range, and obtaining a preliminary assessment of the potential response characteristics with the drug, the better to design subsequent phase II trials.

THE PHASE I/II INTERFACE

Selection of Patient Populations

Targeted therapies would be expected to have clear means of defining susceptible patient populations. Vemurafenib (PLX4032) has astounding activity in its target population of *BRAF*-mutant melanoma (21), and preclinical studies provide a compelling rationale as to why the drug might not be effective, or even be deleterious in patients without this molecular lesion (22). The initial phase I/II trial showed a dose relationship for target inhibition in tumor, a clear relationship of response to the presence of a *BRAF* mutation, and striking shrinkage of melanoma (23). In CRC, this agent was much less effective in response rates (only 1 of 19), though in retrospect the PFS data for BRAF-mutant CRC, which has been found to be associated with very poor survival, may be encouraging after all (24). A greater understanding of potential mechanisms

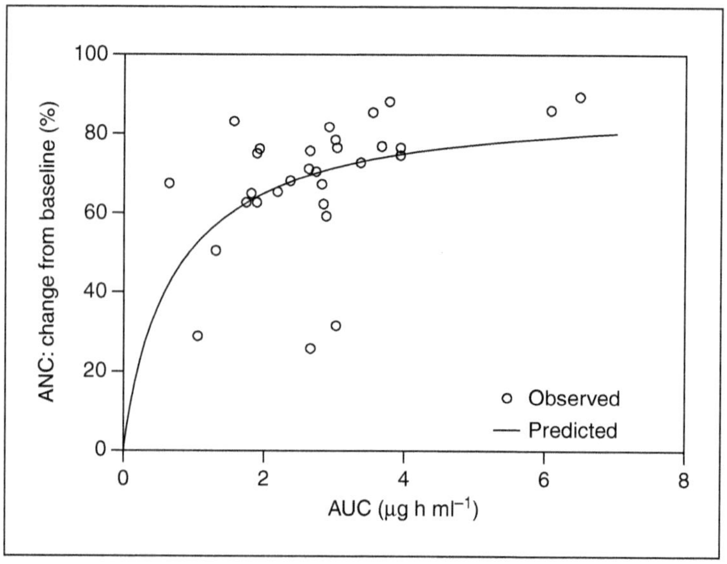

FIGURE 12.1A An excellent, well-predictable dose-response relationship between plasma drug level and neutropenia, seen in a phase I trial of PD0332991. AUC, area under curve; ANC, absolute neutrophil count. Reproduced from Br J Cancer. 2011. 104:1862-8.

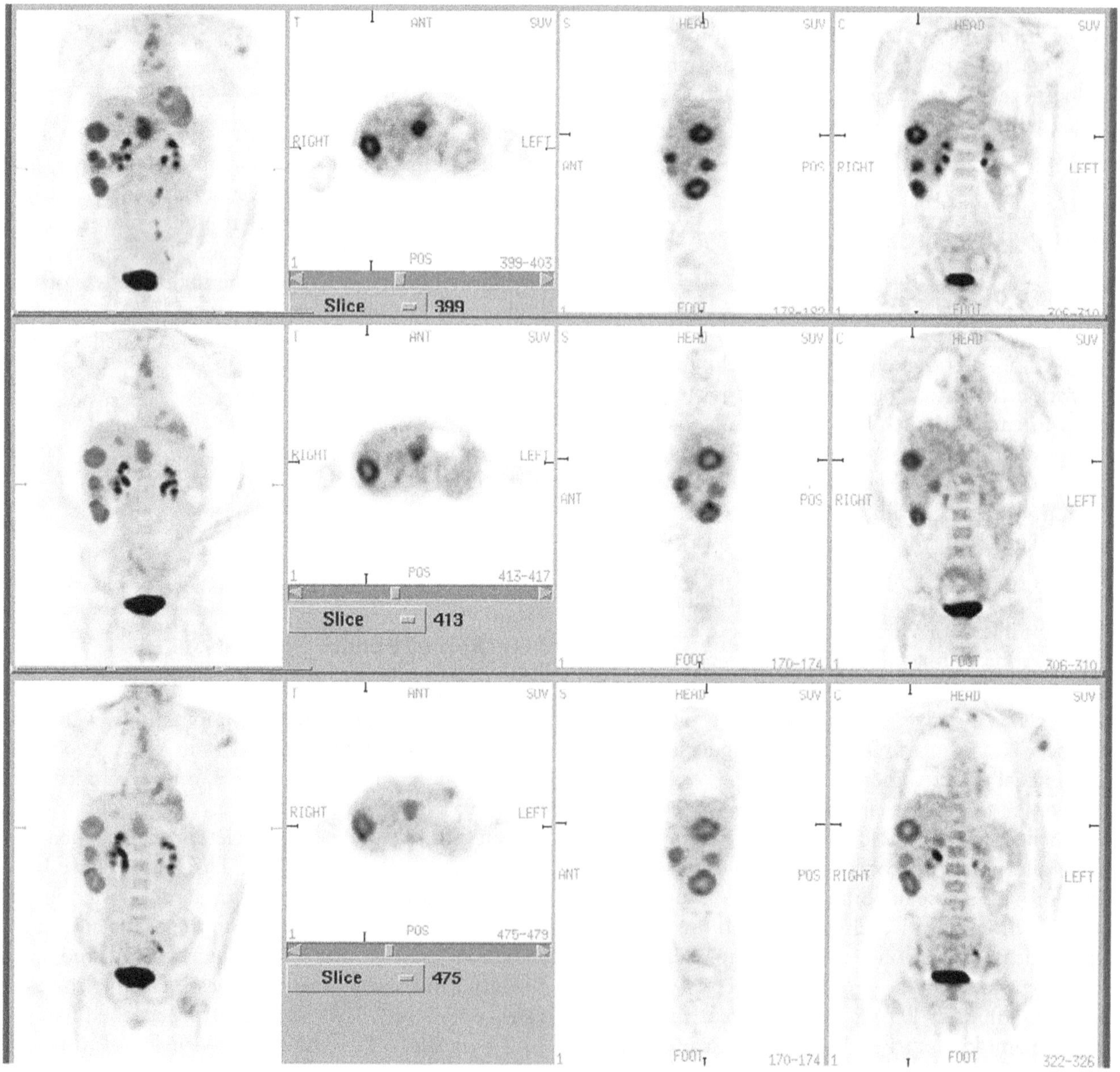

FIGURE 12.1B Serial positron emission tomography (PET) showing response to therapy in tumor metastases—a potential surrogate biomarker of response.

of resistance, including activation of EGFR signaling, has led to a proposed trial with inhibitors of this axis. This example serves to emphasize that a molecular lesion alone cannot be the basis for inferring activity, and that responses are likely to be disease-specific for many targeted therapies.

Initial Evidence of Response

By testing target- and patient-level effects, early evidence of response to the test drug can be sought. While traditional response parameters, such as progression-free and overall survival, take a long time to accumulate, the early phase trials utilize alternative methods to identify response signals. Metabolic imaging (FDG-PET, FLT-PET), tissue evaluation (complete or major pathologic response, serum target protein levels, autophagic vesicle counts, neovascularization density analyses), pathway analyses (phospho-protein assays), and genomic analyses (microarray-based gene expression, DNA methylation quantification) are some such methods.

An imaging intervention of great interest is glutamine-PET, to quantify uptake of the amino acid into tumor cells. Recent developments in tumor metabolism show that oncogene activation can alter metabolic profiles in cells. While many cells depend on glucose for energy requirements, some tumors, especially those with dysregulated myc signaling, rely more on glutamine as a source, and specific approaches to targeting c-myc are in development (25). Among them is an epigenetic approach to inhibition of BET signaling, which can downregulate c-myc expression in tumor models, with potent and selective antitumor activity (26). Clinical trials are being designed to target myc-expressing tumors, to incorporate both FDG-PET and glutamine-PET as PD markers to establish target inhibition. In CRCs, PET biomarkers, though widely used in the clinic to follow response, have not been developed to a level at which they could inform treatment selection, nor even treatment strategy, such as early detection of resistant disease.

In the expansion phase of phase I/II trials, testing may concentrate on specific disease or subtype populations to help define groups most likely to benefit and to help validate biomarkers. If a drug is active at this point, sample collection from the early phase II trials may begin to establish a database from which molecular profiles of responding patients may emerge. *K-ras* mutation and resistance to anti-EGFR molecules is a good example, though it did not emerge during the early development of the drugs. It could have, though, if the technology at the time of the development of cetuximab had been what it is today. Using such technology, drugs are being tested increasingly in subpopulations defined by genomics. For example, inhibitors of the PI3Kinase arm of the EGFR pathway are being tested in patients whose tumors specifically harbor mutations in the PI3Kinase arm molecules (NCT01501604, NCT01277757). As these trials proceed, assays of several molecules in the EGFR and related pathways are being done, to allow refinement of patient selection and validation of biomarkers.

FUTURE PHASE I TRIALS—WHAT WE SHOULD TRY TO LEARN

Role of PK

The advent of biologic agents in the treatment of cancer necessitates refinement of traditional PK assumptions and methods. Small molecules generally behave like traditional chemotherapeutic agents; however, monoclonal antibodies may not do so. Being large molecules, with specific targets in the body, the latter have special PK features. They do not diffuse from blood to peripheral tissues; rather, they extravasate by convection (27). They are distributed variably in tissues, depending on target antigen concentrations, and may be eliminated by nonlinear (concentration-dependent, akin to endogenous IgG, usually the case for antibodies targeting cell surface antigens, such as cetuximab for EGFR) or linear (concentration-independent, usually the case for antibodies targeting plasma antigens, such as bevacizumab for VEGF) clearance rates (28). Moreover, they usually have long half-lives, of the order of several days. These characteristics require nuanced evaluation of PK–PD relationships. Preclinical modeling may help in this evaluation as well, such as in the case of cetuximab (29). In addition, binding of an antibody to its intended target can affect the PK–PD relationship; this is termed target-mediated drug disposition (TMDD), and can be used to study the behavior of monoclonal antibodies in vivo (30).

Refinement of PD Markers

As mentioned above, novel methods of assessing PDs are being tested in early phase drug development. Since many newer biologic agents lead to disease control without effecting overt tumor size changes, traditional RECIST criteria for assessing response are sometimes not the most revealing. In some cases, especially with immunotherapeutic agents such as ipilimumab, an early progression of disease may be apparent on imaging, but leading to eventual disease control (31). In such cases, refining methods to assess drug activity is an important objective. Plasma assays (apoptosis markers, autophagic vesicle counts), tissue assays (angiogenic markers, target antigen stains), imaging using novel metabolic intermediates (glutamine-PET), circulating tumor cells, and so on, are some such methods.

Genomics

Genetic and epigenetic changes, among the hallmarks of a cancer cell, are attractive targets for drug development. Mutations in genes, copy number changes, methylation of DNA, histone acetylation, and so on, are some of the changes that can occur. Identifying these changes as drivers of disease and/or therapeutic targets can be studied in various ways, starting with whole-genome assays and moving on to specific gene/pathway analyses. Subsets of disease may have varying genetic profiles, and it is clearly the case in CRC. *K-ras* mutations render the EGFR antibodies ineffective in this disease, and alterations in molecules of the EGFR signaling pathway lead to different clinical outcomes (32,33). Mechanistic proof of drug efficacy or inefficacy is emerging from bench studies (34), and such analyses in tumor tissues can lead to sophisticated drug development in early phase trials.

REFERENCES

1. Ling J, Zhou H, Jiao Q, Davis HM. Interspecies scaling of therapeutic monoclonal antibodies: initial look. *J Clin Pharmacol.* 2009;49(12):1382–1402.
2. Ducongé J, Fernández-Sánchez E, Alvarez D. Interspecies scaling of the monoclonal anti-EGF receptor ior EGF/r3 antibody disposition using allometric paradigm: is it really suitable? *Biopharm Drug Dispos.* 2004;25(4):177–186.
3. Parulekar WR, Eisenhauer EA. Phase I trial design for solid tumor studies of targeted, non-cytotoxic agents: theory and practice. *J Natl Cancer Inst.* 2004;96(13):990–997.
4. Eisenhauer EA, O'Dwyer PJ, Christian M, Humphrey JS. Phase I clinical trial design in cancer drug development. *J Clin Oncol.* 2000;18(3):684–692.
5. Le Tourneau C, Lee JJ, Siu LL. Dose escalation methods in phase I cancer clinical trials. *J Natl Cancer Inst.* 2009;101(10):708–720.
6. Kummar S, Doroshow JH, Tomaszewski JE, Calvert AH, Lobbezoo M, Giaccone G; Task Force on Methodology for the Development of Innovative Cancer Therapies (MDICT). Phase 0 clinical trials: recommendations from the Task Force on Methodology for the Development of Innovative Cancer Therapies. *Eur J Cancer.* 2009;45(5):741–746.
7. Faivre S, Delbaldo C, Vera K, et al. Safety, pharmacokinetic, and antitumor activity of SU11248, a novel oral multitarget tyrosine kinase inhibitor, in patients with cancer. *J Clin Oncol.* 2006;24(1):25–35.
8. Motzer RJ, Hutson TE, Olsen MR, et al. Randomized phase II trial of sunitinib on an intermittent versus continuous dosing schedule as first-line therapy for advanced renal cell carcinoma. *J Clin Oncol.* 2012;30(12):1371–1377.
9. Weber J. Ipilimumab: controversies in its development, utility and autoimmune adverse events. *Cancer Immunol Immunother.* 2009;58(5):823–830.
10. Carter BZ, et al. Antagonizing IAPs by SMAC mimetic TL32711 induces apoptosis in AML cells including AML stem/progenitor cells alone and in combination with chemotherapy. *Blood.* 2011;118(21):Abstract 66.
11. Rodón J, Saura C, Dienstmann R, et al. Molecular prescreening to select patient population in early clinical trials. *Nat Rev Clin Oncol.* 2012;9(6):359–366.
12. Baselga J, Albanell J, Ruiz A, et al. Phase II and tumor pharmacodynamic study of gefitinib in patients with advanced breast cancer. *J Clin Oncol.* 2005;23(23):5323–5333.
13. Folprecht G, Tabernero J, Köhne CH, et al. Phase I pharmacokinetic/pharmacodynamic study of EKB-569, an irreversible inhibitor of the epidermal growth factor receptor tyrosine kinase, in combination with irinotecan, 5-fluorouracil, and leucovorin (FOLFIRI) in first-line treatment of patients with metastatic colorectal cancer. *Clin Cancer Res.* 2008;14(1):215–223.
14. Tabernero J, Rojo F, Calvo E, et al. Dose- and schedule-dependent inhibition of the mammalian target of rapamycin pathway with everolimus: a phase I tumor pharmacodynamic study in patients with advanced solid tumors. *J Clin Oncol.* 2008;26(10):1603–1610.
15. Baselga J, Cortés J, Kim SB, et al.; CLEOPATRA Study Group. Pertuzumab plus trastuzumab plus docetaxel for metastatic breast cancer. *N Engl J Med.* 2012;366(2):109–119.
16. Baselga J, Campone M, Piccart M, et al. Everolimus in postmenopausal hormone-receptor-positive advanced breast cancer. *N Engl J Med.* 2012;366(6):520–529.
17. Tabernero J, Cervantes A, Rivera F, et al. Pharmacogenomic and pharmacoproteomic studies of cetuximab in metastatic colorectal cancer: biomarker analysis of a phase I dose-escalation study. *J Clin Oncol.* 2010;28(7):1181–1189.
18. Flaherty KT, Lorusso PM, Demichele A, et al. Phase I, dose-escalation trial of the oral cyclin-dependent kinase 4/6 inhibitor PD 0332991, administered using a 21-day schedule in patients with advanced cancer. *Clin Cancer Res.* 2012;18(2):568–576.
19. Schwartz GK, LoRusso PM, Dickson MA, et al. Phase I study of PD 0332991, a cyclin-dependent kinase inhibitor, administered in 3-week cycles (Schedule 2/1). *Br J Cancer.* 2011;104(12): 1862–1868.
20. Perini RF, et al. Phase II/pharmacodynamic trial of PD0332991 in patients with breast, colon, germ cell, and epithelial tumors containing amplification of CCND1. *J Clin Oncol.* 2011;29(15s):3088.
21. Chapman PB, Hauschild A, Robert C, et al.; BRIM-3 Study Group. Improved survival with vemurafenib in melanoma with BRAF V600E mutation. *N Engl J Med.* 2011;364(26):2507–2516.
22. Poulikakos PI, Zhang C, Bollag G, Shokat KM, Rosen N. RAF inhibitors transactivate RAF dimers and ERK signalling in cells with wild-type BRAF. *Nature.* 2010;464(7287):427–430.
23. Flaherty KT, Puzanov I, Kim KB, et al. Inhibition of mutated, activated BRAF in metastatic melanoma. *N Engl J Med.* 2010;363(9): 809–819.
24. Kopetz S, et al. PLX4032 in metastatic colorectal cancer patients with mutant BRAF tumors. *J Clin Oncol.* 2010;28(15s):3534.
25. Liu W, Le A, Hancock C, et al. Reprogramming of proline and glutamine metabolism contributes to the proliferative and metabolic responses regulated by oncogenic transcription factor c-MYC. *Proc Natl Acad Sci USA.* 2012;109(23):8983–8988.
26. Mertz JA, Conery AR, Bryant BM, et al. Targeting MYC dependence in cancer by inhibiting BET bromodomains. *Proc Natl Acad Sci USA.* 2011;108(40):16669–16674.
27. Keizer RJ, Huitema AD, Schellens JH, Beijnen JH. Clinical pharmacokinetics of therapeutic monoclonal antibodies. *Clin Pharmacokinet.* 2010;49(8):493–507.
28. Mould DR, Green B. Pharmacokinetics and pharmacodynamics of monoclonal antibodies: concepts and lessons for drug development. *BioDrugs.* 2010;24(1):23–39.
29. Luo FR, Yang Z, Dong H, et al. Correlation of pharmacokinetics with the antitumor activity of Cetuximab in nude mice bearing the GEO human colon carcinoma xenograft. *Cancer Chemother Pharmacol.* 2005;56(5):455–464.
30. Levy G. Pharmacologic target-mediated drug disposition. *Clin Pharmacol Ther.* 1994;56(3):248–252.
31. Saenger YM, Wolchok JD. The heterogeneity of the kinetics of response to ipilimumab in metastatic melanoma: patient cases. *Cancer Immun.* 2008;8:1.
32. Karapetis CS, Khambata-Ford S, Jonker DJ, et al. K-ras mutations and benefit from cetuximab in advanced colorectal cancer. *N Engl J Med.* 2008;359(17):1757–1765.
33. De Roock W, Claes B, Bernasconi D, et al. Effects of K-ras, BRAF, NRAS, and PIK3CA mutations on the efficacy of cetuximab plus chemotherapy in chemotherapy-refractory metastatic colorectal cancer: a retrospective consortium analysis. *Lancet Oncol.* 2010;11(8):753–762.
34. Prahallad A, Sun C, Huang S, et al. Unresponsiveness of colon cancer to BRAF(V600E) inhibition through feedback activation of EGFR. *Nature.* 2012;483(7387):100–103.

13 Management of Systemic Treatment-Induced Toxicities

MAXWELL T. VERGO
AXEL GROTHEY
JULIA MINOCHA
JONATHAN COTLIAR

INTRODUCTION

Systemic treatment for colorectal cancer (CRC) has clearly improved outcome for patients including survival and quality of life. Therapy also has the potential to result in significant toxicities that require intervention. This chapter will focus on some of the common adverse events experienced by CRC patients receiving systemic therapies including diarrhea, neurotoxicity secondary to oxaliplatin, EGFR associated cutaneous toxicities and hand and foot syndrome.

DIARRHEA

Diarrhea can be life-threatening when associated with chemotherapy (1) as well as impact on patient-reported quality of life during and after treatment has completed (2). With modern day combination chemotherapy or chemoradiation therapy, diarrhea is common occurring in about 60%–70% of patients including up to 16% with grade 3 to 4 toxicity (Table 13.1). Over 50% of patients require dose modification of their chemotherapy in CRC due to diarrhea including 11% with grade 1 to 2 toxicity, highlighting the importance of aggressive management to help maintain dose intensity of the chemotherapy (3). In one retrospective analysis of 63 CRC patients admitted to the hospital for supportive care, the mortality rate of 4.8% was reported (4). Therefore, this is an important symptom for practicing oncologists to feel comfortable managing.

In this section, we aim to review etiologies and predisposing factors for diarrhea and provide a comprehensive approach to work up and management including a review of the literature for existing first and second-line antidiarrheal agents.

Etiologies and Predisposing Factors

Etiologies of diarrhea in CRC should be considered prior to initiation of a clinical response. In particular, reversible etiologies need to be explored and corrected. Dietary, medication, nonmalignant syndromes, and infectious etiologies (Table 13.2) must be considered either as primary causes of diarrhea or as exacerbating factors with chemotherapy-induced diarrhea (CID; 5–7). In general, dietary modifications are warranted and nonessential contributing medications should be discontinued. Work up for infectious diarrhea is usually guided by presentation with fever and when diagnosed should be managed with targeted antibiotic therapy.

The major etiologies of diarrhea in CRC include both CID and radiation induced diarrhea (for rectal cancer patients in particular). Although the mechanism of CID is not well elucidated and likely varies from one chemotherapeutic agent to the next, 5-fluorouracil (5-FU) is felt to damage rapidly dividing crypt cells in the intestinal epithelium as well as affecting digestive enzymatic action leading to both a malabsorptive and osmotic diarrhea (5). Predisposing factors for CID in CRC include female sex, older age (65 or order), and poor performance status (greater than or equal to 2; 8–10). In addition, chemotherapy-specific risk factors include toxicity associated with cycle 1 of therapy (risk of CID declines over time, arguing for weekly monitoring between cycle 1 and 2), chemotherapy cycle length greater than 3 weeks, and coexisting neutropenia (11).

There is hope that molecular biomarkers will help predict patients with an increased risk of severe (grade 3–5) toxicity. Currently, polymorphisms of uridine diphosphate glucuronosyltransferase 1A1 (UGT1A1) and deficiency of dihydropyrimidine dehydrogenase (DPD), for irinotecan and 5-FU, respectively, are two of the most widely evaluated markers.

UGT1A1 is responsible for the clearance of SN-38, the main active metabolite of irinotecan, and the homozygous UGT1A1*28 7/7 polymorphism (7 TA base pair repeats in the promoter region of both genes) present in about 10% of the population has been associated with hematological toxicity, but not consistently with GI toxicity or diarrhea. A large population-based study revealed no significant

Table 13.1 Reports of Grade 1 to 2 and Grade 3 to 4 Toxicity From Diarrhea Reported in Major Clinical Trials in CRC

Chemotherapy Regimen	Grade 1 to 2 Toxicity (%)	Grade 3 to 4 Toxicity (%)
Infusional 5-FU/LV (26)	38.5	5.3
Bolus 5-FU/LV (27)	39.5	25.6
Capecitabine* (28)	35	11
Weekly Irinotecan (29)	46	36
Irinotecan every 3 weeks (29)	57	19
Cetuximab (30)	NA	1.7
Panitumumab (31)	20	1
FOLFIRI (27)	55.2	13
FOLFOX (26)	46.9	11.9
FOLFIRI + cetuximab (32)	NA	15.7
FOLFIRI + panitumumab (33)	43	14
FOLFOX + cetuximab (34)	NA	8
FOLOX + panitumumab (35)	NA	18
Radiation + infusional 5FU (36)	72	2
Radiation + capecitabine (36)	58	4

*1250 mg/m^2 by mouth twice daily dosing.

5-FU, 5-fluorouracil; LV, leucovorin; NA, not available; FOLFIRI, 5FU + irinotecan; FOLFOX, 5FU + oxaliplatin.

Table 13.2 Etiologies of Diarrhea in CRC Patients

Etiology	Examples
Dietary	Lactose containing foods*
	Caffeine consumption
	Spicy foods
	Fatty/fried foods
	Cruciferous vegetables
	High carbohydrate content**
	High osmolar supplements
	Sorbitol containing products (like sugar free gum)
	High fiber foods
	Alcohol consumption
Medications	Antiacids with magnesium
	Antibiotics (especially macrolides)
	Bile salts
	Lactulose
	Colchicine***
	Potassium chloride
	Prokinetic agents (such as metoclopromide)****
	Nonsteroidal anti-inflammatory drugs
	H2 blockers
	Proton pump inhibitors
Nonmalignant syndromes	Constipation with overflow diarrhea
	Malabsorptive syndromes
	Hyperthyroidism
	Inflammatory bowel disease
	Irritable bowel syndrome
Infectious	*Clostridia difficile*
	Salmonella
	Escherichia coli
	Campylobacter
	Other infectious colitis

*Protracted diarrhea causes transient loss of lactase activity in the large colon leading to functional lactase intolerance.
**These are not properly absorbed and cause an osmotic diarrhea.
***Greater than 20% incidence of diarrhea.
****Greater than 10% incidence of diarrhea.

relationship between the UGT1A1*28 7/7 polymorphism and diarrhea grade 3 to 4 toxicity in 214 evaluable patients (12). In addition, there is a poor positive predictive value of 0.24 in pooled data from three studies that reported a positive correlation between the polymorphism and diarrhea (13).

DPD is responsible for the catabolism of 5-FU to fluoro-5, 6-dihydrouracil (FUH_2) and is the rate-limiting and major step and in elimination of 5-FU (and capecitabine, which is a prodrug of 5-FU; 14). Clinically, either DPD activity (via peripheral mononuclear cells; 15) or the DPD gene mutation IVS14+1G>A, the most common clinically significant mutation (16), have been associated with 5-FU-related toxicity including neurotoxicity, neutropenia, mucositis, and diarrhea (17,18). DPD activity is preferred since this appears to detect more clinically relevant toxicities compared with DPD gene mutation analysis (19). There are no prospective data available in regard to DPD deficiency for predicting 5-FU related toxicity and the prevalence of DPD deficiency in a general CRC population is low (17). Therefore, it may be best utilized only in patients after severe 5-FU-related toxicity raising a clinical suspicion for DPD deficiency as confirmation as the prevalence of deficiency in this group can be as high as 24% (18).

Lastly, measurement of the 5-FU area under the curve (AUC) has been linked with grade 2 to 4 toxicity in colorectal patients receiving the Mayo bolus regimen (5-FU 425 mg/m^2 + leucovorin 20 mg/m^2 bolus days 1–5 every 28 days) but only for the first cycle since appropriate clinically based dose reductions minimized grade 2 to 4 toxicity in later cycles (20). Tolerable dose escalations have been shown in CRC patients guided by AUC, but there are no data comparing the efficacy of this strategy with standard dosing (21). At this time, it is not clear that AUC dosing of 5-FU allows for improved tolerability or efficacy over standard dosing and dose adjustment.

Clinical Assessment and Management

In the initial assessment of a CRC patient receiving chemotherapy who presents with diarrhea, it is essential for the physician to both properly grade the severity of the diarrhea and to classify it as "uncomplicated" or "complicated" as these measures will ultimately determine the appropriate clinical response (see Tables 13.3 and 13.4, respectively). Complicated diarrhea consists of either CTCAE v4.03 grade 3 to 4 diarrhea or patients who present with a "GI syndrome" consisting of severe diarrhea, nausea, vomiting, anorexia, and abdominal cramping with accompanying severe dehydration, neutropenia, fever, and electrolyte imbalances (22). Recognition of complicated diarrhea is essential to prevent significant morbidity or mortality from CID.

A proposed clinical algorithm has been developed and modified by an expert panel in 2002 (Figure 13.1) and this will serve as a guide for the discussion here for management and treatment decisions.

Uncomplicated diarrhea is generally managed with a combination of oral hydration, dietary modification, "low dose" loperamide (4 mg followed by 2 mg every 4 hours or after every unformed stool; maximum 16 mg/day), and holding cytotoxic chemotherapy until symptoms have resolved. It should be noted that in a double-blind crossover study design for patients with chronic diarrhea, although diphenoxylate reduced the stool frequency similarly to loperamide, it was less effective at producing solid stool and reducing urgency/incontinence as well as causing more central nervous system effects (23). Although we do not have studies in patients with CID, this has led to recommendations of loperamide as a first-line agent. Newer preparations of diphenoxylate combined with atropine have not been evaluated formally against loperamide. Loperamide is continued until diarrhea has stopped for 12 hours, but patients receiving radiation should continue on loperamide for the duration of their radiation course as the diarrhea is not anticipated to stop prior to this.

Persistent uncomplicated diarrhea for greater than 12 to 24 hours on low-dose loperamide requires escalation

Table 13.3 Common Toxicity Criteria (V4.03) for Diarrhea

Adverse Event	Grade 1	Grade 2	Grade 3	Grade 4	Grade 5
Diarrhea	Increase of less than 4 stools per day over baseline; mild increase in ostomy output compared to baseline	Increase of 4 to 6 stools per day over baseline; moderate increase in ostomy output compared to baseline	Increase of greater than or equal to 7 stools per day over baseline; incontinence; hospitalization indicated; severe increase in ostomy output compared to baseline; limiting self-care ADL*	Life-threatening consequences; urgent intervention indicated	Death

*Self-care ADL refers to bathing, dressing and undressing, feeding self, using the toilet, taking medications, and not be bedridden.

Adapted from the National Cancer Institute, evs.nci.nih.gov/ftp1/CTCAE/CTCAE_4.03_2010-06-14_QuickReference_5x7.pdf, accessed December 21 2011.

Table 13.4 Classification of Diarrhea as Complicated or Uncomplicated Using CTCAE V4.03 and Other Clinical Signs and Symptoms

	Uncomplicated Diarrhea	Complicated Diarrhea
CTCAE v4.03 Grading signs and symptoms	1 to 2 No complicating signs/symptoms	3 to 4 Cramping Nausea/vomiting (greater than or equal to grade 2) Decreased performance status Fever Sepsis Neutropenia Frank bleeding Dehydration

Adapted from Benson (22).

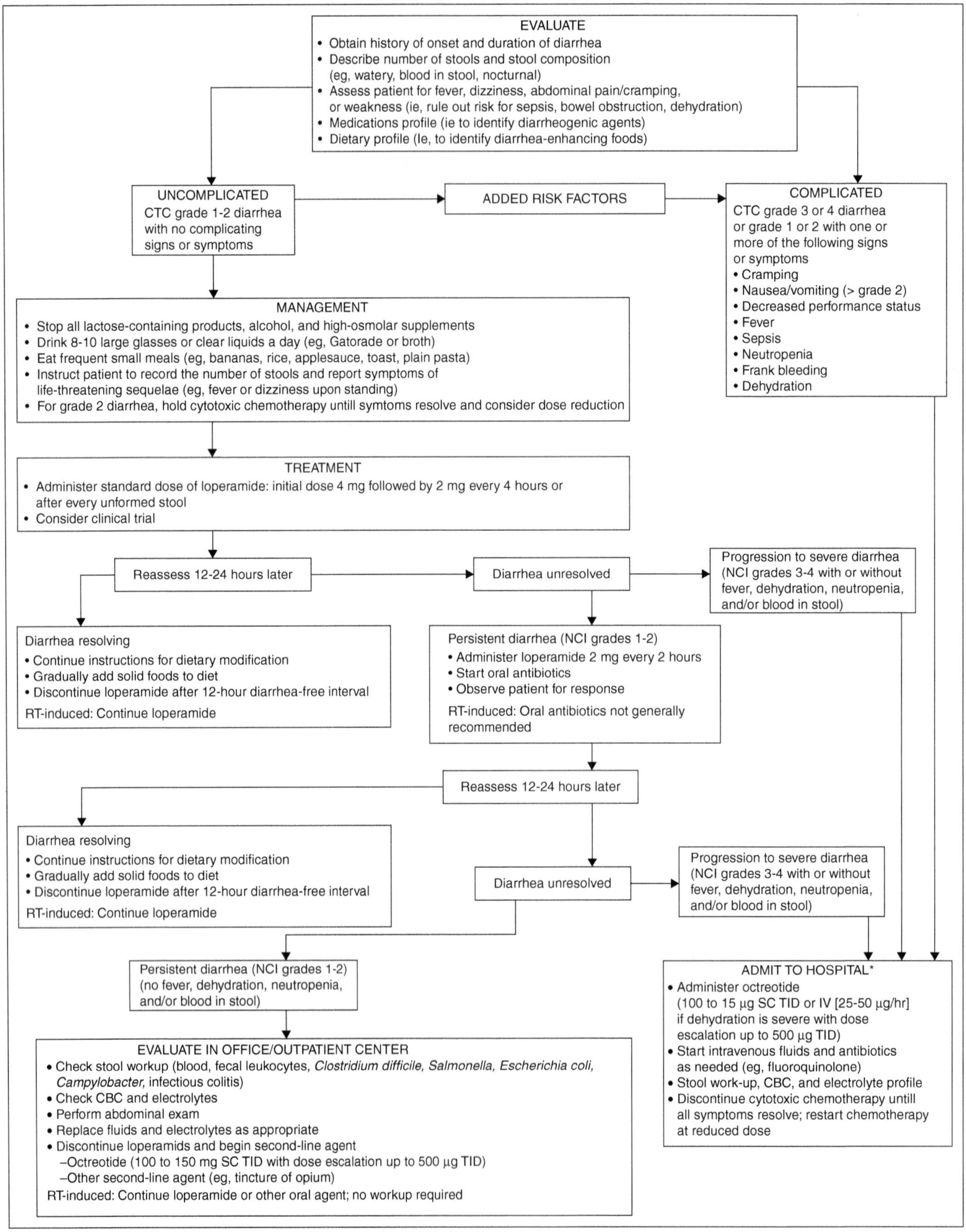

FIGURE 13.1 Expert panel proposed chemotherapy-treatment induced diarrhea management and treatment algorithm.

CTC, common toxicity criteria; NCI, National Cancer Institute; RT, radiotherapy; SC, subcutaneous; tid, three times a day; IV, intravenous; CBC, complete blood count; CID, chemotherapy-induced diarrhea.

of loperamide to "high-dose" (2 mg every 2 hours; maximum of 24 mg/day). Patients receiving high-dose irinotecan (400–600 mg/m^2) started this high-dose loperamide with their first diarrhea episode (median time to onset was 6 days) and continued it until 12 hours of no diarrhea or 3 days of continued nonstop loperamide intake. Only 1 out of 17 patients required admission for diarrhea for treatment failure and 80% were able to tolerate three or more cycles of high-dose irinotecan (24). In addition to high-dose loperamide, oral antibiotics are also recommended at this time for patients not undergoing radiation therapy for a presumed infectious etiology (1). Persistent uncomplicated diarrhea for 48 hours or more requires an office visit for stool cultures and studies, blood count and electrolyte monitoring, physical exam, potential intravenous fluids, cessation of loperamide, and initiation of second-line antidiarrheal agents (Table 13.5; 22).

Of particular note, a large double-blinded, placebo-controlled, randomized study (RTOG 0315) utilized octreotide depot formulation at 30 mg monthly and did not find a significant difference from placebo in terms of grade 2 to 4 diarrhea (49% placebo vs 44% octreotide; $P = .21$; 25). Given that the antidiarrheal mechanism of action for octreotide includes slowing intestinal transit time, increasing intestinal water reabsorption, and decreased intestinal secretions, it is understandable that it failed to control diarrhea being generated from an insult to the most distal portion of the GI tract.

Complicated diarrhea may be present from the start of the diarrheal episode, but occasionally uncomplicated diarrhea can become complicated. In either situation, the algorithm is much more aggressive including admission to the hospital to expedite the workup and treatment as this has a much higher rate of morbidity and mortality compared to uncomplicated diarrhea. Upon admission, the patient is worked up for the etiology of the diarrhea (complete blood count, electrolyte profile, stool studies and cultures), started immediately on intravenous fluids with careful attention to rehydrating and matching

Table 13.5 Second-Line Antidiarrheal Agents After Failure of Loperamide Including Suggested Dosing and Summarized Evidence

Agent	Suggested Dosing	Summarized Evidence
Octreotide*	100–500 mcg SC TID or 30 to 40 mg depot IM every 28 days	92% RR for patients with grade 3–4 diarrhea refractory to loperamide (37) 90% vs 61% CR of diarrhea (500 mcg vs 100 mcg SC TID; $P < .05$) in loperamide refractory patients (38) Reduced CID by greater than or equal to 2 grades in 89% of drug resistant disease (39) Nonsignificant trend for less severe diarrhea, less IVFs, less unscheduled visits in 40 mg vs 30 mg depot (40)
Tincture of opium*	Deodorized tincture (10 mg/mL) 10–15 drops PO every 3 to 4 hours or paregoric/camphorated tincture (0.4 mg/mL) 1 tsp (5 mL) in water PO every 3 to 4 hours	Expert opinion (41)
Budesonide	9 PO daily (days 2 through 5 or 7)	No difference in phase III double-blind RCT, but more loperamide used in placebo and trends for less duration and frequency of diarrhea in budesonide (42)
Lomotil	2.5–5 mg PO every 6–8 hours (maximum 20 mg per day)	Expert opinion (41)
Glutamine	6 g PO TID (days -5 through +10)	Less loperamide needed in double-blind RCT (favoring glutamine), nonsignificant trend in lower AUC of diarrhea (43)
Probiotics	Lactobacillus rhamnosis GG (1–2 × 10^{10} PO per day)	RCT revealing less grade 3/4 diarrhea (22% vs 37%; $P = .03$), less abdominal discomfort, less hospital care, less chemotherapy reductions (44)
Activated charcoal	Charcodote 5 mL of 1000 mg/25 mL aqueous solution PO TID (days—1 through 2)	Patient served as control and found less grade 3/4 diarrhea (7% vs 25%), more grade 0 diarrhea (46% vs 21%), higher median planned dose (98% vs 70%), and less loperamide use (25% vs 54%) although insufficient power (45)
COX-2 inhibition	400 mg PO BID	Two RCTs both concluded no significant difference in diarrhea toxicity with irinotecan based regimens (46,47)

*Supported by expert consensus panel (Benson [22]).

SC, subcutaneous; TID, three times a day; RR, response rate; CR, complete resolution; CID, chemotherapy induced diarrhea; IVFs, intravenous fluids; PO, by mouth; RCT, randomized controlled trial; AUC, area under the curve.

the diarrheal output, potential intravenous antibiotics (depending on the clinical suspicion), and starting octreotide as frontline therapy. Subcutaneous or intravenous octreotide are recommended in the acute setting as depot octreotide given intramuscularly can take up to 2 weeks to take therapeutic effect. Starting doses are similar to second-line dosing for uncomplicated diarrhea, 100 to 150 mcg subcutaneously every 8 hours. Hospitalized patients have intravenous access to start octreotide as a continuous infusion usually starting around 25 to 50 mcg/hr. Lastly, complicated diarrhea almost certainly requires a decrease in chemotherapy dose intensity. Due to this, there is a push to develop strategies that prevent complicated diarrhea to allow improved dose intensity and hopefully both improved patient reported and disease centered outcomes.

Current clinical trials for impacting diarrhea in CRC focus on utilizing probiotics, improving predictive biomarkers, and trials with new agents (ie, calcium aluminosilicate).

Summary and Conclusion

CID is a significant issue in CRC due to the use of 5-FU, irinotecan, and the EGFR inhibitors. This can lead to worsened patient quality of life, increased patient morbidity and mortality, and effect dose intensity of chemotherapy which may impact disease-free survival or disease-control rates.

Predictive markers are not yet ready to be incorporated into standard care. We need more prospective data with the hope that a particular biomarker could have an adequate positive predictive value to allow us to prevent CID by either using targeted therapies or more tailored dosing strategies.

Classifying patients by the grade of their diarrhea and by the presence of the GI syndrome can help practitioners manage CID in an efficacious and streamlined fashion using the algorithm that has been previously developed. Loperamide and octreotide remain well-supported standards for the management of CID, but we need a larger repertoire of effective antidiarrheal agents especially with the emergence of new therapeutic agents. In addition, there are gaps in our knowledge still. For example, is there a viable way to prevent or better treat chemoradiation-induced diarrhea? Or is the best strategy actually to stop loperamide when starting a second-line agent? Could there be a synergistic or additive effect to adding a second agent as we do for management of constipation? Lastly, do we need to further understand the mechanisms by which each cytotoxic agent causes diarrhea and be more targeted in our approach to management of this challenging adverse effect?

■ OXALIPLATIN-INDUCED NEUROTOXICITY

Chemotherapy-induced sensory neurotoxicity occurs in the majority of patients undergoing treatment with oxaliplatin for CRC. Oxaliplatin improves survival in patients with CRC in the adjuvant and palliative setting, but its use is associated with both acute neuropathy and chronic sensory neurotoxicity, which can be persistent for a subset of patients and can have significant impact on quality of life. The acute sensory toxicity, an oxaliplatin-associated adverse event, is transient and develops concurrent with oxaliplatin administration. Chronic sensory neuropathy, in contrast, develops with cumulative doses and routinely becomes the limiting factor in the total dose of oxaliplatin that patients can tolerate. Since treatment options for established chemotherapy-induced peripheral neurotoxicity are limited, the emphasis in clinical practice should focus on prevention.

Oxaliplatin is an integral part of the management of CRC in the adjuvant and advanced treatment setting. Oxaliplatin was added to adjuvant treatment regimens after results from three large randomized phase III trials comparing its addition to standard 5-FU/leucovorin (5-FU/LV) therapy (48–50). The pivotal and standard-setting phase III trial, the Multicenter International Study of Oxaliplatin/5-Fluorouracil/Leucovorin in the Adjuvant Treatment of Colon Cancer (MOSAIC), found that oxaliplatin added to 5-FU/LV led to a 23% improvement in 3-year disease-free survival (DFS). Updated results of the MOSAIC trial revealed that the improvement in 3-year DFS translated into an overall survival (OS) benefit at 6 years (51).

The inclusion of oxaliplatin in standard chemotherapy for advanced CRC was established following results from the phase III intergroup trial N9741 that compared FOLFOX4, bolus 5-FU/LV plus irinotecan (IFL) and irinotecan plus oxaliplatin (IROX) as first-line therapy for patients with advanced CRC (52). Patients treated with FOLFOX4 experienced a median progression-free survival (PFS) of 8.7 months and an OS of 19.5 months, which was significantly longer than either infusional IFL or IROX. Based on results of N9741, FOLFOX became the standard of care for the first-line treatment of advanced CRC across the United States and in many other countries. Due to current strategies to incorporate biologic agents into treatment for advanced CRC, such as bevacizumab and antiepidermal growth factor-receptor (anti-EGFR) antibodies, patients are receiving systemic therapy for longer periods of time. The need for strategies to prevent and/or reduce the neurotoxic effects of oxaliplatin continues to grow to maximize outcomes for patients. In this section, we will discuss evidence-based strategies for managing chemotherapy-induced sensory neuropathy associated with oxaliplatin in patients undergoing treatment for CRC.

■ OXALIPLATIN-INDUCED PERIPHERAL NEUROPATHY

There are several main classes of peripheral neuropathy associated with oxaliplatin treatment: cold-induced acute neuropathy, cumulative sensory neurotoxicity, muscle-spasms, and delayed sensory neurotoxicity (coasting) which manifests after discontinuation of oxaliplatin therapy. During or shortly after treatment with oxaliplatin, 85%–95% of patients develop acute neurosensory changes. Acute neuropathy commonly includes perioral, or distal paresthesias and dysesthesias, which are commonly triggered or exacerbated by exposure to cold. Paralaryngeal dysesthesias occur in 1%–2% of patients and although patients sense that they have difficulty breathing or swallowing, this is not due to actual laryngeal obstruction and is limited to sensory phenomenon. Less often, patients might experience myotonic spasms, especially in the jaw or hands. Acute sensory changes are transient in nature and can last several hours to days. It has been suggested that the mechanism underlying these sensory changes is due to a deregulation of the neural sodium ion channels (53,54). Oxalate, released from oxaliplatin, could chelate calcium and cause an influx of sodium ions followed by hyperexcitability.

Chronic sensory neurotoxicity changes associated with oxaliplatin consist of peripheral nerve paresthesias or dysesthesias and sometimes a neuropathic pain syndrome. These symptoms become more pronounced with cumulative doses of oxaliplatin and can advance to being persistent throughout treatment cycles. This peripheral neuropathy eventually interferes with daily functions, including buttoning clothes, writing, and handling small objects. At this stage, the symptoms meet the National Cancer Institutes Common Toxicity Criteria (NCI-CTC) definition of grade 3 neurotoxicity (Table 13.6). The effects of chronic sensory neuropathy from oxaliplatin are likely due to an accumulation of platinum in the cells of the dorsal root ganglion (55,56).

In the MOSAIC trial, 92% of patients reported peripheral sensory neuropathy of any grade during adjuvant treatment (48). At the end of treatment, 31.6% had moderate sensory loss and paresthesias (grade 2) and 12.4% of patients had neuropathy severe enough to interfere with function (grade 3). The majority of the neurotoxicity was reversible, with 4.8% and 3.4% of patients having residual grade 2 neuropathy at 1 and 1.5 years, respectively. Of patients with grade 3 neuropathy, symptoms persisted in 1.1% and 0.5% of patients at 1 year and 1.5, years after chemotherapy. Similarly, in the NSABP C-07 trial with a

■ Table 13.6 National Cancer Institute Common Terminology Criteria for Adverse Events Version 4.0

Adverse Event	Grade 1	Grade 2	Grade 3	Grade 4	Grade 5
Acneiform rash (papulopustular eruption)	Papules and/or pustules covering less than 10% BSA, which may or may not be associated with pruritus or pain	Papules and/or pustules covering 10%–30% BSA, which may or not be associated with pruritus or pain; associated with psychosocial impact; limiting instrumental ADL	Papules and/or pustules covering greater than 30% BSA, which may or may not be associated with pruritus or pain; limiting self-care ADL; associated with local superinfection with oral antibiotics indicated	Papules and/or pustules covering any % BSA, which may or may not be associated with pruritus or pain, and are associated with extensive superinfection with IV antibiotics indicated; life-threatening consequences	Death
Dry skin (xerosis)	Covering less than 10% BSA and no associated erythema or pruritus	Covering 10%–30% BSA with erythema or pruritus; limiting instrumental ADL	Covering greater than 30% BSA and associated with pruritus; limiting self-care ADL		
Pruritus	Mild or localized; topical intervention indicated	Intense or widespread; intermittent; skin changes from scratching; oral intervention indicated; limiting instrumental ADL	Intense or widespread; constant; limiting self-care ADL or sleep; oral corticosteroid or immunosuppressive therapy indicated		

(Continued)

■ **Table 13.6** *(Continued)*

Adverse Event	Grade 1	Grade 2	Grade 3	Grade 4	Grade 5
Radiation dermatitis	Faint erythema or dry desquamation	Moderate to brisk erythema; patchy moist desquamation, mostly confined to skin folds and creases; moderate edema	Moist desquamation in areas other than skin folds and creases; bleeding induced by minor trauma or abrasion	Life-threatening consequences; skin necrosis or ulceration of full-thickness dermis; spontaneous bleeding from involved site; skin graft indicated	Death
Nail infection (paronychia)	Localized, local intervention indicated	Oral intervention indicated	IV antibiotic, antifungal, or antiviral intervention indicated; radiologic or operative intervention indicated		
Palmar—plantar erythrodysesthesia syndrome (hand-foot syndrome)	Minimal skin changes (erythema, edema, or hyperkeratosis) without pain	Skin changes (peeling, blisters, bleeding, edema, or hyperkeratosis) with pain, limiting instrumental ADLs	Severe skin changes (peeling, blisters, bleeding, edema, or hyperkeratosis) with pain, limiting self-care ADLs		

ADL, actvities for daily living; BSA, body surface area.

lower target overall cumulative dose of oxaliplatin administered, 0.5% of patients had grade 3 neurosensory toxicity at 12 months (57). The median time to resolution of grade 3 sensory neurotoxicity was previously noted to be 13 weeks (58).

Peripheral sensory neuropathy in the advanced disease setting was evaluated in a toxicity analysis of N9741 (59). Of the 696 patients who were randomized to FOLFOX4, 63% discontinued therapy for reasons other than tumor progression, most commonly neurotoxicity and myelosuppression. The median time to development of grade 2 and 3 neurotoxicity was 5 and 6 months, respectively. Time-to-treatment response was 2.2 months. Interestingly, the time-to-treatment failure was 5.8 months compared to time to tumor progression of 9.3 months. Of patients who developed grade 2 or 3 neurotoxicity, 43% and 74% discontinued treatment for that reason.

The development of peripheral sensory neuropathy increases with cumulative dose of oxaliplatin. At the cumulative dose of 780 to 850 mg/m^2, 15% of patients have grade 3 neurotoxicity, increasing to 50% at the cumulative dose of 1170 mg/m^2 (60). At cumulative doses of greater than 1000 mg/m^2, there have been reports of atypical neurotoxicities including the development of Lhermitte's sign and urinary retention (61). Tumor response typically occurs by a cumulative dose of 700 mg/m^2, before the majority of patients will experience grade 3 peripheral sensory neurotoxicity.

It is important to note that peripheral sensory neurotoxicity symptoms can worsen after completion of therapy. This "coasting" phenomenon, is estimated to occur in approximately 10%–15% of patients (60). Additionally, patients may develop an exacerbation of their neuropathy after surgery, potentially attributed to high concentrations of intraerythrocytic oxaliplatin and hemolysis intraoperatively (62). This might have implications for patients undergoing neoadjuvant therapy for advanced CRC.

Clinical Management of Oxaliplatin-Induced Peripheral Neuropathy

The mainstays of management of chemotherapy-induced sensory neuropathy (CIPN) are prevention, both nonpharmacologic and pharmacologic in nature, and symptomatic management and treatment of established CIPN (63). It is difficult to alleviate symptoms once CIPN occurs, and thus particular emphasis has been placed on prevention.

Prevention of Sensory Neuropathy (Table 13.7)

Steps to minimize the effects of the acute sensory neuropathy can be made by both the patient and clinician. It is important that patients are counseled regarding choices in lifestyle that can minimize any acute neurosensory symptoms. Patients should avoid cold temperatures, in their environments and in their food, as it can trigger pharyngolaryngeal dysesthesias.

Individuals with pre-existing neuropathy are at greater risk for developing CIPN and should be identified prior to treatment (64). A careful history should be taken to identify patients who may have existing nerve damage such as those with diabetes mellitus, prior exposure to neurotoxic agents, alcohol abuse, or inherited neuropathy. For these patients, extremely close monitoring for neurologic toxicities is recommended to prevent a functionally disabling neuropathy (65). Initial pharmacogenomic studies have identified patients with a polymorphism in GSTP1 (V105I), a gene encoding glutathione-S-transferase, a detoxifying enzyme, to be at higher risk of developing early onset of neurotoxicity, but these data require further validation in subsequent studies (66).

Drug regimen modification is a common strategy to prevent chronic peripheral neurotoxicity from oxaliplatin (63). The individual's associated risk for developing peripheral sensory neurotoxicity and the cumulative oxaliplatin dose the patient has received must be kept in mind. Adjuvant therapy is administered with curative intent efforts should be made to maintain the dose intensity whenever possible. The authors of the MOSAIC study recommend dose reduction or discontinuation of oxaliplatin when paresthesias or functional impairment persist between cycles (51).

With the exception of neoadjuvant or conversion therapy (aimed at "converting" a patient from unresectable to resectable status), treatment in the advanced disease setting is considered palliative and emphasis is not placed on strict adherence to a particular dose-intense regimen. Oxaliplatin breaks have been investigated as a way to maintain the antitumor effects of the drug while minimizing neurotoxicity. Along these lines, paralaryngeal dysesthesias may be prevented by prolonging the oxaliplatin administration time (up to 4–6 hours) and thereby avoiding high peak oxaliplatin plasma concentrations (67).

Intermittent administration of oxaliplatin, or the stop-and-go strategy, was investigated in the OPTIMOX trials (68,69). The OPTIMOX1 trial randomized patients with advanced CRC to treatment with either FOLFOX4 (bolus and infusional 5-FU plus oxaliplatin 85 mg/m^2) given until disease progression or unacceptable toxicity, or FOLFOX7 (infusional 5-FU plus oxaliplatin 130 mg/m^2) for six cycles followed by maintenance 5-FU until disease progression and then reintroduction of FOLFOX7 for six cycles (68). Outcome measures of efficacy were comparable in FOLFOX4- and FOLFOX7-treated patients in terms of response rate (58.5% vs 59.2%), PFS (9.0 vs 8.7 months; P = .04) and OS (19.3 vs 21.2 months; HR, 0.93; P = .49). However, the rate of grade 3 neurotoxicity was higher in patients who received FOLFOX4, albeit not statistically significant (17.9% vs 13.3%; P = .12). The lack of statistical significance for the difference in neurotoxicity overall could have been related to the fact that the absolute oxaliplatin dose administered with each cycle was higher with FOLFOX7. However, patients treated with FOLFOX7 who were not given oxaliplatin from cycle 7 through 18 had reduced grade 3 neurotoxicity in this period. The results from OPTIMOX1 demonstrated that breaks in oxaliplatin with reintroduction at a future point does not compromise the efficacy of oxaliplatin in terms of survival and reduces the incidence of cumulative grade 3 neurotoxicity.

Based on the results of the large randomized phase II OPTIMOX2 trial, complete breaks from chemotherapy are not recommended as a default for all patients (69).

Table 13.7 Clinically Relevant Approaches in the Prevention of Oxaliplatin-Induced Sensory Neurotoxicity (sNT)

Approach	Effect on Neurotoxicity	Effect on Efficacy	Comment
Adjuvant Setting			
Dose reduction or omission of oxaliplatin when grade 2 sNT occurs	Can prevent further worsening of sNT	Not clear, likely minimal after cycle 9, the median number of cycles in MOSAIC	Reflects common clinical practice
Planned administration of a reduced number (eg, 6 instead of 12) of oxaliplatin containing cycles	Limits development of oxaliplatin-induced sNT	Unclear	This approach is currently being tested in various international phase III trials
Use of IV Ca/Mg	Early data suggest decreased sNT	No decreased antitumor activity in the advanced disease setting	Data from confirmatory phase III trial pending
Advanced Disease Setting			
Intermittent use of oxaliplatin ("stop-and-go")	Documented decrease in sNT	No reduced efficacy in terms of RR, PFS, and OS	Considered standard of care in clinical practice

This study compared the OPTIMOX1 regimen with six cycles of FOLFOX7 followed by a complete chemotherapy holiday and the reintroduction of FOLFOX7 at disease progression (OPTIMOX2). Median PFS was not statistically different between OPTIMOX2 and OPTIMOX1 (29 vs 36 weeks; $P = .08$). Notwithstanding, median OS was significantly reduced for patients who had chemotherapy-free intervals on OPTIMOX2 (18.9 vs 24.6 months; $P = .05$). Therefore, complete chemotherapy-free intervals are not recommended as default when using the strategy of intermittent oxaliplatin administration.

The intermittent administration of oxaliplatin in combination with bevacizumab in patients with untreated metastatic CRC was investigated in the Combined Oxaliplatin Neurotoxicity Prevention Trial (CONcePT; 70). Patients were randomized to receive continuous or intermittent modified FOLFOX7 (oxaliplatin 85 mg/m^2, LV 200 mg/m^2, 5FU 2,400 mg/m^2 × 46 h) plus bevacizumab with or without calcium and magnesium (Ca/Mg). In the intermittent arm, patients with stable disease after eight cycles of FOLFOX plus bevacizumab began to maintenance therapy with infusional 5-FU/LV plus bevacizumab. After eight cycles of maintenance therapy, oxaliplatin was re-introduced. Time-to-treatment failure was significantly longer in patients receiving the intermittent oxaliplatin schedule (5.6 vs 4.2 months; HR, 0.58; $P = .0025$). Interestingly, a longer PFS for the intermittent oxaliplatin arm was observed as well as a reduction of severe neurotoxicity (10% vs 24%) when compared to the continuous oxaliplatin arm. The concept of an induction-maintenance therapy approach with targeted agents is being further investigated in ongoing clinical trials (71,72).

As previously mentioned, it has been suggested that oxalate released from oxaliplatin as it enters the nerve cell could mediate at least some of the neurotoxic effects from oxaliplatin. Oxalate is able to chelate calcium, which can interfere with the proper function of calcium gated sodium channels of the nerve cell and lead to a disruption of sensory perception. This proposed mechanism is the basis for investigating the potential of infusional Ca/Mg in reducing the neurotoxic effects of oxaliplatin.

A retrospective cohort study of patients treated with oxaliplatin-based therapy for advanced CRC evaluated 96 patients who received infusion of calcium gluconate (1 g) and magnesium sulfate (1 g) before and after oxaliplatin compared to those who did not. The Ca/Mg group had few patients who discontinued therapy due to neuropathy compared to controls (4% vs 31%; $P < .001$) and less neuropathy at the end of treatment (20% vs 45%; $P = .003$). Additionally, patients who received Ca/Mg had significantly less acute neurotoxicity and a more rapid recovery of their neuropathy at the end of treatment. There was no compromise in the efficacy of the oxaliplatin-based therapy with Ca/Mg. The neuroprotective effect of Ca/Mg administered before and after FOLFOX therapy was also supported by results of a randomized, double-blind, placebo-controlled study in patients with early stage CRC (73). Patients undergoing adjuvant therapy for CRC were randomized to receive FOLFOX with or without Ca/Mg, and those who had received Ca/Mg experienced significantly delayed time to onset of grade 2 sensory neurotoxicity. Unfortunately, the trial stopped accrual prematurely at about 50% of the accrual goal when initial data from the CONcePT trial erroneously suggested that the use of Ca/Mg interfered with the antitumor activity of FOLFOX. To help definitively clarify the role of Ca/Mg in the prevention of oxaliplatin-induced neurotoxicity, a randomized phase III trial has been recently been completed that compared the addition of Ca/Mg before and after oxaliplatin, Ca/Mg before oxaliplatin, or placebo to FOLFOX adjuvant therapy for CRC. Unfortunately, this definitive trial showed no benefit for the use of IV Ca/Mg against oxaliplatin-induced neurotoxicity. (cite Loprinzi C, et al., ASCO 2013).

Xaliproden has also been investigated as a potential neuroprotectant for its ability to mimic the effects of nerve growth factor and its role as a serotonin 5-HT1A receptor agonist (60). A phase III trial of 649 patients undergoing treatment for advanced CRC randomized patients to receive FOLFOX4 with or without xaliproden (74). Xaliproden was associated with a 39% reduction in the probability of grade 3 to 4 CIPN and there was no decrease in efficacy of FOLFOX4 when combined with xaliproden. However, efficacy of xaliproden was not apparent until patients received 650 to 700 mg cumulative oxaliplatin dose. Xaliproden also failed to impact grades 1 to 2 CIPN and had no effect on the acute, cold-induced neuropathy associated with oxaliplatin. Clinical development of xaliproden as neuroprotectant has been abandoned.

Treatment of Established CIPN

Multiple agents have been investigated for their role in the management of CIPN. Unfortunately, there is a paucity of well-conducted clinical trials designed for this area of research. As a result, there has been limited success in establishing effective treatment options for these patients.

One strategy that produced modest results under investigation was the topical application of a novel combination of agents for established CIPN (75). A randomized, double-blind, placebo-controlled trial was implemented to assess the combination of baclofen 10 mg, amitriptyline HCL 40 mg, and ketamine 20 mg in a pluronic lecithin organogel (BAK) as a topical gel in patients with a score greater than or equal to 5 on a 0-to-10 neurotoxicity scale. Numbness, tingling, pain, and motor function were evaluated. Patients treated with BAK had a modest but significant improvement in the motor subscale. There were no related systemic toxicities from the agents.

Venlaflaxine, an antidepressant that functions by inhibiting the uptake of serotonin and norepinephrine, has also been assessed as a potential treatment agent for oxaliplatin-induced neuropathy (Table 13.8). In a randomized, double-blind study, the EFFOX trial, 48 patients experiencing acute neurotoxicity were treated with either venlafaxine 50 mg 1 hour prior oxaliplatin infusion and venlafaxine extended release 37.5 mg twice daily from day 2 to day 11 or placebo (76). Based on a numeric rating scale for pain intensity, patients treated with venlaflaxine had full relief of symptoms at a higher rate than those who received placebo (31.3% vs 5.3%; P = .03). Although venlaflaxine treatment was associated with no grade 3/4 toxicity, a high rate of grade 1 to 2 nausea (43.1%) and asthenia (39.2%) was noted. The authors suggested that a possible mechanism of action for venlaflaxine's activity in treating oxaliplatin-induced neurosensory toxicity is a protective effect against oxaliplatin-induced oxidative stress.

Another antidepressant that might be effective in ameliorating the neuropathic pain associated with oxaliplatin is duloxetine (Table 13.8). A large placebo-controlled phase III trial of duloxetine 60 mg in 231 patients with a CIPN pain score (Brief Pain Inventory-Short Form) of greater than 4/10 due to taxane or platinum treatment (about 59% were oxaliplatin-treated) suggested its efficacy in controlling pain from neurotoxicity (77). There was a significantly larger change in pain score reported by patients who received duloxetine than in those who received placebo (mean change score = −1.09 vs−0.33; P = .004). In addition, no difference in the efficacy was noted in patients who were treated with taxane or platinating agents. A significant increase in grade 2+ fatigue was found in patients who had received duloxetine (11% vs 3%; P = .029). Results of this trial were similar to those from an earlier open-label pilot study that found an improvement in oxaliplatin-induced peripheral neuropathy reported in patients after treatment with duloxetine (78).

At the current time, the best management strategy for oxaliplatin related neurotoxicity is prevention. Dose modifications in the adjuvant setting and intermittent oxaliplatin administration in the advanced setting are valid options for reducing the likelihood of severe neurotoxicity. Pharmacologic agents that can act as neuroprotectants are eagerly sought and are being tested in prospective trials, but at this point in time none of the investigated agents including IV CaMg can be considered standard of care. Larger, randomized trials are needed to evaluate treatment options for established CIPN.

■ EPIDERMAL GROWTH FACTOR-RECEPTOR INHIBITORS AND CRC

Molecularly targeted therapies for the treatment of CRC are widely used. The epidermal growth factor-receptor inhibitors (EGFRi) cetuximab and panitumumab are anti-EGFR monoclonal antibodies. EGFR is heavily expressed in the skin and its appendages including keratinocytes in the basal and suprabasal layers of the epidermis, outer layers of the hair follicle, pilosebaceous and eccrine sweat glands (79,80). EGFR mediates multiple keratinocyte functions including proliferation, differentiation, migration and survival (81). Inhibition of the receptor commonly leads to cutaneous toxicities such as papulopustular rash, hair changes, radiation dermatitis enhancement, pruritus, mucositis, skin xerosis/fissures, and paronychia. These side effects have been shown to have a profound impact on patients' health-related quality of life (QOL) and may interfere with treatment adherence (82). Pre-emptive treatment has been shown to reduce the incidence of skin toxicities and lessen the QOL impairment (83).

Papulopustular Eruption

During the first weeks of therapy, a papulopustular eruption is the most clinically significant cutaneous toxicity associated with EGFRi. The earliest signs of the eruption can occur 5 to 7 days after initiation of the drug. The incidence of papulopustular eruptions is exceedingly high, 76%–88% of patients treated with cetuximab and up to 95% of those treated with panitumumab (84). In this patient population males and those older than 70 years of age are at higher risk. Severe eruptions are seen in 10%–17% of patients (85). Some studies have demonstrated that treatment response rate and survival time may positively correlate with the presence or severity of the papulopustular rash (86,87). The eruption is characterized by pruritic tender erythematous papules and pustules on areas with a high density of pilosebaceous units including the scalp,

■ Table 13.8 Treatment of Oxaliplatin-Induced Sensory Neurotoxicity (sNT) With Benefit in Randomized Placebo-Controlled Trials

Intervention	Clinical Effect	Comments
Venlaflaxine	Small, 48-patient placebo-controlled trial suggests decreased sNT as assessed by pain scale	Awaits confirmation in further clinical trials
Duloxetine	Larger, 135-patient placebo-controlled trial shows moderate effect on painful sNT	No detrimental effect on treatment efficacy noted; effect on paresthesias and dysethesias unclear

face, neck, chest, and back (Figure 13.2). In severe cases, it can develop into confluent plaques with pustules, hemorrhagic crust, ulcerations, or eschars (88). Secondary skin infection with Staphylococcus species can occur. The rash peaks in weeks 4 to 6 and decreases in severity after 6 to 8 weeks. Histopathologic analysis reveals intrafollicular collections of neutrophils and perifollicular lymphocytes. In contrast to acne vulgaris, no comedones are seen.

Recent guidelines set forth by the MASCC Skin Toxicity Study Group include preventive management unless contraindicated with application of a class IV topical corticosteroid (eg, hydrocortisone 1% cream) with moisturizer and sunscreen twice daily combined with a tetracycline antibiotic such as doxycycline or minocycline for the first 6 to 8 weeks of therapy (83,89). Doxycycline has a more favorable side effect profile; however, it is photosensitizing, so minocycline may be preferable in seasons or locations with high UV exposure. For moderate to severe eruptions higher potency topical corticosteroids such as hydrocortisone 2.5% cream, alclometasone 0.05% cream, or fluocinonide 0.05% cream twice daily are recommended. Topical antibiotics including clindamycin and low-oral isotretinoin (20–30 mg/day) have been shown to be effective (90,91). Topical retinoids and calcineurin inhibitors have not been shown to be efficacious for the papulopustular eruption (89,92). Aggressive treatment is recommended to maintain adherence to cancer therapy.

Xerosis

Xerosis results from EGFRi-induced abnormal keratinocyte differentiation and deterioration of the stratum corneum. Onset is later and is usually noted 4 to 8 weeks into treatment. Almost half of patients taking cetuximab will experience xerosis and the incidence is lower in those taking panitumumab. Patients that are older, those previously treated with cytotoxic agents, or patients with a history of atopic dermatitis are at higher risk (93). Dry skin may be accompanied by asteatotic dermatitis, fissuring on the fingertips (Figure 13.3), palms and soles, and/or superinfection.

Patients should be educated on good dry skin care, including proper bathing techniques, liberal use of emollients, avoidance of extreme temperatures and sun exposure, and choosing skin care products without fragrance or irritants. Patients should bathe with lukewarm water and avoid hot water, use mild moisturizing soaps or bath oils, and avoid over bathing. Bathing should be immediately followed by application of emollients. For severe xerosis, petrolatum-based ointments may be used. If asteatotic dermatitis develops medium- to high-potency topical steroids such as triamcinolone acetonide 0.1% should be added. Fissured skin on the palms and soles should be protected with gloves and socks. Fissures can be sealed with cyanoacrylate liquid glues to alleviate pain, reduce infection, and aid in healing (93). Bathing once weekly for 10 minutes in a diluted bleach bath made with one half-cup of bleach in a full tub of water (approximately 6 gallons of warm water) can reduce the incidence of skin infection. Topical or oral antibiotics are indicated in the event of superinfection.

Pruritus

Pruritus is experienced by approximately 50% of patients treated with EGFRi and often accompanies the papulopustular eruption and xerosis. Treatment of the concomitant dermatitis or xerosis when present should be optimized. Nonsedating, second-generation antihistamines (eg, loratidine, cetirizine, fexofenadine) during the daytime and first-generation antihistamines (eg, hydroxyzine and diphenhydramine) at night time are recommended. Antiepileptics such as gabapentin and pregabalin should be considered second-line therapies, given their antipruritic properties. Gabapentin has been shown to reduce itch in the setting

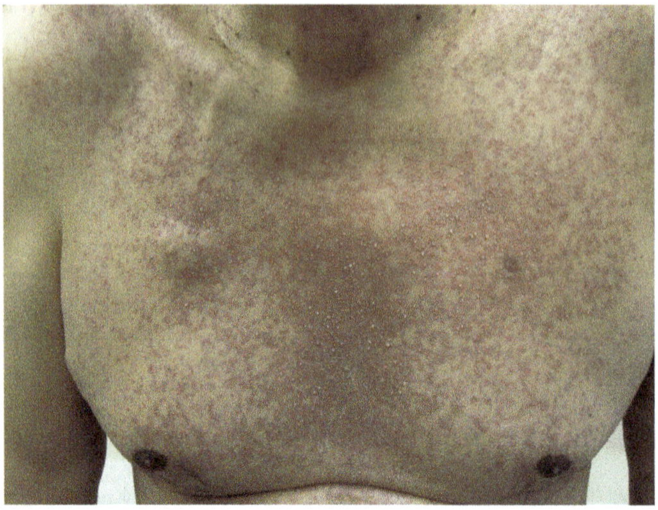

FIGURE 13.2 Papulopustular eruption on the chest.

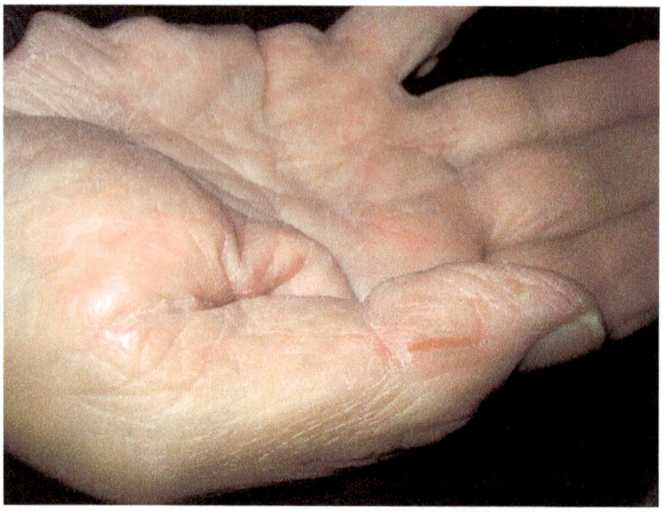

FIGURE 13.3 Xerosis of the palm with skin fissure on the first digit.

of other dermatologic conditions (94). A recent case report demonstrated the beneficial effects of pregabalin on cetuximab-related itch (95). Aprepitant, a neurokinin-1 receptor antagonist indicated for chemotherapy-induced nausea and vomiting, has been efficacious for the treatment of erlotinib-induced pruritus; however, it may inhibit cytochrome P-450 3A4 and increase levels of erlotinib (96–98). Careful evaluation of potential drug-drug interactions must be done when considering this therapy. Other oral agents such as doxepin and topical agents such as menthol and pramoxine containing products can also be considered.

Hair Changes

Hair changes secondary to EGFRi therapy include facial hypertrichosis, eyelash trichomegaly, and nonscarring alopecia of the scalp, in addition to the scarring alopecia that may result from the papulopustular eruption. Facial hypertrichosis and trichomegaly, lengthening and curling of the eyelashes and eyebrows, begins after 1 to 2 months of therapy and continues for the duration of therapy (84). Unwanted facial hair may be treated with hair removal techniques including depilatories, waxing, eflornithine cream, laser hair removal, or electrolysis. Trichomegaly can be uncomfortable and lead to ocular problems such as corneal scarring (99). Regular trimming of eyelashes with referral to an ophthalmologist for persistent problems is recommended. Patchy nonscarring alopecia typically begins after 2 to 3 weeks of therapy and may progress to diffuse alopecia with long-term treatment. Hair often regrows after cessation of therapy. Supportive measures including education and cosmetic solutions should be offered to patients. The use of topical minoxidil in the setting of EGFRi has not been studied but may provide some benefit; however, caution should be used as this may worsen facial hypertrichosis and pruritus and potentiate scalp irritation.

Radiation Dermatitis

Concomitant administration of EGFRi with radiation therapy may increase the severity of radiation dermatitis (100,101). Radiotherapy treatment courses should take into account EGFRi therapy and attempt to minimize the delivered dose to the epidermis while maintaining efficacy. Standard prophylactic measures to reduce radiation dermatitis should be utilized including gentle washing and drying of the skin within the radiation portal prior to treatment. Topical emollients and dressings should not be applied shortly before radiation treatment because they can increase the radiation dose to the epidermis. In the event of acute radiation dermatitis severe enough to cause bullae or erosions, drying pastes, gels, and hydrophilic dressings can be used in moist areas. Short courses of high-potency topical steroids may be used for grade 2 or 3 radiation dermatitis. Physicians should maintain a low threshold for initiating antibiotic treatment of suspected skin superinfection, especially in the setting of concomitant chemotherapy and neutropenia. If an EGFRi-related papulopustular eruption develops within the irradiated field, management guidelines depend on the grade of radiation dermatitis. In the setting of grade 0 or 1 radiation dermatitis, the aforementioned recommendations for treatment of the EGFRi-associated papulopustular eruption should be followed. If grade 2 or higher radiation dermatitis is present the recommendations for treating the radiation dermatitis should be followed (102).

Nail Changes

Nail changes may develop after 2 or more months of exposure in 17%–25% of patients treated with cetuximab or panitumumab (103,104). Paronychia, inflammation of the nail fold, and periungual pyogenic granulomata are the most common findings. Secondary changes such as onychodystrophy or onycholysis may result from nail matrix damage. Paronychia is characterized by tender, edematous, and sometimes purulent inflammation of the nail folds (Figure 13.4). Both fingernails and toenails may be affected. Superinfection may occur and culturing of drainage is recommended. Periungual pyogenic granulomata are friable vascular neoplasms on the lateral nail folds. Treatment guidelines focus on minimizing trauma, preventing superinfection, and removing excess granulation tissue when pain or bleeding is excessive. Topical silver nitrate may be helpful for severe pyogenic granulomata. Paronychia can be treated with topical corticosteroids and low-dose oral tetracyclines as anti-inflammatory agents (105,106). Diluted bleach or white vinegar soaks can reduce the incidence of superinfection. In cases of paronychia associated with severe pain, partial or complete nail avulsion may be necessary.

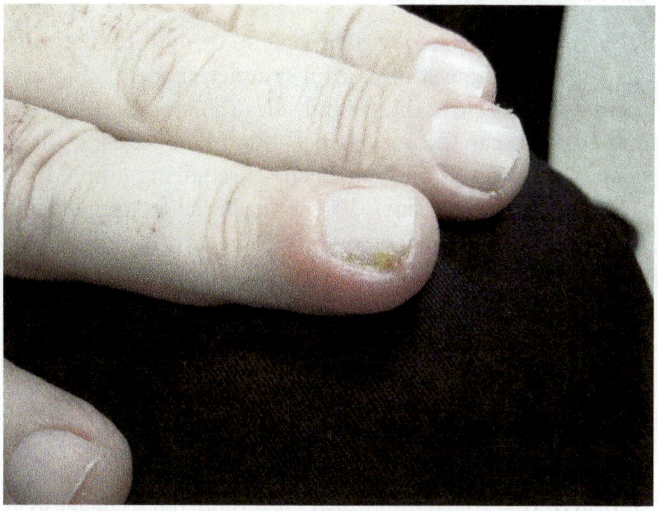

FIGURE 13.4 Periungual erythema, edema, and purulent drainage characteristic of paronychia.

Oral Complications

Oral complications are uncommon in patients treated with EGFRi as monotherapy. Mucositis is the most frequently reported side effect and is often seen in patients receiving concomitant chemotherapy. Good oral care is the best preventive measure. It is important to monitor for secondary oral infections (eg, candidiasis, herpes simplex).

■ HAND-FOOT SYNDROME FROM DRUGS USED IN CRC

Hand-foot syndrome (HFS) is a localized skin eruption associated with the use of several chemotherapeutic agents in the treatment of CRC, namely pyrimidine analogs 5-FU and capecitabine.

Nomenclature

Toxic erythema of chemotherapy is now regarded as the preferred nomenclature when describing a variety of adverse cutaneous reactions to traditional chemotherapeutic agents such as alkylating agents, antimetabolites, and anthracyclines (107). This term was suggested to help unify what had previously been very confusing for practitioners when reporting specific skin reactions that developed during the course of cancer therapy. HFS has been referred to in the medical literature by a variety of other names, among them acral erythema, erythrodysesthesia syndrome and palmar-plantar erythema. HFS is currently recognized as a specific reaction subtype of toxic erythema of chemotherapy. This is not to be confused with hand-foot skin reaction (HFSR), a more recently described entity distinct from HFS, but clinically similar (108). HFSR is associated with multikinase inhibitors such as sorafenib and sunitinib.

Clinical Presentation

HFS is characterized by a prodrome of dysesthesia, with the subsequent onset of painful symmetric edema and erythema of the palms, digits, and soles (Figure 13.5); blisters and erosions can also develop. Though HFS rarely leads to hospitalization (109), tissue necrosis requiring amputation (110,111) and secondary bacterial superinfection leading to death has been reported (108). More importantly, HFS causes significant derangements in quality of life (112), and given the estimated incidence of HFS of 28%–74% (113) in patients treated with capecitabine, HFS is likely to become a factor with respect to a patient's ability to complete cancer therapy. Luckily, it has been estimated that nearly 80% of patients with HFS present with NCI Grade I toxicity (114).

The onset of HFS can occur within 24 hours of the initiation of therapy, but has also been reported to develop as late as 10 months; factors related to onset include higher peak plasma levels and total cumulative dose of medication (113–115). Capecitabine-associated HFS typically appears within the first 3 cycles of treatment (116) and worsens in subsequent cycles (117).

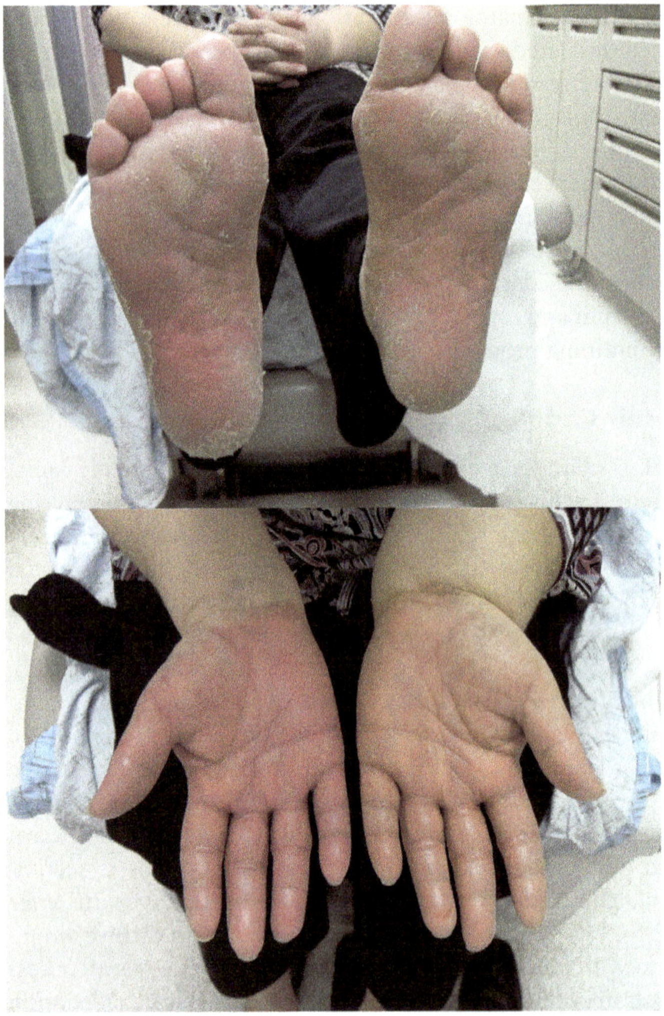

FIGURE 13.5 Hand-foot syndrome causing erythema and edema of the palms and soles.

Skin biopsies taken from patients with HFS demonstrate hyperkeratosis, parakeratosis, and epidermal spongiosis. Focal vacuolization of the basal cell layer along with ectatic dermal blood vessels and a mild perivascular lymphohistiocytic infiltrate can also be seen (114,118,119).

Pathophysiology

Although the exact mechanism remains unknown, HFS is felt to develop as a result of direct toxicity of the chemotherapeutic agents to cutaneous structures (114,120). It has been hypothesized that these agents accumulate in eccrine sweat ducts, which leads to epidermal damage, and explains the distinct anatomic location of HFS, as acral sites are dense in eccrine glands (118,121). There is also evidence that overexpression of cyclooxygenase 2 in the skin during chemotherapy leads to inflammation and the development of HFS (117,118).

Mechanical pressure on the palms and soles as a result of normal activities of daily living may also play a role in the development of HFS. Such activities have been postulated to lead to capillary damage and subsequent toxic injury to the skin of the hands and feet (115). Thymidine phosphorylase, which helps to activate capecitabine in vivo, is more prevalent on the palms of the hands, as compared to the dorsal surface, and has also been implicated in the pathogenesis of HFS (122).

Treatment

Dose reduction or cessation of the offending agent is the only effective treatment for HFS, and resolution of skin lesions typically ensues within 2 weeks of discontinuation (114). For those patients on capecitabine with NCI grade 2 or 3 HFS, per the package insert, treatment should be held until improvement to grade 0 or 1.

Several interventions can be attempted for symptomatic relief of HFS as a means to help ensure patient adherence to cancer therapy. These interventions are largely anecdotal and include counseling patients to minimize mechanical trauma to hands and feet, avoidance of tight-fitting shoes, socks and gloves, and minimization of exposures to excessive amounts of heat (113,123,124). Elevation of hands and feet (125) and regional cooling with ice packs may also be beneficial, the latter technique allowing for vasoconstriction in an attempt to minimize exposure to toxic metabolites of drugs that cause HFS at target sites (126). Being mindful of any derangement of kidney function for patients placed on capecitabine (and adjusting dose accordingly) can also help to decrease the risk of HFS (113,127).

Topical emollients such as petrolatum-lanolin based ointments haven proven effective in the prevention and treatment of HFS, and patients should be counseled about their liberal use throughout the day (109,125). Topical anesthetic agents and cold compresses can provide symptomatic relief of burning and pain (113,125). High-potency topical steroids are helpful in cases where pruritus is the predominant symptom.

A variety of systemic medications have been used in an attempt to abate the symptoms associated with HFS, including pyridoxine (128–131), celecoxib (132), and oral vitamin E (109). A randomized, double-blinded trial with pyridoxine 200 mg given daily failed to show any benefit in the prophylaxis or treatment of HFS (133). However, given its appealing safety profile and anecdotal evidence of efficacy, pyridoxine is still widely used. The use of celecoxib has been demonstrated to attenuate the incidence and severity of HFS for patients with metastatic CRC (132). Transdermal nicotine patches have also been used to help prevent HFS (134).

Vigilance with respect to early identification of skin superinfection is vital. The development of honey-colored crusting, frank purulence, malodor, or systemic symptoms such as fever and chills should warrant affected areas to be swabbed for bacterial and fungal culture, as well as a low threshold for further evaluation and treatment for systemic infection. Appropriate oral and/or intravenous antibacterial therapy should be initiated in an expeditious manner for those patients with skin superinfection.

■ REFERENCES

1. Rothenberg ML, Meropol NJ, Polpin EA, et al. Mortality associated with irinotecan plus bolus fluorouracil/leucovorin: summary findings of an independent panel. *J Clin Oncol.* 2001; 19:3801–3807.
2. Jensen L, Herrmann A, Stegmaier C, et al. Health-related quality of life during the 10 years after diagnosis of colorectal cancer: a population-based study. *J Clin Oncol.* 2011;29:3263–3269.
3. Arbuckle RB, Huber SL, Zacker C. The consequences of diarrhea occurring during chemotherapy for colorectal cancer: A retrospective study. *Oncologist.* 2000;5:250–259.
4. Dranitsaris G, Maroun J, Shah A. Estimating the cost of illness in colorectal cancer patients who were hospitalized for severe chemotherapy-induced diarrhea. *Can J Gastroenterol.* 2005;19:83–87.
5. Saltz LB. Understanding and managing chemotherapy-induced diarrhea. *J Support Onc.* 2003;1:35–46.
6. Schiller LR. Nutrition management of chronic diarrhea and malabsorption. *Nutr Clin Pract.* 2006;21:34–39.
7. Abraham B, Sellin JH. Drug-induced diarrhea. *Curr Gastroenterol Rep.* 2007;9:365–372.
8. Stein BN, Petrelli NJ, Douglass HO, et al. Age and sex are independent predictors of 5-fluorouracil toxicity. Analysis of a large scale phase III trial. *Cancer.* 1995;75:11–17.
9. Sloan JA, Goldenberg RM, Sargent DJ, et al. Women experience greater toxicity with fluorouracil-based chemotherapy for colorectal cancer. *J Clin Oncol.* 2010;20:1491–1498.
10. Dranitsaris G, Shah A, Spirovski B, et al. Severe diarrhea in patients with advanced-stage colorectal cancer receiving FOLFOX or FOLFIRI chemotherapy: the development of a risk prediction tool. *Clin Colorectal Cancer.* 2007;6:367–373.
11. Maroun JA, Anthony LB, Blais N, et al. Prevention and management of chemotherapy-induced diarrhea in patients with colorectal cancer: a concensus statement by the Canadian Working Group on Chemotherapy-Induced Diarrhea. *Curr Oncol.* 2007;14:13–20.
12. Shulman K, Cohen I, Barnett-Griness O, et al. Clinical implications of ugt1a1*28 genotype testing in colorectal cancer patients. *Cancer.* 2011;117:3156–3162.
13. Deeken JF, Slack R, Marshall JL. Irinotecan and uridine diphosphate glucoronosyltransferase 1a1 pharmacogenetics: to test or not to test, that is the question. *Cancer.* 2008;113:1502–1510.
14. Heggie GD, Sommadossi JP, Cross DS, et al. Clinical pharmacokinetics of 5-fluorouracil and its metabolites in plasma, urine, and bile. *Cancer Res.* 1987;47:2203–2206.
15. Chazal M, Etienne MC, Renee N, et al. Link between dihydropyrimidine dehydrogenase activity in peripheral blood mononuclear cells and liver. *Clin Cancer Res.* 1996;2:507–510.
16. van Kuilenburg ABP. Dihydropyrimidine dehydrogenase and the efficacy and toxicity of 5-fluorouracil. *Eur J Cancer.* 2004;40:939–950.
17. Raida M, Schwabe W, Hausler P, et al. Prevalence of a common point mutation in the dihydropyrimidine dehydrogenase (DPD) gene within the 5'-splice donor site of intron 14 in patients with severe 5-fluorouracil (5-FU) related toxicity compared with controls. *Clin Cancer Res.* 2001;7:2832–2839.
18. Milano G, Etienne MC, Pierrefite V, et al. Dihydropydrimidine dehydrogenase deficiency and fluorouracil related toxicity. Br J Cancer. 1999;79:627–630.
19. van Kuilenberg ABP, Muller EWW, Haasjes J, et al. Clinical implications of dihydropyrimidine dehydrogenase (DPD) deficiency in patients with severe 5-fluorouracil-associated toxicity:

identification of new mutations in the DPD gene. *Clin Cancer Res.* 2000;6:4705–4712.
20. Grucella M, Crepaldi G, Barile C, et al. Pharmacokinetic and demographic markers of 5-fluorouracil toxicity in 181 patients on adjuvant therapy for colorectal cancer. *Ann Oncol.* 2006;17:1656–1660.
21. Ychou M, Duffour J, Kramar A, et al. Individual 5-FU dose adaption in metastatic colorectal cancer: results of a phase II study using a bimonthly pharmacokinetically intensified LV5FU2 regimen. *Cancer Chemother Pharmacol.* 2003;52:282–290.
22. Benson AB III, Ajani JA, Catalano RB, et al. Recommended guidelines for the treatment of cancer treatment-induced diarrhea. *J Clin Oncol.* 2004;22:2918–2926.
23. Palmer KR, Corbett CL, Holdsworth CD. Double-blind cross-over study comparing loperamide, codeine, and diphenoxylate in the treatment of chronic diarrhea. *Gastroenterology.* 1980;79:1272–1275.
24. Abigerges D, Armand JP, Chabot GG, et al. Irinotecan (CPT-11) high-dose escalation using intensive high-dose loperamide to control diarrhea. *J Natl Cancer Inst.* 1994;86:446–449.
25. Zachariah B, Gwede CK, James J, et al. Octreotide acetate in prevention of chemoradiation-induced diarrhea in anorectal cancer: randomized RTOG trial 0315. *J Natl Cancer Inst.* 2010;102:547–556.
26. de Gramant A, Figer A, Seymour M, et al. Leucovorin and fluorouracil with or without oxaliplatin as first line treatment in advanced colorectal cancer. *J Clin Oncol.* 2000;18:2938–2947.
27. Douillard JY, Cunningham D, Roth AD, et al. Irinotecan combined with fluorouracil alone as first-line treatment for metastatic colorectal cancer: a multicentre randomized trial. *Lancet.* 2000;355:1041–1047.
28. Twelves C, Wong A, Nowack MP, et al. Capecitabine as adjuvant treatment for stage III colon cancer. *N Engl J Med.* 2005;352:2696–2704.
29. Fuchs CS, Moore MR, Harker G, et al. Phase III Comparison of Two Irinotecan Dosing Regimens in Second-Line Therapy of Metastatic Colorectal Cancer. *J Clin Oncol.* 2003;21:807–814.
30. Cunningham D, Humblet Y, Siena S, et al. Cetuximab monotherapy and cetuximab plus irinotecan in irinotecan refractory metastatic colorectal cancer. N Engl J Med. 2004;351:337–345.
31. Van Cutsem E, Peeters M, Siena S, et al. Open label phase iii of panitumumab plus best supportive care compared with best supportive care alone in patients with chemotherapy-refractory metastatic colorectal cancer. J Clin Oncol. 2005;25:1658–1664.
32. Van Cutsem E, Kohne C-H, Hitre E, et al. Cetuximab and chemotherapy as initial treatment for metastatic colorectal cancer. N Engl J Med. 2009;360:1408–1417.
33. Peeters M, Price TJ, Cervantes A, et al. Randomized phase iii study of panitumumab with fluorouracil, leucovorin, and irinitecan (folfiri) compared with folfiri alone as second-line treatment in patients with metastatic colorectal cancer. J Clin Oncol. 2010;2028:4706–4713.
34. Bokemeyer C, Bondarenko I, Makhsan A, et al. Fluorouracil, Leucovorin, and Oxaliplatin With and Without Cetuximab in the First-Line Treatment of Metastatic Colorectal Cancer. J Clin Oncol. 2008;27:663–671.
35. Douillard J-Y, Siena S, Cassidy J, et al. Randomized phase iii trial of panitumumab with infusional fluorouracil, leucovorin, and oxaliplatin (folfox4) versus folfox4 alone as first-line treatment in patient with previously untreated metastatic colorectal cancer: the prime study. J Clin Oncol. 2010;28:4697–4705.
36. Das P, Lin EH, Bhatia S, et al. Preoperative chemoradiotherapy with capecitabine versus protracted infusion 5-fluorouracil for rectal cancer: a matched-paired analysis. Int J Radiation Oncology Biol Phys. 2006;66:1378–1383.
37. Barbounis V, Koumakis G, Vassilomanolakis M, et al. Control of irinotecan-induced diarrhea by octreotide after loperamide failure. *Support Care Cancer.* 2001;9:258–260.
38. Goumas P, Naxakis S, Christopoulou A, et al. Octeotide acetate in the treatment of fluorouracil-induced diarrhea. *The Oncologist.* 1998;3:50–53.
39. Bhattacharya S, Vijayasekar C, Worlding J, et al. Octreotide in chemotherapy induced diarrhea in colorectal cancer: a review article. *Acta Gastroenterol Belg.* 2009;72:289–295.
40. Rosenoff SH, Gabrail NY, Conklin R, et al. A multicenter, randomized trial of long-acting octreotide for the optimum prevention of chemotherapy-induced diarrhea: results of the STOP trial. *J Support Oncol.* 2006:4:289–294.
41. Kinnear DG. Drugs used in the symptomatic treatment of diarrhea. *Canad Med Ass J* 1964;91:971–972.
42. Karthaus M, Ballo H, Abenhardt W, et al. Prospective, double-blind, placebo-controlled, multicenter, randomized phase iii study with orally administered budesonide for prevention of irinotecan (cpt-11)-induced diarrhea in patients with advanced colorectal cancer. *Oncology* 2005;68:326–332.
43. Daniele B, Perrone F, Gallo C, et al. Oral glutamine in the prevention of fluorouracil induced intestinal toxicity: a double blind, placebo controlled, randomised trial. *Gut* 2001:48:28–33.
44. Osterlund P, Ruotsalainen T, Korpela R, et al. Lactobacillus supplementation for diarrhoea related to chemotherapy of colorectal cancer: a randomised study. *Br J Cancer* 2007;97:1028–1034.
45. Michael M, Brittain M, Nagai J, et al. Phase II study of activated charcoal to prevent irinotecan-induced diarrhea. *J Clin Oncol.* 2004;22:4410–4417.
46. Maiello E, Giuliani F, Gebbia V, et al. FOLFIRI with or without celecoxib in advanced colorectal cancer: a randomized phase II study of the Gruppo Oncologico dell'Italia Meridionale (GOIM). *Ann Oncol.* 2006;17(suppl 7):vii55–59.
47. Kohne CH, De Greve J, Hartmann JT, et al. Irinotecan combined with infusional 5-fluorouracil/folinic acid or capecitabine plus celecoxib or placebo in the first-line treatment of patients with metastatic colorectal cancer. EORTC study 40015. *Ann Oncol.* 2008;19:920–926.
48. Andre T, Boni C, Mounedji-Boudiaf L, et al. Oxaliplatin, fluorouracil, and leucovorin as adjuvant treatment for colon cancer. *N Engl J Med.* 2004;350(23):2343–2351.
49. Kuebler JP, Wieand HS, O'Connell MJ, et al. Oxaliplatin combined with weekly bolus fluorouracil and leucovorin as surgical adjuvant chemotherapy for stage II and III colon cancer: results from NSABP C-07. *J Clin Oncol.* 2007;25(16):2198–2204.
50. Haller D, Cassidy J, Tabernero J, et al. Efficacy findings from a randomized phase III trial of capecitabine plus oxaliplatin versus bolus 5-FU/LV for stage III colon cancer (NO16968): No impact of age on disease-free survival (DFS). Paper presented at: 2010 Gastrointestinal Cancers Symposium 2010; Orlando.
51. Andre T, Boni C, Navarro M, et al. Improved overall survival with oxaliplatin, fluorouracil, and leucovorin as adjuvant treatment in stage II or III colon cancer in the MOSAIC trial. *J Clin Oncol.* 2009;27(19):3109–3116.
52. Goldberg RM, Sargent DJ, Morton RF, et al. A randomized controlled trial of fluorouracil plus leucovorin, irinotecan, and oxaliplatin combinations in patients with previously untreated metastatic colorectal cancer. *J Clin Oncol.* 2004;22(1):23–30.
53. Gamelin E, Gamelin L, Bossi L, Quasthoff S. Clinical aspects and molecular basis of oxaliplatin neurotoxicity: current management and development of preventive measures. *Semin Oncol.* 2002;29(5 Suppl 15):21–33.
54. Wilson RH, Lehky T, Thomas RR, Quinn MG, Floeter MK, Grem JL. Acute oxaliplatin-induced peripheral nerve hyperexcitability. *J Clin Oncol.* 2002;20(7):1767–1774.
55. Lehky TJ, Leonard GD, Wilson RH, Grem JL, Floeter MK. Oxaliplatin-induced neurotoxicity: acute hyperexcitability and chronic neuropathy. *Muscle Nerve.* 2004;29(3):387–392.
56. Verstappen CC, Heimans JJ, Hoekman K, Postma TJ. Neurotoxic complications of chemotherapy in patients with cancer: clinical signs and optimal management. *Drugs.* 2003;63(15):1549–1563.
57. Land SR, Kopec JA, Cecchini RS, et al. Neurotoxicity from oxaliplatin combined with weekly bolus fluorouracil and leucovorin as surgical adjuvant chemotherapy for stage II and III colon cancer: NSABP C-07. *J Clin Oncol.* 2007;25(16):2205–2211.

58. de Gramont A, Figer A, Seymour M, et al. Leucovorin and fluorouracil with or without oxaliplatin as first-line treatment in advanced colorectal cancer. *J Clin Oncol.* 2000;18(16):2938–2947.
59. Green E, Sargent DJ, Goldberg RM, Grothey A. Detailed analysis of oxaliplatin-associated neurotoxicity in Intergroup trial N9741; Program and abstracts of the American Society of Clinical Oncology 2005 Gastrointestinal Cancers Symposium; January 27–29, 2005;Hollywood, Florida (Abstract #182).
60. Grothey A. Clinical management of oxaliplatin-associated neurotoxicity. *Clin Colorectal Cancer.* 2005;5(Suppl 1):S38-S46.
61. Taieb S, Trillet-Lenoir V, Rambaud L, Descos L, Freyer G. Lhermitte sign and urinary retention: atypical presentation of oxaliplatin neurotoxicity in four patients. *Cancer.* 2002;94(9):2434–2440.
62. Gornet JM, Savier E, Lokiec F, Cvitkovic E, Misset JL, Goldwasser F. Exacerbation of oxaliplatin neurosensory toxicity following surgery. *Ann Oncol.* 2002;13(8):1315–1318.
63. Windebank AJ, Grisold W. Chemotherapy-induced neuropathy. *J Peripher Nerv Syst.* 2008;13(1):27–46.
64. Quasthoff S, Hartung HP. Chemotherapy-induced peripheral neuropathy. *J Neurol.* 2002;249(1):9–17.
65. Chaudhry V, Chaudhry M, Crawford TO, Simmons-O'Brien E, Griffin JW. Toxic neuropathy in patients with pre-existing neuropathy. *Neurology.* 2003;60(2):337–340.
66. Grothey A, McLeod HL, Green EM, et al. Glutathione S-transferase P1 I105V (GSTP1 I105V) polymorphism is associated with early onset of oxaliplatin-induced neurotoxicity. *ASCO Meeting Abstracts.* 2005;23(16 suppl):3509-.
67. Extra JM, Marty M, Brienza S, Misset JL. Pharmacokinetics and safety profile of oxaliplatin. *Semin Oncol.* 1998;25(2 Suppl 5):13–22.
68. Tournigand C, Cervantes A, Figer A, et al. OPTIMOX1: a randomized study of FOLFOX4 or FOLFOX7 with oxaliplatin in a stop-and-Go fashion in advanced colorectal cancer–a GERCOR study. *J Clin Oncol.* 2006;24(3):394–400.
69. Maindrault-Goebel FLG, Chibaudel B, et al. Final results of OPTIMOX2, a large randomized phase II study of maintenance therapy of chomtherapy-free intervals (CFI) after FOLFOX in patients with metastatic colorectal cancer (MRC): a GERCOR study. *J Clin Oncol.* 2007;ASCO Annual Meeting Proceeds Part I. Vol 25, No 18S (June 20 Supplement):4013.
70. Grothey A, Hart L, Rowland K, et al. Intermittent oxaliplatin administration improves time-to-treatment failure in metastatic colorectal cancer: final results of the phase III CONcePT trial. *J Clin Oncol.* 2008;American Society of Clinical Oncology (May 20 supplement).
71. a study of avastin (bevacizumab) plus crossover fluoropyrimidine-based chemotherapy in patients with metastatic colorectal cancer. http://clinicaltrials.gov/ct2/show/NCT00700102?term=AIO0504&rank=1. Accessed on February 12, 2010.
72. (GERCOR) GCMeO. Combination chemotherapy and bevacizumab with or without erlotinib in treating patients with metastatic colorectal cancer that cannot be removed by surgery. http://clinicaltrials.gov/ct/show/NCT00265824?order=2. Accessed on February 12, 2010.
73. Nikcevich DA, Grothey A, Sloan JA, et al. Effect of intravenous calcium and magnesium (IV CaMg) on oxaliplatin-induced sensory neurotoxicity (sNT) in adjuvant colon cancer: results of the phase III placebo-controlled, double-blind NCCTG trial N04C7. *J Clin Oncol. 2008;26(May 20 suppl):abstr 4009*
74. Cassidy J, Bjarnason GA, Hickish T, et al. Randomized double-blind (DB) placebo (Plcb) controlled phase III study assessing the efficacy of xaliproden (X) in reducing the cumulative peripheral sensory neuropathy (PSN) induced by the oxaliplatin (Ox) and 5-FU/LV combination (FOLFOX4) in first-line treatment of patients (pts) with metastatic colorectal cancer (MCRC). *J Clin Oncol.* ASCO Annual Meeting Proceedings Part I. Vol 24, No. 18S (June 20 Supplement), 2006:3507
75. Barton DL, Wos E, Qin R, et al. A randomized controlled trial evaluating a topical treatment for chemotherapy-induced neuropathy: NCCTG trial N06CA. *J Clin Oncol.* 2009 (suppl; abstr 9531);*27:15s*
76. Durand JP, Brezault C, Goldwasser F. Protection against oxaliplatin acute neurosensory toxicity by venlafaxine. *Anticancer Drugs.* 2003;14(6):423–425.
77. Smith EML, Pang H, Cirrincione C, et al. CALGB 170601: A phase III double-blind trial of duloxetine to treat painful chemotherapy-induced peripheral neuropathy (CIPN). *ASCO Meeting Abstracts.* 2012;30(18 suppl):CRA9013.
78. Yang YH, Lin JK, Chen WS, et al. Duloxetine improves oxaliplatin-induced neuropathy in patients with colorectal cancer: an open-label pilot study. *Support Care Cancer.* 2012;20(7): 1491–1497.
79. Nanney LB, Magid M, Stoscheck CM, King LE, Jr. Comparison of epidermal growth factor binding and receptor distribution in normal human epidermis and epidermal appendages. *J Invest Dermatol.* 1984;83(5):385–393.
80. Nanney LB, Stoscheck CM, King LE, Jr., Underwood RA, Holbrook KA. Immunolocalization of epidermal growth factor receptors in normal developing human skin. *J Invest Dermatol.* 1990;94(6):742–748.
81. Jost M, Huggett TM, Kari C, Boise LH, Rodeck U. Epidermal growth factor receptor-dependent control of keratinocyte survival and Bcl-xL expression through a MEK-dependent pathway. *J Biol Chem.* 2001;276(9):6320–6326.
82. Wagner LI, Lacouture ME. Dermatologic toxicities associated with EGFR inhibitors: the clinical psychologist's perspective. Impact on health-related quality of life and implications for clinical management of psychological sequelae. *Oncology (Williston Park).* 2007;21(11 Suppl 5):34–36.
83. Lacouture ME, Mitchell EP, Piperdi B, et al. Skin toxicity evaluation protocol with panitumumab (STEPP), a phase II, open-label, randomized trial evaluating the impact of a pre-emptive skin treatment regimen on skin toxicities and quality of life in patients with metastatic colorectal cancer. *J Clin Oncol.* 2010;28(8):1351–1357.
84. Balagula Y, Garbe C, Myskowski PL, et al. Clinical presentation and management of dermatological toxicities of epidermal growth factor receptor inhibitors. *Int J Dermatol.* 2011;50(2):129–146.
85. Lacouture ME, Anadkat MJ, Bensadoun RJ, et al. Clinical practice guidelines for the prevention and treatment of EGFR inhibitor-associated dermatologic toxicities. *Support Care Cancer.* 2011;19(8):1079–1095.
86. Lenz HJ, Van Cutsem E, Khambata-Ford S, et al. Multicenter phase II and translational study of cetuximab in metastatic colorectal carcinoma refractory to irinotecan, oxaliplatin, and fluoropyrimidines. *J Clin Oncol.* 2006;24(30):4914–4921.
87. Lievre A, Bachet JB, Boige V, et al. K-ras mutations as an independent prognostic factor in patients with advanced colorectal cancer treated with cetuximab. *J Clin Oncol.* 2008;26(3):374–379.
88. Heidary N, Naik H, Burgin S. Chemotherapeutic agents and the skin: an update. *J Am Acad Dermatol.* 2008;58(4):545–570.
89. Scope A, Agero AL, Dusza SW, et al. Randomized double-blind trial of prophylactic oral minocycline and topical tazarotene for cetuximab-associated acne-like eruption. *J Clin Oncol.* 2007;25(34):5390–5396.
90. Vezzoli P, Marzano AV, Onida F, et al. Cetuximab-induced acneiform eruption and the response to isotretinoin. *Acta Derm Venereol.* 2008;88(1):84–86.
91. Gutzmer R, Werfel T, Mao R, Kapp A, Elsner J. Successful treatment with oral isotretinoin of acneiform skin lesions associated with cetuximab therapy. *Br J Dermatol.* 2005;153(4):849–851.
92. Scope A, Lieb JA, Dusza SW, et al. A prospective randomized trial of topical pimecrolimus for cetuximab-associated acnelike eruption. *J Am Acad Dermatol.* 2009;61(4):614–620.
93. Hu JC, Sadeghi P, Pinter-Brown LC, Yashar S, Chiu MW. Cutaneous side effects of epidermal growth factor receptor inhibitors: clinical presentation, pathogenesis, and management. *J Am Acad Dermatol.* 2007;56(2):317–326.

94. Yesudian PD, Wilson NJ. Efficacy of gabapentin in the management of pruritus of unknown origin. *Arch Dermatol.* 2005;141(12):1507–1509.
95. Porzio G, Aielli F, Verna L, et al. Efficacy of pregabalin in the management of cetuximab-related itch. *J Pain Symptom Manage.* 2006;32(5):397–398.
96. Leveque D. Aprepitant for erlotinib-induced pruritus. *N Engl J Med.* 2010;363(17):1680–1681; author reply 1681.
97. Mir O, Blanchet B, Goldwasser F. More on aprepitant for erlotinib-induced pruritus. *N Engl J Med.* 2011;364(5):487.
98. Vincenzi B, Tonini G, Santini D. Aprepitant for erlotinib-induced pruritus. *N Engl J Med.* 2010;363(4):397–398.
99. Lane K, Goldstein SM. Erlotinib-associated trichomegaly. *Ophthal Plast Reconstr Surg.* 2007;23(1):65–66.
100. Tejwani A, Wu S, Jia Y, Agulnik M, Millender L, Lacouture ME. Increased risk of high-grade dermatologic toxicities with radiation plus epidermal growth factor receptor inhibitor therapy. *Cancer.* 2009;115(6):1286–1299.
101. Bonner JA, Harari PM, Giralt J, et al. Radiotherapy plus cetuximab for squamous-cell carcinoma of the head and neck. *N Engl J Med.* Feb 9 2006;354(6):567–578.
102. Bernier J, Bonner J, Vermorken JB, et al. Consensus guidelines for the management of radiation dermatitis and coexisting acne-like rash in patients receiving radiotherapy plus EGFR inhibitors for the treatment of squamous cell carcinoma of the head and neck. *Ann Oncol.* 2008;19(1):142–149.
103. Eames T, Grabein B, Kroth J, Wollenberg A. Microbiological analysis of epidermal growth factor receptor inhibitor therapy-associated paronychia. *J Eur Acad Dermatol Venereol.* 2010;24(8):958–960.
104. Giusti RM, Shastri KA, Cohen MH, Keegan P, Pazdur R. FDA drug approval summary: panitumumab (Vectibix). *Oncologist.* 2007;12(5):577–583.
105. Shu KY, Kindler HL, Medenica M, Lacouture M. Doxycycline for the treatment of paronychia induced by the epidermal growth factor receptor inhibitor cetuximab. *Br J Dermatol.* 2006;154(1):191–192.
106. Tosti A, Piraccini BM, Ghetti E, Colombo MD. Topical steroids versus systemic antifungals in the treatment of chronic paronychia: an open, randomized double-blind and double dummy study. *J Am Acad Dermatol.* 2002;47(1):73–76.
107. Bolognia JL, Cooper DL, Glusac EJ. Toxic erythema of chemotherapy: a useful clinical term. *J Am Acad Dermatol.* 2008;59(3):524–529.
108. Hoesly FJ, Baker SG, Gunawardane ND, Cotliar JA. Capecitabine-induced hand-foot syndrome complicated by pseudomonal superinfection resulting in bacterial sepsis and death: case report and review of the literature. *Arch Dermatol.* 2011;147(12):1418–1423.
109. Kara IO, Sahin B, Erkisi M. Palmar-plantar erythrodysesthesia due to docetaxel-capecitabine therapy is treated with vitamin E without dose reduction. *Breast.* 2006;15(3):414–424.
110. Guenova E, Weber HO, Voykov B, et al. Palmar-plantar erythrodysesthesia secondary to sunitinib treatment resulting in necrotic foot syndrome aggravated by background diabetic vascular disease. *Arch Dermatol.* 2008;144(8):1081–1082.
111. Palaia I, Angioli R, Bellati F, Basile S, Rabitti C, Panici PB. Distal phalange necrosis: a severe manifestation of palmar plantar erythrodysesthesia. *American J Obstet Gynaecol.* 2006;195(4):e1–2.
112. Sibaud V, Dalenc F, Chevreau C, et al. HFS-14, a specific quality of life scale developed for patients suffering from hand-foot syndrome. *The oncologist.* 2011;16(10):1469–1478.
113. Gressett SM, Stanford BL, Hardwicke F. Management of hand-foot syndrome induced by capecitabine. *Journal of oncology pharmacy practice: official publication of the International Society of Oncology Pharmacy Practitioners.* Sep 2006;12(3):131–141.
114. Nagore E, Insa A, Sanmartin O. Antineoplastic therapy-induced palmar plantar erythrodysesthesia ('hand-foot') syndrome. Incidence, recognition and management. *Am J Clin Dermatol.* Jul-Aug 2000;1(4):225–234.
115. Lipworth AD, Robert C, Zhu AX. Hand-foot syndrome (hand-foot skin reaction, palmar—plantar erythrodysesthesia): focus on sorafenib and sunitinib. *Oncology.* 2009;77(5):257–271.
116. Heo YS, Chang HM, Kim TW, et al. Hand-foot syndrome in patients treated with capecitabine-containing combination chemotherapy. *J Clin Pharmacol.* 2004;44(10):1166–1172.
117. Janusch M, Fischer M, Marsch W, Holzhausen HJ, Kegel T, Helmbold P. The hand-foot syndrome–a frequent secondary manifestation in antineoplastic chemotherapy. *Eur J Dermatol: EJD.* 2006;16(5):494–499.
118. Clark AS, Vahdat LT. Chemotherapy-induced palmar-plantar erythrodysesthesia syndrome: etiology and emerging therapies. *Supportive cancer therapy.* 2004;1(4):213–218.
119. Gordon KB, Tajuddin A, Guitart J, Kuzel TM, Eramo LR, VonRoenn J. Hand-foot syndrome associated with liposome-encapsulated doxorubicin therapy. *Cancer.* 1995;75(8):2169–2173.
120. Beldner M, Jacobson M, Burges GE, Dewaay D, Maize JC, Jr., Chaudhary UB. Localized palmar-plantar epidermal hyperplasia: a previously undefined dermatologic toxicity to sorafenib. *The oncologist.* 2007;12(10):1178–1182.
121. Jacobi U, Waibler E, Schulze P, et al. Release of doxorubicin in sweat: first step to induce the palmar-plantar erythrodysesthesia syndrome? *Annals of oncology: official journal of the European Society for Medical Oncology / ESMO.* 2005;16(7):1210–1211.
122. Milano G, Etienne-Grimaldi MC, Mari M, et al. Candidate mechanisms for capecitabine-related hand-foot syndrome. *Br J Clin Pharmacol.* 2008;66(1):88–95.
123. Lacouture ME, Wu S, Robert C, et al. Evolving strategies for the management of hand-foot skin reaction associated with the multitargeted kinase inhibitors sorafenib and sunitinib. *The oncologist.* 2008;13(9):1001–1011.
124. Chu D, Lacouture ME, Fillos T, Wu S. Risk of hand-foot skin reaction with sorafenib: a systematic review and meta-analysis. *Acta Oncol.* 2008;47(2):176–186.
125. Saif MW. Capecitabine and hand-foot syndrome. *Expert Opin Drug Saf.* 2011;10(2):159–169.
126. Mangili G, Petrone M, Gentile C, De Marzi P, Vigano R, Rabaiotti E. Prevention strategies in palmar-plantar erythrodysesthesia onset: the role of regional cooling. *Gynecol Oncol.* 2008;108(2):332–335.
127. Poole C, Gardiner J, Twelves C, et al. Effect of renal impairment on the pharmacokinetics and tolerability of capecitabine (Xeloda) in cancer patients. *Cancer Chemother Pharmacol.* 2002;49(3):225–234.
128. Yoshimoto N, Yamashita T, Fujita T, et al. Impact of prophylactic pyridoxine on occurrence of hand-foot syndrome in patients receiving capecitabine for advanced or metastatic breast cancer. *Breast Cancer.* 2010;17(4):298–302.
129. Mortimer JE, Anderson I. Weekly fluorouracil and high-dose leucovorin: efficacy and treatment of cutaneous toxicity. *Cancer Chemother Pharmacol.* 1990;26(6):449–452.
130. Fabian CJ, Molina R, Slavik M, Dahlberg S, Giri S, Stephens R. Pyridoxine therapy for palmar-plantar erythrodysesthesia associated with continuous 5-fluorouracil infusion. *Invest New Drugs.* 1990;8(1):57–63.
131. Chalermchai T, Tantiphlachiva K, Suwanrusme H, Voravud N, Sriuranpong V. Randomized trial of two different doses of pyridoxine in the prevention of capecitabine-associated palmar-plantar erythrodysesthesia. *Asia-Pacific journal of clinical oncology.* 2010;6(3):155–160.
132. Lin E, Morris JS, Ayers GD. Effect of celecoxib on capecitabine-induced hand-foot syndrome and antitumor activity. *Oncology (Williston Park).* 2002;16(12 Suppl No 14):31–37.
133. Kang YK, Lee SS, Yoon DH, et al. Pyridoxine is not effective to prevent hand-foot syndrome associated with capecitabine therapy: results of a randomized, double-blind, placebo-controlled study. *J Clin Oncol.* 2010;28(24):3824–3829.
134. Kingsley EC. 5-Fluorouracil dermatitis prophylaxis with a nicotine patch. *Ann Intern Med.* 1994;120(9):813.

14 *Radiation Palliative Care*

HANNAH YOON

WILLIAM SMALL, JR.

STEPHEN LUTZ

■ SYMPTOM MANAGEMENT OF RADIATION PALLIATIVE CARE

Brief Historical Perspective

The concept of hospice and palliative care dates back to the Middle Ages when monastic hospices provided care and comfort for pilgrims seeking refuge (1). In the modern era, Dame Cicely Saunders, a physician who originally trained as a nurse and social worker, helped establish the first modern hospice with St. Christopher's Hospice in London in 1967. Palliative care is defined by the World Health Organization as health care that improves quality of life, relieves pain, and provides spiritual and psychosocial support for terminally ill patients (2). Hospice in the United States is a subset of palliative care defined by the Hospice Medicare Benefit, which provides symptom management for patients whose prognosis is documented to be less than 6 months. The potential value of hospice for some patients may go unrealized, however, because of hospice referrals, which are made inappropriately late in the disease course. For example, studies have shown that 37% of patients referred to hospice die within 1 week.

The establishment of an interdisciplinary team is integral to the administration of palliative care. According to the National Comprehensive Cancer Network (NCCN) guidelines, screening for palliative care includes examining for uncontrolled symptoms, moderate/severe distress related to cancer diagnosis and treatment, severe comorbidity, life-expectancy of less than 12 months, patient and family concerns regarding disease trajectory of decision making, and requests for palliative care consult (3). Referrals to specialists for pain and symptom control and improved functional status include interventional radiology, anesthesia, orthopedics, radiation oncology, medical oncology, rehabilitation, and surgical oncology. Medical social workers are also a vital asset to the team, especially when dealing with financial issues (1).

Disease Trajectory in Rectal Cancer

There are greater than 40,000 new cases of rectal cancer annually in the United States, and about 30% of these patients present with metastatic disease at the time of their first diagnosis (4). Of the remaining patients, nearly 40% will suffer a local recurrence and will need palliative management of local symptoms (5). So, in total, up to half of patients who present with rectal cancer will eventually require palliative therapy at some point in the disease course either because of symptoms from local disease or metastases (6). Patients with asymptomatic recurrence or metastases are best managed with chemotherapy (7). Palliative options for local disease include surgical resection, surgical diversion, endoscopic stenting, radiotherapy, radiochemotherapy, and laser or argon photocoagulation. The choice for palliative treatment of local disease depends both upon patient-related factors such as age, performance status, and comorbid conditions as well as tumor-related factors such as size and location of the disease.

A myriad of symptoms may arise due to colon cancer. These include abdominal pain, nausea, vomiting, unintentional weight loss, change in bowel habits, bleeding, and bowel obstruction. Metastatic involvement of the sacral plexus by colorectal cancer (CRC)can cause pain and neurologic dysfunction, with higher pain scores negatively correlated with overall survival (8). Tumor may also spread via penetration of the bowel wall into adjacent organs and structures, leading to symptoms related to dysfunction of those organs (9). Spread can also occur via lymph nodes, as smooth metastatic nodules of pericolic or perirectal fat, or vascular invasion as irregularly shaped nodules in fat. Distant metastases most commonly occur in the liver and lung (Table 14.1).

Overview

The ability of radiation to relieve symptoms from cancer was realized soon after the discovery of the x-ray by Roentgen in 1895. The first two to three decades following that discovery saw radiation treatments given either as a single large dose or a small number of fairly large doses. The subsequent understanding that normal tissues might repair themselves more efficiently than cancer cells led to

Table 14.1 Palliative Sites and Management

Liver	Resection if possible, otherwise neoadjuvant chemotherapy (FOLFIRI or FOLFOX or CapeOx) ± bevacizumab ± cetuximab or panitumumab, and re-evaluation for resection; otherwise, can also consider hepatic arterial infusion of chemotherapy or arterial radioembolization with yttrium-90 microspheres, radiofrequency ablation (RFA) and conformal external beam radiotherapy
Lung	Resection if possible, otherwise neoadjuvant chemotherapy (FOLFIRI or FOLFOX or CapeOx) ± bevacizumab ± cetuximab or panitumumab, and re-evaluation for resection, or conformal external beam radiotherapy
Abdominal/peritoneal	If nonobstructing, chemotherapy. If obstructed, colonic resection, diverting colostomy, bypass of impending obstruction, or stenting
Rectal	Chemotherapy and palliative radiotherapy

Adapted from (3).

the current standard of delivering 30 to 40 smaller doses from 1.8 to 2.0 Gy for patients treated with curative intent. The use of a single 8 Gy dose or a small number of 3.0 to 5.0 Gy fractions may still be used for patients treated with palliative intent, an approach termed hypofractionation.

Data from studies show that 15%–50% of patients treated with radiotherapy are managed with palliative, rather than curative intent, with that described variation depending on referral patterns, geographic location, and differences in what clinicians deem as "palliative" (10). Nevertheless, 50% of cancer patients do receive palliative radiotherapy at some point during their disease trajectory (8). About one-quarter of palliative radiotherapy is delivered to relieve symptoms from newly diagnosed primary tumors, while around three-quarters is delivered for patients who have locally recurrent or metastatic disease. The most common indication for palliative radiotherapy is to relieve symptomatic bone metastases, though two-thirds of palliative radiotherapy is delivered for symptoms other than bone pain (8). Radiotherapy offers palliation that may be superior to chemotherapy because of its shorter duration of delivery and mild, self-limiting side effects, which involve only the treated volume of tissue (8). The cost of palliative radiotherapy is comparable or superior to other medical costs such as systemic chemotherapy, drugs, or surgery.

However, the cost of radiotherapy may be too high for patients in hospice programs that provide care at rates of approximately $130 per day. Survey results have shown that although the majority of hospice professionals feel that radiotherapy is an important part of palliative care, less than 3% of hospice patients actually received radiotherapy (11). Barriers to care in addition to cost of treatment include transportation difficulty, short life expectancy, and lack of awareness or education regarding the potential benefits of radiotherapy. Only 50% of hospice professionals feel comfortable identifying indications for palliative radiotherapy in their patients, while, alternatively, less than 10% of palliative care professionals view radiation oncologists as part of the palliative care team (12).

SYMPTOM MANAGEMENT OF RECTAL CANCER

Stage IV Disease at Presentation

The role of primary resection for Stage IV rectal carcinoma remains undefined. Certain findings correlate with unresectability, including: sciatic nerve pain, bilateral ureteral obstruction, fixation to the lateral pelvic side wall, sacral involvement above the level of S2, bilateral lymphedema, multiple peritoneal metastases, or metastases fixed to vital organs. The presence of any of these circumstances would suggest a low likelihood of achieving a margin-negative resection and suggest a potential for significant postoperative morbidity (13).

The reported rate of mechanical obstruction in patients with rectal cancer at their time of disease presentation varies from 10% to about 25% (14,15). Surgical intervention may include resection of the tumor or a diverting procedure to bypass the obstructing lesion. Patients who require surgery on an emergent rather than elective basis have been shown to have higher local recurrence rates and shorter survival, so the preferred operation for a patient with an acute presentation of bowel obstruction is a diverting colostomy (15). One study has suggested that emergency decompressive surgery may be associated with a mortality rate of 20%, a postoperative complication rate of 50%, and a greater chance that patients will require permanent colostomy than would be true in the setting of an elective procedure (16).

The time required to heal following a surgery suggests that a patient should only undergo palliative resection if they have a life expectancy of 6 months or more (17–20). Palliative resection types may include low anterior resection (LAR), abdominoperineal resection (APR), Hartmann procedure, or pelvic exenteration. The choice among these surgeries depends upon both patient and tumor factors. For tumors that reside sufficiently far away from the anal canal, either an LAR or Hartmann procedure would be considered reasonable. The LAR may help to maintain normal bowel function, while the Hartmann procedure with colostomy placement might better serve the needs of a patient who has previously received high dose radiotherapy to the site which would serve as the anastomosis for the LAR (21). An APR procedure is the preferred method of resection for any rectal cancer that invades the anus (22). The pelvic exenteration procedure may cause significant morbidity and prolonged healing times, however, and as such is not commonly employed in the palliative setting (23). Some have suggested that a palliative endoscopic trans-anal resection might be appropriate for some patients who present with metastatic disease but who also require treatment of local symptoms of rectosigmoid cancer (24).

While diverting colostomy can allow for a resolution in obstructive symptoms, stoma placement can cause deleterious effects such as skin irritation, leakage, bowel prolapse, pain, necrosis, and retraction in up to one-third of patients who undergo a diverting colostomy (25). One-quarter to one-third of patients describe that their quality of life has been significantly negatively impacted following the placement of a stoma. So, one must also consider the potential usefulness of radiotherapy in this setting. Palliative radiotherapy is a local modality that is helpful in cases of locally advanced rectal cancer that cause pain, rectal bleeding, tenesmus, and rectal obstruction. Pelvic radiotherapy is commonly delivered through a three-field technique with the patient lying in a prone position, though it is feasible to spare normal adjacent structures through the use of intensity modulated radiotherapy (IMRT; 9).

As study from Princess Margaret Hospital showed excellent palliative results. In 84 patients who received greater than 45 Gy, 89% reported palliation of pain, 79% reported bleeding cessation, 71% reported resolution of mass effect, 50% reported improvement in rectal discharge, and 22% reported resolution of urologic symptoms in the 6 to 8 weeks after completion of treatment (26). In a separate study from Thomas Jefferson University, 65% reported resolution of pain, 100% reported resolution of bleeding, and 24% reported resolution of mass effect with duration of relief lasting 8 to 10 months after treatment (27). One study showed that a regimen of 30 Gy in six fractions twice per week, over a total of 3 weeks, with continuous infusion 5-fluorouracil chemotherapy was effective in controlling pain up to 90% with acceptable toxicity (28). Approximately, 66% of patients did not require subsequent colostomy placement for their locally advanced disease. Radiation therapy has been shown to provide about a 75% rate of relief of pain and bleeding with a mean duration of symptom response of 6 to 9 months in this patient group (29).

Radiation therapy is also very useful in the treatment of colorectal metastases, especially those that cause symptoms due to spread to the bony skeleton or brain (30,31). Recent efforts have also focused on the ability of stereotactic body radiation therapy to relieve symptoms from metastases of the liver. There are some circumstances when palliative radiotherapy should be avoided, however. Patient-related situations where clinicians should counsel against the use of radiotherapy include when death is imminent, when there is a plethora of symptoms, and when the patient may be unable to give informed consent. Treatment-related barriers to radiotherapy include scenarios when retreatment exceeds normal tissue radiation tolerance or where it requires an inconveniently lengthy course. Health care system-related issues include unavailability of a nearby radiotherapy facility, the lack of specialized technology such as stereotactic radiotherapy, or an ineffective coordination between radiotherapy and palliative medicine (8).

Improvements in chemotherapy efficacy for patients with metastatic CRC have improved both overall survival and quality of life for this patient population. Still, there are very little data available to evaluate the improvements in local symptom control following radiotherapy combined with these newer chemotherapy agents. One recent single-institutional study described favorable symptom response and minimal side effects following chemoradiotherapy for patients with pelvic symptoms from CRC (32). The authors suggested that the only variable that noticeably improved outcomes was a biologically equivalent dose (BED) greater than 40 Gy10. Researchers at the M. D. Anderson Cancer Center examined the possibility that chemoradiotherapy might relieve symptoms and obviate the need for colostomy placement in patients who presented with synchronous distant metastases from rectal cancer (33). The report from Crane et al showed that 94% of patients receiving pelvic radiotherapy had complete resolution of pelvic symptoms, with 2-year pelvic symptom-free survival of 82%. Concurrent 5-fluorouracil-based chemotherapy was administered concurrently with radiotherapy to doses including 30 Gy in 6 fractions, 35 Gy in 14 fractions, or 45 Gy in 25 fractions. Some of the patients also underwent pelvic resection, hepatic metastatectomy, or additional rounds of systemic chemotherapy. The chemoradiotherapy group had a colostomy-free survival rate of 79%, while the group that also had pelvic surgery exhibited higher rates of pelvic tumor control and overall survival. Predictors for worse survival included pelvic pain at presentation, a biologically equivalent radiotherapy dose below 35 Gy, and poorly differentiated tumor.

The use of self-expanding metal stents (SEMS) may provide successful palliation without further intervention, or they may provide temporary relief while transitioning to an elective surgical resection or other local therapy. SEMS may be placed into a lightly sedated patient with the aid of fluoroscopy, endoscopy, or both (34). Stents vary in length and diameter, and they can therefore be chosen to best fit the specific clinical situation. Stents often become fixed in place by causing pressure necrosis into the tumor itself (35). Stent placement has been shown to relieve obstruction greater than 90% of the time with a mean duration of relief of 106 days (34). The main cause of stent failure was an inability to pass the guidewire beyond the obstructing lesion during the initial placement procedure. SEMS placement for a low-lying rectal lesion, within 3 cm of the anorectal ring, is contraindicated because patients may subsequently suffer intractable anal pain, tenesmus, or incontinence (36). The potential complications of stent placement may include bleeding, malposition, or occlusion in the acute phase as well as stent migration, bleeding, pain, incontinence, or perforation in the late phase (37–41). Still, the comparable outcomes and side effect profiles of stent use vs surgical resection suggest that it may provide an excellent option for many patients who present with obstruction due to locally advanced or recurrent rectal cancer (42).

For patients in whom neither stent placement nor surgical excision are feasible, the combination of laser ablation plus intraluminal high dose rate brachytherapy radiation may prove effective for relieving the effects of colonic obstruction (43). Laser treatment may create its intended effects by either promoting coagulative necrosis or by directly vaporizing tumor cells. The neodymium yttrium argon garnet laser (Nd:YAG) is the most commonly used laser in this setting. Endoscopic laser ablation of rectal lesions may achieve improvement in rectal bleeding at a rate of 80%–90% following two to five treatment sessions (44,45). The side effect rates of laser ablation occur at a rate of 2%–15% and may include perforation requiring laparotomy. An alternative method for fulgurating bleeding vessels is the use of Argon plasma coagulation (APC) which has a theoretical advantage of lower perforation risk than Nd:YAG treatment because of a limited depth of penetration of only 2–3 mm (44).

Locally Recurrent Disease

The rate of postoperative local recurrence for patients with rectal carcinoma has historically been found to be around 10%–25% (46–48). One study suggested that the local symptoms from incurable rectal cancer included obstruction (42%), rectal bleeding (37%), pain or rectal discharge (16%), or no symptoms (5%; 49). For those patients with locally recurrent disease, no evidence for distant metastases, and a reasonable performance status, curative surgery provides improved survival, quality of life, and patient well-being when compared to noncurative surgery or a nonsurgical approach (50). Still, only 20%–30% of patients are able to undergo surgery with curative intent in the setting of locally recurrent rectal cancer (51). For the majority of patients with locally recurrent rectal cancer who cannot undergo surgery with curative intent, the data have shown that neither survival nor quality of life are significantly improved with noncurative surgery vs nonsurgical interventions (51–55).

A recent review of 106 articles dealing with treatment of locally recurrent rectal cancer found no randomized trials but confirmed that surgery may improve local control and perhaps survival for this patient group (56). The authors conclude that improvements in surgical technique have allowed for greater choices in reconstructive surgery, and they note that an R0 resection is a favorable prognostic indicator. Still, they do admit that the morbidity of the surgical approach for these patients may be significant. They also recommend clinical algorithms that include interdisciplinary care to help determine proper management of this patient group.

It is feasible to effectively and safely reirradiate patients with locally recurrent rectal cancer (57). A patient group that had originally been treated with a median dose of 50.4 Gy received reirradiation with concurrent 5-fluorouracil-based chemotherapy to an additional 34.8 Gy with the goal of alleviating recurrent symptoms. The median time between treatment courses was 19 months, and the median cumulative dose was 85.8 Gy. One-third of the patients also had surgical resection following their reirradiation. The median survival times were 26 months for the entire group, while the median survival for those who underwent surgery was 44 months. Grade 3 acute toxicity measured about 15% while late complications were noted in about 20% of those treated.

Alternatively, a retrospective study from Korea suggests that patients with locally recurrent rectal cancer treated with chemoradiotherapy may have an average life expectancy of nearly 5 years either with or without surgical resection (58). These patients received a mean dose of 54.6 Gy, and their survival did correlate with the severity of symptoms present at the time of local recurrence.

Patients with limited treatment options because of previous radiotherapy or surgery have been treated with isolated pelvic perfusion of chemotherapy drugs to the length of rectum involved with tumor by using a simplified balloon-occlusion technique (59). Additionally, some small series of patients with recurrent rectal carcinomas have been shown to have improvements in Brief Pain Inventory (BPI) scores following the use of radiofrequency ablation (RFA; 60).

Last Weeks of Life

The final weeks of life for patients with CRC may cause several challenges for their caregivers. Uncontrolled disease in the pelvis requires detailed attention to a pain medicine regimen. Nausea and vomiting caused by obstruction must be managed with antiemetics and/or a nasogastric tube to relieve pressure in the alimentary tract. As patients become increasingly disinterested with food, their family should be counseled against placement of a nasogastric or percutaneous gastric feeding tube. Anorexia commonly accompanies the dying process, so once a feeding tube is placed the family might suffer unnecessary emotional stress when the patient's death becomes imminent and they must decide whether to discontinue its use.

■ CONCLUSIONS

Palliative radiotherapy for patients who have CRC is time efficient and cost effective in relieving symptoms. It remains underutilized due to a combination of cost and lack of education of staff and physicians regarding the available resources, but when used properly, it is a crucial modality in palliating symptoms in terminally ill patients with CRC.

■ REFERENCES

1. Singer M, Furlani C. Palliative care for metastatic disease. In: Tagian AG, Smith BL, Erban JK, eds. *Breast Cancer: A Multidisciplinary Approach to Diagnosis and Management.* New York, NY: 2010;221–228.
2. World Health Organization. Palliative care definition. Available at www.who.int/cancer/palliative/en.
3. NCCN Clinical Practice Guidelines: Palliative Care: Available at www.nccn.org.
4. Jemal A, Siegel R, Ward E, et al. Cancer statistics 2009. *CA Cancer J Clin.* 2009;59:225–249.
5. Rothenberger C. Palliative therapy of rectal cancer. Overview: epidemiology, indications, goals, extent, and nature of work-up. *J Gastrointest Surg.* 2004;8:259–261.
6. Van Custem E, Oliveira J. Advanced colorectal cancer: ESMO clinical recommendations for diagnosis, treatment and follow-up. *Ann Oncol.* 2009;20 (Supp 4):61–63.
7. Engstrom P, Arnoletti J, Benson A, et al. NCCN clinical practice guidelines in oncology: rectal cancer. *J Natl Compr Canc Netw.* 2009;7:838–881.
8. Lutz S, Chow EL, Hartsell WF, Konski AA. A review of hypofractionated palliative radiotherapy. *Cancer.* 2007;1–9.
9. Minsky, BD, Welton, ML, Venook, AP. Cancer of the rectum. In: Hoppe RT, Phillips TL, Roach M, eds. *Leibel and Phillips Textbook of Radiation Oncology.* Philadelphia, PA: 2010:851–869.
10. Coia LR. Palliative radiation therapy in the United States. *Can J Oncol.* 1996;6 Suppl 1:62–69.
11. Lutz S, Spence C, Chow E, Janjan N, Connor S. Survey on use of palliative radiotherapy in hospice care. *J Clin Oncol.* 2004;22(17):3581–3585.
12. McCloskey S, Tao M, Rose C, et al. National survey of perspectives of palliative radiation therapy: role, barriers, and needs. *Cancer J.* 2007;13:130–137.
13. Bouchard P, Efron J. Management of recurrent rectal cancer. *Ann Surg Oncol.* 2010;17:1343–1356.
14. Alvarez J, Baldonedo R, Bear I, et al. Presentation, treatment, and multivariate analysis of risk factors for obstructive and perforative colorectal carcinoma. *Am J Surg.* 2005;190:376–382.
15. Phang P, MacFarlane J, Taylor R, et al. Effect of emergent presentation on outcome from rectal cancer management. *Am J Surg.* 2003;185:450–454.
16. Leitman I, Sullivan J, Brams D, et al. Multivariate analysis of morbidity and mortality from the initial surgical management of obstructing carcinoma of the colon. *Surg Gynecol Obstet.* 1992;174:513–518.
17. Wasserberg N, Kaufman H. Palliation of colorectal cancer. *Surg Oncol.* 2007;16:299–310.
18. Rosen S, Buell J, Yoshida A, et al. Initial presentation with stage IV colorectal cancer: how aggressive should we be? *Arch Surg.* 2000;135:530–534.
19. Law W, Chu K. Outcomes of resection of stage IV rectal cancer with mesorectal excision. *J Surg Oncol.* 2006;93:523–528.
20. Sigurdsson H, Korner H, Dahl O, et al. Palliative surgery for rectal cancer in a national cohort. *Colorectal Dis.* 2008;10:336–343.
21. Hassan I, Larson D, Cima, et al. Long-term functional and quality of life outcomes after coloanal anastomosis for distal rectal cancer. *Dis Colon Rectum.* 2006;49:1266–1274.
22. Fazio V. Indications and surgical alternatives for palliation of rectal cancer. *J Gastrointest Surg.* 2004;8:262–265.
23. Nishio M, Sakakura C, Nagata T, et al. Outcomes of total pelvic exenteration for colorectal cancer. *Hepatogastroenterology.* 2009;56:1637–1641.
24. Donohoe C, Brannigan A, O'Connell P. Palliative endoscopic trans-anal resection of advanced rectosigmoid carcinoma. *Ir J Med Sci.* 2011;180:541–544.
25. Pittman J, Rawl S, Schmidt C, et al. Demographic and clinical factors related to ostomy complications and quality of life in veterans with an ostomy. *J Wound Ostomy Continence Nurs.* 2008;35:493–503.
26. Brierley J, Cummings B, Wong C, et al. Adenocarcinoma of the rectum treated by radical radiation therapy. *Int J Radiat Oncol Biol Phys.* 31;2:255–259.
27. Mohiuddin M, Marks G, Marks J. Long term results of re-irradiation for patients with recurrent rectal carcinoma. *Cancer.* 2001;95:1144–1150.
28. Janjan NA, Breslin T, Lenzi R, et al. Avoidance of colostomy placement in advanced colorectal cancer with twice weekly hypofractionated radiation plus continuous infusion 5-fluorouracil. *J Pain Symptom Management.* 2000;20:266–72.
29. Salts L. Palliative management of rectal cancer: the roles of chemotherapy and radiation therapy. *J Gastrointest Surg.* 2004;8:274–276.
30. Lutz S, Berk L, Chang E, et al. Palliative radiotherapy for bone metastases: An ASTRO evidence-based guideline. *Int J Radiat Oncol Biol Phys.* 2011;79:965–76.
31. Tsao M, Rades D, Wirth A, et al. Radiotherapeutic and surgical management for brain metastasis/es: An ASTRO evidence based guideline. (in press).
32. Bae S, Won P, Choi D, et al. Palliative radiotherapy in patients with a symptomatic pelvic mass of metastatic colorectal cancer. *Radiation Oncology.* 2011;6:52.
33. Crane C, Janjan N, Abbruzzese J, et al. Effective pelvic symptom control using initial chemoradiation without colostomy in metastatic rectal cancer. *Int J Radiat Oncol Biol Phys.* 2001;49:107–116.
34. Watt A, Faragher I, Griffin T, et al. Self-expanding metallic stents for relieving malignant colorectal obstruction: a systematic review. *Ann Surg.* 2007;246:24–30.
35. Baron T. Indications and results of endoscopic rectal stenting. *J Gastrointest Surg.* 2004;8:266–269.
36. Hunerbein M, Krause M, Moesta K, et al. Palliation of malignant rectal obstruction with self-expanding metal stents. *Surgery.* 2005;137:42–47.
37. Faragher I, Chaitowitz I, Stupart D. Long-term results of palliative stenting or surgery for incurable obstructing colon cancer. *Colorectal Dis.* 2008; 10, 668–672.
38. Biondo S, Pares D, Frago R, et al. Large bowel obstruction: predictive factors for postoperative mortality. *Dis Colon Rectum.* 2004; 47, 1889–1897.
39. Scoggins C, Meszoely I, Blanke C, et al. Nonoperative management of primary colorectal cancer in patients with state IV disease. *Ann Surg Oncol.* 1999;6:651–657.
40. Ogunbiyi O, McKenna K, Birnbaum E, et al. Aggressive surgical management of recurrent rectal cancer–is it worthwhile? *Dis Colon Rectum.* 1997;40:150–155.

41. Garcia-Aguilar J, Cromwell J, Marra C, et al. Treatment of locally recurrent rectal cancer. *Dis Colon Rectum*. 2001;44:1743–1748.
42. Ptok H, Marusch F, Steinert R, et al. Incurable stenosing colorectal carcinoma: endoscopic stent implantation or palliative surgery? *World J Surg*. 2006;30:1481–1487.
43. Tam T, Mukherjee S, Farrell T, et al. Endoscopic brachytherapy for obstructive colorectal cancer. *Brachytherapy*. 2009;8:313–317.
44. Kimmey M. Endoscopic methods (other than stents) for palliation of rectal carcinoma. J *Gastrointest Surg*. 2004;8:270–273.
45. Rao V, Al-Mukhtar A, Rayan F, et al. Endoscopiclaser ablation of advanced rectal carcinoma—a DGH experience. *Colorectal Dis*. 2005;7:58–60.
46. Rao A, Kagan A, Chan P, et al. Patterns of recurrence following curative resection alone for adenocarcinoma of the rectum and sigmoid colon. *Cancer*. 1981;48:1492–1495.
47. Pilipshen S, Heilweil M, Quan S, et al. Patterns of pelvic recurrence following definitive resections of rectal cancer. *Cancer*. 1984;53:1354–1362.
48. Douglass H, Moertel C, Mayer R, et al. Survival after postoperative combination treatment of rectal cancer. *N Engl J Med*. 1986;315:1294–1295.
49. Courtney E, Raja A, Leicester R. Eight years experience of high-powered endoscopic diode laser therapy for palliation of colorectal carcinoma. *Dis Colon Rectum*. 2005;48:845–850.
50. You Y, Habiba H, Chang G, et al. Prognostic value of quality of life and pain in patients with locally recurrent rectal cancer. *Ann Surg Oncol*. 2011;18:989–996.
51. Nielsen M, Laurberg S, Holm T. Current management of locally recurrent rectal cancer. *Colorectal Dis*. 2009;13:732–742.
52. Palmer G, Martling A, Cedermark B, et al. A population-based study on the management and outcome in patients with locally recurrent rectal cancer. *Ann Surg Oncol*. 2007;14:447–454.
53. Hahnloser D, Nelson H, Gunderson L, et al. Curative potential of multimodality therapy for locally recurrent cancer. *Ann Surg*. 2003;237:502–508.
54. Miner T, Jaques D, Paty P, et al. Symptom control in patients with locally recurrent rectal cancer. *Ann Surg Oncol*. 2003;10:72–79.
55. Miller A, Cantor S, Peoples G, et al. Quality of life and cost effectiveness analysis of therapy for locally recurrent rectal cancer. *Dis Colon Rectum*. 2000;43:1695–1701.
56. Mirnezami A, Sagar P, Kavanagh D, et al. Clinical algorithms for the surgical management of locally recurrent rectal cancer. *Dis Colon Rectum*. 2010;53:1248–1257.
57. Mohiuddin M, Marks G, Marks J. Long-Term Results of Reirradiation for Patients with Recurrent Rectal Carcinoma. *Cancer*. 2002;95:1144–1150.
58. Lee J, Kim D, Kim S, et al. Clinical outcomes of chemoradiotherapy for locally recurrent rectal cancer. *Radiat Oncol*. 2011;6:51.
59. Wanebo H, DiSiena M, Begossi G, et al. Isolated chemotherapeutic perfusion of pelvis as neoadjuvant or palliative therapy for advanced cancer of the rectum. *Ann Surg Oncol*. 2008;15:1107–16.
60. Belfiore G, Tedeschi E, Ronza F, et al. CT-guided radiofrequency ablation of recurrent rectal cancer. *Am Journal of Roentgenol*. 2009;192:137–141.

15 Multidisciplinary Approach to Quality of Life

JOHN M. SALSMAN
DAVID CELLA
MAXWELL T. VERGO
SUSAN E. YOUNT

■ HEALTH-RELATED QUALITY OF LIFE

Over the past two decades, health-related quality of life (HRQL) has gained in importance in oncology overall. Due to the often chronic and/or incurable nature of cancer, the toxicity of new treatments and the resulting impact on HRQL, it can be as important as efficacy outcomes. A debilitated HRQL status can jeopardize a patient's ability or willingness to complete a treatment regimen, thereby also affecting its efficacy. HRQL assessment may also aid in establishing a response in the absence of conventional endpoints, such as measurable tumor shrinkage.

HRQL differs from classical toxicity ratings in two important ways: (a) HRQL incorporates more aspects of function (eg, mood, affect, social well-being) than those attributed to treatment; and (b) the focus is on the patient's perspective, not a clinician rating (1). There is wide consensus that HRQL is both subjective and multidimensional, and has been defined as "the extent to which one's usual or expected physical, emotional and social well-being are affected by a medical condition or its treatment" (1). Assessment of HRQL involves a multidimensional approach to quantification of subjective variables: physical, functional, social, emotional, and spiritual well-being, where physical well-being reflects disease symptoms and treatment side effects; functional well-being reflects a patient's ability to perform activities of daily living and role performance; social/family well-being reflects the quality of relationships and communication with family members; emotional well-being reflects a wide range of psychological impacts of disease and treatment side effects; and spiritual well-being reflects the degree to which patients find comfort and peace from their spiritual beliefs when coping with their illness. Symptoms are also an integral component of HRQL (2). Oncology patients experience many disease- and treatment-related symptoms, and most patients, especially those with advanced disease, experience 11.5 symptoms on average (3). All commonly used HRQL questionnaires in oncology include self-reported symptoms, including concerns specific to the disease site. For example, colorectal cancer (CRC) patients are asked about items such as appetite, bowel control, stomach-related problems, weight loss, body image, and abdominal swelling or cramping (4).

HRQL assessment in oncology clinical practice has been used to help monitor disease and treatment, detect physical or psychosocial problems, and improve care. Routine HRQL assessment may also help guide treatment planning and decision making, which could, in turn, improve patient HRQL (5). The few empirical studies that have investigated this practice have yielded equivocal results, with some reporting improved detection of and communication about patients' symptoms and concerns following HRQL assessment (6–9). Importantly, positive effects on patient satisfaction and patient-reported health status have also been noted (7). While some studies have provided evidence that adequate HRQL assessment alone can have salutary treatment effects (7–10), others have suggested that providing feedback of assessment results to providers is a key ingredient to success in improving HRQL. In fact, some have suggested that providing clinicians with information about not only what patients' HRQL scores are but what to do with the information obtained, such as guideline-based treatment recommendations, may be necessary for the demonstration of consistently positive results (5,11,12).

Measuring HRQL

There are many questionnaires available to measure HRQL of people with cancer; this summary will highlight the most pertinent to CRC patients' clinical care. The process of selecting a measure is often driven by many considerations, including the purpose of the study, the patient-reported endpoint(s) selected to address the study's purpose, the content of items in the questionnaire, and the validity of the questionnaire (13). Measures of HRQL in oncology can be categorized as generic, cancer specific, or symptom specific. Generic measures (often described as health-profile type instruments) are often used in general populations to assess a wide range of domains applicable to a variety of health states, conditions, and diseases. They are particularly useful in conducting general survey research on health and comparing different disease states. Examples of such measures include the Medical Outcomes Study Short Form Health Survey (SF-36; 14–16), Nottingham Health Profile (17), and Sickness Impact Profile (18,19). The SF-36 is one of the most widely used generic health questionnaires. It measures eight domains of physical function, social function, role limitations due to physical problems, role limitations due to emotional problems, vitality, bodily pain, emotional health, and general health. In addition, two higher-order summary scores can be calculated: Physical Component Summary and Mental Component Summary. Higher scores reflect improved HRQL. The SF-36 has been extensively validated and is widely used in various outpatient settings to measure functional status.

There are also general cancer-specific measures that focus on broad, yet clinically relevant issues and a few symptoms. Such measures allow for group comparisons as well as help assess overall impact of disease and treatment on HRQL. However, because general measures focus on broader HRQL issues, they tend to lack sensitivity to specific changes in the impact of cancer for individual patients (20). On the other hand, disease-specific tools focus on detailed symptom assessment and are responsive to changes in important concerns relevant to the patient group being studied, but they do not easily allow for comparisons between disease groups. A more complete approach is to combine both generic and disease-specific measures to capture the overall HRQL of patients without compromising sensitivity to changes in disease-specific issues. Such a modular approach, which utilizes a generic core questionnaire assessing broader HRQL concepts, supplemented with shorter disease-specific and symptom-specific measures, has become more practical. Examples include the European Organization for Research and Treatment of Cancer (EORTC) QLQ-C30 (21) and the Functional Assessment of Cancer Therapy-General (FACT-G; 22), both of which entail a general core questionnaire to assess overall HRQL (eg, QLQ-C30, FACT-G) that can be supplemented with a site-specific symptom module or subscale to address additional concerns specific to that cancer population. The following are three specific examples relevant to patients with CRC: EORTC QLQ-CR29, FACT-C, and National Comprehensive Cancer Network/ FACT-Colorectal Symptom Index (NFCSI).

The EORTC QLQ-C30 is a general 30-item questionnaire designed for cancer patients. It evaluates five HRQL domains (physical, role, cognitive, emotional, and social); several symptoms (fatigue, pain, nausea, vomiting, dyspnea, sleep disturbance, appetite, constipation, diarrhea); and global health/HRQL. All items are rated on a 4-point Likert-type scale from "not at all" to "very much"; the global scale is a numerical 7-point Likert-type scale representing a continuum from "very poor" to "excellent." High functioning and global scale scores and low symptom scores reflect better functioning and lower symptom distress. The EORTC QLQ-C30 has demonstrated good reliability and validity in various large, international cancer populations and is available in many languages (23). The CR29 is a 29-item module supplementing the QLQ-C29 core questionnaire designed to assess impact of treatment on symptoms specifically relevant to CRC patients.

The Functional Assessment of Chronic Illness Therapy (FACIT) measurement system is a collection of HRQL questionnaires targeted to the management of chronic illness. "FACIT" was adopted as the formal name in 1997 to reflect expansion of the familiar FACT questionnaires into other chronic illnesses and conditions. The FACT-G (22) is easy to complete (5–10 min) and has demonstrated reliability, validity, and sensitivity to change. It is written at or below the sixth grade reading level. The FACT-G is considered appropriate for use with patients with any form of cancer and has also been used and validated in other chronic illness conditions. The FACT-G (now version 4) is a 27-item compilation of general questions divided into four primary domains: physical well-being (PWB), social/ family well-being (SWB), emotional well-being (EWB), and functional well-being (FWB). Validation of the core measure has allowed for evolution of multiple disease, treatment, condition, and other targeted questionnaires. For instance, the FACT-Colorectal (FACT-C; 24) is comprised of the FACT-G plus the CRC Subscale (CCS), consisting of seven CRC-specific concerns (ie, stomach swelling or cramps, losing weight, bowel control, food digestion, diarrhea, appetite, body image).

The Trial Outcome Index (TOI) is yet another scoring option for the FACT-C and is a sum of the PWB, FWB, and CCS subscales. The TOI-C has been shown to be an efficient summary index of physical/functional outcomes and is, therefore, a common endpoint used in clinical trials because it is responsive to change in physical/functional outcomes, sometimes more than a total (overall) multidimensional aggregated score. The FACT-C, CCS, and TOI-C have been shown to be valid, reliable, and responsive to change (24).

Effective symptom management begins with accurate symptom assessment (25). The EORTC QLQ-C30/CR29 and the FACT-C include an assessment of some common symptoms associated with CRC (3,21,22). However, brief tumor-specific symptom measures are needed, and, in particular, measures that are psychometrically acceptable and based on both patient and health care provider input to ensure clinical relevance. Such measures should be sensitive to the impact of drug therapy (26), thereby serving clinical, research, and regulatory purposes.

In 2003, we conducted a comprehensive survey of physician and nurse experts at 17 National Comprehensive Cancer Network (NCCN) member institutions to examine the priority symptoms endorsed by oncology experts (27). Using questions from the FACT measurement system and data from this survey of experts, we constructed tumor-specific indexes comprised of the most important symptoms and concerns to monitor in evaluating treatment for nine advanced cancers, including colorectal. The results of this survey demonstrated good agreement between expert physicians and nurses on the relative importance of symptoms in this survey. However, patient input was not obtained, and patient ratings of symptom relevance and severity often differ from those of providers (25,28,29–32), especially regarding psychological symptoms and concerns (33,34). Thus, there remained the possibility that the symptom indexes did not capture the full range of patient priority symptoms.

Therefore, we sought to identify patients' highest priority cancer symptoms for an expanded range of advanced cancers, including colorectal, compare their priority ratings with those of oncology experts, and construct brief symptom indexes utilizing the combined input (ie, physicians, nurses, patients) to assess these symptoms and concerns. The methodology used was similar to that used with clinical experts (27) and has been reported on elsewhere (35). In addition, physician expert input was obtained as to which symptoms associated with each of 11 diseases are considered to be disease-related vs treatment-related. Patient-completed FACT HRQL questionnaires specific to their disease provided data for a preliminary validation of the symptom indexes. The following focuses exclusively on the development and preliminary validation of the NFCSI.

Participants in this study included 50 adult patients diagnosed with advanced CRC and physicians who treat patients with CRC. Patients must have had prior experience with chemotherapy for at least two cycles (1 month for noncyclical chemotherapy) and were recruited from a subset of NCCN member institutions as well as community support agencies to balance preferences of patients from tertiary referral centers with patients seen in the community.

A subset of 29 patients was asked to respond to an open-ended question soliciting the full range of their experience receiving drug treatment for their illness and asking them to list the most important symptoms or concerns to monitor when assessing the value of drug treatment for their illness. Patients were then asked to rate, using a 0 to 10 scale, how important each symptom or concern was to them. Next, patients were asked to complete a symptom/concern checklist that included 26 items nominated by clinician experts from the FACT-C questionnaire, identical to that administered to NCCN providers previously (27). In a two-step process, patients were first asked to select no more than 10 symptoms or concerns that they felt were "the most important symptoms or concerns to monitor when assessing the value of drug treatment for advanced CRC" and then asked to select, from the 10 symptoms/concerns nominated as "the most important," up to five as "the very most important." Space was provided for respondents to write in symptoms or concerns not already listed. Patients then completed the FACT-C (24).

The sample of 50 advanced colorectal patients had a median age of 57 years. Slightly over half of the sample was female (54%) and was predominantly White (90%), and well educated (76% with some college or college degree); equal percentages were employed full time, on disability or retired (26%). Using the Eastern Cooperative Oncology Group [ECOG] performance status rating [PSR] 5-point scale (0 = no symptoms, 1 = some symptoms but does not require bedrest during the waking day, 2 = requires bedrest for less than 50% of the waking day, 3 = requires bedrest for more than 50% of the waking day, 4 = unable to get out of bed), most (54%) patients reported normal activity with some symptoms.

Items retained in the final symptom index were derived from patients' spontaneous reports in response to an open-ended question (eg, fatigue, nausea, neuropathy including numbness/tingling, temperature sensitivity, treatment efficacy/side effects, diarrhea, hair loss, appetite, and constipation); their nominations of the top 10 most important symptom/concerns selected from a checklist (eg, fatigue, ability to enjoy life, being content with the quality of one's life, nausea, ability to work, appetite, feeling ill, being able to enjoy things for fun, sleeping well, and worry about their condition worsening); their nominations of the top five very most important symptoms/concerns from the checklist (eg, fatigue, ability to enjoy life, being content with the quality of one's life, nausea, control over bowels, and diarrhea); and patient write-in symptoms/concerns on the checklist. The final NFCSI was composed of 19 symptoms/concerns (see Table 15.1). Eleven of the 19 were retained because they met the threshold of being selected by patients as among their top five "very most important" symptoms to monitor at a rate exceeding chance. Three additional symptoms (pain, weight loss, swelling or cramps in stomach area) were not rated by patients as among their top five concerns but were endorsed by providers in the previous NCCN FACT study (27). Four additional symptoms were spontaneously reported by at least 21% of patients as significant concerns (numbness and tingling, temperature sensitivity, treatment effects, hair loss) and were retained in the index. One symptom (fatigue) was spontaneously reported at a rate substantially greater than other symptoms (48%), so a second fatigue item ("I feel fatigued") from the FACIT measurement system was added to complement the "I have a lack of energy" item.

Ten physician experts in CRC rated symptoms and concerns as disease-related, treatment-related, both or neither. Nine of the symptoms were considered disease-related symptoms and comprise the Disease-Related Symptoms (DRS) subscale. Eight were considered treatment-related

Table 15.1 NCCN/FACT Colorectal Symptom Index-19 (NFCSI-19)

Subscale	Item
DRS	I have a lack of energy
	I have pain
	I am losing weight
	I have swelling or cramps in my stomach area
	I feel fatigued
	Because of my physical condition, I have trouble meeting the needs of my family
	I worry that my condition will get worse
	I have a good appetite
	I am sleeping well
TSE	I have nausea
	I am bothered by hair loss
	I have control of my bowels
	I have diarrhea
	I am bothered by constipation
	I have numbness or tingling in my hands
	I have pain in my hands or feet when I am exposed to cold temperatures
	I am bothered by side effects of treatment
F/WB	I am able to enjoy life
	I am content with the quality of my life right now

DRS, disease-related symtoms; TSE, treatment-related side effects; F/WB, function and well-being subscale.

and comprise the Treatment-Related Side Effects (TSE) subscale. Two items were thought to reflect general function and well-being (F/WB) and were so categorized. Table 15.1 includes all 19 items of the NFCSI-19.

Four of the items on the NFCSI-19 were not in the FACT-C ("I feel fatigued," "I am bothered by constipation," "I have numbness and tingling in my hands," and "I have pain in my hands or feet when I am exposed to cold temperatures"). Thus, preliminary analyses of the symptom index included only 15 of the 19 items in the index ("NFCSI-15"). The 15-item version of the NFCSI showed good internal consistency, with a Cronbach's alpha of 0.86. Associations between the NFCSI and FACT-C scale and subscale scores were evaluated with Spearman correlations. The NFCSI-15 was highly correlated with the PWB subscale (r = 0.90), FWB subscale (r = 0.77), CCS (r = 0.82), FACT-G total (r = .83), FACT-C total (r = .90), and TOI (r = 0.96), all $P < .0001$. The NFCSI-15 was significantly but less strongly associated with the EWB subscale (r = 0.51; $P < .0001$) and SWB subscale (r = 0.33; $P < .05$). Similarly, the NFCSI-DRS was significantly associated with all FACT-G/C subscale and total scores (range r = 0.48–0.89; $P < .001$) except for the SWB subscale. The NFCSI-TSE and F/WB were significantly associated with all subscales and total score (range, r = 0.30–0.87; $P < .05$). The NFCSI contains five PWB items, three FWB items, and one EWB item, which could produce inflated correlations due to redundancy. However, even after redundant items were removed, correlations were lower but remained significant (range, r = 0.46–0.74). Similar patterns of correlations, albeit lower in magnitude, were found for the NFCSI-DRS, and NFCSI-TSE.

As further preliminary evidence of the NFCSI's validity, we examined its ability to discriminate patients based on ECOG PSR. Because of a small sample size in the PSR = 3 group, the PSR = 2 and 3 groups were collapsed. For all NFCSI subscales, the scores across PSR groups were in the expected direction, that is, patients with the lowest PSR (ie, best performance status) had the highest NFCSI scores (ie, better symptom status). The NFCSI-15 ($F[2,47]$ = 14.27; P = .0001), NFCSI-DRS ($F[2,47]$ = 16.63; P = .0001), NFCSI-TSE ($F[2,47]$ = 7.02; P = .002) and NFCSI-F/WB ($F[2,47]$ = 4.77; P =.01) all significantly discriminated patients in the three ECOG PSR groups. Interestingly, some studies of patients with advanced CRC have shown that HRQL appears to be a stronger predictor of overall survival than performance status ratings provided by clinicians thus underscoring the importance of obtaining HRQL data (36,37).

Preliminary validation analyses suggest that the NFCSI-19 represents a psychometrically acceptable brief symptom index for advanced CRC, with good internal consistency and evidence of construct validity. While preliminary results appear encouraging, this index awaits more extensive validation in patient populations with advanced CRC. If a clinician or researcher was interested in measuring both multidimensional HRQL as well as symptoms, it is possible to score the NFCSI-19 index from an administration of the FACT-C (34 items). Because the NFCSI-19 includes four items not present in the FACT-C, deriving a symptom index score from the FACT-C requires that the 15 NFCSI items be scored and then prorated to a full 19-item index. This is accepted as standard methodology in the FACIT measurement system and has been demonstrated to be superior compared to other methods of handling "missing" data (38).

Disease-specific symptom assessment has a potentially key role in evaluating patient-related endpoints in clinical trials and in clinical care. In addition to representing an efficient and clinically-relevant means of obtaining information related to the symptom component of QOL, it may also clarify a treatment's toxicity, potential palliative benefit, or need to make a change in the patient's clinical management (39). In evaluating the efficacy of new chemotherapeutic agents, the ability to demonstrate the amelioration of symptoms specific to a given tumor may represent efficacy in achieving a meaningful patient outcome. Thus, a brief tumor-specific tool to assess symptomatology, such as the NFCSI-19, serves an important role in clinical care.

A diagnosis of CRC and subsequent treatments can impact multiple dimensions of HRQL and sexual functioning is often one of the dimensions adversely affected. Both men and women report problems such as changes in level of sexual activity, a lack of sexual enjoyment, and alterations in body image following treatment for CRC (40–43). Overall, problems with sexual functioning appear to be more pronounced for younger patients and females with CRC (44). The variety in the nature of sexual difficulties reported can be attributed, in part, to the multiple modalities used to treat CRC (45) as well as methodological differences across studies, including the approaches used to assess and define sexual dysfunction and the timing and type of assessments (46). This could be alleviated, in part, through the use of more targeted measures to assess self-reports of sexual functioning, such as the International Index of Erectile Dysfunction (IIEF; 47), the Female Sexual Function Index (FSFI; 48), and/or the Patient-Reported Outcomes Measurement Information System (PROMIS) Sexual Function Item Banks (49–51).

The IIEF is a 15-item self-report measure developed to assess sexual function in men and the psychometric properties are well-established. The IIEF yields scores for five domains: sexual desire, erectile function, orgasmic function, intercourse satisfaction, and overall satisfaction. The measure has been used to evaluate sexual function in CRC patients (52–54).

The FSFI is a 19-item self-report measure developed to assess female sexual function and the psychometric properties are also well-established. The FSFI yields an overall score and six domain scores: desire, arousal, lubrication, orgasmic capacity, dyspareunia, and sexual satisfaction. The measure has been used to evaluate sexual function in CRC patients (52,53,55).

The PROMIS (www.nihpromis.org) Sexual Function measures include 11 scales or items pools addressing multiple domains of sexual functioning, including global satisfaction with sex life, interest in sexual activity, erectile function, and orgasm, among others.

Education and counseling about sexual dysfunction after treatment for CRC should be provided at diagnosis and throughout treatment and follow up as needed to facilitate realistic expectations and enhance patient adaptation. More complex and severe problems may require combined medical and psychological therapies, but relatively simple sexual problems can frequently be managed by providing information and strategies for behavior change (46). In addition, the supportive and positive attitude of patients, partners have been particularly helpful in overcoming anxiety about physical intimacy for sexually active patients with ostomies (56). We will discuss in more detail the sexual dysfunction specific for extent of disease and in relation to treatment received later in this chapter.

Interpretation of HRQL Scores

The interpretation of scores generated from HRQL instruments is not necessarily straightforward. For instance, if HRQL is measured on 0 to 100 scale and a 5-point improvement is demonstrated in a group of patients, without a criterion with which to judge the change, a clinician or researcher may be uncertain as to whether this improvement is meaningful. Similarly, the HRQL of control and intervention arms in a randomized trial may differ significantly based on statistical comparisons, but the differences may not be clinically or subjectively meaningful to patients. In the late 1980s and early 1990s, methods for determining the magnitude of change in health outcome that should be considered meaningful began appearing in the literature (57–60). These included both distribution-based and anchor-based methods. Distribution-based methods rely on statistical distributions of HRQL scores, and include effect size, responsiveness index, reliable change index, and standard error of measurement (SEM). Anchor-based methods include cross-sectional or longitudinal differences in HRQL scores that are compared or anchored to clinically familiar and relevant indicators (eg, global rating of change, performance status). The terminology for referring to these meaningful changes in scores is varied but will be referred to here as "minimally important differences" (MID), which is defined as "the smallest difference in scores in the domain of interest that patients perceive as important, either beneficial or harmful, and that would lead the clinician to consider a change in the patient's management." Because no single method for identifying MIDs is sufficient, it is recommended that multiple strategies be used simultaneously (61).

A conservative estimate for an MID is frequently cited as being approximately one-half of a standard deviation, which is equivalent to an effect size of 0.5 (62). In some cases, this may overestimate the true MID, so this guideline may be most appropriately applied in situations where instrument-specific MID data are lacking. We advocate for identifying plausible ranges of MIDs rather than an individual number to account for variability across samples and settings. For an individual patient, the recommendation is to use the large end of the range; for average group scores, using the smaller end is optimal for measurement error management. MIDs have been calculated for the FACT-C and its subscales and are two to three points for the CCS, four to six points for the TOI-C, and five to eight points for FACT-C total score.

HRQL Issues Based Upon Extent of Disease and Treatment

The 5-year relative survival rate for CRC has increased from 51% for individuals diagnosed in the mid-1970s, to 65% for cases diagnosed in 2001 to 2007 (62). For localized disease, the 5-year survival rate is 91%, but only 37%

of CRC patients diagnosed between 2000 and 2007 had localized-stage disease. In contrast, the 5-year survival rates for patients diagnosed at the regional and distant stage are 70% and 11%, respectively (63). The introduction of newer cytotoxic chemotherapeutic and biologic agents for metastatic CRC have increased median survival time from 10 months to over 20 months (64,65), offering promise of continued improvements in survival rates for those with advanced CRC. With over half of all CRC patients surviving at least 5 years, HRQL parallels quantity of life as an important outcome.

Patients with CRC are affected by their disease and/or its treatment in at least four different domains of HRQL (see Table 15.2 for an overview of common issues): physical function (eg, urgency to defecate, frequent/irregular bowel movements, gas, fecal leakage, diarrhea, constipation; 42,44,66); social functioning (eg, social activities hampered by urgency and/or frequency of bowel movements or gas; 66); sexual functioning (erectile dysfunction, ejaculatory impotence, incapability of orgasm in men; dyspareunia, diminished orgasm, less frequent intercourse in women; 42,43,67); and emotional distress, including the potential double stigma of cancer and colostomy (68,69). Relative to patients with rectal cancer, the HRQL of patients with colon cancer has been relatively understudied. There is some evidence that 6 weeks after open curative surgery for CRC, HRQL scores for patients with colon cancer have been shown to be marginally better than those for patients with rectal cancer; additional factors independently influencing HRQL at 6 weeks include: age younger than 65 years, poor ECOG performance status, stoma, diarrhea, and constipation (70). Because the HRQL issues for patients with CRC tend to differ based on extent of disease and treatment, we will consider these separately.

■ LOCALIZED DISEASE (STAGES I–III COLON AND RECTAL CANCER)

Surgical Procedures

Studies exploring HRQL associated with treatment for early stage colon and rectal cancer have focused on laparoscopic vs conventional open surgery for cure. Individual large randomized trials comparing the two types of surgery have not shown significant differences in morbidity (71–74). The literature confirms fewer postoperative complications from laparoscopic surgery as well as other advantages (less blood loss, less postoperative pain, shorter length of stay, gains in cosmesis, less disability, quicker recovery of alimentary functions; 71,75–81). The short-term benefits of laparoscopic surgery have been shown to extend to older patients as well (82).

■ **Table 15.2** Most Common Disease and Treatment-Related HRQL Issues in CRC

	Local and Locally Advanced	Recurrent/Metastatic
Colon Cancer		
Disease-related	Potential obstruction or bleeding	Intestinal obstruction, perforation, bleeding/anemia, abdominal mass, pain, weight loss, fatigue, peritonitis, poor appetite, sleep dysfunction, anxiety, difficulties with activities of daily living
Treatment-related	Short-term benefits of laparoscopic vs open surgery: less blood loss, less postoperative pain, shorter length of stay, gains in cosmesis, less morbidity and disability, quicker recovery of alimentary functions; GI toxicity (diarrhea, nausea, anorexia, stomatitis), anemia, and neutropenia	Diarrhea or constipation, hair loss, neutropenia, hand-foot syndrome, neuropathy, fatigue, muscle weakness and loss of tone, dizziness, nausea, poor appetite, weight loss, depression, anxiety, abdominal cramping, and skin toxicities (which impact emotional and social functioning)
Rectal cancer		
Disease-related	Fatigue, poor body image, emotional issues, sleep dysfunction, fear of recurrence, gastrointestinal problems, anxiety, depression, and urinary, bowel and sexual dysfunction, bleeding, pain	Intractable pain, fatigue, poor appetite, weight loss, sleep dysfunction, bleeding, peritonitis, bowel dysfunction and chronic pelvic sepsis, difficulties with activities of daily living, and anxiety
Treatment-related	Fatigue, pain, and reduced physical activity (for the first few postoperative months); bowel dysfunction (fecal incontinence, tenesmus, diarrhea), dysuria, and sexual dysfunction	Nausea, hair loss, diarrhea or constipation, neutropenia, hand-foot syndrome, dysuria, sexual dysfunction, neuropathy, fatigue, muscle weakness and loss of tone, dizziness, poor appetite, weight loss, depression, anxiety, and skin toxicities (which impact emotional and social functioning)

Surgery is also the primary treatment modality for localized rectal cancer, which may be combined with preoperative radiotherapy or adjuvant chemotherapy or both (83). Surgery is potentially curative but is associated with short- and long-term detriments in HRQL. For the first few months postoperatively, fatigue, pain, and reduced physical activity are common. However, the many adverse effects of disease and its treatment can also be long standing and include continued fatigue, poor body image, emotional issues, sleep dysfunction, fear of recurrence, GI problems, sensory neuropathy, anxiety, depression, and urinary, bowel, and sexual dysfunction (83,84). In the elderly, these problems can be compounded by multiple comorbidities (85). Distal location of rectal cancer has also been associated with worse HRQL. Compared with patients treated for upper and middle rectal cancer, patients with cancer in the lower rectal third had worse HRQL scores, a higher frequency of abdominoperineal excision with permanent stoma, and worse body image problems, sexual problems, and outlook on their future (86). Distal cancer was also associated with more postoperative complications and need for re-operation and interventional treatment, resulting in poor anorectal and sexual function. Many patients, especially rectal cancer patients, may need to adapt to life with a permanent or temporary stoma (44,70).

Patients With Ostomies

These patients are almost exclusively distal rectal cancer patients with the exception of patients who have an ostomy placed as a palliative procedure for initial or subsequent bowel obstruction. Several studies have shown that ostomies are associated with multiple HRQL difficulties. The impact of having an ostomy on HRQL may include psychological problems (87–89), problems with appearance (90), skin or leakage complications (91), difficulty paying for supplies (92), and interference with work, sporting, and recreational activities (93). In particular, lower social HRQL scores may reflect the impact of the disease and treatment on employment, leisure pursuits, and sexual function (66,94). While some research suggests that comorbidities play a greater role in predicting HRQL than having an ostomy (95) compared to patients without an ostomy, several studies describe patients with an ostomy as having significantly worse HRQL (66,94,96–98).

That said, other studies provide a more equivocal picture of the impact of having an ostomy on HRQL. As already noted, for most CRC patients and survivors the presence of an ostomy can have detrimental effects on HRQL. However, detailed results are inconclusive. In a study of 5-year survivors of rectal cancer, participants with an ostomy reported worse global health status, poorer physical and role functioning, more body image and sexual functioning problems, and worse fatigue, dyspnea, and appetite loss than patients without an ostomy (99). In comparison, a separate study of long-term survivors of rectal cancer used the same HRQL instrument (the EORTC QLQ-C30) and only found significantly worse physical functioning scores in survivors with an ostomy (100). The authors speculated that the extended period posttreatment (participants were an average of 15 years postsurgery) provided opportunity to adapt to having an ostomy and thus led to insignificant differences between many of the HRQL subscale scores. Similarly, Ramsey et al (101) noted that in a sample of CRC survivors 3 years postdiagnosis, an ostomy did not appear to affect overall HRQL significantly, and a study by Bekkers et al (102) found that both stoma and nonstoma patients experienced similar levels of psychosocial problems 4 years after surgery. Moreover, Rauch et al found that rectal cancer patients who had an ostomy reported better HRQL than those with an anastomosis (103). So in some cases, an ostomy may be a preferred option for enhancing HRQL.

It should be noted the impact on HRQL of having an ostomy may vary by gender. Krouse et al (104) reported that male and female rectal cancer survivors with ostomies both reported worse social HRQL compared to control participants, but the effect on other domains varied. Male survivors reported slightly better overall HRQL scores whereas female survivors reported clinically meaningful and significantly worse psychological HRQL. In addition, female survivors reported worse scores in seven of eight HRQL domains as well as worse mental and physical composite scores of the SF-36 compared to controls. For younger females (less than 75 years of age), an ostomy had a greater impact on physical well-being compared to older females. In a qualitative study of long-term CRC survivors with ostomies, Grant et al (105) described similar findings; both men and women identified challenges with sexuality and intimacy but women described more specific psychological and social issues than men.

Adapting to and learning how to manage an ostomy can be difficult, with the first postoperative year being particularly challenging (102). For long-term CRC survivors (greater than 5 years since diagnosis), living with an ostomy is comparable to managing other chronic care issues related to cancer's effects and epitomizes the blending of problems and challenges with solutions and adaptation that represent the complexity of life with a chronic illness or disability (106). Effective strategies for managing the challenges of an ostomy exist and may help minimize the adverse impact on HRQL. For example, preoperative psychological preparation may reduce anxiety and stress to aid recovery (107), and enhancing patient self-efficacy may also ease the burden of an ostomy (108). Supportive spouses and significant others can be particularly helpful in coping with an ostomy (88), and for patients who have the option, ostomy reversal may also improve HRQL (96).

Sexual Function After Surgery

Surgical intervention has been associated with worsening sexual function for both males and females. In a large, randomized trial comparing patients with operable rectal cancer who either underwent radiotherapy prior to surgery or surgery followed by selective postoperative chemoradiotherapy for patients with a positive circumferential resection margin, results suggested that for male patients, sexual dysfunction was the main adverse effect of surgery (not radiotherapy), and this dysfunction persisted to the 3-year follow-up assessment (109). Sexual dysfunction is better documented in men than in women after surgery and includes erectile and ejaculatory dysfunction, including retrograde and loss of or alterations in ejaculation (86,109–111). Impotence rates vary from 15%–92% but are decreasing due to newer surgical techniques (112). Similarly, women report a number of problems including: decreased libido or sexual desire, dyspareunia, and changes in vaginal lubrication, arousal, and frequency of orgasm after abdominoperineal resection for rectal cancer (52,111,113).

Symms et al noted the presence of an ostomy for males is associated with lower rates of sexual activity and higher erectile dysfunction (114). This, in turn, may be associated with poorer social and psychological HRQL. Patients with an ostomy are more likely to have negative feelings about their body appearance, which can lead to less intimacy and greater isolation (90).

Adjuvant Chemotherapy

Adjuvant treatment can introduce significant treatment-related adverse effects. Adjuvant chemotherapy with intravenous fluorouracil (5-FU) and leucovorin (LV) has been shown to prolong disease-free survival and overall survival (115). However, one-third of those patients will develop a recurrence within 5 years (115). Adverse events associated with 5-FU and levamisole or LV are well-documented and include GI toxicity (diarrhea, nausea, anorexia, stomatitis), anemia, and neutropenia, which are experienced during the 6 months of therapy but not long-term afterward (97,116). Oxaliplatin-based regimens are associated with neurotoxicity, which limits its use at higher doses and is cumulative. These effects are often severe and debilitating and significantly negatively impact HRQL (117,118). The neuropathic adverse effects are seen as soon as 3 months into chemotherapy and include acute (cold-induced dysesthesias and parasthesias of the upper extremities and face, cold hypersensitivity, jaw tightness, pharyngolaryngeal dysesthesia, muscle spasms, fasciculations, voice changes, and ocular pain) and chronic (peripheral stocking and glove pattern axonal sensory neuropathy) symptoms. In a randomized trial of calcium (Ca) and magnesium (Mg) to reduce the adverse effects of oxaliplatin, 41% of patients who did not receive Ca/Mg continued to report chronic sensory neuropathy 1 year later (119). Physical therapy, gait and balance training, and patient education on maintaining a safe environment may be required to enhance physical performance and avoid injury for patients with chronic sensory neuropathy. Patients typically have difficulties with activities of daily living and also experience significant psychological effects including depression, anxiety, a sense of isolation, and frustration.

Studies have also examined the ability of elderly patients to tolerate adjuvant chemotherapy, and results have been mixed. For example, one study of patients 70 years and older showed no survival benefit when using an unplanned subset analysis (120), while another study reviewing observational data sources and randomized controlled trials showed improved overall survival for patients receiving adjuvant therapy (121). While some have suggested that chronological age alone should not be a factor in treatment decision making because patients 70 years and older do not report more side effects or decrements in HRQL (122), others have noted that older patients do typically report worse toxicity but not to a degree that warrants emergency room visits or hospitalizations (123).

Chemoradiation Therapy and Rectal Cancer

Preoperative chemoradiotherapy prior to total mesorectal excision is now considered standard care for locally advanced mid-low rectal cancer, resulting in a significant reduction in 5-year local recurrence rates of 6%–8% (RR, 0.46; 95% CI, 0.26–0.82; 124,125) Studies have shown that patients treated for locally advanced rectal cancer report good overall HRQL, but these patients still report symptoms and functional limitations (eg, bowel dysfunction, fecal incontinence, sexual dysfunction) many years after the diagnosis (103,124–126). Preoperative radiotherapy arms have been shown to have a significant increase in the level of fecal incontinence at 2-years post-randomization. There were no differences between arms or time points in terms of overall physical function or HRQL. Additional side effects of pelvic radiation therapy include tenesmus, diarrhea, dysuria during therapy, with chemotherapy treatment having an additive effect (97).

Sexual dysfunction is better documented in men than in women and includes erectile dysfunction and ejaculatory dysfunction (86,109,110). However, Mannaerts et al found a 50% reduction in the preoperative ability to achieve orgasm for both men and women who received multimodality treatment for rectal cancer (127). In addition, women have reported experiencing dyspareunia, pain interfering with sexual pleasure, fear of stool leakage, and vaginal dryness secondary to pelvic radiation (128).

Late adverse effects have been found in a significant proportion of patients being followed for a median of 8.8 years after surgery for rectal cancer (86). With a median age of 61 and an overall survival rate of 48.1%, anorectal dysfunction, small bowel obstruction, and male sexual dysfunction were, not surprisingly, significantly more common among those who had neoadjuvant chemoradiotherapy. Long-term survivors (median greater than 13 years) reported that receiving adjuvant chemoradiotherapy, a permanent stoma and lower-third rectal carcinoma were associated with significantly worse HRQL outcomes.

Survivorship

Due in part to earlier detection of and improved treatment for CRC, more people are surviving cancer and living longer. The increase in the number of CRC survivors highlights the importance of examining the late and long-term effects of treatment as well as changes in HRQL over time. To date, studies that have examined the relationship between time since diagnosis and HRQL have found positive associations and the overall HRQL of CRC survivors has typically been quite good relative to the general population (98,129,130). For example, Schag et al (131) found improvements in HRQL associated with longer time since diagnosis in a sample of colon cancer patients, with the most notable improvements occurring in the psychosocial domain of HRQL. Similarly, Ramsey et al (101) found the negative impact of CRC on HRQL was most evident in the first 2 to 3 years after diagnosis before HRQL scores improved and then stabilized at a relatively high level. This finding was evident for patients across all disease stages except for those with Stage IV disease and is not surprising since patients are being told the first few years after diagnosis is a time with the highest chance of recurrence and are seeing oncologists every 3 months.

Despite the overall improvement of HRQL scores over time for CRC survivors, some problems may remain. Specifically, physical and psychological problems may continue despite a reduction in illness-related demands or patients' psychological adjustment to the disease. Pain, functional well-being, and social well-being may be affected to varying degrees across all stages and times post-diagnosis (101). Some CRC survivors also report slightly poorer physical HRQL than the general population and worse depression scores as well as long-term symptoms such as bowel problems and distress secondary to their cancer (129). Comparable findings from a qualitative study of long-term colon cancer survivors noted that their predominant HRQL complaints were problems with low energy and with sexual and bowel functioning (132). In a recent study of CRC survivors 4 years postdiagnosis, the most commonly reported symptoms were "fatigue" (23%), "negative feelings about body appearance" (14%), "diarrhea" (13%), and "constipation" (7%). Since this study was conducted before oxaliplatin was a standard treatment approach, chronic neuropathy was not commonly reported. Although the absolute prevalence of reported symptoms was fairly low, a significant percentage of respondents attributed lingering health issues to their cancer and its treatment; concerns most frequently endorsed included "worry about health" (24%), "physical discomfort" (19%), and "activity limitations" (15%; 90).

The long-term and late effects of being diagnosed with and treated for CRC vary across demographic and clinical factors, highlighting the impact on HRQL and thus the special needs of particular groups of CRC survivors. CRC survivors of low socioeconomic status appear to be at particular risk for poorer outcomes. Low income status has been associated with poorer outcomes for pain, ambulation, and social and emotional well-being compared to CRC survivors with higher income status (101). In a systematic review of long-term (greater than 5 years) CRC survivors, Jansen et al (129) found younger age, lower income, a higher body mass index, and a higher number of comorbidities were associated with poorer HRQL. In contrast, having a larger social network (eg, number of close friends or relatives and participation in community organizations) was associated with better HRQL, particularly with mental HRQL (133). Mixed results were reported regarding the question of whether the presence of a stoma has a detrimental effect on HRQL. In sum, despite an overall good HRQL, CRC survivors have specific physical and psychological problems that may include pain, fatigue, and concerns about bowel function or a possible recurrence. By identifying those subgroups of survivors at risk of poorer outcomes, providers may be able to intervene more rapidly to provide support and minimize the potential adverse impact on HRQL. More prospective studies are needed to further delineate the trajectory and predictors of HRQL for CRC survivors.

■ LOCALLY RECURRENT AND METASTATIC DISEASE

Local Recurrence

Local recurrence of rectal cancer remains a challenging significant problem and is associated with intractable pelvic or sciatic pain, bleeding, bowel dysfunction, and chronic pelvic sepsis, as well as a diminished HRQL and an extremely poor prognosis (109,134,135). Treatment options are often limited by previous pelvic irradiation, surgery, and/or systemic therapy (136,137). Surgical salvage with curative intent is typically feasible in only 20%–30% of patients with locally recurrent rectal cancer, with 5-year overall survival rates for margin-negative resections ranging from 9%–43% (138). Bowel, urinary, and sexual function and lifestyle can be permanently altered, and prolonged rehabilitation may be required after discharge (139). Curative surgery has been shown to offer prolonged survival and maintenance of HRQL compared to noncurative and nonsurgical treatment, but long-term survivors experienced significant pain (140). Palliative radiation therapy may be appropriate treatment for patients with symptomatic metastases in the bone, brain or presacral space as well as uncontrolled bleeding that is not amenable to surgery.

Metastatic Disease

Among those who are diagnosed with locally advanced rectal cancer, surgical treatment has historically resulted in an overall survival between 40% and 60%, but the addition of neoadjuvant chemoradiation with 5-FU has seen an improvement in overall survival between 65% and 75% (141). Unfortunately, 15%–20% of patients with colorectal malignancies will present with metastatic disease at the time of diagnosis (142–144). A small proportion of patients will have potentially resectable hepatic metastases, but the majority will have unresectable disease (145). The rate of progression of metastatic CRC is variable, but for those who forego all treatment, the median survival is 6 to 9 months from time of diagnosis; the overall 5-year survival rate for metastatic CRC is 12% (146). Patients with advanced CRC will be faced with a variety of disease-related physical and psychological concerns (eg, obstruction, bleeding, perforation, pain, weight loss, fatigue), all of which diminish HRQL (147,148). The purpose of the palliative interventions is to provide relief from local and systemic symptoms and to improve the HRQL of the patient's remaining life. Interventions may be directed at urgent complications (eg, obstruction or perforation) or chronic symptoms (eg, anemia, fatigue, weight loss due to disease burden; 147). Patients with advanced CRC are often significantly debilitated because of underlying disease, so tolerance to adverse side effects and complications of therapy is reduced. With improvements in length of life from additional therapeutic options, it is critical to be able to inform patients about the HRQL with each therapeutic option.

Treatment options for advanced CRC include chemotherapeutic, surgical, and advanced endoscopic interventions. Chemotherapy can improve HRQL by reducing symptom burden or it can diminish HRQL as a result of therapy-related toxicities. While 5-FU has been a mainstay of palliative chemotherapy regimens, additional and more potent and effective agents have been added to the armamentarium for advanced disease (147). We previously covered associated toxicity and HRQL issues with 5-FU and oxaliplatin based therapy (so-called FOLFOX), but in this section we will cover other agents that are active only in the metastatic or recurrent setting. While these newer agents have resulted in improved median survival times when added to 5-FU, in some cases they have also been associated with more significant toxicities and side effects that have adversely impacted HRQL. For cytotoxic chemotherapeutic agents, such as irinotecan, diarrhea and neutropenia are the most common grade 3 and 4 toxicities (149). Oral capecitabine is associated with less neutropenia but a higher incidence of hand-foot syndrome and diarrhea than 5-FU (150,151).

Newer biologic agents for treatment of metastatic CRC can be classified as antivascular endothelial growth factor (anti-VEGF) agents (eg, bevacizumab) or antiepidermal growth factor receptor (EGFR) agents (cetuximab, panitumumab; 149). However, even with the recent advances in treatment of metastatic CRC provided by targeted agents, most patients will eventually die of their disease, so the goals of therapy remain delaying disease progression, controlling symptoms, and maintaining HRQL for as long as possible (152,153). More research is needed about the symptom burden and resulting HRQL for patients receiving VEGF agents, but EGFR agents are associated with significant skin toxicities, including pruritus, acneiform dermatitis, skin desquamation, paronychia, skin fissures, pustular rash, skin infection, skin ulceration, and local infections (154,155). While rarely life threatening, they do impact HRQL and place the patient at risk for infection, leading to inconsistent EGFR inhibitor administration, which may affect clinical outcomes (156–158). Panitumumab monotherapy, which is approved for chemorefractory wild-type *K-ras* metastatic CRC, was shown, in combination with best supportive care, to result in less deterioration in HRQL, as measured by the NFCSI (27), compared with best supportive care alone (159). However, skin toxicity occurred in 90% of patients in the panitumumab group vs 9% in best supportive care. These skin toxicities also impact physical symptoms, emotional state and social functioning, with women, those 55 to 65 years of age, and patients with partial remission reporting worst HRQL (160). Thus, management of skin toxicities is vital to ensure dose intensity and to maintain patients' HRQL. More severe skin toxicity from panitumumab has been associated with higher rather than lower HRQL scores; this has also been observed with cetuximab and may reflect awareness by patients that skin rash is indicative of response to therapy, which could help them cope with challenging side effects (161,162).

Of note, EGFR inhibitors are used in combination with traditional cytotoxic chemotherapy. In a randomized trial of panitumumab in combination with first-line chemotherapy for metastatic CRC, there was evidence of a higher incidence of skin toxicity, diarrhea, and hypomagnesemia but these toxicities were effectively managed and, consistent with other studies, an association between skin toxicity and efficacy was observed (163). In a randomized phase III trial of panitumumab with second-line chemotherapy, adverse events were generally comparable across the study arms with the exception of known toxicities associated with anti-EGFR therapy (eg, skin toxicity and hypomagnesemia; 164). Studies examining the addition of cetuximab to chemotherapy have found similar findings. In a randomized trial of cetuximab with irinotecan, fluorouracil, and leucovorin (FOLFIRI), the incidence rates of grade 3 or 4 diarrhea and skin reactions were significantly higher with cetuximab, but were generally manageable (165). A randomized study of cetuximab with FOLFOX found that cetuximab was generally well tolerated with the most common adverse events of any grade being skin and subcutaneous tissue disorders (90%) and GI disorders (78%) in the cetuximab plus chemotherapy group (166). The authors also concluded that there was no evidence that cetuximab increased the frequency or severity of the known toxicities of oxaliplatin and 5-FU or vice versa. In sum, the added toxicity of panitumumab or cetuximab used in combination with traditional chemotherapy for metastatic CRC should be weighed against the potential average survival benefit, and further research is needed to identify the impact on multiple dimensions of HRQL.

The main presenting symptoms of patients who undergo palliative surgery for CRC are rectal bleeding and anemia or intestinal obstruction associated with a change in bowel habits, abdominal pain, and/or peritonitis (167). One-third of patients with CRC present with near or complete bowel obstruction (168). Patients with metastatic disease presenting with symptomatic bowel obstruction caused by their primary tumor have traditionally undergone either laparotomy for resection of primary tumor, intestinal bypass, or a nonfunctioning stoma to alleviate obstructing symptoms. The colostomy is the most widely utilized procedure for CRC palliation, but this treatment itself is associated with significant morbidity and negative effects on HRQL, especially in frail, elderly patients (169). Surgery is associated with significant postoperative morbidity (20%–30%) and mortality (5%–12%), with the most common complication being wound infection (147). Surgical treatment decisions for advanced disease tend to be based on numerous factors, such as patient age, comorbidities, aggressiveness of tumor biology, response to chemotherapy, the local extent of disease, and severity of patient symptoms (170). There is consensus regarding surgical intervention for palliation of symptoms such as bleeding, perforation, or obstruction, but resection in asymptomatic patients with advanced disease is not indicated due to potential morbidity and mortality risks. Patients with Stage IV incurable CRC who are not candidates for surgery may benefit from endoscopic palliation, including laser therapy and self-expanding metallic stents (169). However, stenting has a significant incidence of malfunction. Laser therapy can successfully provide symptomatic relief for patients with bleeding, mucus discharge, or tenesmus.

■ CONCLUSIONS

HRQL is a multidimensional concept that includes self-reported symptoms, functional abilities, and physical, mental, social, and spiritual health perceptions. When measuring HRQL among CRC patients, the EORTC QLQ-C30 and the FACT-G are two of the most commonly used cancer-specific measures and may be supplemented with disease-specific modules for more targeted assessment of CRC-specific concerns (ie, EORTC QLQ-CR29, FACT-C). In addition, the newly developed NFCSI-19 represents a psychometrically acceptable brief symptom index for advanced CRC, useful for evaluating patient-related endpoints in clinical trials and clinical care. HRQL issues for patients with CRC tend to be site- and stage-specific and may include several disease-related (eg, fatigue, pain, changes in appetite) and treatment-related (eg, nausea, hair loss, neuropathy) factors. Long-term survivors of CRC typically report good overall HRQL, but pain, fatigue, and significant disruptions in emotional, sexual, and bowel functioning may persist. Survivors with ostomies may be particularly prone to body image and sexual dysfunction concerns. The assessment and management of sexual dysfunction in men and women treated for CRC should be standard practice throughout treatment and in survivorship. Similarly, HRQL assessment should be an integral part of clinical practice and may provide critical insight into the advantages and disadvantages of various treatment options not provided by traditional endpoints. Future research should focus on clinical applications of HRQL outcomes, including the benefit of routine HRQL assessment and subsequent impact on patient-provider communication and shared decision-making. By linking HRQL outcomes to clinical benchmarks and quality of care, the HRQL for CRC patients and survivors may be better understood, maintained, and ultimately enhanced.

■ REFERENCES

1. Cella D. Quality of Life. In: Breitbart W, Holland JC, Jacobsen PB, et al. eds. *Psycho-oncology*. New York, NY: Oxford University Press; 1998:1135–1146.
2. Aronson N, Melilli L, Cella D, Gondek K. Time to symptomatic progression: an emerging clinical trial endpoint in oncology. *J Clin Oncol*. 2007;25(18s):709s.
3. Portenoy RK, Thaler HT, Kornblith AB, et al. Symptom prevalence, characteristics and distress in a cancer population. *Qual Life Res*. 1994;3(3):183–189.
4. Yost KJ, Cella D, Chawla A, et al. Minimally important differences were estimated for the Functional Assessment of Cancer Therapy-Colorectal (FACT-C) instrument using a combination of distribution- and anchor-based approaches. *J Clin Epidemiol*. 2005;58(12):1241–1251.
5. Davis KM, Cella D. Assessing quality of life in oncology clinical practice: a review of barriers and critical success factors. *J Clin Outcomes Manag*. 2002;9(6):327–332.
6. Detmar SB, Muller MJ, Schornagel JH, Wever LD, Aaronson NK. Health-related quality-of-life assessments and patient-physician communication: a randomized controlled trial. *JAMA*. 2002;288(23):3027–3034.
7. Velikova G, Booth L, Smith AB, et al. Measuring quality of life in routine oncology practice improves communication and patient well-being: a randomized controlled trial. *J Clin Oncol*. 2004;22(4):714–724.

8. McLachlan SA, Allenby A, Matthews J, et al. Randomized trial of coordinated psychosocial interventions based on patient self-assessments versus standard care to improve the psychosocial functioning of patients with cancer. *J Clin Oncol.* 2001;19(21):4117–4125.
9. Rubenstein LV, McCoy JM, Cope DW, et al. Improving patient quality of life with feedback to physicians about functional status. *J Gen Intern Med.* 1995;10(11):607–614.
10. Hayes SC, Nelson RO, Jarrett RB. The treatment utility of assessment. A functional approach to evaluating assessment quality. *Am Psychol.* 1987;42(11):963–974.
11. Rosenbloom SK, Victorson DE, Hahn EA, Peterman AH, Cella D. Assessment is not enough: a randomized controlled trial of the effects of HRQL assessment on quality of life and satisfaction in oncology clinical practice. *Psychooncology.* 2007;16(12):1069–1079.
12. Velikova G, Brown JM, Smith AB, Selby PJ. Computer-based quality of life questionnaires may contribute to doctor-patient interactions in oncology. *Br J Cancer.* 2002;86(1):51–59.
13. Webster K, Cella D, Yost K. The Functional Assessment of Chronic Illness Therapy (FACIT) Measurement System: properties, applications, and interpretation. *Health Qual Life Outcomes.* 2003;1:79.
14. Ware JE Jr, Sherbourne CD. The MOS 36-item short-form health survey (SF-36). I. Conceptual framework and item selection. *Med Care.* 1992;30(6):473–483.
15. McHorney CA, Ware JE Jr, Raczek AE. The MOS 36-Item Short-Form Health Survey (SF-36): II. Psychometric and clinical tests of validity in measuring physical and mental health constructs. *Med Care.* 1993;31(3):247–263.
16. McHorney CA, Ware JE Jr, Lu JF, Sherbourne CD. The MOS 36-item Short-Form Health Survey (SF-36): III. Tests of data quality, scaling assumptions, and reliability across diverse patient groups. *Med Care.* 1994;32(1):40–66.
17. Hunt S, McKenna S, McEwen J, Williams J, Papp E. The Nottingham Health Profile: subjective health status and medical consultations. *Soc Sci Med.* 1981;55(2):301–311.
18. Bergner M, Bobbitt RA, Pollard WE, Martin DP, Gilson BS. The sickness impact profile: validation of a health status measure. *Med Care.* 1976;14(1):57–67.
19. Bergner M, Bobbitt RA, Carter WB, Gilson BS. The Sickness Impact Profile: development and final revision of a health status measure. *Med Care.* 1981;19(8):787–805.
20. Soni MK, Cella D. Quality of life and symptom measures in oncology: an overview. *Am J Manag Care.* 2002;8(18 Suppl):S560–S573.
21. Aaronson NK, Ahmedzai S, Bergman B, et al. The European Organization for Research and Treatment of Cancer QLQ-C30: a quality-of-life instrument for use in international clinical trials in oncology. *J Natl Cancer Inst.* 1993;85(5):365–376.
22. Cella DF, Tulsky DS, Gray G, et al. The Functional Assessment of Cancer Therapy scale: development and validation of the general measure. *J Clin Oncol.* 1993;11(3):570–579.
23. Whistance RN, Conroy T, Chie W, et al.; European Organisation for the Research and Treatment of Cancer Quality of Life Group. Clinical and psychometric validation of the EORTC QLQ-CR29 questionnaire module to assess health-related quality of life in patients with colorectal cancer. *Eur J Cancer.* 2009;45(17):3017–3026.
24. Ward WL, Hahn EA, Mo F, Hernandez L, Tulsky DS, Cella D. Reliability and validity of the Functional Assessment of Cancer Therapy-Colorectal (FACT-C) quality of life instrument. *Qual Life Res.* 1999;8(3):181–195.
25. Naughton M, Homsi J. Symptom assessment in cancer patients. *Curr Oncol Rep.* 2002;4(3):256–263.
26. Kong SX, Gandhi SK. Methodologic assessments of quality of life measures in clinical trials. *Ann Pharmacother.* 1997;31(7–8):830–836.
27. Cella D, Paul D, Yount S, et al. What are the most important symptom targets when treating advanced cancer? A survey of providers in the National Comprehensive Cancer Network (NCCN). *Cancer Invest.* 2003;21(4):526–535.
28. Strömgren AS, Groenvold M, Sorensen A, Andersen L. Symptom recognition in advanced cancer. A comparison of nursing records against patient self-rating. *Acta Anaesthesiol Scand.* 2001;45(9):1080–1085.
29. Brunelli C, Costantini M, Di Giulio P, et al. Quality-of-life evaluation: when do terminal cancer patients and health-care providers agree? *J Pain Symptom Manage.* 1998;15(3):151–158.
30. Justice AC, Rabeneck L, Hays RD, Wu AW, Bozzette SA. Sensitivity, specificity, reliability, and clinical validity of provider-reported symptoms: a comparison with self-reported symptoms. Outcomes Committee of the AIDS Clinical Trials Group. *J Acquir Immune Defic Syndr.* 1999;21(2):126–133.
31. Nekolaichuk CL, Bruera E, Spachynski K, MacEachern T, Hanson J, Maguire TO. A comparison of patient and proxy symptom assessments in advanced cancer patients. *Palliat Med.* 1999;13(4):311–323.
32. Stephens RJ, Hopwood P, Girling DJ, Machin D. Randomized trials with quality of life endpoints: are doctors' ratings of patients' physical symptoms interchangeable with patients' self-ratings? *Qual Life Res.* 1997;6(3):225–236.
33. Lampic C, Nordin K, Sjoeden PO. Agreement between cancer patients and their physicians in the assessment of patient anxiety at follow-up visits. *Psychooncology.* 1995;4(4):301–310.
34. Passik SD, Dugan W, McDonald MV, Rosenfeld B, Theobald DE, Edgerton S. Oncologists' recognition of depression in their patients with cancer. *J Clin Oncol.* 1998;16(4):1594–1600.
35. Cella D, Rosenbloom SK, Beaumont JL, et al. Development and validation of 11 symptom indexes to evaluate response to chemotherapy for advanced cancer. *J Natl Compr Canc Netw.* 2011;9(3):268–278.
36. Earlam S, Glover C, Fordy C, Burke D, Allen-Mersh TG. Relation between tumor size, quality of life, and survival in patients with colorectal liver metastases. *J Clin Oncol.* 1996;14(1):171–175.
37. Maisey NR, Norman A, Watson M, Allen MJ, Hill ME, Cunningham D. Baseline quality of life predicts survival in patients with advanced colorectal cancer. *Eur J Cancer.* 2002;38(10):1351–1357.
38. Fairclough DL, Cella DF. Functional Assessment of Cancer Therapy (FACT-G): non-response to individual questions. *Qual Life Res.* 1996;5(3):321–329.
39. Chang VT, Hwang SS, Feuerman M, Kasimis BS. Symptom and quality of life survey of medical oncology patients at a veterans affairs medical center: a role for symptom assessment. *Cancer.* 2000;88(5):1175–1183.
40. Sideris L, Zenasni F, Vernerey D, et al. Quality of life of patients operated on for low rectal cancer: impact of the type of surgery and patients' characteristics. *Dis Colon Rectum.* 2005;48(12):2180–2191.
41. Guren MG, Eriksen MT, Wiig JN, et al.; Norwegian Rectal Cancer Group. Quality of life and functional outcome following anterior or abdominoperineal resection for rectal cancer. *Eur J Surg Oncol.* 2005;31(7):735–742.
42. Lewis WG, Holdsworth PJ, Stephenson BM, Finan PJ, Johnston D. Role of the rectum in the physiological and clinical results of coloanal and colorectal anastomosis after anterior resection for rectal carcinoma. *Br J Surg.* 1992;79(10):1082–1086.
43. Santangelo ML, Romano G, Sassaroli C. Sexual function after resection for rectal cancer. *Am J Surg.* 1987;154(5):502–504.
44. Sprangers MA, Taal BG, Aaronson NK, te Velde A. Quality of life in colorectal cancer. Stoma vs. nonstoma patients. *Dis Colon Rectum.* 1995;38(4):361–369.
45. Hassan I, Cima RR. Quality of life after rectal resection and multimodality therapy. *J Surg Oncol.* 2007;96(8):684–692.
46. Donovan KA, Thompson LM, Hoffe SE. Sexual function in colorectal cancer survivors. *Cancer Control.* 2010;17(1):44–51.
47. Rosen RC, Riley A, Wagner G, Osterloh IH, Kirkpatrick J, Mishra A. The international index of erectile function (IIEF): a multidimensional scale for assessment of erectile dysfunction. *Urology.* 1997;49(6):822–830.

48. Rosen R, Brown C, Heiman J, et al. The Female Sexual Function Index (FSFI): a multidimensional self-report instrument for the assessment of female sexual function. *J Sex Marital Ther.* 2000;26(2):191–208.
49. Jeffery DD, Tzeng JP, Keefe FJ, et al. Initial report of the cancer Patient-Reported Outcomes Measurement Information System (PROMIS) sexual function committee: review of sexual function measures and domains used in oncology. *Cancer.* 2009;115(6):1142–1153.
50. Fortune-Greeley AK, Flynn KE, Jeffery DD, et al.; PROMIS Sexual Function Domain Committee. Using cognitive interviews to evaluate items for measuring sexual functioning across cancer populations: improvements and remaining challenges. *Qual Life Res.* 2009;18(8):1085–1093.
51. Flynn KE, Jeffery DD, Keefe FJ, et al. Sexual functioning along the cancer continuum: focus group results from the Patient-Reported Outcomes Measurement Information System (PROMIS®). *Psychooncology.* 2011;20(4):378–386.
52. Hendren SK, O'Connor BI, Liu M, et al. Prevalence of male and female sexual dysfunction is high following surgery for rectal cancer. *Ann Surg.* 2005;242(2):212–223.
53. Liang JT, Lai HS, Lee PH, Chang KJ. Laparoscopic pelvic autonomic nerve-preserving surgery for sigmoid colon cancer. *Ann Surg Oncol.* 2008;15(6):1609–1616.
54. Sartori CA, Sartori A, Vigna S, Occhipinti R, Baiocchi GL. Urinary and sexual disorders after laparoscopic TME for rectal cancer in males. *J Gastrointest Surg.* 2011;15(4):637–643.
55. Rodrigues AC, Teixeira R, Teixeira T, Conde S, Soares P, Torgal I. Impact of pelvic radiotherapy on female sexuality. *Arch Gynecol Obstet.* 2012;285(2):505–514.
56. Rozmovits L, Ziebland S. Expressions of loss of adulthood in the narratives of people with colorectal cancer. *Qual Health Res.* 2004;14(2):187–203.
57. Guyatt G, Walter S, Norman G. Measuring change over time: assessing the usefulness of evaluative instruments. *J Chronic Dis.* 1987;40(2):171–178.
58. Kazis LE, Anderson JJ, Meenan RF. Effect sizes for interpreting changes in health status. *Med Care.* 1989;27(3 Suppl):S178–S189.
59. Jacobson NS, Truax P. Clinical significance: a statistical approach to defining meaningful change in psychotherapy research. *J Consult Clin Psychol.* 1991;59(1):12–19.
60. Kraemer HC. Reporting the size of effects in research studies to facilitate assessment of practical or clinical significance. *Psychoneuroendocrinology.* 1992;17(6):527–536.
61. Guyatt GH, Osoba D, Wu AW, Wyrwich KW, Norman GR; Clinical Significance Consensus Meeting Group. Methods to explain the clinical significance of health status measures. *Mayo Clin Proc.* 2002;77(4):371–383.
62. Norman GR, Sloan JA, Wyrwich KW. Interpretation of changes in health-related quality of life: the remarkable universality of half a standard deviation. *Med Care.* 2003;41(5):582–592.
63. Howlader N, Noone AM, Krapcho M, et al. *SEER Cancer Statistics Review, 1975–2008.* Bethesda, MD: National Cancer Institute; 2011.
64. Meulenbeld HJ, Creemers GJ. First-line treatment strategies for elderly patients with metastatic colorectal cancer. *Drugs Aging.* 2007;24(3):223–238.
65. Grothey A, Sugrue MM, Purdie DM, et al. Bevacizumab beyond first progression is associated with prolonged overall survival in metastatic colorectal cancer: results from a large observational cohort study (BRiTE). *J Clin Oncol.* 2008;26(33):5326–5334.
66. Williams NS, Johnston D. The quality of life after rectal excision for low rectal cancer. *Br J Surg.* 1983;70(8):460–462.
67. Devlin HB, Plant JA, Griffin M. Aftermath of surgery for anorectal cancer. *Br Med J.* 1971;3(5771):413–418.
68. Fain SN, Patin CS, Morgenstern L. Use of a mechanical suturing apparatus in low colorectal anastomosis. *Arch Surg.* 1975;110(9):1079–1082.
69. Heald RJ. Towards fewer colostomies–the impact of circular stapling devices on the surgery of rectal cancer in a district hospital. *Br J Surg.* 1980;67(3):198–200.
70. Wilson TR, Alexander DJ, Kind P. Measurement of health-related quality of life in the early follow-up of colon and rectal cancer. *Dis Colon Rectum.* 2006;49(11):1692–1702.
71. Clinical Outcomes of Surgical Therapy Study Group. A comparison of laparoscopically assisted and open colectomy for colon cancer. *N Engl J Med.* 2004;350(20):2050–2059.
72. Guillou PJ, Quirke P, Thorpe H, et al.; MRC CLASICC trial group. Short-term endpoints of conventional versus laparoscopic-assisted surgery in patients with colorectal cancer (MRC CLASICC trial): multicentre, randomised controlled trial. *Lancet.* 2005;365(9472):1718–1726.
73. Jayne DG, Guillou PJ, Thorpe H, et al.; UK MRC CLASICC Trial Group. Randomized trial of laparoscopic-assisted resection of colorectal carcinoma: 3-year results of the UK MRC CLASICC Trial Group. *J Clin Oncol.* 2007;25(21):3061–3068.
74. Veldkamp R, Kuhry E, Hop WC, et al.; COlon cancer Laparoscopic or Open Resection Study Group (COLOR). Laparoscopic surgery versus open surgery for colon cancer: short-term outcomes of a randomised trial. *Lancet Oncol.* 2005;6(7):477–484.
75. Schwenk W, Haase O, Neudecker J, Müller JM. Short term benefits for laparoscopic colorectal resection. *Cochrane Database Syst Rev.* 2005;(3):CD003145.
76. Tjandra JJ, Chan MK. Systematic review on the short-term outcome of laparoscopic resection for colon and rectosigmoid cancer. *Colorectal Dis.* 2006;8(5):375–388.
77. Fingerhut A, Ata T, Chouillard E, Alexakis N, Veyrie N. Laparoscopic approach to colonic cancer: critical appraisal of the literature. *Dig Dis.* 2007;25(1):33–43.
78. Noel JK, Fahrbach K, Estok R, et al. Minimally invasive colorectal resection outcomes: short-term comparison with open procedures. *J Am Coll Surg.* 2007;204(2):291–307.
79. Abraham NS, Byrne CM, Young JM, Solomon MJ. Meta-analysis of non-randomized comparative studies of the short-term outcomes of laparoscopic resection for colorectal cancer. *ANZ J Surg.* 2007;77(7):508–516.
80. Leung KL, Kwok SP, Lam SC, et al. Laparoscopic resection of rectosigmoid carcinoma: prospective randomised trial. *Lancet.* 2004;363(9416):1187–1192.
81. Abraham NS, Young JM, Solomon MJ. Meta-analysis of short-term outcomes after laparoscopic resection for colorectal cancer. *Br J Surg.* 2004;91(9):1111–1124.
82. Allardyce RA, Bagshaw PF, Frampton CM, et al.; Australasian Laparoscopic Colon Cancer Study Group. Australasian Laparoscopic Colon Cancer Study shows that elderly patients may benefit from lower postoperative complication rates following laparoscopic versus open resection. *Br J Surg.* 2010;97(1):86–91.
83. Gujral S, Avery KN, Blazeby JM. Quality of life after surgery for colorectal cancer: clinical implications of results from randomised trials. *Support Care Cancer.* 2008;16(2):127–132.
84. Gray NM, Hall SJ, Browne S, et al. Modifiable and fixed factors predicting quality of life in people with colorectal cancer. *Br J Cancer.* 2011;104(11):1697–1703.
85. Koroukian SM, Xu F, Bakaki PM, Diaz-Insua M, Towe TP, Owusu C. Comorbidities, functional limitations, and geriatric syndromes in relation to treatment and survival patterns among elders with colorectal cancer. *J Gerontol A Biol Sci Med Sci.* 2010;65(3):322–329.
86. Hoerske C, Weber K, Goehl J, Hohenberger W, Merkel S. Long-term outcomes and quality of life after rectal carcinoma surgery. *Br J Surg.* 2010;97(8):1295–1303.
87. Thomas C, Turner P, Madden F. Coping and the outcome of stoma surgery. *J Psychosom Res.* 1988;32(4–5):457–467.
88. Krouse RS, Grant M, Rawl SM, et al. Coping and acceptance: the greatest challenge for veterans with intestinal stomas. *J Psychosom Res.* 2009;66(3):227–233.

89. Thomas C, Madden F, Jehu D. Psychological effects of stomas–I. Psychosocial morbidity one year after surgery. *J Psychosom Res.* 1987;31(3):311–316.
90. Schneider EC, Malin JL, Kahn KL, Ko CY, Adams J, Epstein AM. Surviving colorectal cancer: patient-reported symptoms 4 years after diagnosis. *Cancer.* 2007;110(9):2075–2082.
91. Pittman J, Rawl SM, Schmidt CM, et al. Demographic and clinical factors related to ostomy complications and quality of life in veterans with an ostomy. *J Wound Ostomy Continence Nurs.* 2008;35(5):493–503.
92. Coons SJ, Chongpison Y, Wendel CS, Grant M, Krouse RS. Overall quality of life and difficulty paying for ostomy supplies in the Veterans Affairs ostomy health-related quality of life study: an exploratory analysis. *Med Care.* 2007;45(9):891–895.
93. Matthiessen P, Hallböök O, Rutegård J, Simert G, Sjödahl R. Defunctioning stoma reduces symptomatic anastomotic leakage after low anterior resection of the rectum for cancer: a randomized multicenter trial. *Ann Surg.* 2007;246(2):207–214.
94. MacDonald LD, Anderson HR. Stigma in patients with rectal cancer: a community study. *J Epidemiol Community Health.* 1984;38(4):284–290.
95. Jain S, McGory ML, Ko CY, et al. Comorbidities play a larger role in predicting health-related quality of life compared to having an ostomy. *Am J Surg.* 2007;194(6):774–9; discussion 779.
96. Engel J, Kerr J, Schlesinger-Raab A, Eckel R, Sauer H, Hölzel D. Quality of life in rectal cancer patients: a four-year prospective study. *Ann Surg.* 2003;238(2):203–213.
97. DeCosse JJ, Cennerazzo WJ. Quality-of-life management of patients with colorectal cancer. *CA Cancer J Clin.* 1997;47(4):198–206.
98. Dunn J, Lynch B, Aitken J, Leggett B, Pakenham K, Newman B. Quality of life and colorectal cancer: a review. *Aust N Z J Public Health.* 2003;27(1):41–53.
99. Fucini C, Gattai R, Urena C, Bandettini L, Elbetti C. Quality of life among five-year survivors after treatment for very low rectal cancer with or without a permanent abdominal stoma. *Ann Surg Oncol.* 2008;15(4):1099–1106.
100. Pollack J, Holm T, Cedermark B, et al. Late adverse effects of short-course preoperative radiotherapy in rectal cancer. *Br J Surg.* 2006;93(12):1519–1525.
101. Ramsey SD, Andersen MR, Etzioni R, et al. Quality of life in survivors of colorectal carcinoma. *Cancer.* 2000;88(6):1294–1303.
102. Bekkers MJ, van Knippenberg FC, van Dulmen AM, van den Borne HW, van Berge Henegouwen GP. Survival and psychosocial adjustment to stoma surgery and nonstoma bowel resection: a 4-year follow-up. *J Psychosom Res.* 1997;42(3):235–244.
103. Rauch P, Miny J, Conroy T, Neyton L, Guillemin F. Quality of life among disease-free survivors of rectal cancer. *J Clin Oncol.* 2004;22(2):354–360.
104. Krouse RS, Herrinton LJ, Grant M, et al. Health-related quality of life among long-term rectal cancer survivors with an ostomy: manifestations by sex. *J Clin Oncol.* 2009;27(28):4664–4670.
105. Grant M, McMullen CK, Altschuler A, et al. Gender differences in quality of life among long-term colorectal cancer survivors with ostomies. *Oncol Nurs Forum.* 2011;38(5):587–596.
106. McMullen CK, Hornbrook MC, Grant M, et al. The greatest challenges reported by long-term colorectal cancer survivors with stomas. *J Support Oncol.* 2008;6(4):175–182.
107. Rust J. Care of patients with stomas: the pouch change procedure. *Nurs Stand.* 2007;22(6):43–47.
108. Bekkers MJ, van Knippenberg FC, van den Borne HW, van Berge-Henegouwen GP. Prospective evaluation of psychosocial adaptation to stoma surgery: the role of self-efficacy. *Psychosom Med.* 1996;58(2):183–191.
109. Stephens RJ, Thompson LC, Quirke P, et al. Impact of short-course preoperative radiotherapy for rectal cancer on patients' quality of life: data from the Medical Research Council CR07/National Cancer Institute of Canada Clinical Trials Group C016 randomized clinical trial. *J Clin Oncol.* 2010;28(27):4233–4239.
110. Pucciarelli S, Del Bianco P, Efficace F, et al. Patient-reported outcomes after neoadjuvant chemoradiotherapy for rectal cancer: a multicenter prospective observational study. *Ann Surg.* 2011;253(1):71–77.
111. Havenga K, Maas CP, DeRuiter MC, Welvaart K, Trimbos JB. Avoiding long-term disturbance to bladder and sexual function in pelvic surgery, particularly with rectal cancer. *Semin Surg Oncol.* 2000;18(3):235–243.
112. Keating JP. Sexual function after rectal excision. *ANZ J Surg.* 2004;74(4):248–259.
113. Bergman B, Nilsson S, Petersén I. The effect on erection and orgasm of cystectomy, prostatectomy and vesiculectomy for cancer of the bladder: a clinical and electromyographic study. *Br J Urol.* 1979;51(2):114–120.
114. Symms MR, Rawl SM, Grant M, et al. Sexual health and quality of life among male veterans with intestinal ostomies. *Clin Nurse Spec.* 2008;22(1):30–40.
115. Wolmark N, Rockette H, Fisher B, et al. The benefit of leucovorin-modulated fluorouracil as postoperative adjuvant therapy for primary colon cancer: results from National Surgical Adjuvant Breast and Bowel Project protocol C-03. *J Clin Oncol.* 1993;11(10):1879–1887.
116. Wolmark N, Bryant J, Smith R, et al. Adjuvant 5-fluorouracil and leucovorin with or without interferon alfa-2a in colon carcinoma: National Surgical Adjuvant Breast and Bowel Project protocol C-05. *J Natl Cancer Inst.* 1998;90(23):1810–1816.
117. Tofthagen C. Surviving chemotherapy for colon cancer and living with the consequences. *J Palliat Med.* 2010;13(11):1389–1391.
118. Grothey A. Oxaliplatin-safety profile: neurotoxicity. *Semin Oncol.* 2003;30(4 Suppl 15):5–13.
119. Grothey A, Nikcevich DA, Sloan JA, et al. Intravenous calcium and magnesium for oxaliplatin-induced sensory neurotoxicity in adjuvant colon cancer: NCCTG N04C7. *J Clin Oncol.* 2011;29(4):421–427.
120. Yothers G, O'Connell MJ, Allegra CJ, et al. Oxaliplatin as adjuvant therapy for colon cancer: updated results of NSABP C-07 trial, including survival and subset analyses. *J Clin Oncol.* 2011;29(28):3768–3774.
121. Sanoff HK, Carpenter WR, Martin CF, et al. Comparative effectiveness of oxaliplatin vs non-oxaliplatin-containing adjuvant chemotherapy for stage III colon cancer. *J Natl Cancer Inst.* 2012;104(3):211–227.
122. Ades S. Adjuvant chemotherapy for colon cancer in the elderly: moving from evidence to practice. *Oncology (Williston Park, NY).* 2009;23(2):162–167.
123. Sanoff HK, Carpenter WR, Freburger J, et al. Comparison of adverse events during 5-fluorouracil versus 5-fluorouracil/oxaliplatin adjuvant chemotherapy for stage III colon cancer: a population-based analysis. *Cancer.* 2012;118(17):4309–4320.
124. Sauer R, Becker H, Hohenberger W, et al.; German Rectal Cancer Study Group. Preoperative versus postoperative chemoradiotherapy for rectal cancer. *N Engl J Med.* 2004;351(17):1731–1740.
125. Bosset JF, Collette L, Calais G, et al.; EORTC Radiotherapy Group Trial 22921. Chemotherapy with preoperative radiotherapy in rectal cancer. *N Engl J Med.* 2006;355(11):1114–1123.
126. Bujko K, Nowacki MP, Nasierowska-Guttmejer A, Michalski W, Bebenek M, Kryj M. Long-term results of a randomized trial comparing preoperative short-course radiotherapy with preoperative conventionally fractionated chemoradiation for rectal cancer. *Br J Surg.* 2006;93(10):1215–1223.
127. Mannaerts GH, Schijven MP, Hendrikx A, Martijn H, Rutten HJ, Wiggers T. Urologic and sexual morbidity following multimodality treatment for locally advanced primary and locally recurrent rectal cancer. *Eur J Surg Oncol.* 2001;27(3):265–272.
128. Bambrick M, Fazio VW, Hull TL, Pucel G. Sexual function following restorative proctocolectomy in women. *Dis Colon Rectum.* 1996;39(6):610–614.

129. Jansen L, Koch L, Brenner H, Arndt V. Quality of life among long-term (>5 years) colorectal cancer survivors–systematic review. *Eur J Cancer.* 2010;46(16):2879–2888.
130. Gall CA, Weller D, Esterman A, et al. Patient satisfaction and health-related quality of life after treatment for colon cancer. *Dis Colon Rectum.* 2007;50(6):801–809.
131. Schag CA, Ganz PA, Wing DS, Sim MS, Lee JJ. Quality of life in adult survivors of lung, colon and prostate cancer. *Qual Life Res.* 1994;3(2):127–141.
132. Phipps E, Braitman LE, Stites S, Leighton JC. Quality of life and symptom attribution in long-term colon cancer survivors. *J Eval Clin Pract.* 2008;14(2):254–258.
133. Sapp AL, Trentham-Dietz A, Newcomb PA, Hampton JM, Moinpour CM, Remington PL. Social networks and quality of life among female long-term colorectal cancer survivors. *Cancer.* 2003;98(8):1749–1758.
134. Sasson AR, Sigurdson ER. Management of locally advanced rectal cancer. *Surg Oncol.* 2000;9(4):193–204.
135. Esnaola NF, Cantor SB, Johnson ML, et al. Pain and quality of life after treatment in patients with locally recurrent rectal cancer. *J Clin Oncol.* 2002;20(21):4361–4367.
136. Bakx R, Visser O, Josso J, Meijer S, Slors JF, van Lanschot JJ. Management of recurrent rectal cancer: a population based study in greater Amsterdam. *World J Gastroenterol.* 2008;14(39):6018–6023.
137. Palmer G, Martling A, Cedermark B, Holm T. A population-based study on the management and outcome in patients with locally recurrent rectal cancer. *Ann Surg Oncol.* 2007;14(2):447–454.
138. Bedrosian I, Giacco G, Pederson L, et al. Outcome after curative resection for locally recurrent rectal cancer. *Dis Colon Rectum.* 2006;49(2):175–182.
139. Rodriguez-Bigas MA, Chang GJ, Skibber JM. Barriers to rehabilitation of colorectal cancer patients. *J Surg Oncol.* 2007;95(5):400–408.
140. You YN, Habiba H, Chang GJ, Rodriguez-Bigas MA, Skibber JM. Prognostic value of quality of life and pain in patients with locally recurrent rectal cancer. *Ann Surg Oncol.* 2011;18(4):989–996.
141. Vergo M, Nimeiri H, Benson A. Adjuvant chemotherapy after neoadjuvant chemoradiation and surgery: a quest to improve survival for stage II and III rectal cancer. *Curr Colorectal Cancer Rep.* 2009;5(3):151–157.
142. Rosen SA, Buell JF, Yoshida A, et al. Initial presentation with stage IV colorectal cancer: how aggressive should we be? *Arch Surg.* 2000;135(5):530–4; discussion 534.
143. Fong Y, Kemeny N, Paty P, Blumgart LH, Cohen AM. Treatment of colorectal cancer: hepatic metastasis. *Semin Surg Oncol.* 1996;12(4):219–252.
144. Mella J, Biffin A, Radcliffe AG, Stamatakis JD, Steele RJ. Population-based audit of colorectal cancer management in two UK health regions. Colorectal Cancer Working Group, Royal College of Surgeons of England Clinical Epidemiology and Audit Unit. *Br J Surg.* 1997;84(12):1731–1736.
145. Martin R, Paty P, Fong Y, et al. Simultaneous liver and colorectal resections are safe for synchronous colorectal liver metastasis. *J Am Coll Surg.* 2003;197(2):233–41; discussion 241.
146. Jemal A, Siegel R, Xu J, Ward E. Cancer statistics, 2010. *CA Cancer J Clin.* 2010;60(5):277–300.
147. Hassan I, Cima RC, Sloan JA. Assessment of quality of life outcomes in the treatment of advanced colorectal malignancies. *Gastroenterol Clin North Am.* 2006;35(1):53–64.
148. Amersi F, Stamos MJ, Ko CY. Palliative care for colorectal cancer. *Surg Oncol Clin N Am.* 2004;13(3):467–477.
149. Goldberg RM. Advances in the treatment of metastatic colorectal cancer. *Oncologist.* 2005;10(Suppl 3):40–48.
150. Scheithauer W, McKendrick J, Begbie S, et al.; X-ACT Study Group. Oral capecitabine as an alternative to i.v. 5-fluorouracil-based adjuvant therapy for colon cancer: safety results of a randomized, phase III trial. *Ann Oncol.* 2003;14(12):1735–1743.
151. Van Cutsem E, Hoff PM, Harper P, et al. Oral capecitabine vs intravenous 5-fluorouracil and leucovorin: integrated efficacy data and novel analyses from two large, randomised, phase III trials. *Br J Cancer.* 2004;90(6):1190–1197.
152. Wiseman LR, Lyseng-Williamson KA. Management of metastatic colorectal cancer: defining the role of capecitabine. *Dis Manage Health Outcomes.* 2005;13(2):137–149.
153. Tappenden P, Jones R, Paisley S, Carroll C. Systematic review and economic evaluation of bevacizumab and cetuximab for the treatment of metastatic colorectal cancer. *Health Technol Assess.* 2007;11(12):1–128, iii.
154. Hynes NE, Lane HA. ERBB receptors and cancer: the complexity of targeted inhibitors. *Nat Rev Cancer.* 2005;5(5):341–354.
155. Segaert S, Tabernero J, Chosidow O, et al. The management of skin reactions in cancer patients receiving epidermal growth factor receptor targeted therapies. *J Dtsch Dermatol Ges.* 2005;3(8):599–606.
156. Wagner LI, Lacouture ME. Dermatologic toxicities associated with EGFR inhibitors: the clinical psychologist's perspective. Impact on health-related quality of life and implications for clinical management of psychological sequelae. *Oncology (Williston Park, NY).* 2007;21(11 Suppl 5):34–36.
157. Eilers RE Jr, Gandhi M, Patel JD, et al. Dermatologic infections in cancer patients treated with epidermal growth factor receptor inhibitor therapy. *J Natl Cancer Inst.* 2010;102(1):47–53.
158. Boone SL, Rademaker A, Liu D, Pfeiffer C, Mauro DJ, Lacouture ME. Impact and management of skin toxicity associated with anti-epidermal growth factor receptor therapy: survey results. *Oncology.* 2007;72(3–4):152–159.
159. Odom D, Barber B, Bennett L, et al. Health-related quality of life and colorectal cancer-specific symptoms in patients with chemotherapy-refractory metastatic disease treated with panitumumab. *Int J Colorectal Dis.* 2011;26(2):173–181.
160. Andreis F, Rizzi A, Mosconi P, et al. Quality of life in colon cancer patients with skin side effects: preliminary results from a monocentric cross sectional study. *Health Qual Life Outcomes.* 2010;8:40.
161. Peeters M, Siena S, Van Cutsem E, et al. Association of progression-free survival, overall survival, and patient-reported outcomes by skin toxicity and K-ras status in patients receiving panitumumab monotherapy. *Cancer.* 2009;115(7):1544–1554.
162. Romito F, Giuliani F, Cormio C, Tulipani C, Mattioli V, Colucci G. Psychological effects of cetuximab-induced cutaneous rash in advanced colorectal cancer patients. *Support Care Cancer.* 2010;18(3):329–334.
163. Douillard JY, Siena S, Cassidy J, et al. Randomized, phase III trial of panitumumab with infusional fluorouracil, leucovorin, and oxaliplatin (FOLFOX4) versus FOLFOX4 alone as first-line treatment in patients with previously untreated metastatic colorectal cancer: the PRIME study. *J Clin Oncol.* 2010;28(31):4697–4705.
164. Peeters M, Price TJ, Cervantes A, et al. Randomized phase III study of panitumumab with fluorouracil, leucovorin, and irinotecan (FOLFIRI) compared with FOLFIRI alone as second-line treatment in patients with metastatic colorectal cancer. *J Clin Oncol.* 2010;28(31):4706–4713.
165. Van Cutsem E, Köhne CH, Hitre E, et al. Cetuximab and chemotherapy as initial treatment for metastatic colorectal cancer. *N Engl J Med.* 2009;360(14):1408–1417.
166. Bokemeyer C, Bondarenko I, Makhson A, et al. Fluorouracil, leucovorin, and oxaliplatin with and without cetuximab in the first-line treatment of metastatic colorectal cancer. *J Clin Oncol.* 2009;27(5):663–671.
167. Law WL, Chan WF, Lee YM, Chu KW. Non-curative surgery for colorectal cancer: critical appraisal of outcomes. *Int J Colorectal Dis.* 2004;19(3):197–202.
168. Deans GT, Krukowski ZH, Irwin ST. Malignant obstruction of the left colon. *Br J Surg.* 1994;81(9):1270–1276.
169. Wasserberg N, Kaufman HS. Palliation of colorectal cancer. *Surg Oncol.* 2007;16(4):299–310.
170. McCahill LE, Krouse RS, Chu DZ, et al. Decision making in palliative surgery. *J Am Coll Surg.* 2002;195(3):411–22; discussion 422.

16 Racial Disparities in Colorectal Cancer

EDITH MITCHELL

Colorectal cancer (CRC) is the most common malignancy in the gastrointestinal tract and the fourth leading cause of cancer deaths worldwide. In the United States, it is estimated that 142,820 patients will be diagnosed in 2013 and 50,830 will be unfortunately succumb to the disease (1). While colon cancer death rates have decreased in the United States by approximately 30% over the last three decades differences in mortality rates exists between reported statistics among populations. Multiple studies have demonstrated that African American patients have a less favorable prognosis and have higher mortality rates than do whites with CRC (2–15).

A review of data from the Surveillance, Epidemiology, and End Results (SEER) Program for the years 1992 to 1997 showed significant disparities in 5-year relative survival rates for all stages of CRC, with overall survival rates of 60.2% for whites and 51.2% for Blacks (2). The differences in mortality rates has been to a number of factors, the most significant of which is suggested as a more advanced stage of disease at the time of diagnosis. However, multiple other potential factors exist, including lack of access to and utilization of health care system resources, presence of comorbid diseases and other active medical conditions, aggressiveness of tumors, tolerance of treatment, and tumor response to treatment. The end result is that African Americans experience a higher incidence of colon and rectal cancer and are more likely to die of the disease (3–15).

Because there was a similar distribution among stages for whites and blacks during this time period, this SEER report further provided evidence of a worse 5-year survival for blacks for overall survival, but for each stage of the disease–localized, regional and metastatic disease. There was no information in these reports identifying differences in aggressiveness of tumors or other characteristics of inherent tumor biology. Additionally, treatment parameters received by patients were not delineated and therefore the potential role of therapeutic impact as a potential contributor to disparities among minority groups was not defined (2).

Using SEER data, Robbins et al evaluated racial disparities in stage-specific CRC mortality rates from 1985 to 2008 and examined whether this mortality pattern varied according to stage at diagnosis. This report identified the main outcome measure as stage-specific mortality rates by race from the nine original SEER regions from 1985 to 1987 to 2006 to 2008 and demonstrated that CRC mortality rates decreased for each stage in both blacks and whites, however, the declines were smaller in the black population for every stage of the disease. This was especially true for metastatic and distant-stage disease. While the mortality for localized stage decreased 30.3% over this time period in whites, the declined in blacks was 13.2%. For regional disease stage, declines were 48.5% in whites compared to 34% in blacks. For distant stage the gap was even greater with declines of 32.6% in whites compared to 4.6% in blacks. As a result of these data, the black/white ratio increased from 1.17 (95% CI, 0.98 to 1.39) to 1.41 (95% CI, 1.21 to 1.63) for localized disease, from 1.03 (95% CI, 0.93 to 1.14) to 1.30 (95% CI, 1.17 to 1.44) for regional-stage disease, and from 1.21 (95% CI, 1.10 to 1.34) to 1.72 (95 % CI, 1.58 to 1.86) for distant-stage disease. The evidence clearly demonstrates that the disparity in distant-stage deaths accounted for approximately 60% of the overall differences in black/white mortality. Thus, implying that increased efforts in prevention of CRC and detection of the disease at earlier stages could improve treatment outcomes in African Americans and potentially impact the worsening black/white disparities trend (16).

While a significantly larger proportion of black patients present with advanced stage disease, several studies have demonstrated that even after controlling for tumor stage at diagnosis, black patients have worse survival than whites. In addition, after adjusting for other factors such as poverty, lack of access to care, socioeconomic factors, treatment differences, there is no concrete rationale that clearly explains survival differences or treatment outcomes. Studies indicate that African Americans undergo surveillance screening less frequently than Caucasians, have a predominance of right-sided tumors and have more extensive and later stage disease and thus a worse prognosis at the time of diagnosis. Additionally, differences in treatment exist with fewer African Americans receiving postoperative adjuvant chemotherapy after resection of colon cancer or radiotherapy during rectal cancer treatment.

This review will outline and summarize details of differences that exist between minority populations and Caucasians and reports contributing factor such as surveillance and screening trends, molecular and biologic characteristics, and prognosis and treatment.

COLORECTAL SURVEILLANCE AND SCREENING

Surveillance evaluations for CRC are accomplished less frequently in African Americans than other racial or ethnic groups (12). Contributing factors are believed to include knowledge and cultured beliefs, education and awareness of screening tests, physician recommendations for screening modalities, as well as level of education and socioeconomic status (3–18).

James et al reported an analysis of colon cancer screening in African Americans in North Carolina and indicated that screening was negatively associated with fecal occult blood testing and sigmoidoscopy, whereas, there was a positive association with sigmoidoscopy and colonoscopy (17).

Schroy et al reported a lower knowledge and understanding of CRC in African Americans (19). In a large qualitative study Palmer et al reported that adherence to screening guidelines was positivity related to knowledge of the disease and benefits of screening as well as physician recommendation and insurance status (20).

Because evidence did not clearly delineate whether the disproportionately higher incidence and mortality from CRC among blacks compared with whites reflected inherent differences in CRC susceptibility or health care utilization, the results of 60,572 non-Hispanic white and black participants in the Prostate, Lung, colorectal, and Ovarian (PLCO) Cancer Screening Trial who underwent trial-sponsored screening flexible sigmoidoscopy (FSG) without biopsy at baseline. Subjects with abnormalities were then referred for diagnostic evaluations. This report demonstrated that 23.9% of whites and 25.5% of blacks had abnormal findings, with 72.5% of whites and 62.6% of blacks undergoing diagnostic colonoscopy within one year. The diagnostic procedure revealed no statistically significant differences by race in the incidence of pathological findings that included adenoma, advanced adenoma, high grade dysplasia or villous histology in adenomas less than10mm, or colorectal. The overall results demonstrated a substantially lower rate of follow-up of abnormalities detected during screening among blacks compared to whites, but no differences in identifiable colorectal neoplasia. As a result of these data, these authors suggested that health care utilization, or lack thereof, may play a greater role in CRC racial disparity than biology of the disease (20).

In evaluation of racial disparities and barriers to colorectal screening in participants in a rural survey, physician recommendation for colorectal screening had the strongest association with individuals being current on screening (22–26). Other reports have endorsed this opinion and emphasized the importance of increasing public service advertisements as means of addressing the racial gap in mortality rates (27–42).

Based on incidence and mortality rates the American College of Gastroenterologists issued new guidelines to health care providers regarding screening of African Americans for colon cancer. This report indicates that African Americans should be screened for CRC beginning at age 45, five years earlier than other populations, in response to findings of earlier onset of disease coupled with higher incidence and mortality rates (42). Furthermore, colonoscopy was recommended as the initial screening procedure for African Americans because of the high incidence of right-sided cancers and polyps (42).

COLORECTAL DISEASE STATUS

In a large study of information obtained from screening colonoscopies in asymptomatic men and women from 67 centers, Lieberman et al reported that blacks were more likely to have one or more polyps larger than 9 mm than whites.

Among 5,464 African Americans and 80,061 whites, approximately 8% of African Americans had one or more polyps larger than 9 mm while only 6% of whites have similar findings. Overall, in the gender analyses, African American women demonstrated a 62% greater risk of having a polyp greater than 9 mm than whites and African American men had a 16% greater risk (43).

Multiple studies have reported differences in location and sites of tumors within the colon. Blacks are more likely to have proximal colon cancer than distal blacks are less likely than whites to have localized disease at the time of diagnosis (44).

DECREASING INCIDENCE AND MORTALITY

CRC incidence rates in the United States decreased from 1975 to 2009 (2). The substantial decline in incidence rates has been attributed mainly to increased utilization of screening modalities in asymptomatic individuals with detection and removal of precancerous polyps (15, 44,57). Others tend to agree with this finding (58–71). Estimates of new CRC cases among African Americans for 2013 indicate that CRC is the third leading cause of cancer incidence in women and men and account for 10%

of cancers in men and 11% in women (Figure 16.1 from DeSantis et al 121). These authors further indicated that cancers of the colon and rectum further account for the third leading cause of cancer deaths in both men and women (Figure 16.2 from DeSantis et al 121).

There has been a continuous and consistent decline in CRC incidence rates of 2.4% per year in men and 2.2% per year in women since 1998 (72).

Nonhereditary sporadic CRC occurs more frequently and at a younger age in African Americans, suggesting

Leading Sites of New Cancer Cases Among African Americans - 2013 Estimates

Males			Females		
Prostate	35,430	37%	Breast	27,060	33%
Lung & Bronchus	13,110	14%	Lung & Bronchus	10,980	13%
Colon & Rectum	9,280	10%	Colon & Rectum	8,830	11%
Kidney	4,400	5%	Uterine Corpus	5,690	7%
Liver & Intrahepatic Bile Duct	3,270	3%	Thyroid	3,850	5%
Hon-Hodgkin Lymphoma	2,960	3%	Kidney	3,030	4%
Pancreas	2,670	3%	Pancreas	2,930	4%
Oral Cavity & Pharynx	2,460	3%	Non-Hodgkin Lymphoma	2,590	3%
Urinary Bladder	2,380	2%	Myeloma	2,170	3%
Leukemia	2,220	2%	Uterine Cervix	2,060	3%
All Sites	94,540		All Sites	82,080	

FIGURE 16.1 Leading sites of new cancer cases among African Americans, 2013. (Adapted from DeSantis et al [121].)

Leading Sites of Cancer Deaths Among African Americans - 2013 Estimated

Males			Females		
Lung & Bronchus	9,430	29%	Lung & Bronchus	6,830	21%
Prostate	4,980	15%	Breast	6,080	19%
Colon & Rectum	3,600	11%	Colon & Rectum	3,250	10%
Liver & Intrahepatic Bile Duct	2,240	7%	Pancreas	2,390	7%
Pancreas	2,110	6%	Uterine Corpus	1,500	5%
Stomach	1,100	3%	Ovary	1,330	4%
Leukemia	1,040	3%	Myeloma	940	3%
Myeloma	950	3%	Leukemia	890	3%
Esophagus	900	3%	Liver & Intrahepatic Bile Duct	830	3%
Kidney	820	2%	Stomach	760	2%
All Sites	32,970		All Sites	31,910	

FIGURE 16.2 Leading sites of cancer deaths among African Americans, 2013. (Adapted from DeSantis et al [121].)

that there may be a potential in risk and other factors contributing to initiation and/or promotion of disease development. Deaths from CRC are higher in African American men and women than in any other ethnic or racial group. While the pathogenesis and etiology of these striking disparities have not been delineated, because of the overall diagnosis in African Americans at a younger age, the American college of Gastroenterology has recommended earlier screening with colonoscopies at 45 years of age rather than the 50 years included in other clinical guidelines (42). It is assumed that earlier screening intervention may detect colon cancer at an earlier stage or other colon abnormalities and allow for more effective treatment and improved therapeutic outcomes (15,73).

PROGNOSTIC FACTORS IN AFRICAN AMERICANS

While mortality rates declined in both Caucasians and African Americans the rates for blacks are higher and thus the gap has overall increased (77–81). Gomez et al reported socioeconomic status accounted for most of the observed differences in the likelihood of death Stage III colon cancer and Stage II and III rectal cancer. Additionally, while comorbidities did not appear to contribute, however other treatment, including surgery, irradiation, and chemotherapy accounted for same difference in outcomes and all cause mortality. Other studies have confirmed socioeconomic status as an important factor in determining prognosis in CRC among ethnic and minority populations (81).

Multiple studies have demonstrated more advanced stage at the time of diagnosis of CRC in African Americans, than in Caucasians (82–86). Furthermore, Blacks are more likely to be diagnosed at a younger age and with more advanced disease with rectal cancer when compared to whites (91). Similar findings have also been reported by others (92–99). In a study of in-hospital mortality in the State of Maryland, Ahuya et al reported that African Americans were more likely to present more advanced symptoms and life-threatening events at diagnosis of CRC than whites. Furthermore, African Americans were more likely to die during hospitalization than whites and this factor was independent of socioeconomic status (100).

Differences in tumor grade at the time of diagnosis have varied. In an extensive analysis of differences in tumor grade and aggressiveness of CRC among black and white, Chen et al reported that blacks were less likely to be diagnosed with poorly differentiated histopathology when compared to whites (OR = 0.44; 95% CI 0.22–0.88) or with lymphoid reaction (OR = 0.49; 95% CI 0.26 – 0.90). There were no differences in vascular and lymphatic vessel invasion, mucinous histology, or tumoral necrosis. This was statistically significant after adjustments for age, sex, metropolitan area, socioeconomic status, body mass index, and health care access. These authors suggested that there were other factors that contributed to outcomes disparities (101).

MOLECULAR AND GENE EXPRESSION

While much research on colon cancer disparities has focused on epidemiology and socioeconomic issues as contributing factors to the disparities that exist among specific populations, with most data indicating differences between black and whites, research also supports the role of genetic and biological factors (101–110). Using SNP for incidence of microsatellite instability and level of gene methylation, Ashktorab et al reported on genetic differences between African Americans and Caucasians with CRC. In this study, they evaluated gene expression of P16, hMLH1, and hMSHS2 and inactivation by hypermethylation of their respective promoter regions, thereby abrogating cellular regulation of proliferation and repair mechanisms. Five markers, D2S123, D5S346, D17S250, BAT25, and BAT26, were utilized to evaluate microsatellite instability and P16 and hMLH1 promoter methylation evaluated by bisulfite modification of DNA methylation specific PCR. Expression of hMLH1 and hMSH2 were evaluated by immunohistochemistry. Matched normal and tumor colon cancer specimen from 51 African American patients were examined. Results demonstrated that 43% of the tumors showed microsatellite instability-high (MSI-H), 53% were microsatellite (MSS), and 4% were microsatellite instability-low (MSI-L). The majority of the MSI-H patients were female and had tumors located in the proximal colon and well differentiated mucinous histopathology. P16 promoter methylation was present in 40% of tumors with 33% of these being MSI-H. The hML1 promoter was methylated in 85% of the tumors with 87% of these being MSI-H. Compared to the U.S. Caucasian population, these authors report that the prevalence of MSI-H CRV was two-to-threefold higher and mismatch repair genes similar (106). Sylvester et al (123) reported no differences in MSI or BRAF, however, African Americans with tumors demonstrating MSS or MSI-L had a higher proportion of *K-ras* mutations than Caucasians (34% vs 23%, $P = .048$). Thus, indicating that the distribution of factors influencing chemotherapy selection may play a role in survival disparities (122). Jovov et al performed gene expression profiling of CRCs and normal tissue from 43 African Americans and 43 Caucasians matched by stage using Agilent human whole genome 4x44k cDNA arrays and analyses by Significance Analysis of Microarrays (SAM), tenfold cross validation, and Ingenuity Pathway

Analysis (IPA). Results demonstrated that 95 genes were differentially expressed between African Americans and Caucasians and that the most frequently expressed pathways were related to inflammation and immune response. Furthermore, expression of 10 genes could predict ethnicity with 94% accuracy. Thus, implicating that gene expression and variability in susceptibility to inflammation may influence disparities in CRC outcomes (107)

Further analyses of the 9,741 study revealed variations in pharmacogenomics parameters with UGT1A1 6/7 and 7/7 polymorphisms more commonly observed in African Americans and UGT1A1 6/6 more frequently found in Caucasians (P = .0082). Other findings included ERCC2-d A/A and A/B more common in Caucasians and ERCC2-d B/B more frequent in African Americans (P=.0002), the absence of GSTM1–0 in Caucasians and present in African Americans, and xrcc1-r399q C/C more frequent in African Americans than Caucasians CP=0.0006 (109).

■ THERAPIES OF CRC

Differences in treatment outcomes among black and white patients have been reported and thus may be a contributing factor to outcomes disparities. In Figure 16.3 the 5-year relative survival rates for CRC are given (from DeSantis et al 121). A comparison of incidence rates between African Americans and whites is given in Figure 16.4 (from DeSantis et al 121). Furthermore, these authors have demonstrated that African Americans present with later stage disease in Figure 16.5 (from DeSantis et al 121). In a study of surgical treatment of rectal cancer the rate of sphincter-ablation was 37% for white compared to 43% for blacks (91, 95). Other studies have also reported difference in extent of treatment between black and white patients, usually with poorer outcomes for blacks (96–102). Other studies reveal similar outcomes in minority populations when there is uniformity in care. Among patients treated on five serially conducted, randomized clinical trials of the National Surgical Adjuvant Breast and Bowel Project (NSABP) Dignam et al reported recurrence-free survival, disease-free survival and survival using statistical modeling to account for differences in patient and disease characteristics between the groups. This study was particularly important since the randomized clinical trial setting. There were similarities in disease stage and a uniform treatment plan between blacks and whites. The results from this study demonstrated that the stage of disease and number of involved lymph nodes were similar between African American and Caucasian patients in each trial. Overall the combined trials, an 8% (95% [CI] = -6%–25%; P = .27) excess risk of colon cancer recurrence that was not statistically significant was observed for blacks. However, blacks experienced statistically significantly poorer survival with a 21% (95% CI = 6% -37%; P = .004) greater risk of death. The conclusions from this study indicated that while overall survival

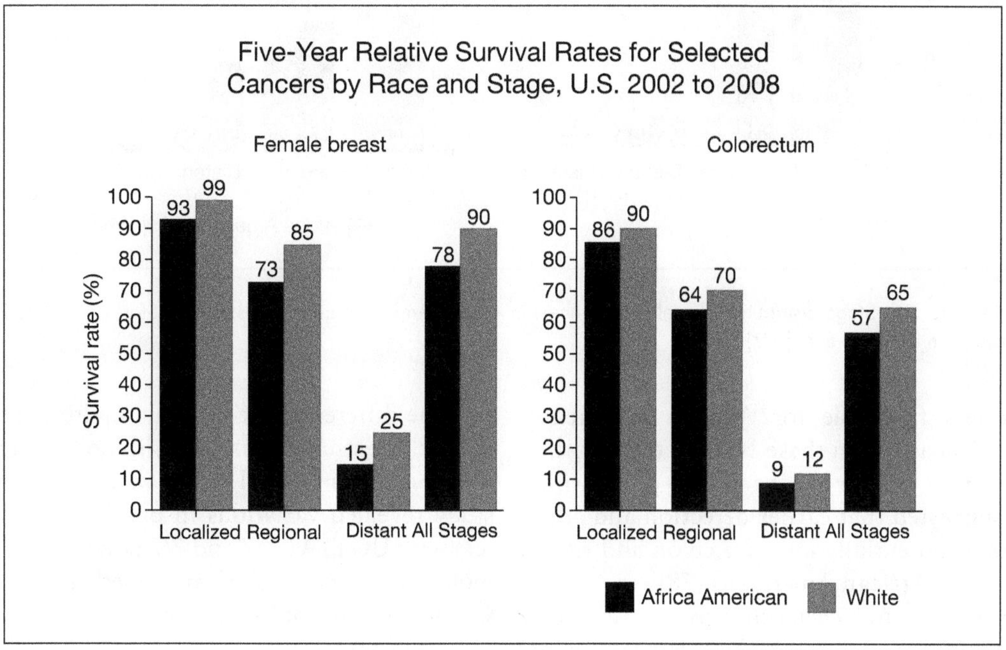

FIGURE 16.3 Five-year relative survival rates for breast and colorectal cancer. (Adapted from DeSantis et al [121].)

Comparison of Cancer Incidence Rates Between African Americans and Whites in U.S. 2005-2009

	Males			
Cancer	African American Rate	White Rate	Difference	Rate Ratio
Myeloma	13.6	6.6	7.0	2.06
Stomach	16.3	8.4	7.9	1.94
Colorectum	65.1	52.8	12.3	1.23
Prostate	228.8	140.3	88.5	1.63
Breast	1.9	1.3	0.6	1.40

FIGURE 16.4 Comparison of death rates between African Americans and whites, United States, 2005 to 1009. (Adapted from DeSantis et al [121].)

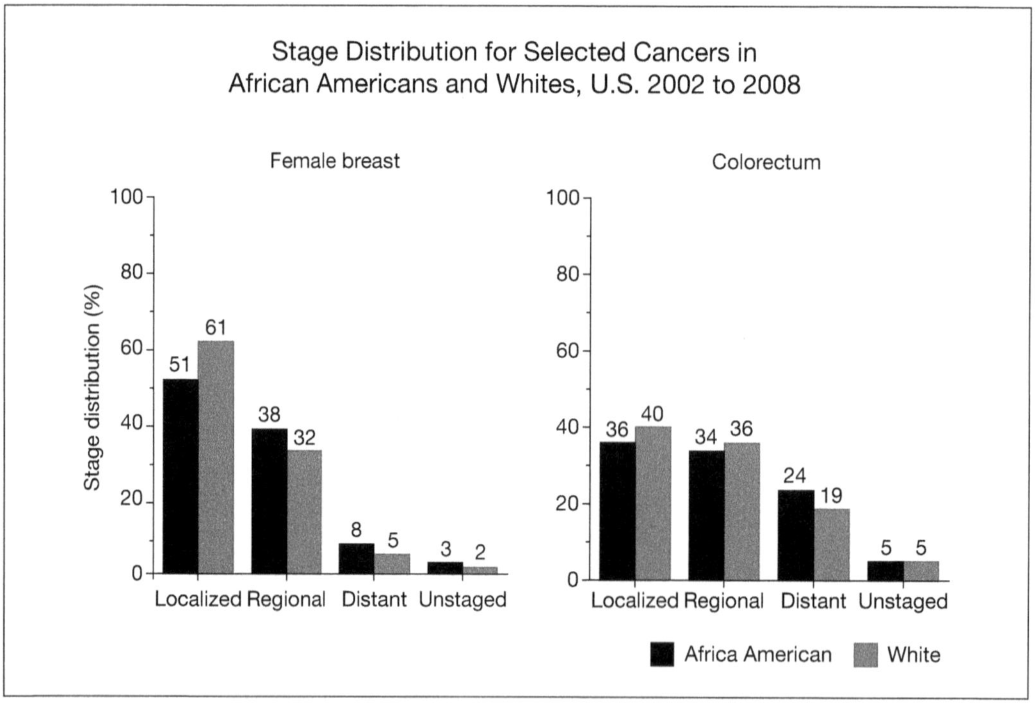

FIGURE 16. 5. Stage distribution for selectec cancers in African American and whites, United States, 2002 to 2008. (Adapted from DeSantis et al [121].)

prognosis was less favorable for African Americans compared with Caucasians in these NSABP trials, other outcomes were more similar to the whole population. These authors suggested that earlier detection and adjuvant therapy could potentially improve colon and rectal cancer prognosis for African Americans (78).

Racial variations to chemotherapy have been reported (111). Goldberg et al reported differences among Caucasians (41%) and African Americans (30%) to the chemotherapy regimens FOLFOX, IROX, or IFL.

The differences existed in a multivariate analysis and for each treatment arm, but with no differences in disease progression or overall survival. Further analyses of this study revealed variations in pharmacogenomics parameters with UGT1A1 6/7 and 7/7 polymorphisms more commonly observed in African Americans and xrcc1-r399q C/C more frequent in African Americans than Caucasians CP = 0.0006 (109).

In this, ECOG 3200 study of bevacizumab, FOLFOX, or the combination as second-line chemotherapy in patients with metastatic disease, African Americans were found to have lower response rates (10.2% vs 11.88%, P = 0.03) and overall survival (10.2 mo vs 11.2 mo, P=0.03), but no significant difference in progression-free survival (4.2 mo vs 5.0 mo; 112). Other reports of treatment differences and outcomes reveal varying results and conclusions (113–117).

■ OTHER CONSIDERATIONS

Other disease entities have been evaluated in association with CRC (118–120). In a retrospective cohort design study, the association between type 2 diabetes mellitus, colorectal cancer and subsites of the colon in African Americans and European Americans in South Carolina were studied. Individuals who had type 2 diabetes mellitus were more likely to be diagnosed with colon cancer than those without the disease and this association was higher in African Americans (118).

The association of Vitamin D deficiency was investigated with excess risk for CRC for blacks in the Third National Health and Nutrition Examination Survey (NHANES III) that was performed during the period 1988 to 1994. The results of this study indicated that black race and a history of CRC predicted CRC mortality. Vitamin D deficiency further contributed to CRC mortality when incorporated into the model. This led to the conclusion that Vitamin D deficiency was a contributing factor to the disparity of excess CRC mortality in African Americans (120).

■ CONCLUSIONS

It is well recognized that CRC mortality rates have declined, but for each stage of the disease the decrease in deaths is less for African Americans. Less is known about other minority populations because of a lack of data. Multiple factors may contribute to risks such as smoking, obesity, consumption of processed and red meat, and alcohol. Biological factors, including histopathology, stage of disease earlier age of onset, more aggressive and later stage disease in African Americans.

To address the trends, it is imperative that screening of asymptomatic individuals is imperative to intervene and provide therapy at an earlier stage.

■ REFERENCES

1. Siegel R, Naihadham D, Jemal A. Cancer Statistics, 2013. *CA Cancer J Clin.* 2013;63:11–30.
2. Ries LA, Kosary CL, Hankey BF, Miller BA, Edwards BK, eds. *SEER cancer statistics review,* 1973–1995. Bethesda (MD): National Cancer Institute; 1998.
3. Zimmerman RK, Tabbarah M, Trauth J, Nowalk MP, Ricci EM. Predictors of lower endoscopy use among patients at three inner-city neighborhood health centers. *J Urban Health.* 2006;83:221–230.
4. Etzioni DA, Yano EM, Rubenstein LV, Lee ML, Ko CY, Brook RH, Parkerton PH, Asch SM. Measuring the quality of colorectal cancer screening: the importance of follow-up. *Dis Colon Rectum.* 2006;49:1002–1010.
5. Holmes-Rovner M, Williams GA, Hoppough S, Quillan L, Butler R, Given CW. Colorectal cancer screening barriers in persons with low income. *Cancer Pract.* 2002;10:240–247.
6. Peterson NB, Murff HJ, Fowke JH, Cui Y, Hargreaves M, Signorello LB, Blot WJ. Use of colonoscopy and flexible sigmoidoscopy among African Americans and whites in a low-income population. *Prev Chronic Dis.* 2008;5:A28.
7. Peterson NB, Murff HJ, Ness RM, Dittus RS. Colorectal cancer screening among men and women in the United States. *J Womens Health (Larchmt).* 2007;16:57–65.
8. James TM, Greiner KA, Ellerbeck EF, Feng C, Ahluwalia JS. Disparities in colorectal cancer screening: a guideline-based analysis of adherence. *Ethn Dis.* 2006;16:228–233.
9. Vlahov D, Ahern J, Vazquez T, et al. Racial/ethnic differences in screening for colon cancer: report from the New York Cancer Project. *Ethn Dis.* 2005;15:76–83.
10. Janz NK, Wren PA, Schottenfeld D, Guire KE. Colorectal cancer screening attitudes and behavior: a population-based study. *Prev Med.* 2003;37:627–634.
11. Shokar NK, Carlson CA, Weller SC. Prevalence of colorectal cancer testing and screening in a multiethnic primary care population. *J Community Health.* 2007;32:311–323.
12. Shokar NK, Carlson CA, Weller SC. Factors associated with racial/ethnic differences in colorectal cancer screening. *J Am Board Fam Med.* 2008;21:414–426.
13. Zhao BB, Kilbourne B, Stain SC, et al. Racial disparities and trends in use of colorectal procedures among Tennessee elderly (1996–2000). *Ethn Dis.* 2006;16:412–420.
14. Ries LA, Wingo PA, Miller DS, et al. The annual report to the nation on the status of cancer, 1973–1997, with a special section on colorectal cancer. *Cancer.* 2000;88:2398–2424.
15. Edwards BK, Ward E, Kohler BA et al. Annual report to the nation on the status of cancer, 1975–2006, featuring colorectal cancer trends and impact of interventions (risk factors, screening and treatment) to reduce future rates. *Cancer.* 2010;116(3):544–573.
16. Robbins AS, Siegel RL, and Jemal A. Racial disparities in stage-specific colorectal cancer mortality rates from 1985 to 2008. *J Clin Oncology.* 2011;30:401–405.
17. James AS, Campbell MK, Hudson MA. Perceived barriers and benefits to colon cancer screening among African Americans in North Carolina: how does perception relate to screening behavior? *Cancer Epidemiol Biomarkers Prev.* 2002;11:529–534.
18. Lawsin C, DuHamel K, Weiss A, Rakowski W, Jandorf L. Colorectal cancer screening among low-income African Americans in East Harlem: a theoretical approach to understanding barriers and promoters to screening. *J Urban Health.* 2007;84:32–44.
19. Schroy PC 3rd, Glick JT, Robinson PA, Lydotes MA, Evans SR, Emmons KM. Has the surge in media attention increased public awareness about colorectal cancer and screening? *J Community Health.* 2008;33:1–9.
20. Palmer RC, Midgette LA, Dankwa I. Colorectal cancer screening and African Americans: findings from a qualitative study. *Cancer Control.* 2008;15:72–79.
21. Laiyemo AO, Doubeni CA, Pinsky PF, et al. Race and colorectal disparities: health care utilization versus cancer susceptibilities. *J Natl Cancer Institute.* 2010;102(8):538–546.
22. Greiner KA, Born W, Nollen N, Ahluwalia JS. Knowledge and perceptions of colorectal cancer screening among urban African Americans. *J Gen Intern Med.* 2005;20:977–983.
23. Katz ML, James AS, Pignone MP, et al. Colorectal cancer screening among African American church members: a qualitative and quantitative study of patient-provider communication. *BMC Public Health.* 2004;4:62.

24. Taylor V, Lessler D, Mertens K, et al. Colorectal cancer screening among African Americans: the importance of physician recommendation. *J Natl Med Assoc.* 2003;95:806–812.
25. Lipkus IM, Lyna PR, Rimer BK. Colorectal cancer risk perceptions and screening intentions in a minority population. *J Natl Med Assoc.* 2000;92:492–500.
26. Frank D, Swedmark J, Grubbs L. Colon cancer screening in African American women. *ABNF J.* 2004;15:67–70.
27. Coughlin SS, Thompson TD, Seeff L, Richards T, Stallings F. Breast, cervical, and colorectal carcinoma screening in a demographically defined region of the southern U.S. *Cancer.* 2002;95:2211–2222.
28. O'Malley AS, Forrest CB, Feng S, Mandelblatt J. Disparities despite coverage: gaps in colorectal cancer screening among Medicare beneficiaries. *Arch Intern Med.* 2005;165:2129–2135.
29. Shih YC, Zhao L, Elting LS. Does Medicare coverage of colonoscopy reduce racial/ethnic disparities in cancer screening among the elderly? *Health Aff (Millwood).* 2006;25:1153–1162.
30. Rajapaksa RC, Macari M, Bini EJ. Racial/ethnic differences in patient experiences with and preferences for computed tomography colonography and optical colonoscopy. *Clin Gastroenterol Hepatol.* 2007;5:1306–1312.
31. McMahon LF Jr, Wolfe RA, Huang S, Tedeschi P, Manning W Jr, Edlund MJ. Racial and gender variation in use of diagnostic colonic procedures in the Michigan Medicare population. *Med Care.* 1999;37:712–717.
32. Murff HJ, Peterson NB, Fowke JH, et al. Colonoscopy screening in African Americans and Whites with affected first-degree relatives. *Arch Intern Med.* 2008;168:625–631.
33. Murff HJ, Peterson NB, Greevy RA, Shrubsole MJ, Zheng W. Early initiation of colorectal cancer screening in individuals with affected first-degree relatives. *J Gen Intern Med.* 2007;22:121–126.
34. Griffith KA, McGuire DB, Royak-Schaler R, Plowden KO, Steinberger EK. Influence of family history and preventive health behaviors on colorectal cancer screening in African Americans. *Cancer.* 2008;113:276–285.
35. Rawl SM, Champion VL, Scott LL, et al. A randomized trial of two print interventions to increase colon cancer screening among first-degree relatives. *Patient Educ Couns.* 2008;71:215–227.
36. Dolan NC, Ferreira MR, Fitzgibbon ML et al. Colorectal cancer screening among African-American and white male veterans. *Am J Prev Med.* 2005;28:479–482.
37. Kelly KM, Dickinson SL, Degraffinreid CR, Tatum CM, Paskett ED. Colorectal cancer screening in 3 racial groups. *Am J Health Behav.* 2007;31:502–513.
38. Schenck AP, Klabunde CN, Davis WW. Racial differences in colorectal cancer test use by Medicare consumers. *Am J Prev Med.* 2006;30:320–326.
39. Fisher DA, Dougherty K, Martin C, Galanko J, Provenzale D, Sandler RS. Race and colorectal cancer screening: a population-based study in North Carolina. *N C Med J.* 2004;65:12–15.
40. Fisher DA, Jeffreys A, Coffman CJ, Fasanella K. Barriers to full colon evaluation for a positive fecal occult blood test. *Cancer Epidemiol Biomarkers Prev.* 2006;15:1232–1235.
41. McAlearney AS, Reeves KW, Dickinson SL, et al. Racial differences in colorectal cancer screening practices and knowledge within a low-income population. *Cancer.* 2008;112:391–398.
42. Rex DK, Johnson DA, Anderson JC, et al. Colorectal cancer screening. *Am J Gastroenterology.* 2009;104:739–750.
43. Lieberman DA, Holub JL, Moravec MD, Eisen GM, Peters D, Morris CD. Prevalence of colon polyps detected by colonoscopy screening in asymptomatic black and white patients. *JAMA.* 2008;300:1417–1422.
44. Phillips KA, Liang SY, Ladabaum U, et al. Trends in colonoscopy for colorectal screening. *Med Care.* 2007;45(2):160–167.
45. Shavers VL. Racial/ethnic variation in the anatomic subsite location of in situ and invasive cancers of the colon. *J Natl Med Assoc.* 2007;99:733–748.
46. Thornton JG, Morris AM, Thornton JD, Flowers CR, McCashland TM. Racial variation in colorectal polyp and tumor location. *J Natl Med Assoc* 2007;99:723–728.
47. Francois F, Park J, Bini EJ. Colon pathology detected after a positive screening flexible sigmoidoscopy: a prospective study in an ethnically diverse cohort. *Am J Gastroenterol.* 2006;101:823–830.
48. Cheng X, Chen VW, Steele B, et al. Subsite-specific incidence rate and stage of disease in colorectal cancer by race, gender, and age group in the United States, 1992–1997. *Cancer.* 2001;92:2547–2554.
49. Irby K, Anderson WF, Henson DE, Devesa SS. Emerging and widening colorectal carcinoma disparities between Blacks and Whites in the United States (1975–2002). *Cancer Epidemiol Biomarkers Prev.* 2006;15:792–797.
50. Mostafa G, Matthews BD, Norton HJ, Kercher KW, Sing RF, Heniford BT. Influence of demographics on colorectal cancer. *Am Surg.* 2004;70:259–264.
51. Nelson RL, Dollear T, Freels S, Persky V. The relation of age, race, and gender to the subsite location of colorectal carcinoma. *Cancer.* 1997;80:193–197.
52. Nelson RL, Persky V, Turyk M. Carcinoma in situ of the colorectum: SEER trends by race, gender, and total colorectal cancer. *J Surg Oncol.* 1999;71:123–129.
53. Devesa SS, Chow WH. Variation in colorectal cancer incidence in the United States by subsite of origin. *Cancer.* 1993;71:3819–3826.
54. Matanoski G, Tao XG, Almon L, Adade AA, Davies-Cole JO. Demographics and tumor characteristics of colorectal cancers in the United States, 1998–2001. *Cancer.* 2006;107:1112–1120.
55. Shipp MP, Desmond R, Accortt N, Wilson RJ, Fouad M, Eloubeidi MA. Population-based study of the geographic variation in colon cancer incidence in Alabama: relationship to socioeconomic status indicators and physician density. *South Med J.* 2005;98:1076–1082.
56. Haas JS, Earle CC, Orav JE, Brawarsky P, Neville BA, Williams DR. Racial segregation and disparities in cancer stage for seniors. *J Gen Intern Med.* 2008;23:699–705.
57. Cress RD, Morris C, Ellison GL, Goodman MT. Secular changes in colorectal cancer incidence by subsite, stage at diagnosis, and race/ethnicity, 1992–2001. *Cancer.* 2006;107:1142–1152.
58. Theuer CP, Taylor TH, Brewster WR, Anton-Culver H. Gender and race/ethnicity affect the cost-effectiveness of colorectal cancer screening. *J Natl Med Assoc.* 2006;98:51–57.
59. Fairley TL, Cardinez CJ, Martin J, et al. Colorectal cancer in U.S. adults younger than 50 years of age, 1998–2001. *Cancer.* 2006;107:1153–1161.
60. Agrawal S, Bhupinderjit A, Bhutani MS, et al. Colorectal cancer in African Americans. *Am J Gastroenterol.* 2005;100:515–523; discussion 514.
61. Satia-Abouta J, Galanko JA, Martin CF, Potter JD, Ammerman A, Sandler RS. Associations of micronutrients with colon cancer risk in African Americans and whites: results from the North Carolina Colon Cancer Study. *Cancer Epidemiol Biomarkers Prev.* 2003;12:747–754.
62. Sansbury LB, Millikan RC, Schroeder JC, Moorman PG, North KE, Sandler RS. Use of nonsteroidal antiinflammatory drugs and risk of colon cancer in a population-based, case-control study of African Americans and Whites. *Am J Epidemiol.* 2005;162:548–558.
63. Satia-Abouta J, Galanko JA, Potter JD, Ammerman A, Martin CF, Sandler RS. Associations of total energy and macronutrients with colon cancer risk in African Americans and Whites: results from the North Carolina colon cancer study. *Am J Epidemiol.* 2003;158:951–962.
64. O'Keefe SJ, Chung D, Mahmoud N, et al. Why do African Americans get more colon cancer than Native Africans? *J Nutr.* 2007;137:175S–182S.
65. Fulgoni V 3rd, Nicholls J, Reed A, Buckley et al. Dairy consumption and related nutrient intake in African-American adults and children in the

United States: continuing survey of food intakes by individuals 1994–1996, 1998, and the National Health And Nutrition Examination Survey 1999–2000. *J Am Diet Assoc.* 2007;107:256–264.

66. Huang K, Sandler RS, Millikan RC, Schroeder JC, North KE, Hu J. GSTM1 and GSTT1 polymorphisms, cigarette smoking, and risk of colon cancer: a population-based case-control study in North Carolina (United States). *Cancer Causes Control.* 2006;17:385–394.
67. Slattery ML, Herrick J, Wolff RK, Caan BJ, Potter JD, Sweeney C. CDX2 VDR polymorphism and colorectal cancer. *Cancer Epidemiol Biomarkers Prev.* 2007;16:2752–2755.
68. KekuT,MillikanR,WorleyK,etal.5,10-Methylenetetrahydrofolate reductase codon 677 and 1298 polymorphisms and colon cancer in African Americans and whites. *Cancer Epidemiol Biomarkers Prev.* 2002;11:1611–1621.
69. Goodman JE, Bowman ED, Chanock SJ, Alberg AJ, Harris CC. Arachidonate lipoxygenase (ALOX) and cyclooxygenase (COX) polymorphisms and colon cancer risk. *Carcinogenesis.* 2004;25:2467–2472.
70. Peters U, McGlynn KA, Chatterjee N, et al. Vitamin D, calcium, and vitamin D receptor polymorphism in colorectal adenomas. *Cancer Epidemiol Biomarkers Prev.* 2001;10:1267–1274.
71. Piffath TA, Whiteman MK, Flaws JA, Fix AD, Busht TL. Ethnic differences in cancer mortality trends in the US, 1950–1992. *Ethn Health.* 2001;6:105–119.
72. Minardi AJ Jr, Sittig KM, Zibari GB, McDonald JC. Colorectal cancer in the young patient. *Am. J Surg.* 1998;64:849–853.
73. Petitjean A, Achatz MI, Borresen-Dale AL, Hainaut P, Olivier M. TP53mutationsinhumancancers:functionalselectionandimpacton cancer prognosis and outcomes. *Oncogene.* 2007;26:2157–2165.
74. Irby K, Anderson WF, Henson DE, Devesa SS. Emerging and widening colorectal carcinoma disparities between blacks and whites in the United States (1975–2002). *Cancer Epidemiol. Biomarkers Prev.* 2009;18(6):1695–1698.
75. AxtellLM,MyersMH.Contrastsinsurvivalofblackandwhitecancer patients, 1960–73. *J Natl Cancer Inst.* 1978;60:1209–1215.
76. Miller BA, Kolonel LN, Bernstein L, Young JL Jr, Swanson GM, West D, eds. *Racial/Ethnic Patterns of Cancer in the United States 1988–1992.* Bethesda (MD): National Institutes of Health, National Cancer Institute; 1996 Report No.: DHHS Publ No. (NIH) 96.
77. Bach PB, Schrag D, Brawley OW, Galaznik A, Yakren S, Begg CB. Survival of blacks and whites after a cancer diagnosis. *JAMA.* 2002;287:2106–2113.
78. Dignam JJ, Ye Y, Colangelo L, et al. Prognosis after rectal cancer in blacks and whites participating in adjuvant therapy randomized trials. *J Clin Oncol.* 2003;21:413–420.
79. Du XL, Fang S, Vernon SW, et al. Racial disparities and socioeconomic status in association with survival in a large population-based cohort of elderly patients with colon cancer. *Cancer.* 2007;110:660–669.
80. Mayberry RM, Coates RJ, Hill HA, et al. Determinants of black/white differences in colon cancer survival. *J Natl Cancer Inst.* 1995;87:1686–1693.
81. Gomez SL, O'Malley CD, Stroup A, Shema SJ, Satariano WA. Longitudinal, population-based study of racial/ethnic differences in colorectal cancer survival: impact of neighborhood socioeconomic status, treatment and comorbidity. *BMC Cancer.* 2007;7:193.
82. Du XL, Meyer TE, Franzini L. Meta-analysis of racial disparities in survival in association with socioeconomic status among men and women with colon cancer. *Cancer.* 2007;109:2161–2170.
83. Marcella S, Miller JE. Racial differences in colorectal cancer mortality. The importance of stage and socioeconomic status. *J Clin Epidemiol.* 2001;54:359–366.
84. Chien C, Morimoto LM, Tom J, Li CI. Differences in colorectal carcinoma stage and survival by race and ethnicity. *Cancer.* 2005;104:629–639.
85. Le H, Ziogas A, Lipkin SM, Zell JA. Effects of socioeconomic status and treatment disparities in colorectal cancer survival. *Cancer Epidemiol Biomarkers Prev.* 2008;17:1950–1962.
86. Kinsey T, Jemal A, Liff J, Ward E, Thun M. Secular trends in mortality from common cancers in the United States by educational attainment, 1993–2001. *J Natl Cancer Inst.* 2008;100:1003–1012.
87. Alexander D, Chatla C, Funkhouser E, Meleth S, Grizzle WE, Manne U. Postsurgical disparity in survival between African Americans and Caucasians with colonic adenocarcinoma. *Cancer.* 2004;101:66–76.
88. Alexander D, Jhala N, Chatla C, et al. High-grade tumor differentiation is an indicator of poor prognosis in African Americans with colonic adenocarcinomas. *Cancer.* 2005;103:2163–2170.
89. Wudel LJ Jr, Chapman WC, Shyr Y, et al. Disparate outcomes in patients with colorectal cancer: effect of race on long-term survival. *Arch Surg.* 2002;137:550–554; discussion 554–556.
90. Ayanian JZ, Zaslavsky AM, Guadagnoli E, et al. Patients' perceptions of quality of care for colorectal cancer by race, ethnicity, and language. *J Clin Oncol.* 2005;23:6576–6586.
91. Morris AM, Billingsley KG, Baxter NN, Baldwin LM. Racial disparities in rectal cancer treatment: a population-based analysis. *Arch Surg.* 2004;139:151–155; discussion 156.
92. Doubeni CA, Field TS, Buist DS, et al. Racial differences in tumor stage and survival for colorectal cancer in an insured population. *Cancer.* 2007;109:612–620.
93. Demissie K, Oluwole OO, Balasubramanian BA, Osinubi OO, August D, Rhoads GG. Racial differences in the treatment of colorectal cancer: a comparison of surgical and radiation therapy between Whites and Blacks. *Ann Epidemiol.* 2004;14:215–221.
94. Rogers SO, Ray WA, Smalley WE. A population-based study of survival among elderly persons diagnosed with colorectal cancer: does race matter if all are insured? (United States). *Cancer Causes Control.* 2004;15:193–199.
95. Morris AM, Wei Y, Birkmeyer NJ, Birkmeyer JD. Racial disparities in late survival after rectal cancer surgery. *J Am Coll Surg.* 2006;203:787–794.
96. Govindarajan R, Shah RV, Erkman LG, Hutchins LF. Racial differences in the outcome of patients with colorectal carcinoma. *Cancer.* 2003;97:493–498.
97. Jessup JM, Stewart A, Greene FL, Minsky BD. Adjuvant chemotherapy for stage III colon cancer: implications of race/ethnicity, age, and differentiation. *JAMA.* 2005;294:2703–2711.
98. Morris AM, Billingsley KG, Hayanga AJ, Matthews B, Baldwin LM, Birkmeyer JD. Residual treatment disparities after oncology referral for rectal cancer. *J Natl Cancer Inst.* 2008;100:738–744.
99. Baldwin LM, Dobie SA, Billingsley K, et al. Explaining black-white differences in receipt of recommended colon cancer treatment. *J Natl Cancer Inst.* 2005;97:1211–1220.
100. Potosky AL, Harlan LC, Kaplan RS, Johnson KA, Lynch CF. Age, sex, and racial differences in the use of standard adjuvant therapy for colorectal cancer. *J Clin Oncol.* 2002;20:1192–1202.
101. Ahuja N, Chang D, Gearhart SL. Disparities in colon cancer presentation and in-hospital mortality in Maryland: a ten-year review. *Ann Surg Oncol.* 2007;14:411–416.
102. Chen VW, Fenoglio-Preiser CM, Wu XC, et al. Aggressiveness of colon carcinoma in blacks and whites. National Cancer Institute Black/White Cancer Survival Study Group. *Cancer Epidemiol Biomarkers Prev.* 1997;6:1087–1093.
103. Ikenaga M, Tomita N, Sekimoto M et al. Use of microsatellite analysis in young patients with colorectal cancer to identify those with hereditary non polyposis colorectal cancer. *J Surg Oncol.* 2002;79:157–165 (2002).
104. Berg M, Danielsen SA, Ahlquist T et al. DNA sequence profiles of colorectal cancer critical gene set K-ras–BRAF–PIK3CA–PTEN–TP53 related disease at onset. *PLoS ONE5.* 2010;(11):e13978 (2010).
105. Lothe RA, Peltomaki P, Meling GI et al. Genomic instability in colorectal cancer: relationship to clinicopathological variables and family history. *Cancer Res.* 1993;53:5849–5452.
106. Popat S, Huber R, Houlston RS. Systematic review of microsatellite instability and colorectal cancer prognosis. *J Clin Oncol.* 2005;23:609–618.

107. Ashktorab H, Smoot DT, Carethers JM, et al. High incidence of microsatellite instability in colorectal cancer from African Americans. *Clinical Cancer Res.* 2003;9:1112–1117.
108. Jovov B, Araujo-Perez F, Sigel CS et al. Differential Gene Expression between African and European American Colorectal Cancer Patients. *PLoS ONE7.* 2012;(1):e30168.
109. Kumar K, Brim H, Giardello F et al. Distinct BRAF (V600E) and K-ras mutation in high microsatellite instability sporadic colorectal cancer in African Americans. *Clin Cancer Res.* 2009:15(4):1155–1161.
110. McLeod HL, Parodi L, Sargent J, Marsh et al. UGT1A1*28 toxicity and outcome in advanced colorectal cancer: Results from trial N9741. 2006 ASCO Annual Meeting Abstract No. 3520.
111. Koshiji M, Kumamoto K, Morimura K, et al. Correlation of N-myc downstream-regulated gene 1 expression with clinical outcomes of colorectal cancer patients of different race/ethnicity. *World J Gastroenterol.* 2007;13:2803.
112. Goldberg RM, McLeod HL, Sargent DJ Morton RF, et al. Genetic polymorphisms, toxicity, and response rate in African Americans (AA) with metastatic colorectal cancer (MCRC) compared to Caucasians (C) when treated with IFL, FOLFOX or IROX in Intergroup N9741. 2006 ASCO Annual Meeting Abstract No. 3503.
113. Catalano PJ, Mitchell EP, Giantonio BJ, Meropol NJ, Benson AB. Outcomes of African Americans and Caucasians treated with bevacizumab, FOLFOX4 or the combination in patients with metastatic colorectal cancer (MCRC): Results from the Eastern Coooperative Oncology Group Study E3200. 2007 ASCO Annual Meeting Abstract No. 4100.
114. Potosky AL, Harlan LC, Kaplan RS, et al. Age, sex, and racial differences in the use of standard adjuvant therapy for colorectal cancer. *J Clin Oncol.* 2002; 20(5):1192–1202.
115. Dobie SA, Baldwin LM, Dominitz JA, Matthews B, Billingsley K, Barlow W. Completion of therapy by Medicare patients with stage III colon cancer. *J Natl Cancer Inst.* 2006;98:610–619.
116. McGory ML, Zingmond DS, Sekeris E, Bastani R, Ko CY. A patient's race/ethnicity does not explain the underuse of appropriate adjuvant therapy in colorectal cancer. *Dis Colon Rectum.* 2006;49:319–329.
117. McCollum AD, Catalano PJ, Haller DG, et al. Outcomes and toxicity in African-American and Caucasian patients in a randomized adjuvant chemotherapy trial for colon cancer. *J Natl Cancer Inst.* 2002;94:1160–1167.
118. Mattison LK, Fourie J, Desmond RA, Modak A, Saif MW, Diasio RB. Increased prevalence of dihydropyrimidine dehydrogenase deficiency in African Americans compared with Caucasians. *Clin Cancer Res.* 2006;12:5491–5495.
119. Cavicchia PP, Adams SA, Steck SE, et al. Racial disparities in colorectal cancer by type 2 diabetes mellitus status. *Cancer Causes Control.* 2013;24 (2): 277–285.
120. Hu FB, Manson JE, Liu S, Hunter D, et al. Prospective study of adult onset diabetes mellitus (type 2) and risk of colorectal cancer in women. *J Natl Cancer Inst.* 1999;91(6):542–547.
121. Fiscella K, Winters P, Tancredi D, et al. Racial disparity in death from colorectal cancer. a randomized adjuvant chemotherapy trial for colon cancer. *J Natl Cancer Institute.* 2002;94:1160–1167.
122. DeSantis C, Naishadham D, Jemal A. Cancer statistics for African Americans, 2013. *Ca Cancer J Clin.* 2013;63:151–166.
123. Sylvester BE, Huo D, Khramtsov A, et al. Molecular analysis of colorectal tumors from a diverse cohort at a single institution. *Clin Cancer Res.* 2012;18(2):350–359.

17 Models of Care Delivery

JULIA TROSMAN
CHRISTINE WELDON

Delivery of care to patients with colorectal cancer (CRC) is a complex challenging process involving multiple specialties in a variety of settings. Many of these challenges are common to the U.S. health care system (1), and to oncology in general (2), but unique issues exist in the care for CRC patients (3,4). This chapter describes the challenges of CRC care delivery and reviews how the emerging and evolving care delivery models may apply to that care. We offer a view of a future CRC delivery model, and suggest how care providers may prepare for it. The chapter is concluded with a case study, provided by Patrick J. Flynn, of how some of the care models may be implemented in the community setting.

CHALLENGES OF CRC CARE DELIVERY—A PERFECT STORM?

In the last two decades, oncology medicine has seen tremendous scientific advances, but it also found itself in a "perfect storm" of challenges for care providers, patients, and payers. Several interrelated trends contribute to these challenges and underscore the need to modernize care delivery models.

Fragmentation of Care Delivery

Scientific advancements drove both a higher degree of oncology specialization, and a need for more coordinated participation of multiple disciplines in cancer care. As specialties organized into clinical domains (eg, surgery, medical oncology, radiology), coordination across domains became more difficult. A CRC patient may receive care from over a dozen domains: gastroenterology; surgery; medical oncology; radiology; radiation oncology; diagnostics/pathology; primary care; co-morbidity care (eg, cardiology); genetic counseling; supportive care (psychosocial therapy, nutrition, etc); palliative care, disease management (eg, from a health plan), and others. The care domains serving one patient may exist within different care settings, organizations, and geographies. For example, a rectal cancer patient may receive surgery in an academic institution, radiation treatment in a local hospital and adjuvant chemotherapy in a local private oncology practice.

Resulting Gaps

- Disconnect of care decisions and care plans across providers. Each domain serving a CRC patient may create a care plan, but there is rarely one integrated plan; care decisions are not aligned across domains. Domains are often involved in care of one patient sequentially, rather than concurrently. Joint decision making occurs ad hoc rather than planned.
- Lack of the overall physician "quarterback." Although there is often a physician directing care for a given patient within a specific domain, no one typically oversees patient care and aligns medical decisions across domains from the beginning throughout the care continuum.
- Lack of patient-level coordination. Faced with fragmentation, patient and family are compelled to "shuttle" between care domains, reconcile care decisions from multiple physicians, and coordinate their own care. There is a need to focus coordination around the patient as he/she receives care across multiple care events and domains in the care continuum.

These gaps may be especially pronounced in CRC, with a predominantly older patient population who are covered by Medicare. Medicare, in contrast to many private health plans, does not provide disease management services, leaving patients to deal with care fragmentation on their own.

Personalization of Care

Personalization of care is driven by several converging trends: (a) development of biomarkers that allow tailoring treatment to patient biological traits; (b) expansion of treatment options for a specific condition; (c) increased patient education and awareness. Personalized care requires shared decision making which weighs both clinical factors and patient preferences. In CRC, there are a number of decisions that require the patient to participate in shared decision making, such as the decision to use gene expression profile tests for Stage II colon cancer patients to assess the probably of recurrence and assist in treatment decisions (5).

Resulting Gaps

- Lack of an effective delivery model for personalized care and shared decision making. Care personalization and shared decision making requires substantial physician time, which is difficult to devote under cost pressures. To deliver truly personalized care, patient preferences need to be established, recorded, and used by all providers involved. There is currently no framework or capability to support this need.
- Lack of support for patient education. Personalized care is contingent upon an informed and active patient. CRC patients may not have access to sufficient education and support resources, which exist in other cancers, such as breast cancer, where numerous patient advocacies provide peer counseling and other support.

Inadequate Provider Reimbursement Model

The current oncology reimbursement model emerged in the 1970s. It combines the fee-for-service payment for cognitive services (common to the rest of health care) with "buy-and-bill" reimbursement for infusion therapeutics, which is based on a drug markup (a component unique to oncology and a limited number of other specialties). The "buy-and-bill" reimbursement historically has been a substantial source of revenue for oncology providers, while the fee-for-service component has not kept pace with growing costs of care (6). For example, it may not consistently reimburse supportive care (eg, psychosocial counseling) and genetic counseling (eg, related to Lynch syndrome). Historically, oncology practices utilized the drug markup revenue to subsidize the services that are not directly reimbursed. However, the recent moves by Medicare and private insurers to limit the markup on infusion drugs (7) challenge the ability of providers to sustain these and other services (6,8).

Resulting Gap

The reimbursement system creates barriers to contemporary CRC care. Care providers strive to deliver appropriate care, but they often do this despite the inherent disincentives and barriers of the reimbursement system. The impact of reimbursement on treatment decisions was demonstrated in studies by Jacobson et al (9,10). Oral therapies that have been introduced in recent years in colorectal and other cancers are an important example of misaligned reimbursement: they are not subject to buy-and-bill reimbursement, and there may be a disincentive to prescribe them versus infusion drugs.

Escalating Costs of Oncology Care

Oncology is considered one of the most expensive areas of health care, and CRC is the second largest source of cancer expenditures (11). The cost containment efforts by private and public payers have escalated in the recent years and are expected to continue in the future. Changes in Medicare reimbursement of infusion drugs resulted in net reduction of provider revenues (8,12) driving consolidation of oncology providers and a trend toward hospital-based oncology care. As population aging contributes to the rise of cancer incidents, the cost pressures for payers and providers may further intensify.

Resulting Gaps

- Lack of a mechanism to contain costs without compromising care. Oncology providers may not have financial resources to continue offering services that are now subsidized by the buy-and-bill model. As part of cost containment, patient out-of-pocket costs increase, creating an incentive for patients to compromise or avoid care.
- Capacity and viability challenges. The trends described above, coupled with predicted shortage of oncologists, aging population, and related increase in CRC incidents, will likely pose provider capacity shortage and risk to organizational viability of cancer providers.

■ DO EMERGING DELIVERY MODELS ADDRESS CHALLENGES?

In the last two decades, a number of solutions for oncology care delivery have emerged or have been adapted from chronic disease and primary care. The impact of these models on patient outcomes, cost of care, or coordination gaps has not been demonstrated beyond small trials or single institution experiences, although larger studies are underway. Here we describe several key examples of the models relevant to oncology care delivery, and offer an opinion whether they address the current gaps (Table 17.1).

Patient Navigation Models

Background

Patient navigation (the assessment and alleviation of barriers to adequate health care by a specifically trained

Table 17.1 Summary of Emerging Care Models and Their Impact on Current Gaps

	Current Gaps and Needs						
Model	Disconnect of Care Decisions and Care Plans Across Providers	Lack of the Overall Physician "Quarterback"	Lack of Patient-Level Coordination	Need to Personalize Care	Need Right Incentives for Right Care and Coordination	Escalating Care Costs	Oncology Practice Viability and Capacity
Patient navigator models			++	+			+
Multidisciplinary care models (meetings, teams, clinics)	+	+	+			+–	–
Medical home models	–	++	+	+	+	+–	–
Risk/reward sharing payment models (eg, ACO, bundled payment)	+–		+–		+	+–	+–

++, model addresses the gap; +, model partially addresses the gap; +–, the impact is unknown and may be positive or negative; –, negative impact; Blank, model does not address the gap.

person) emerged in the 1990s from the need to reduce cancer care disparities by helping the patient navigate the maze of fragmented health care (13). The navigation models are now widely adopted in oncology care, with the common feature of a "go-to" person working with and on behalf of the patient to satisfy the patient's care-coordination needs. There is a large variability in who plays this role (eg, a nurse, a social worker, or a trained lay person), what aspects of care the navigator helps to coordinate (eg, logistical or clinical) and how the role is financed (eg, funded by a charity or budgeted by a care organization;14–17).

Advantages and Limitations

Patient navigation is one of the few models that directly address the gap in patient-level care coordination and education. Its support of the patient in shared decision making is especially relevant for CRC patients, who reported in a study that they valued information support from a navigator above logistical and other services (18). Patient navigation may moderately contribute to practice capacity, as navigators take on functions that would be otherwise performed by a nurse or a physician. A key limitation of the navigation models is that while they help patients navigate the care "maze," they do not improve the maze itself. It is typically not the duty of a navigator to ensure that physicians communicate with each other regarding a specific patient, or that the care plans from different domains for a single patient are aligned. In fact, a study shows that navigators struggle when put between the physicians and the patient, or when faced with the patient's medical dilemmas (19). Another limitation is a navigator may be effective within a medical center, but have limited reach to help patients beyond the organizational walls, eg, in transitioning to a private oncology practice that may not have its own navigator function. And finally, the navigator service is currently not reimbursed, and its sustainability is subject to availability of charity funds or to the willingness of care organizations to internally fund this function. It is not clear whether patient navigation ultimately helps to contain and/or reduce net care costs.

Multidisciplinary Decision Models

Background

The multidisciplinary (MD) decision models emerged in 1990s in chronic care from models such as the Chronic Care Model (20,21) and were adopted in oncology to address the disconnect among care domains, decisions, and care plans. These models may take several forms: (a) MD meetings (ie, tumor boards)—the most common form; (b) MD teams which include MD meetings, development of a coherent care plan, and consultations from several domains in one patient visit; (c) MD clinics—a more formal organization of MD teams and meetings, which may include physician remuneration for participation, and a patient navigator who helps the patient with downstream care. The MD models vary widely in their features, such as which cancers are included, whether and how community providers are included, and whether and how patients are included in decision making (22–28).

Advantages and Limitations

MD models are reported to overcome the coordination gaps, align care decisions, and develop care plans across domains, especially during the diagnosis and initial care planning. Consultations from multiple disciplines in one patient visit improve patient-level coordination, and patient satisfaction (27,29). However, other advantages of MD models are subject to institutional implementation, eg, they may or may not include a navigator helping the patient with downstream care; and may or may not consider patients returning for follow up. Thus, downstream care decisions may lack the multidisciplinary approach. Few institutions establish the formal role of lead physician, or quarterback, to oversee downstream care. MD models typically do not include patients in the MD meetings, which may limit their support for care personalization and shared decision making (30,31). MD models may be complex and expensive to set up and operate (28,32,33), potentially adding to the costs of care and negatively impacting the organizational care capacity. Typically designed around face-to-face meetings and co-located consultations, these models may not use the physicians' time efficiently (24,27,34) and could become impractical and cost prohibitive if rolled out beyond large institutions (32). Until asynchronous and remote "virtual" team communication is feasible, these models may not become a reality for community oncology where 85% of cancer care is delivered.

Medical Home Models

Background

In response to fragmentation in primary care, attrition of primary care physicians and escalating costs of chronic disease, it has been proposed to establish a "Medical Home" model. In this model, a personal primary care physician is the focal point of care for a patient, with the responsibility to coordinate care for a patient across subspecialists, hospitals, and other domains and settings. In 2007, the American Academy of Family Physicians, the American Academy of Pediatrics, the American College of Physicians, and the American Osteopathic Association developed joint principles of the Patient Centered Medical Home, which include: personal physician; physician directed medical practice; coordinated and integrated care; quality and safety; enhanced access; and appropriate payment (35). To address specialty care, the authors of the model suggested additional principles of how medical home models may transition to an oncologist, using CRC as an example (36). Some oncology practices have also established and described themselves as an oncology medical home (37,38). Although there is little data on effectiveness of the medical home models, they have been embraced by health systems and public and private payers who have conducted a number of demonstration projects in primary care.

Advantages and Limitations

Key advantages of the medical home model, if applied to CRC delivery, include a formalized physician quarterback and formal reimbursement for improved care coordination. Oncology medical home has the potential to facilitate patients' experiences across domains and patients' participation in care decisions, but it will require further development, such as inclusion of a navigator, making the metrics more patient-oriented, providing a framework for effective patient involvement in care, and improving the reimbursement model (39). A key limitation of the model is the lack of a framework to facilitate patient transition across domains: The suggested approach to develop agreements between providers involved in transition may in fact cause friction in provider relationships and increase provider burden (40,41). Additionally, complex patients with significant comorbidities (common in CRC) may require that other specialists (eg, diabetes specialists) are equally involved in the care of these patients. A framework for such concurrent involvement and leadership by multiple physicians needs to be developed.

Risk/Reward Sharing Payment Models

Background

Emerging in the mid 2000s, new provider payment models intend to contain rising health care costs while making providers accountable for quality and costs of care. The two most notable examples—Accountable Care Organization (ACO) and episode of care payment models—have received significant attention, such as inclusion in the Patient Protection and Affordable Care Act (HR2490). In contrast to the current fee-for-service reimbursement, provider payment would be predetermined and averaged annually or bundled around an episode of care, effectively shifting the financial risk to the care provider. These models have been proposed for implementation in cancer care, including colorectal care (42,43).

Advantages and Limitations

The proposed models enable care organizations with discretion on how they contain costs, without micromanaging the process. They create incentives for both the adherence to guidelines and for care coordination as dimensions of quality care. Although they do not eliminate the drug bill-and-buy approach, the "capped" payment system may limit the impact of the drug margin incentives on provider care decisions. However, the ability of these models to contain costs is arguable: They will likely drive further consolidation of care providers, and even create health care monopolies who may gain significant negotiation leverage with payers (44). Although the ACO model has been linked to the implementation of medical home, no footprint exists to ensure that the new payment models will support care coordination. Specific to cancer care, these models do not explicitly account for multidisciplinary approaches to care, especially across organizational walls, and may in fact drive a divide between domains if payment distribution is perceived suboptimal. The coordination and personalization of care is left to the discretion of care organizations, which may potentially forego them if faced with significant cost pressures. Safeguards need to be put in place to ensure that care organizations do not avoid providing care to high-cost patients, including CRC patients. Finally, these models drive patients to obtain all care within one care organization, which may not always optimal for all cancer patients.

PREPARING FOR THE FUTURE CANCER DELIVERY MODEL

In the last several decades, many seemingly imminent health care movements lost momentum, reversed themselves, or evolved into a different trend. Although it is difficult to predict how the dynamics described above will develop in the next decade or two, below we hypothesize on the features of the future CRC delivery model and offer considerations for oncology providers. The future scenario and related trends are described below.

1. A need for multidisciplinary decision making and care coordination across provider organizations may intensify. While provider consolidation and transition toward hospital-based care will likely continue, the consolidated entities may not be well integrated, and therefore will require coordination both within and across their boundaries. Additionally, consolidation may be tamed by anti-trust and other concerns, keeping the multidomain, cross-organization care in place.
2. The multidisciplinary care model will evolve into a virtual team led by a "quarterback" physician, include the patient as a team member and be customized to the patient's clinical needs and preferences. These features will be necessitated by several trends: (a) increasingly informed patients will want a choice of how to be involved in care decisions; (b) lack of capacity to provide the full team to every patient will require a "modular" team approach and customization of the team composition to patient subgroups. This may be similar to a "modular" team approach described by Valgus et al (45) where in addition to the base team, there is a roaming team of pharmacist and several other specialists only for patients requiring palliative care.
3. Care team will have an option for asynchronous electronic participation, supported by Health IT. Without this feature, there will be severe shortage of operational capacity and financial resources to broadly implement the contemporary models of cancer care. Current and future information of information technology will support the requirements for privacy and security while facilitating effective sharing of information and joint decision making. However, expanded decision making may lead to a greatly increased amount of extra time required from clinicians. This concern may be partly addressed via a systemic approach to care planning (below).
4. Cancer care will be planned and coordinated using systems engineering methodologies and project management principles. According to the Institute of Medicine, clinical and organizational complexity of cancer care, as well as mounting cost pressures, require that systems engineering principles, used in many other industries, be applied to care planning and delivery (46). However, there is a danger to "over-engineer" medicine, especially in cancer care, which deals with life-threatening disease. One of the systemic tools that may be appropriate for cancer care is the project management discipline. Applying project management principles to cancer care, the virtual care team will have formalized roles to avoid duplication and gaps in care, will be led by the "quarterback" physician as a project manager, and will follow a care plan specifying the sequencing and timing of care events, as well as responsibilities of the team members for each event. This framework will support the notion of provider accountability while serving as an effective communication tool.
5. Cost pressure and risk sharing will continue, making care coordination the financial responsibility of providers. Care delivery improvements will likely be subject to a zero-sum rule, that is, there won't be additional money in the health care system to pay for them, and they will need to be self-paid. Provider quality measurements will be adjusted to include metrics related to the new models.

Considerations for Providers

1. Prepare to work more extensively and effectively with other care providers and domains in a formalized fashion. Start to develop specific relationships with providers who are complementary to your services. For example, medical oncologists may develop specific relationships with gastroenterologists in order to provide comprehensive care, provide referrals, and ultimately develop a multidisciplinary care team—within or across organizations.
2. Become acquainted with systems engineering tools that are being implemented in health care and may be deployed in oncology, eg, six sigma and project management discipline.
3. Identify opportunities where patients may benefit from a lead physician role. Although the role may not

be reimbursed, this will add an important benefit to your patients and will position you well for the evolving multidisciplinary team structure. Determine how to deal with challenges of the current culture of physician's autonomy.

4. Care organizations will need to invest more money and resources into health IT that supports coordination across care sites, beyond the electronic medical record systems. Encourage your organization to improve internal health IT to allow seamless care coordination, including workflow. Develop internal guidelines on how to handle the potential increase in electronic activities both between providers and from the patients.
5. Develop a framework for (a) discussing financial issues with patients and colleagues and (b) for sharing resources with other organizations, both medical and patient advocacies. For example, organizations such as the Patient Advocate Foundation provide some level of co-pay relief to insured patients in need. Find out what organizations support your geographic area. Developing long-term payment plans, and identifying shared payments may be necessary. Develop relationships with safety net providers that will support your patients if they lose insurance and you are no longer able to care for them.

Implementation of Multidisciplinary CRC Care at Abbott Northwestern Hospital, Minneapolis, MN

Community Case Study by Patrick J. Flynn

Our multidisciplinary CRC program has developed over decades to our best practices but is frequently changing as we observe new priorities. We have recognized the importance of an institutional plan to track existing structures, measure results, identify needs, and find solutions. Below, I describe the features of our program and offer considerations, which we found invaluable for successful program implementation and ongoing development.

Program Description

Our urban hospital is a tertiary referral center with over 800 beds that is an academic affiliate with the University of Minnesota Medical School. This may not be typical of other community programs but our program strategies can be adapted to other community based programs by tailoring to the identified goals and strengths. The formation of a Comprehensive Colorectal Program is designed to provide coordinated patient care. The most important component of this coordination has been provided by the nurse coordinator (navigator). This allows the patient to have one "point person" who can be contacted to facilitate interaction with all specialists and services. Physicians and staff are not all employed by single entity but we are all located within a "campus" spanning several blocks. While we considered a model of one clinic with all staff meeting patients and family the logistics and scheduling were not feasible. Patients will, however, frequently meet multiple staff on the same day to coordinate treatment thus speeding care delivery. As referring physicians have become familiar with the program direct contact for new patient referral is often made with the nurse coordinator who schedules the appropriate consultations and gathers the needed records.

The use of regularly scheduled (usually weekly) working tumor conferences has been extraordinarily successful for patient management. Our goal is to present the majority of patients before all definitive therapy has been completed. Review of history, imaging, and pathology often results in changes of the original plans based on new observations or insights. Specific case review also fosters education and participation in clinical trials. The program staff should be encouraged to attend tumor conferences to improve overall care. Input during tumor conferences has resulted in two vital changes to improve our programs. Pathology reports now follow planned templates to be certain of accuracy and content. Discussion of staging and treatment with National Comprehensive Cancer Network (NCCN) guidelines as a point of reference are expected during the patient review.

Research has been a major component of our program with our efforts to include National Cancer Institute funded cooperative group research (member of Metro-Minnesota CCOP since 1983). We have other affiliations, industry, and local research studies that are ongoing. Our most successful model has been to base the study research coordinators in the clinic so they can be as near as possible to patient care activities. This results in improved accrual, patient satisfaction, patient oversight, and staff enthusiasm. The physicians appreciate the ease of contact that near proximity offers.

In addition to treatment of those with newly diagnosed CRC, our program incorporated other services: screening (including identification of individuals with inherited disorders such as Lynch syndrome); surveillance based on NCCN guidelines; genetic counseling; cancer rehabilitation; and survivorship. The incorporation of these added capabilities has taken time but been helpful to our population.

The specific resources available to our program are listed in Table 17.2. There can be others to consider but the number of individuals involved in our Comprehensive Colorectal Program is quite extensive and has grown considerably over more than a decade. Since we are a larger tertiary referral center in a community-based hospital system, this has been made possible.

Table 17.2 Case Study: Physician Specialties in a Multidisciplinary Colorectal Cancer Program

Physician Specialties	Nurses and Practitioners	Ancillary Personnel	Other
Primary care	Nurses	Financial counselor	Tumor registry
Hospitalists	Nurse practitioners	Pharmacy	Philanthropy
Gastroenterology	Physician assistants		Research staff
Medical Oncology	Dieticians		Administrative support
Radiation Oncology	Stomal therapists		
Surgery (Surgical Oncology; Colorectal Surgery; Hepatobiliary Surgery)	Psychosocial		
Imaging and Radiology	Social services		
Rehabilitation Medicine			
Teaching programs (Residents/students)			
Integrative medicine			
Palliative care and hospice			

Patient-centered care experience remains our fundamental goal. To accomplish this goal we use a variety of quality of life instruments to measure and track the outcomes beyond the standard measures of survival and recurrence. We also track referring physician satisfaction and realize this is a key component of ongoing success.

Advice on Program Implementation

- Consult with accreditation programs. For example, the Commission on Cancer (program of the American College of Surgery) has provided accreditation of hospital based cancer programs for decades (www.facs.org). It offers an extremely valuable external list of items for which a program can plan for accreditation.
- Establish institutional goals for the program and obtain executive support. The goal of optimal multidisciplinary care for CRC should be agreed upon and planned. The leaders within the institution need to confirm that support to the program will be provided and implemented. Leadership must then define goals realizing that immediate and long-term issues will arise. It is advisable to begin with recognizing the critical need and identifying some early achieved projects. Building program success is incremental and continuously formed by repeated planned analysis.
- Build the program based on the patient need, not available staff. The realistic analysis of the population base must be obtained to determine program needs and opportunities. This includes determination of the adequate numbers of patients to support the planned strategies, and discussion of potential referral approaches to provide the needed number of patients. The use of personnel to develop underutilized programs can be financially costly and harm motivation and morale. Be careful not to start a program component based on available personnel rather than population needs. The phrase "build it and they will come" works only if enough patients want "it." Use ongoing analysis to determine needed components rather than trying to fulfill everybody's wish list.
- Build an effective referral structure to support patient needs. One of the more difficult tasks to balance is recognizing and facilitating the return of patients to the local care when expertise exists to provide the appropriate treatments. Patients will not always ask if they can receive the appropriate care locally unless we assist in that process with transfer of care. The open recognition of distances and inconvenience to patient and family should be acknowledged in provision of their care. Every comprehensive program should freely acknowledge if options for appropriate more convenient care do exist—referrals should not be only into your program.

■ ACKNOWLEDGMENT

We thank Robin Kate Kelley, MD, for her review and insightful comments.

■ REFERENCES

1. Committee on Quality of Health Care in America, Institute of Medicine. Crossing the Quality Chasm: A New Health System for the 21st Century; 2001.
2. Patlak M, Balogh E, Nass S, Rapporteurs, Medicine Io. Patient-centered cancer treatment planning: improving the quality of oncology care: workshop summary: National Academies Press; 2011.
3. Ayanian JZ, Zaslavsky AM, Guadagnoli E, et al. Patients' perceptions of quality of care for colorectal cancer by race, ethnicity, and language. *J Clin Oncol.* 2005;23(27):6576–6586.
4. Ayanian JZ, Zaslavsky AM, Arora NK, et al. Patients' experiences with care for lung cancer and colorectal cancer: findings from the Cancer Care Outcomes Research and Surveillance Consortium. *J Clin Oncol.* 2010;28(27):4154–4161.

5. National comprehensive Cancer Network. NCCN Clinical Practice Guidlines in Oncology. Colon Cancer. Version 3.2012. www.nccn.org. Accessed 1/20/2012.
6. Nee C. Oncology Drug Management. Atlantic Information Services, Inc., and PharMedQuest. Washington, DC; 2007.
7. Medicare Prescription Drug, Improvement, and Modernizatoin Act of 2033. Public Law 108–173—DEC. 8, 2003. 108th Congress.
8. Siegel J. Impact of the Medicare Prescription Drug Improvement and Modernization Act on the management of colorectal cancer. *Am J Health Syst Pharm.* 2006;63(9 Suppl 2):S18–S21.
9. Jacobson M, O'Malley AJ, Earle CC, Pakes J, Gaccione P, Newhouse JP. Does reimbursement influence chemotherapy treatment for cancer patients? *Health Aff (Millwood).* 2006;25(2):437–443.
10. Jacobson M, Earle CC, Price M, Newhouse JP. How Medicare's payment cuts for cancer chemotherapy drugs changed patterns of treatment. *Health Aff (Millwood).* 2010;29(7):1391–1399.
11. Diagnosis, Prognostic Factors and Treatment Considerations for Colon Cancer. *Managed Care Oncology.* 2011;Quarter 1:1.
12. Buell R, Falconer P, González JL. Economic assessment of the Association of Northern California Oncologists member practices. *J Oncol Pract.* 2011;7(5):295–301.
13. Freeman HP, Muth BJ, Kerner JF. Expanding access to cancer screening and clinical follow-up among the medically underserved. *Cancer Pract.* 1995;3(1):19–30.
14. Steinberg ML, Fremont A, Khan DC, et al. Lay patient navigator program implementation for equal access to cancer care and clinical trials: essential steps and initial challenges. *Cancer.* 2006;107(11):2669–2677.
15. Jandorf L, Fatone A, Borker PV, et al. Creating alliances to improve cancer prevention and detection among urban medically underserved minority groups. The East Harlem Partnership for Cancer Awareness. *Cancer.* 2006;107(8 Suppl):2043–2051.
16. Baquet CR, Mack KM, Mishra SI, et al. Maryland's Special Populations Network. A model for cancer disparities research, education, and training. *Cancer.* 2006;107(8 Suppl):2061–2070.
17. Gabram SG, Lund MJ, Gardner J, et al. Effects of an outreach and internal navigation program on breast cancer diagnosis in an urban cancer center with a large African-American population. *Cancer.* 2008;113(3):602–607.
18. Carroll JK, Humiston SG, Meldrum SC, et al. Patients' experiences with navigation for cancer care. *Patient Educ Couns.* 2010;80(2):241–247.
19. Yosha AM, Carroll JK, Hendren S, et al. Patient navigation from the paired perspectives of cancer patients and navigators: a qualitative analysis. *Patient Educ Couns.* 2011;82(3):396–401.
20. Bodenheimer T, Wagner EH, Grumbach K. Improving primary care for patients with chronic illness. *JAMA.* 2002;288(14): 1775–1779.
21. Bodenheimer T, Wagner EH, Grumbach K. Improving primary care for patients with chronic illness: the chronic care model, Part 2. *JAMA.* 2002;288(15):1909–1914.
22. Ouwens M, Hulscher M, Hermens R, et al. Implementation of integrated care for patients with cancer: a systematic review of interventions and effects. *Int J Qual Health Care.* 2009;21(2):137–144.
23. Wright FC, De Vito C, Langer B, Hunter A; Expert Panel on Multidisciplinary Cancer Conference Standards. Multidisciplinary cancer conferences: a systematic review and development of practice standards. *Eur J Cancer.* 2007;43(6):1002–1010.
24. Gomella LG, Lin J, Hoffman-Censits J, et al. Enhancing prostate cancer care through the multidisciplinary clinic approach: a 15-year experience. *J Oncol Pract.* 2010;6(6):e5–e10.
25. Singh S, Law C. Multidisciplinary reference centers: the care of neuroendocrine tumors. *J Oncol Pract.* 2010;6(6):e11–e16.
26. Gardner TB, Barth RJ, Zaki BI, et al. Effect of initiating a multidisciplinary care clinic on access and time to treatment in patients with pancreatic adenocarcinoma. *J Oncol Pract.* 2010;6(6): 288–292.
27. Bunnell CA, Weingart SN, Swanson S, Mamon HJ, Shulman LN. Models of multidisciplinary cancer care: physician and patient perceptions in a comprehensive cancer center. *J Oncol Pract.* 2010;6(6):283–288.
28. Hammond DB. Multidisciplinary cancer care in a community hospital setting: challenges and rewards. *J Oncol Pract.* 2010;6(6):281–283.
29. Gantos-O'Brien E. A Patient's Perspective on the Multidisciplinary Liver/Pancreas Tumor Clinic: An All-in-One Resort. *J Oncol Pract.* 2010;6(6):292–294.
30. Devitt B, Philip J, McLachlan SA. Team dynamics, decision making, and attitudes toward multidisciplinary cancer meetings: health professionals' perspectives. *J Oncol Pract.* 2010;6(6):e17–e20.
31. Choy ET, Chiu A, Butow P, Young J, Spillane A. A pilot study to evaluate the impact of involving breast cancer patients in the multidisciplinary discussion of their disease and treatment plan. *Breast.* 2007;16(2):178–189.
32. Jury RP, Nadeau L, Wasvary H, Levine R, Robertson J. Implementing a multidisciplinary open-access clinic at a private practice-based community hospital. *J Oncol Pract.* 2010;6(6): e38–e41.
33. Dey P, Bundred N, Gibbs A, et al. Costs and benefits of a one stop clinic compared with a dedicated breast clinic: randomised controlled trial. *BMJ.* 2002;324(7336):507.
34. Chirgwin J, Craike M, Gray C, Watty K, Mileshkin L, Livingston PM. Does multidisciplinary care enhance the management of advanced breast cancer?: evaluation of advanced breast cancer multidisciplinary team meetings. *J Oncol Pract.* 2010;6(6):294–300.
35. American Academy of Family Physicians (AAFP), American Academy of Pediatrics (AAP), American College of Physicians (ACP), American Osteopathic Association (AOA). Joint Principles of the Patient-Centered Medical Home. 2007; http://www.aafp.org/online/etc/medialib/aafp_org/documents/policy/fed/jointprinciplespcmh0207.Par.0001.File.dat/022107medicalhome.pdf. Accessed 1/20/2012.
36. American College of Physicians. The Patient-Centered Medical Home Neighbor: The Interface of the Patient-Centered Medical Home with Specialty/Subspecialty Practices. Philadelphia: American College of Physicians; 2010: Policy Paper. (Available from American College of Physicians, 190 N. Independence Mall West, Philadelphia, PA 19106.). 2010; http://www.acponline.org/advocacy/where_we_stand/policy/pcmh_neighbors.pdf. Accessed 1/15/2012.
37. Sprandio J. Oncology Patient-centered Medical Home and Accountable Cancer Care. *Comm Oncol.* 2010;7(12):8.
38. Eagle D, Sprandio J. A care model for the future: the oncology medical home. *Oncology.* 2011;25(7):571, 575–576.
39. Stange KC, Nutting PA, Miller WL, et al. Defining and measuring the patient-centered medical home. *J Gen Intern Med.* 2010;25(6):601–612.
40. Yee HF Jr. The patient-centered medical home neighbor: A subspecialty physician's view. *Ann Intern Med.* 2011;154(1):63–64.
41. Sinsky CA. The patient-centered medical home neighbor: A primary care physician's view. *Ann Intern Med.* 2011;154(1):61–62.
42. Elkin EB, Bach PB. Cancer's next frontier: addressing high and increasing costs. *JAMA.* 2010;303(11):1086–1087.
43. Bach PB, Mirkin JN, Luke JJ. Episode-based payment for cancer care: a proposed pilot for Medicare. *Health Aff (Millwood).* 2011;30(3):500–509.
44. Richman BD, Schulman KA. A cautious path forward on accountable care organizations. *JAMA.* 2011;305(6):602–603.
45. Valgus J, Jarr S, Schwartz R, Rice M, Bernard SA. Pharmacist-led, interdisciplinary model for delivery of supportive care in the ambulatory cancer clinic setting. *J Oncol Pract.* 2010;6(6):e1–e4.
46. Reid PP, Compton WD, Grossman JH, Fanjiang G. Building a better delivery system: a new engineering/health care partnership: National Academies Press; 2005.

18 Future Directions: Gene Expression Profiling

RICHARD C. TURKINGTON
SANDRA VAN SCHAEYBROECK
PATRICK G. JOHNSTON

■ INTRODUCTION

Throughout the history of modern cancer research the complexity of cancer cell biology has become increasingly apparent. From the initial discoveries of oncogenes and tumor suppressor genes, through to their role in signal transduction pathways and networks, our understanding of the processes governing cancer cell behavior has advanced rapidly. Much of this progress has been fueled by technological advances, such as DNA sequencing and the study of gene copy number, and one of the most powerful techniques is gene expression profiling using microarray analysis (1).

Microarrays use transcript specific probes to profile the expression of tens of thousands of genes simultaneously and so generate large amounts of information relating to the upregulation or suppression of gene expression in a cell (2,3). There are two basic types of arrays. In a two-color (two-channel) array, cDNA from paired samples (eg, cancer vs normal tissue) are labeled with different fluorophores, mixed in equal amounts, and hybridized to the array. This method provides a measure of gene expression in the study sample relative to the reference sample. In a one-color (single-channel) array, the fluorescence intensity for each probe is reported within one sample or condition. The data obtained is normalized to compensate for differences in labeling and hybridization within and between arrays and is filtered according to a set of objective criteria, such as eliminating genes with minimal variance. In this way gene expression profiling generates a list of genes whose expression is either up- or down-regulated and can identify molecular subtypes within a disease, produce gene signatures capable of predicting prognosis or response to treatment and aid in the identification of novel drug targets (Figure 18.1).

One of the first applications of microarray profiling in cancer research was to analyze a large number of tumors and look for patterns of expression within the datasets (4,5). This unsupervised or class discovery approach disregards any prior knowledge of the samples, such as pathological subtype or prognosis, and attempts to classify them according to gene expression alone (Figure 18.2a). This method has been used to identify previously unrecognized disease subtypes and has led to the reclassification of certain tumor types according to gene expression (4,5). Using an unsupervised classification approach, Perou et al subdivided breast cancers into four distinct subtypes based on their gene expression profiles; ER+/luminal-like, basal-like, normal-like, and Erb-B2+ (5). Alternatively, prior information related to the samples, such as response to treatment or prognosis, can be incorporated into the microarray data analysis—a supervised (or class prediction) approach (Figure 18.2b; 6). A major effort has gone into supervised classification approaches to discover gene expression signatures related to overall survival (prognostic biomarkers) or response to standard treatments (predictive biomarkers) in colon cancer. While prognostic biomarkers provide information about a patient's prognosis, irrespective of any treatment given, a predictive biomarker provides information about the effect of therapy given to a patient. Both of these approaches have been used in the classification of colon cancer samples and will be discussed in this chapter.

The wealth of information generated by microarrays can also be utilized in target discovery approaches to link gene expression changes found in disease states to those produced by therapeutic compounds (Figure 18.2). An example is connectivity mapping, which uses pattern-recognition software to pair changes in gene expression to those produced by drug action, providing a powerful target and drug-discovery tool.

■ CLASS DISCOVERY IN COLON CANCER

The use of class discovery techniques has been applied in a number of cancer types and has successfully uncovered new subclasses and redefined disease classification (4,5). Initial efforts to better define a high risk subtype in early

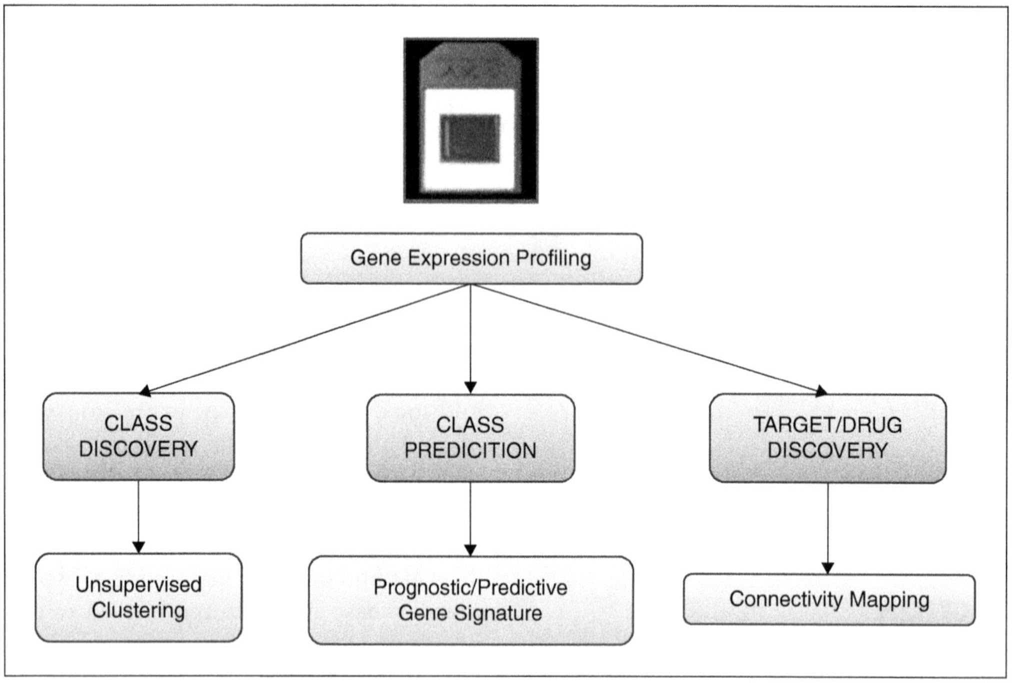

FIGURE 18.1 Applications of gene expression profiling.

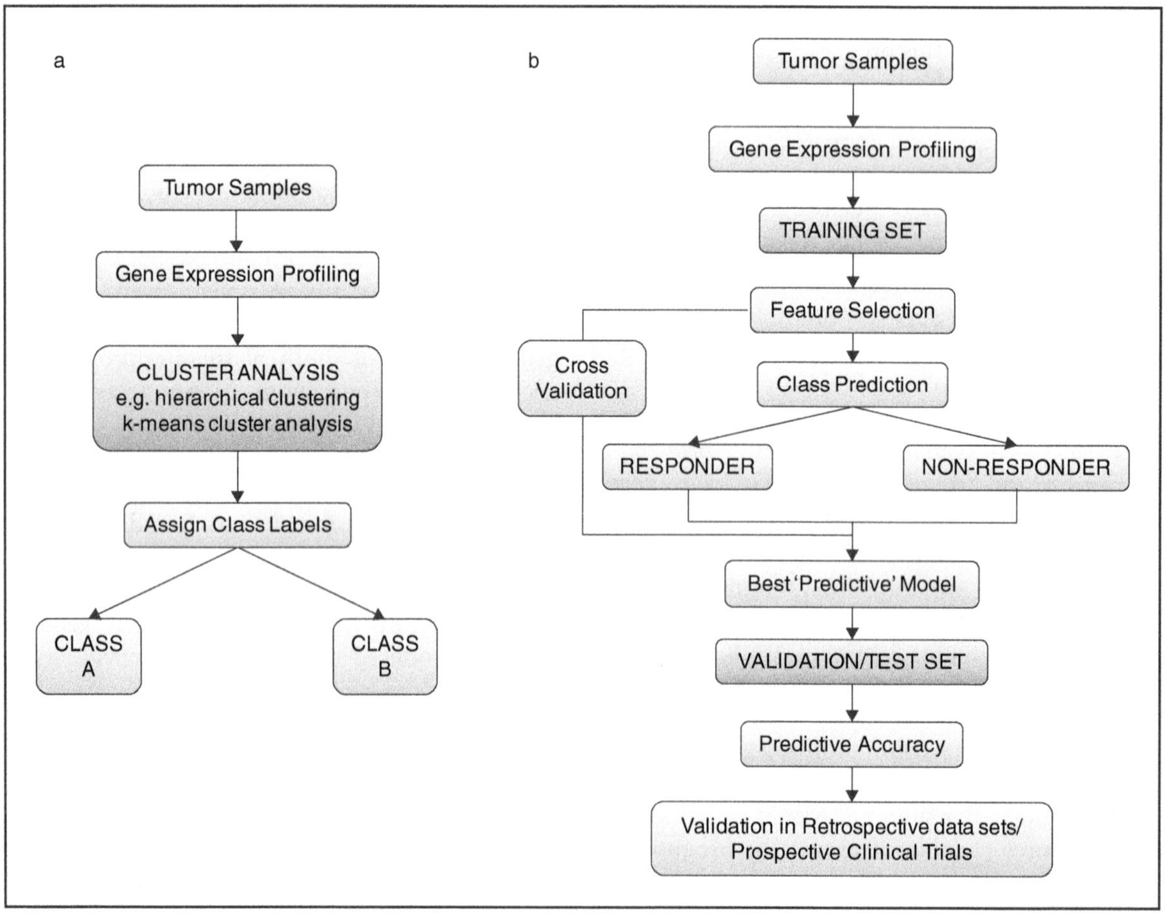

FIGURE 18.2 (a) Unsupervised analysis. Tumor samples are clustered into classes based on similarity of the gene expression profiles. (b) Supervised analysis. Tumor samples are used to train a classifier capable of discriminating between two classes, for example, responder and nonresponder, which is then applied to a validation set to determine predictive assay.

stage colon cancers arose from the discovery that colon tumors were a heterogeneous group and could be divided into subtypes according to molecular alterations and genomic instability.

Tumors displaying microsatellite instability (MSI) account for ~15%–20% of sporadic colon cancers and are predominantly due to epigenetic silencing of *MLH1* by hypermethylation of its promoter region (7). Whereas, over 80% of patients with hereditary nonpolyposis colon cancers (HNPCC or Lynch syndrome) demonstrate MSI due to germline mutations in one or more of the mismatch repair genes *MLH1, MSH2, MSH6* and *PMS2* (8). MSI is more common in early stage disease (22% Stage II, 12% Stage III) compared to the metastatic setting (2% Stage IV) and has been shown to be a significant prognostic marker in Stage II colon cancer (9). Multiple retrospective analyses demonstrate that MSI-H patients have better survival than MSS with a meta-analysis of 32 studies confirming a hazard ratio (HR) for survival of 0.65 (95% CI, 0.59–0.71) for tumors with MSI (10–13). Multivariate analysis of both the QUASAR and PETACC-3 data has also confirmed the prognostic value of MSI status (14,15). The predictive role for MSI is less clear with some studies suggesting that MSI-H patients do not benefit from treatment with 5-FU-based adjuvant chemotherapy while other studies do not detect this association (11,13,16–18).

The most common mechanism of genomic instability, chromosomal instability (CIN), is present in approximately 65%–70% of colorectal cancers (CRCs) and is defined as the presence of structural and numerical chromosomal changes within the tumor cells (19). These tumors are typically MSS and demonstrate the classical adenoma to carcinoma pathway of progression. They acquire mutations in the *APC* gene as well as *K-ras* and *PI3KCA* mutations and loss of chromosomes 18q and 17p. CIN is associated with a worse prognosis and a large meta-analysis of 63 studies demonstrated a HR for death of 1.45 ($P < .001$; 20). A chromosomal abnormality commonly associated with CIN is deletion or loss of heterozygosity (LOH) of chromosome 18q, which is associated with a worse prognosis in colon cancer, but this effect may be stage specific and has not been a universal finding (12,15,21,22).

Gene expression profiling has the ability to examine the underlying genetic changes associated with these broad genomic instability classes and to further reclassify colon cancer into molecular subtypes. Alon et al profiled 40 tumor and 22 normal colon samples alongside two colon cancer cell lines and demonstrated that two-way clustering techniques could separate the normal tissue and cell lines from the tumors and, importantly, subdivide the tumors into classes based on their gene expression (4). Loboda et al profiled 326 colon cancers to define two primary, intrinsic molecular subtypes: epithelial and mesenchymal. These classes could be identified using a cell-line derived epithelial-mesenchymal transition (EMT) signature, suggesting that EMT may be the driving biology behind these two-subgroups and be useful in subclassifying colon cancer (23). A recent study by Popovici et al developed a 64 gene-based classifier capable of detecting *BRAF* mutant tumors with 96% sensitivity and 86% sensitivity (24). Interestingly this study revealed a *BRAF* mutant-like subpopulation of patients (18% of tumors) with no detectable mutations in the *BRAF* gene but a similarly poor prognosis to true *BRAF* mutant patients. This discovery indicates a common biology between *BRAF* mutant and a subset of *BRAF* wild-type tumors and may represent a new subtype, not currently detected by mutation analysis. Apart from these studies there is a need for a large, unbiased examination of the colon cancer transcriptome to define sensitive subpopulations, which could be targeted by novel therapeutic strategies.

■ CLASS PREDICTION IN COLON CANCER

Prognostic and Predictive Biomarkers in Early Stage Colon Cancer

In recent years, there has been much interest in the use of gene expression profiling to identify reliable prognostic and predictive biomarkers in Stages II and III CRC. The overall survival (OS) of patients with colon cancer is closely linked with tumor size (T) and lymph node status (N). Lymph node-negative disease (Stage II) confers an OS at 5 years of approximately 80% with surgery alone (25), with survival declining to 50%–56% for lymph node positive disease (Stage III) and 8.1% for advanced disease with secondary lesions in distant organs (Stage IV; 26,27). The role of adjuvant chemotherapy to reduce the risk of recurrence has been clearly established for Stage III disease where 5-fluorouracil (5-FU)-based chemotherapy was found to reduce mortality by approximately 30% (27–32). The addition of oxaliplatin further increased 5-year disease-free survival (DFS) from 67.4%–73.3% with a resultant improvement in OS at 6 years of 78.5% vs 76% for 5-FU alone (33). However, the situation for Stage II colon cancer is less clear. Numerous studies have demonstrated minimal improvements in DFS or OS with the use of adjuvant chemotherapy (29,34–36). The largest trial, the Quick and Simple and Reliable (QUASAR) study randomized 3239 patients between adjuvant 5-FU-based chemotherapy and chemotherapy alone, of which 91% had Stage II disease (25). A small but significant improvement in OS at 5 years of approximately 3.6% was demonstrated. Considering that 25%–30% of colon cancer patients present with Stage II disease, this means that a large proportion of patients are potentially being exposed to the risks and toxicities of chemotherapy for minimal clinical benefit (37). The ability to distinguish high-risk and low-risk patients within the Stage II population would allow adjuvant chemotherapy to be focused on the patients at a higher risk of recurrence, while sparing other patients the time, toxicity, and expense associated with chemotherapy.

Current clinical guidelines use several clinicopathological criteria to stratify patients into high- and low-risk groups (Table 18.1; 38,39). These include features such as obstructing or perforating tumors, vascular invasion, margin involvement, and inadequate lymph node harvest. The presence of high-risk features is considered an indication for adjuvant chemotherapy but must be weighed against the patient's performance status and comorbidities. These risk factors have arisen from the retrospective subset analysis of clinical trial datasets, such as the Intergroup-0035 trial in which a pooled analysis showed that perforation and obstruction were significantly associated with an increased risk of recurrence (34).

Considering the poor prognosis associated with later-stage disease, there is a clear importance in preventing recurrence. Current clinicopathological risk factors are inadequate and better prognostic and predictive tools are required to allow adjuvant chemotherapy to be focused on the patients who will gain the most benefit.

Gene Expression Profiling–Prognostic Signatures

Multiple studies have attempted to generate prognostic signatures for resected Stage II colon cancer from either tumor or nonneoplastic mucosa (40–48). The interpretation of these trials has been problematic due to small sample size, heterogeneous patient populations, and differing approaches to sample handling and microarray data analysis. Some studies displayed limited validation of the signature in an independent test set and the performance of the signature was not adequately compared with standard clinical and pathological risk factors. Wang et al reported a 23-gene signature developed using microarray profiling of 74 Stage II patients (49). This signature was validated in an independent test set of 36 patients and displayed a positive predictive value of 78%, with further validation performed by an independent group who found a 67% positive predictive value (42). This provided the first instance of a signature being validated by two distinct research groups and indicated the possibility of developing a robust signature that would be widely applicable. Further evidence of the potential value of gene expression profiling to develop prognostic markers in Stage II colon cancer was added by a meta-analysis of 8 patient cohorts comprising 271 patients (50). Pooled analysis demonstrated a sensitivity of 76%, a specificity of 85%, and a likelihood ratio (LR) of 4.7 (95% CI, 3.2–6.8; $P < .00001$) for recurrence or death within 3 years. Despite clear differences in study design and methodology, there was no significant interstudy heterogeneity with different gene signatures predicting similar outcomes. These findings mirror a larger meta-analysis of breast cancer signatures that indicated that many of the signatures produced similar results as they included genes associated with cellular proliferation (51,52). Even though the genes included in each signature may be different, they could be tracking a common biological signal, with each capturing a different aspect of the underlying biology. Subsequently, the focus in both breast and colon cancer moved to the study of larger patient cohorts with adequate external validation and combining signatures with clinical variables in order to provide the best prognostic information. In Stage II colon cancer three gene expression signatures have been developed in recent years and we will discuss each of these.

Table 18.1 Poor Prognostic Features in the National Comprehensive Cancer Network and American Society of Clinical Oncology Guidelines

Poor Prognostic Features
T4 lesion (tumor penetrates to the surface of the visceral peritoneum or directly invades or is adherent to other organs or structures)
Perforation or obstruction
Peri-tumoral lymphovascular invasion
Poorly differentiated histology
Perineural lesion
Less than 12 lymph nodes examined

From (38,39).

Oncotype DX Colon Cancer Assay

The development of the Oncotype DX Colon Cancer test provided a new direction in gene expression-based classifiers (53). Rather than performing supervised analysis of microarray data, researchers at Genomic Health (Redwood City, USA) initially selected 761 candidate genes with potential importance in colon cancer. The resultant signature is based on a predefined biological signal that is hypothesized to be associated with prognosis. The gene expression of the 761 genes was examined in samples obtained from four adjuvant trials: the surgery alone arms of NSABP C-01/C-02 (n = 270), a Cleveland Clinic observational series (n = 765), and two adjuvant 5-FU chemotherapy trials, NSABP C-04 (n = 308), and NSABP C-06 (n = 508). Expression was measured with a Reverse-Transcriptase (RT)-PCR assay using formalin-fixed paraffin embedded (FFPE) tumor samples. Algorithms were derived for a Recurrence Score (RS) based on seven genes, a Treatment Score (TS) based on six genes and five reference genes used to normalize gene expression (Table 18.2).

The prognostic and predictive ability of the Oncotype DX Colon Cancer test was validated in 1436 samples from Stage II colon cancer patients enrolled in the QUASAR trial (Table 18.3; 14). This subset had comparable characteristics to the entire Stage II cohort (n = 2146) and a range of conventional high risk features, including 15% T4 tumors, 30% high grade, and 14% displaying lymphovascular invasion. Notably, the mean number of nodes examined was 11 with harvesting of 12 or more nodes only occurring in 38% of patients, but this was in keeping with standard surgical practice at the time. Application of the RS to the 711 patients in the surgery alone arm stratified them into low-, intermediate-, and high-risk groups with estimated recurrence risks at 3 years of 12%, 18%, and 22%, respectively.

Once the ability of the RS to act as a prognostic marker was established, it was then necessary to control for clinical and pathological factors. Uni- and multivariate Cox Regression analyses were used to assess conventional prognostic factors, such as T stage, grade, and nodes examined, alongside the RS. T4 and MMR deficiency were more significantly associated with recurrence than the RS, leading to efforts to integrate the Oncotype DX Colon RS score with these pathological features. The 11% of patients in the QUASAR validation study with T3 and MSI-H tumors are at low risk of recurrence and so may be considered for observation only (14). Whereas T4/MMR proficient tumors (13% of patients) are at high risk of recurrence and should be considered for adjuvant chemotherapy. The role of the Oncotype DX Colon RS score may be to further stratify the majority of patients (74%) with T3/MMR proficient Stage II disease with the presence of a high RS supporting a recommendation of adjuvant chemotherapy (Figure 18.3). The Oncotype DX Colon Cancer test has recently been validated using patient samples (n = 690) from the CALGB 9581 study of Edrecolomab

Table 18.2 Recurrence and Treatment Score Gene Panel for the Oncotype DX Colon Cancer Assay

Oncotype DX Colon Cancer Assay	Gene	Gene Function
Recurrence score	*Ki-67*	Cell Cycle
	C-MYC	Cell Cycle
	MYBL2	Cell Cycle
	FAP	Stromal
	INHBA	Stromal
	BGN	Stromal
	GADD45B	Early Response
Treatment score	*EFBN2*	Angiogenesis, Migration and cell-cell signaling
	RUNX1	Transcription Factor
	BIK	Apoptosis
	MAD2L1	Cell Cycle
	AXIN2	Wnt Pathway
	HSEP1	Heat Shock
Reference genes	*ATP5E*	
	GPX1	
	PGK1	
	UBB	
	VDAC2	

From (53).

Table 18.3 Comparison of the Primary Characteristics and Validation Results for the Oncotype DX Colon Cancer Assay, ColoPrint, and ColDx

	Oncotype DX Colon Cancer Assay		ColoPrint			ColDX
Tissue	**FFPE**		**Fresh Frozen**			**FFPE**
Assay platform	RT-PCR		Agilent 44K oligonucleotide array			Almac Colorectal Cancer Disease Specific Array
Independent retrospective validation set	QUASAR trial	CALGB 9581	Barcelona set (Stage II only)	Munich set	5 Centre set	12 Centre set
Sample size	1436	690	206	135	320	144
Risk groups	Low (43.7%) Intermediate (30.7%) High (25.6%)	Low (44%) Intermediate (33%) High (22%)	Low (63.2%) High (36.8%)	Low (74%) High (26%)	Low (65%) High (35%)	Low (59%) High (41)%
Recurrence risk (or distant metastasis free survival-DMFS)	Low (12%) at 3 years Intermediate (18%) at 3 years High (22%) at 3 years	Low (13%) at 5 years Intermediate (16%) at 5 years High (21%) at 5 years	Low (90.9%) RFS at 5 years High (73.9%) at 5 years	Low (94.9%) DMFS High (80.5%) DMFS	Low (94%) RFS at 3 years High (79%) RFS at 3 years	Not reported

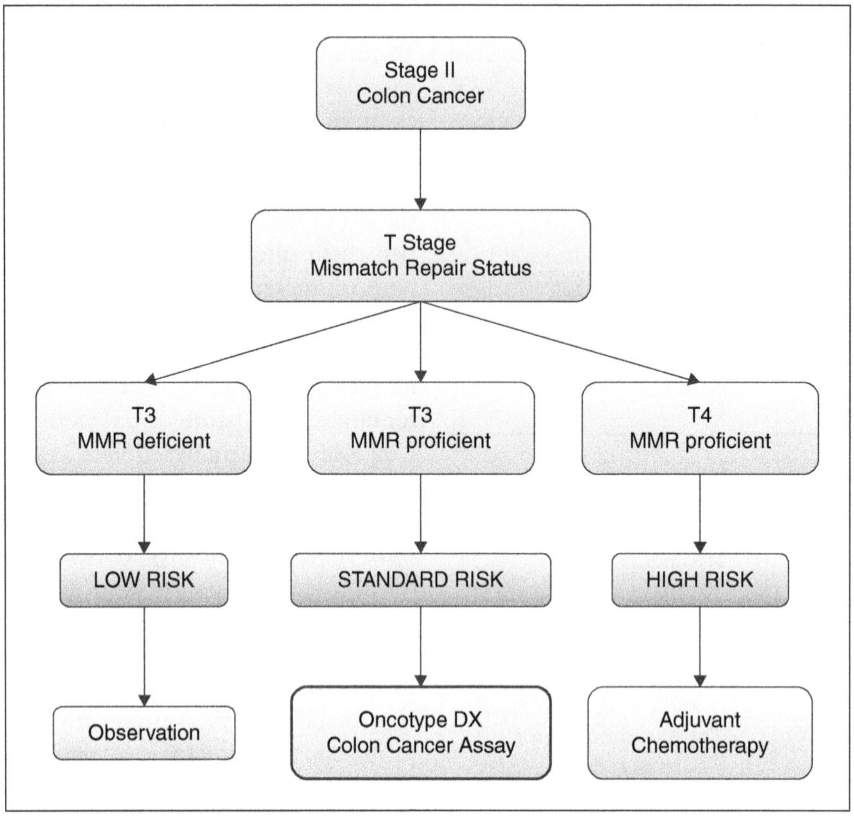

FIGURE 18.3 Integration of the oncotype DX colon cancer assay recurrence score with clinical and pathological risk factors.

(MoAb 17-A) vs surgery alone (54). In a prespecified multivariate analysis of the CALGB 9581 data, RS was significantly associated with recurrence-free interval with 5-year recurrence risks in low-, intermediate-, and high-risk T3/MMR proficient tumors (n = 448) of 13%, 16%, and 21%, respectively. However, T4 stage and MMR deficiency were not associated with recurrence, with the only significant predictor being the RS score (54).

Taking these results together the Oncotype DX Colon Cancer test demonstrates that a prospectively defined gene expression assay is capable of providing information beyond known prognostic factors on recurrence risk in Stage II colon cancer. The use of a RT-PCR-based system allows the score to be derived from FFPE tissue samples, making the test easier to implement in clinical practice. Limitations of the RS primarily relate to the narrow range of recurrence risk between the low- and high-risk groups (12%–22%) when compared to assays in other disease settings, such as the companion Oncotype DX 21 gene signature for breast cancer (low 6.8%, intermediate 14.3%, and high 30.5% risk of recurrence by 10 years; 55). The breast cancer assay is also predictive of the extent of chemotherapy benefit, a feature lacking in the colon test.

ColoPrint

The Netherlands Cancer Institute in collaboration with Agendia BV(Amsterdam) recently developed a prognostic 18-gene signature (ColoPrint; 56). Fresh frozen tissue from 188 Stage I–IV CRC samples were profiled using the Agilent 44K oligonucleotide array and unsupervised hierarchical clustering was performed to reveal three molecular subtypes. The intermediate prognostic group (n = 110) was used to construct a prognostic signature to avoid bias from the other two groups, which had a high proportion of patients with activating *BRAF* V600E mutations. The resultant classifier was then applied to the total training set (n = 188) using a leave-one-out cross validation procedure to define low- and high-risk groups with 5 year distant metastasis-free survival (DMFS) rates of 82% (95% CI, 76%–89%) and 50% (95% CI, 38%–66%) respectively.

Validation of the signature was initially performed in an independent test set of 206 patients collected at the Institut Catala d'Oncologia in Barcelona (Table 18.3) of whom 60% were classified low risk with a 5-year relapse-free survival (RFS) of 87.6% and 40% high risk with a 5-year RFS of 67.2% (56). Further independent validation was performed using 135, Stage-II patients from the Klinikum rechts der Isar, Munich, with 74% classified as low risk (5-year DMFS 94.9%) and 26% high risk (5-year DMFS 80.5%; 57). Multivariate analysis was performed in both studies and the ColoPrint assay was the only significant factor to predict recurrence or the development of distant metastases. Recently results from a combined validation set from 5 independent European centers have confirmed the prognostic capability of the assay (58). The authors propose that ColoPrint identifies the approximately two-thirds of patients who are low risk and may be managed by observation alone.

The ColoPrint signature appears to perform better than standard clinicopathological variables but the requirement for fresh frozen tissue make it more difficult to implement. The small size of the patient cohorts and the lack of randomization of patients between adjuvant chemotherapy and surgery alone means that these results should be interpreted with caution. To address this issue, Agendia is performing the Prospective Study for the Assessment of Recurrence Risk in Stage II Colon Cancer (PARSC trial) in which it is seeking to compare the performance of ColoPrint vs clinical risk assessment in estimating 3- and 5-year relapse rates (59).

ColDx

The most recent prognostic classifier is the 634 transcript ColDx signature developed by Almac Diagnostics (Craigavon, UK; 60). A training set of 215 patients were profiled using the Almac CRC Disease Specific Array (DSA), developed through a combination of high throughput 3'-based sequencing, data mining, and expression analysis (61,62). Crucially, this platform has been optimized for the use of FFPE tissue, abrogating the need for the fresh tumor samples required for other assays. The 634 transcript signature classified the training set into 142 low-risk and 73 high-risk patients and validation in an independent test set of 144 patients demonstrated a HR of 2.53 (95% CI, 1.54–4.15; $P < .001$) for 5-year RFS (Table 18.3).

Univariate and multivariate analyses were used to assess the independence of the signatures from known prognostic factors. The ability of the 634 transcript signature to predict prognosis was significant in both the univariate (HR, 2.53; 95% CI, 1.54–4.15; $P < .001$) and multivariate (HR, 2.55; 95% CI, 1.47–4.42; $P < .001$) analyses, outperforming conventional histopathological factors. Retrospective validation of this signature in a large cohort of Stage II patients from a randomized clinical trial is ongoing.

The ColDx signature combines the depth of information obtained from a microarray platform with the ready availability of FFPE tissue to produce an assay that can be easily applied. The strong prognostic value of the signature, independent of other prognostic factors, and the lack of requirement for individual interpretation are also strengths. However, no information is available on the relationship to MMR status and the lack of a large retrospective validation allows limited assessment of its performance as a prognostic and predictive marker at present.

Other Prognostic Assays in Development

A further prognostic signature to identify the subset of patients who may need oxaliplatin-based adjuvant chemotherapy has been developed using samples from the NSABP C-07 trial. A 33-gene prognostic index was derived from a training set of 478 samples and tested in a validation set of equal size. Two risk groups were defined with 82.6% of low-risk patients recurrence-free at 5 years compared to 64.3% in the high-risk group giving a HR of 2.43 (95% CI, 1.69–3.49; $P < .0001$). A Nanostring multiplex assay for the gene expression signature has been generated with the aim of validating this higher throughput and cheaper assay (63).

Gene expression profiling has also been used to better define existing molecular markers of prognosis. Building on their previous work related to 18q LOH, Watanabe et al have identified a gene signature of the CIN phenotype that has proven to be prognostic in Stage II and III colon cancer. Developing an acceptable definition of CIN has been problematic and the prognostic effect of LOH at different loci has been controversial (15,21,64–66). This signature indicates the potential for the development of a reliable marker of this genomic instability phenotype and so the ability to select high risk early colon cancer patients. Vilar et al used five separate data sets to identify a gene expression signature to distinguish MSI-H from MSS tumors (67). Rather than develop a prognostic classifier they chose to analyze the common gene expression data by connectivity mapping to discover compounds that may be more effective against MSI-H tumors. The connectivity map examines similarities between the query signature and a reference database of gene expression profiles from established cell lines exposed to 164 compounds (68). The correlation between the signature produced by the compound and that found in the query signature is then assessed to identify compounds associated with a particular biological state.

Gene Expression Profiling–Predictive Signatures in Late Stage Colon Cancer

In contrast to the development of prognostic signatures in early stage colon cancer, more limited research activities have gone into predictive assays in the metastatic setting. The development of such a test would allow patients to be spared from the unnecessary time and toxicity of a treatment to which they are unlikely to respond. At present, there are no clinically established biomarkers to predict response to the most commonly used drugs, such as 5-FU, irinotecan, and oxaliplatin. However, small studies have provided proof of principle that the development of predictive gene-based signatures is possible. Del Rio et al developed a 14-gene classifier, derived from profiling 21 primary tumors, which could predict response to irinotecan and 5-FU with an overall accuracy of 95% (69). Sensitivity and specificity were, 92% and 100%, respectively but this signature was not validated in an independent test set but rather in samples derived from the original training set. A further study identified 679 genes that predicted sensitivity to irinotecan and 5-FU and they were derived from a combination of tumor, normal, and metastatic site samples from 13 patients (70). Watanabe et al developed a 27-probe classifier from 40 primary tumor samples to predict response to oxaliplatin and 5-FU chemotherapy (71). The sensitivity and specificity were 78.6% and 100%, respectively, but again this model requires independent validation.

Predictive classifiers of response to epidermal growth factor rate (EGFR) targeted therapy have also been developed. Balko et al used microarray data from 80 metastatic CRC tumors to develop a 26-gene classifier capable of separating samples into high and low risk (72). However, the signature was validated in samples that were present in the original training set and so it will require more extensive validation. A 4-gene RT-PCR based classifier has also been identified by profiling 110 candidate genes in 144 *K-ras* wildtype primary colorectal tumors (73). A recent study by Huang et al selected 74 probesets, representing 33 insulin-like growth factor 1 receptor (IGF-1R) pathway-related genes, to identify markers predictive of benefit from cetuximab in metastatic CRC (74). The IGF-1R pathway shares many downstream effectors with the EGFR pathway and may act in conjunction with EGFR signaling to drive tumor progression.

Johnston et al demonstrated that microarray data obtained from the profiling of colon cancer cell lines can be used to develop gene signatures capable of predicting response to irinotecan/5-FU chemotherapy in clinical samples (75). The resultant 16-gene classifier had an overall accuracy of 75% with a sensitivity and specificity of 81.8% and 66.6%, respectively. This signature demonstrated good separation of samples when applied to 20 pretreatment metastatic liver biopsies, indicating the potential of this approach.

Overall, this group of exploratory studies are limited by small sample numbers, lack of independent validation, and the use of either the primary tumor or biopsies of metastases as the source material. Further work is needed using larger, independently validated data sets to allow a reliable classifier to be developed for use in metastatic CRC.

THE CHALLENGE OF HETEROGENEITY

A central tenet of personalized medicine has been the desire to predict prognosis and response to treatment based on the analysis of a single sample of a patient's tumor. Ideally, a patient would undergo a needle biopsy and enough information could be gained to decide the course of treatment and predict its outcome. However, an important challenge to this ideal is the presence of intra- and intertumor heterogeneity.

Over the last decade, there has been a rapid increase in our ability to study the biology of cancer at multiple levels. From gene copy number to expression profiling, single nucleotide polymorphisms, and next-generation sequencing, each technology has revealed the increasing complexity and heterogeneity of cancer biology. In a thorough examination of four renal cell carcinomas Gerlinger et al performed exome-capture multiregion sequencing, chromosome aberration analysis, ploidy profiling, RNA expression profiling, and immunohistochemical analysis on multiple biopsies from primary tumors and their metastatic sites (76). Of all the somatic mutations detected, 63%–69% were heterogeneous and not present in all the sampled regions of a patient's tumor. Of concern was the finding that a single biopsy revealed only a minority of the chromosomal and genetic changes and so could not be regarded as representative of the entire genomic landscape of the tumor. The study also applied a 110-gene classifier and found that different regions of a single patient's tumor displayed either a good or poor prognosis signature. This study confirms previous findings of intratumor heterogeneity but by combining sequencing with data regarding chromosome alterations and loss of gene function, the authors were able to map the branching evolution of a tumor from its primary lesion through to metastatic sites (77–81). Importantly, some genetic changes found in the primary tumor cells, which form the "trunk" of the phylogenetic tree, remain consistently expressed in all regions of the tumor. Also, some regions of the tumor, and so branches of the evolutionary tree, can have different mutations in the same genes, emphasizing the importance of these genes to tumor growth and development. This phenomenon is referred to as convergent evolution and the identification of these genes, as well as the common "trunk" mutations, may provide an opportunity to identify the core biology of a tumor and so develop more effective biomarkers and therapeutic approaches.

INTEGRATIVE GENOMICS

As outlined above, the genetic landscape of a patient's tumor is markedly heterogeneous and so the problem now arises of how best to capture the fundamental biological signals driving a tumor. Improvements are needed in delineating driver mutations from their passenger changes and so separate the biological signal from the noise. A potential strategy would be to obtain multiple biopsy samples from all primary and metastatic sites but this would be impractical and present significant risk to the patient. Alternatively, we are faced with extracting the greatest amount of biological information from limited tumor samples. Gene expression profiling examines one aspect governing tumor biology but increasingly it is being combined with multiple techniques to gain the greatest depth of insight—a process referred to as integrative genomics (82).

Technological advances over the last several years have rapidly accelerated our ability to examine different aspects of cell function on a genome-wide scale. The study of the role of DNA (genomics), RNA (transcriptomics), transcriptional control (epigenomics), proteins (proteomics), and metabolites (metabolomics) have all lead to a wealth of information but the combination of these methodologies has the potential to be more powerful. Already we are seeing this approach redefining our knowledge of existing disease subtypes with a recent paper by Curtis et al integrating gene expression and copy number analysis to define 10 breast cancer subgroups derived from a discovery set of 997 primary tumors (83). This study further subdivided the previously defined expression-only subgroups to reveal novel driver events of tumorigenesis in these patient groups. Once unsupervised integration has clustered the data from different experiments to identify patient subgroups, this can be used to develop more robust biomarkers. In this way integrating data from multiple techniques may improve the prognostic and predictive performance of existing gene expression classifiers.

In conclusion, gene expression profiling has revolutionized the classification and treatment of colon cancer. From the ability to reclassify the disease into molecular subgroups through to the development of prognostic and predictive tests in all stages of disease this technology has had a profound impact. However, efforts to translate these findings into tangible clinical benefits for patients are in their infancy. By continuing to broaden our understanding of the heterogeneity of cancer through the combination of multiple techniques to examine tumor cell behavior we can advance the role of gene expression profiling in developing novel biomarkers and therapies.

■ REFERENCES

1. Quackenbush J. Microarray analysis and tumor classification. *N Engl J Med.* 2006;354(23):2463–2472.
2. Lipshutz RJ, Morris D, Chee M, et al. Using oligonucleotide probe arrays to access genetic diversity. *BioTechniques.* 1995;19(3):442–447.
3. Schena M, Shalon D, Davis RW, Brown PO. Quantitative monitoring of gene expression patterns with a complementary DNA microarray. *Science.* 1995;270(5235):467–470.
4. Alon U, Barkai N, Notterman DA, et al. Broad patterns of gene expression revealed by clustering analysis of tumor and normal colon tissues probed by oligonucleotide arrays. *Proc Natl Acad Sci USA.* 1999;96(12):6745–6750.
5. Perou CM, Jeffrey SS, van de Rijn M, et al. Distinctive gene expression patterns in human mammary epithelial cells and breast cancers. *Proc Natl Acad Sci USA.* 1999;96(16):9212–9217.
6. Golub TR, Slonim DK, Tamayo P, et al. Molecular classification of cancer: class discovery and class prediction by gene expression monitoring. *Science.* 1999;286(5439):531–537.
7. Thibodeau SN, Bren G, Schaid D. Microsatellite instability in cancer of the proximal colon. *Science.* 1993;260(5109):816–819.
8. Aaltonen LA, Peltomäki P, Leach FS, et al. Clues to the pathogenesis of familial colorectal cancer. *Science.* 1993;260(5109):812–816.
9. Koopman M, Kortman GA, Mekenkamp L, et al. Deficient mismatch repair system in patients with sporadic advanced colorectal cancer. *Br J Cancer.* 2009;100(2):266–273.
10. Gryfe R, Kim H, Hsieh ET, et al. Tumor microsatellite instability and clinical outcome in young patients with colorectal cancer. *N Engl J Med.* 2000;342(2):69–77.
11. Ribic CM, Sargent DJ, Moore MJ, et al. Tumor microsatellite-instability status as a predictor of benefit from fluorouracil-based adjuvant chemotherapy for colon cancer. *N Engl J Med.* 2003;349(3):247–257.
12. Halling KC, French AJ, McDonnell SK, et al. Microsatellite instability and 8p allelic imbalance in stage B2 and C colorectal cancers. *J Natl Cancer Inst.* 1999;91(15):1295–1303.
13. Popat S, Hubner R, Houlston RS. Systematic review of microsatellite instability and colorectal cancer prognosis. *J Clin Oncol.* 2005;23(3):609–618.
14. Gray RG, Quirke P, Handley K, et al. Validation study of a quantitative multigene reverse transcriptase-polymerase chain reaction assay for assessment of recurrence risk in patients with stage II colon cancer. *J Clin Oncol.* 2011;29(35):4611–4619.
15. Roth AD, Tejpar S, Delorenzi M, et al. Prognostic role of K-ras and BRAF in stage II and III resected colon cancer: results of the translational study on the PETACC-3, EORTC 40993, SAKK 60–00 trial. *J Clin Oncol.* 2010;28(3):466–474.
16. Elsaleh H, Iacopetta B. Microsatellite instability is a predictive marker for survival benefit from adjuvant chemotherapy in a population-based series of stage III colorectal carcinoma. *Clin Colorectal Cancer.* 2001;1(2):104–109.
17. Jover R, Zapater P, Castells A, et al.; Gastrointestinal Oncology Group of the Spanish Gastroenterological Association. The efficacy of adjuvant chemotherapy with 5-fluorouracil in colorectal cancer depends on the mismatch repair status. *Eur J Cancer.* 2009;45(3):365–373.
18. Sargent DJ, Marsoni S, Monges G, et al. Defective mismatch repair as a predictive marker for lack of efficacy of fluorouracil-based adjuvant therapy in colon cancer. *J Clin Oncol.* 2010;28(20):3219–3226.
19. Walther A, Johnstone E, Swanton C, Midgley R, Tomlinson I, Kerr D. Genetic prognostic and predictive markers in colorectal cancer. *Nat Rev Cancer.* 2009;9(7):489–499.
20. Walther A, Houlston R, Tomlinson I. Association between chromosomal instability and prognosis in colorectal cancer: a meta-analysis. *Gut.* 2008;57(7):941–950.
21. Watanabe T, Wu TT, Catalano PJ, et al. Molecular predictors of survival after adjuvant chemotherapy for colon cancer. *N Engl J Med.* 2001;344(16):1196–1206.
22. Popat S, Houlston RS. A systematic review and meta-analysis of the relationship between chromosome 18q genotype, DCC status and colorectal cancer prognosis. *Eur J Cancer.* 2005;41(14):2060–2070.
23. Loboda A, Nebozhyn MV, Watters JW, et al. EMT is the dominant program in human colon cancer. *BMC Med Genomics.* 2011;4:9.
24. Popovici V, Budinska E, Tejpar S, et al. Identification of a poor-prognosis BRAF-mutant-like population of patients with colon cancer. *J Clin Oncol.* 2012;30(12):1288–1295.
25 Gray R, Barnwell J, McConkey C, Hills RK, Williams NS, Kerr DJ. Adjuvant chemotherapy versus observation in patients with colorectal cancer: a randomised study. *Lancet.* 2007;370(9604):2020–2029.
26. O'Connell JB, Maggard MA, Ko CY. Colon cancer survival rates with the new American Joint Committee on Cancer sixth edition staging. *J Natl Cancer Inst.* 2004;96(19):1420–1425.

27. Mamounas E, Wieand S, Wolmark N, et al. Comparative efficacy of adjuvant chemotherapy in patients with Dukes' B versus Dukes' C colon cancer: results from four National Surgical Adjuvant Breast and Bowel Project adjuvant studies (C-01, C-02, C-03, and C-04). *J Clin Oncol.* 1999;17(5):1349–1355.
28. André T, Quinaux E, Louvet C, et al. Phase III study comparing a semimonthly with a monthly regimen of fluorouracil and leucovorin as adjuvant treatment for stage II and III colon cancer patients: final results of GERCOR C96.1. *J Clin Oncol.* 2007;25(24):3732–3738.
29. Moertel CG, Fleming TR, Macdonald JS, et al. Levamisole and fluorouracil for adjuvant therapy of resected colon carcinoma. *N Engl J Med.* 1990;322(6):352–358.
30. Laurie JA, Moertel CG, Fleming TR, et al. Surgical adjuvant therapy of large-bowel carcinoma: an evaluation of levamisole and the combination of levamisole and fluorouracil. The North Central Cancer Treatment Group and the Mayo Clinic. *J Clin Oncol.* 1989;7(10):1447–1456.
31. André T, Boni C, Mounedji-Boudiaf L, et al.; Multicenter International Study of Oxaliplatin/5-Fluorouracil/Leucovorin in the Adjuvant Treatment of Colon Cancer (MOSAIC) Investigators. Oxaliplatin, fluorouracil, and leucovorin as adjuvant treatment for colon cancer. *N Engl J Med.* 2004;350(23):2343–2351.
32. Gill S, Loprinzi CL, Sargent DJ, et al. Pooled analysis of fluorouracil-based adjuvant therapy for stage II and III colon cancer: who benefits and by how much? *J Clin Oncol.* 2004;22(10):1797–1806.
33. André T, Boni C, Navarro M, et al. Improved overall survival with oxaliplatin, fluorouracil, and leucovorin as adjuvant treatment in stage II or III colon cancer in the MOSAIC trial. *J Clin Oncol.* 2009;27(19):3109–3116.
34. Moertel CG, Fleming TR, Macdonald JS, et al. Intergroup study of fluorouracil plus levamisole as adjuvant therapy for stage II/Dukes' B2 colon cancer. *J Clin Oncol.* 1995; 13(12):2936–2943.
35. Douillard JY, Bennouna J. Adjuvant chemotherapy for colon cancer: a confusing area! *Ann Oncol.* 2005;16(12):1853–1854.
36. Schippinger W, Samonigg H, Schaberl-Moser R, et al.; Austrian Breast and Colorectal Cancer Study Group. A prospective randomised phase III trial of adjuvant chemotherapy with 5-fluorouracil and leucovorin in patients with stage II colon cancer. *Br J Cancer.* 2007;97(8):1021–1027.
37. Jemal A, Bray F, Center MM, Ferlay J, Ward E, Forman D. Global cancer statistics. *CA Cancer J Clin.* 2011;61(2):69–90.
38 NCCN. Clinical Practice Guidelines in Oncology Colon Cancer. 2012.
39. Benson AB 3rd, Schrag D, Somerfield MR, et al. American Society of Clinical Oncology recommendations on adjuvant chemotherapy for stage II colon cancer. *J Clin Oncol.* 2004;22(16):3408–3419.
40. Garman KS, Acharya CR, Edelman E, et al. A genomic approach to colon cancer risk stratification yields biologic insights into therapeutic opportunities. *Proc Natl Acad Sci USA.* 2008;105(49):19432–19437.
41. Jiang Y, Casey G, Lavery IC, et al. Development of a clinically feasible molecular assay to predict recurrence of stage II colon cancer. *J Mol Diagn.* 2008;10(4):346–354.
42. Barrier A, Boelle PY, Roser F, et al. Stage II colon cancer prognosis prediction by tumor gene expression profiling. *J Clin Oncol.* 2006;24(29):4685–4691.
43. Cavalieri D, Dolara P, Mini E, et al. Analysis of gene expression profiles reveals novel correlations with the clinical course of colorectal cancer. *Oncol Res.* 2007;16(11):535–548.
44. Eschrich S, Yang I, Bloom G, et al. Molecular staging for survival prediction of colorectal cancer patients. *J Clin Oncol.* 2005;23(15):3526–3535.
45. Croner RS, Förtsch T, Brückl WM, et al. Molecular signature for lymphatic metastasis in colorectal carcinomas. *Ann Surg.* 2008;247(5):803–810.
46. Bandrés E, Malumbres R, Cubedo E, et al. A gene signature of 8 genes could identify the risk of recurrence and progression in Dukes' B colon cancer patients. *Oncol Rep.* 2007;17(5):1089–1094.
47. Watanabe T, Kobunai T, Sakamoto E, et al. Gene expression signature for recurrence in stage III colorectal cancers. *Cancer.* 2009;115(2):283–292.
48. Koehler A, Bataille F, Schmid C, et al. Gene expression profiling of colorectal cancer and metastases divides tumours according to their clinicopathological stage. *J Pathol.* 2004;204(1): 65–74.
49. Wang Y, Jatkoe T, Zhang Y, et al. Gene expression profiles and molecular markers to predict recurrence of Dukes' B colon cancer. *J Clin Oncol.* 2004;22(9):1564–1571.
50. Lu AT, Salpeter SR, Reeve AE, et al. Gene expression profiles as predictors of poor outcomes in stage II colorectal cancer: A systematic review and meta-analysis. *Clin Colorectal Cancer.* 2009;8(4):207–214.
51. Wirapati P, Sotiriou C, Kunkel S, et al. Meta-analysis of gene expression profiles in breast cancer: toward a unified understanding of breast cancer subtyping and prognosis signatures. *Breast Cancer Res.* 2008;10(4):R65.
52. Sotiriou C, Wirapati P, Loi S, et al. Gene expression profiling in breast cancer: understanding the molecular basis of histologic grade to improve prognosis. *J Natl Cancer Inst.* 2006;98(4): 262–272.
53. O'Connell MJ, Lavery I, Yothers G, et al. Relationship between tumor gene expression and recurrence in four independent studies of patients with stage II/III colon cancer treated with surgery alone or surgery plus adjuvant fluorouracil plus leucovorin. *J Clin Oncol.* 2010;28(25):3937–3944.
54 Venook AN, Lopatin M, Lee M, et al. Validation of a 12-gene colon cancer recurrence score (RS) in patients (pts) with Stage II colon cancer (CC) from CALGB 9581. *J Clin Oncol.* 2011;29 (suppl):abstr 3518.
55. Paik S, Shak S, Tang G, et al. A multigene assay to predict recurrence of tamoxifen-treated, node-negative breast cancer. *N Engl J Med.* 2004;351(27):2817–2826.
56. Salazar R, Roepman P, Capella G, et al. Gene expression signature to improve prognosis prediction of stage II and III colorectal cancer. *J Clin Oncol.* 2011;29(1):17–24.
57 Rosenberg RM, Simon I, Nitsche U, et al. Independent validation of a prognostic genomic profile (ColoPrint) for stage II colon cancer (CC) patients. *J Clin Oncol.* 2011;29(suppl 4): abstr 358.
58 Tabernero J, Rosenberg R, Nitsche U, et al. Clinical and technical validation of a genomic classifier (ColoPrint) for predicting outcome of patients with stage II colon cancer. *J Clin Oncol.* 2012;30(suppl 4):abstr 384.
59 Salazar R, Glimelius B, Marshall J, et al. The PARSC trial, a prospective study for the assessment of recurrence risk in stage II colon cancer (CC) patients using ColoPrint. *J Clin Oncol.* 2012; 30(suppl 4):abstr 678.
60. Kennedy RD, Bylesjo M, Kerr P, et al. Development and independent validation of a prognostic assay for stage II colon cancer using formalin-fixed paraffin-embedded tissue. *J Clin Oncol.* 2011;29(35):4620–4626.
61. Allen WL, Jithesh PV, Oliver GR, et al. The colorectal cancer disease-specific transcriptome may facilitate the discovery of more biologically and clinically relevant information. *BMC Cancer.* 2010;10:687.
62. Farragher SM, Tanney A, Kennedy RD, Paul Harkin D. RNA expression analysis from formalin fixed paraffin embedded tissues. *Histochem Cell Biol.* 2008;130(3):435–445.
63 Pogue-Geile K, Yothers G, Gavin P, Fumagalli D, Kim C, Colangelo LH, et al. Use of prognostic (prog) gene index and nodal status to identify a subset of stage II and III colon cancer patients (pts) who may not need oxaliplatin (ox)-containing adjuvant chemotherapy. *J Clin Oncol.* 2010;28(15s):abstr 3516.

64. Jen J, Kim H, Piantadosi S, et al. Allelic loss of chromosome 18q and prognosis in colorectal cancer. *N Engl J Med.* 1994;331(4):213–221.
65. Barratt PL, Seymour MT, Stenning SP, et al.; UKCCCR AXIS trial collaborators. Adjuvant X-ray and Fluorouracil Infusion Study. DNA markers predicting benefit from adjuvant fluorouracil in patients with colon cancer: a molecular study. *Lancet.* 2002; 360(9343):1381–1391.
66. Ogino S, Nosho K, Irahara N, et al. Prognostic significance and molecular associations of 18q loss of heterozygosity: a cohort study of microsatellite stable colorectal cancers. *J Clin Oncol.* 2009;27(27):4591–4598.
67. Vilar E, Mukherjee B, Kuick R, et al. Gene expression patterns in mismatch repair-deficient colorectal cancers highlight the potential therapeutic role of inhibitors of the phosphatidylinositol 3-kinase-AKT-mammalian target of rapamycin pathway. *Clin Cancer Res.* 2009;15(8):2829–2839.
68. Lamb J, Crawford ED, Peck D, et al. The Connectivity Map: using gene-expression signatures to connect small molecules, genes, and disease. *Science.* 2006;313(5795):1929–1935.
69. Del Rio M, Molina F, Bascoul-Mollevi C, et al. Gene expression signature in advanced colorectal cancer patients select drugs and response for the use of leucovorin, fluorouracil, and irinotecan. *J Clin Oncol.* 2007;25(7):773–780.
70. Graudens E, Boulanger V, Mollard C, et al. Deciphering cellular states of innate tumor drug responses. *Genome Biol.* 2006;7(3):R19.
71. Watanabe T, Kobunai T, Yamamoto Y, et al. Gene expression signature and response to the use of leucovorin, fluorouracil and oxaliplatin in colorectal cancer patients. *Clin Transl Oncol.* 2011;13(6):419–425.
72. Balko JM, Black EP. A gene expression predictor of response to EGFR-targeted therapy stratifies progression-free survival to cetuximab in K-ras wild-type metastatic colorectal cancer. *BMC Cancer.* 2009;9:145.
73. Baker JB, Dutta D, Watson D, et al. Tumour gene expression predicts response to cetuximab in patients with K-ras wild-type metastatic colorectal cancer. *Br J Cancer.* 2011;104(3):488–495.
74. Huang F, Xu LA, Khambata-Ford S. Correlation between gene expression of IGF-1R pathway markers and cetuximab benefit in metastatic colorectal cancer. *Clin Cancer Res.* 2012;18(4):1156–1166.
75. Allen WL, Coyle VM, Jithesh PV, et al. Clinical determinants of response to irinotecan-based therapy derived from cell line models. *Clin Cancer Res.* 2008;14(20):6647–6655.
76. Gerlinger M, Rowan AJ, Horswell S, et al. Intratumor heterogeneity and branched evolution revealed by multiregion sequencing. *N Engl J Med.* 2012;366(10):883–892.
77. Jones S, Zhang X, Parsons DW, et al. Core signaling pathways in human pancreatic cancers revealed by global genomic analyses. *Science.* 2008;321(5897):1801–1806.
78. Parsons DW, Jones S, Zhang X, et al. An integrated genomic analysis of human glioblastoma multiforme. *Science.* 2008;321(5897): 1807–1812.
79. Sjöblom T, Jones S, Wood LD, et al. The consensus coding sequences of human breast and colorectal cancers. *Science.* 2006; 314(5797):268–274.
80. Varela I, Tarpey P, Raine K, et al. Exome sequencing identifies frequent mutation of the SWI/SNF complex gene PBRM1 in renal carcinoma. *Nature.* 2011;469(7331):539–542.
81. Mardis ER, Ding L, Dooling DJ, et al. Recurring mutations found by sequencing an acute myeloid leukemia genome. *N Engl J Med.* 2009;361(11):1058–1066.
82. Hawkins RD, Hon GC, Ren B. Next-generation genomics: an integrative approach. *Nat Rev Genet.* 2010;11(7):476–486.
83 Curtis C, Shah SP, Chin SF, et al. The genomic and transcriptomic architecture of 2,000 breast tumours reveals novel subgroups. *Nature.* 2012 Apr 18.

19 Development of Targeted Therapies

CHRISTOPHER H. LIEU
S. GAIL ECKHARDT
WELLS A. MESSERSMITH

Investigators first launched the initial modern clinical trials for patients with colorectal cancer (CRC) over 5 decades ago, and since that time, the therapeutics for this disease have evolved considerably. Early trials evaluating surgical and radiation therapy have improved the disease free and overall survival (OS) of patients with early stage disease, while trials evaluating systemic therapy have increased the OS of patients with metastatic disease. Since that time, therapeutics for CRC have been rapidly evolving, and oncologists now have access to several drugs with activity in the first-, second-, and even third-line settings. Targeted agents, such as bevacizumab, cetuximab, and panitumumab have emerged as clinically relevant components of systemic therapy for advanced disease. One of the challenges future investigators face is how to combine new approaches with standards of treatment that have already evolved from older studies.

In this chapter, we will provide a brief historical overview of clinical trials in CRC, we will review promising targets in CRC, and we will discuss potential novel study designs in the adjuvant and metastatic setting.

■ EVOLUTION OF CLINICAL TRIALS IN CRC

Studies involving surgery and radiation have altered the treatment approach in early stage CRC. This is particularly true in rectal cancer where preoperative chemoradiation has led to decreased toxicity and increased sphincter preservation rates (1). In the 1970s and 1980s, numerous trials failed to demonstrate a clear survival benefit for postoperative (adjuvant) chemotherapy. However, in 1988, the National Surgical Adjuvant Breast and Bowel Project (NSABP) published results of a large prospective trial comparing surgery alone with adjuvant immunotherapy with bacilli Calmette-Guérin (BCG) and adjuvant chemotherapy consisting of 5-flurorouracil (5-FU), semustine, and vincristine (2). These findings were the first from a randomized prospective clinical trial to demonstrate that a significant disease-free survival and OS benefit could be achieved with postoperative chemotherapy. Subsequently, numerous studies assessed 5-FU in combination with other modulators (3–6). Adjuvant therapy following surgical resection has evolved following the introduction of newer agents into the clinical arena, including capecitabine and oxaliplatin (7–9). Despite the advances made in pre- and postoperative therapy, it should be noted that significant controversy continues to exist regarding the adjuvant treatment for patients with Stage II disease. Furthermore, no survival advantage has been revealed with the use of irinotecan, bevacizumab, or cetuximab in the adjuvant setting (10–14).

Studies of systemic therapy also began over 50 years ago, and these trials have evolved over time as our knowledge of CRC has advanced. Systemic chemotherapy with 5-FU has been the mainstay of palliative treatment for patients with metastatic disease not amenable to surgical intervention. During the ensuing decades, most trials focused on a variety of 5-FU schedules to determine which schedule was associated with the highest objective response rates. 5-FU has since been combined with irinotecan and oxaliplatin to treat patients with advanced disease (15,16). A novel study has also evaluated the benefit of maintenance therapy as well as a stop-and-go strategy that has changed the clinical practice of treating patients with advanced disease (17,18).

The past 10 years has also seen the advent of monoclonal antibodies to directly target specific proteins critical to intracellular signaling, tumor cell function, or the host–tumor interface. In studies dating back over 30 years, Dr. Judah Folkman demonstrated that tumors could not grow beyond 1 mm without creating new vessels to deliver oxygen and nutrients (19). This observation eventually led to drugs targeting vascular endothelial growth factor (VEGF) including bevacizumab, which was FDA-approved for metastatic CRC in 2004 (20). The monoclonal antibodies, cetuximab and panitumumab, targeting the epidermal growth factor receptor (EGFR) have also been approved in CRC. Interestingly, unplanned retrospective analysis of the CRYSTAL trial revealed that clinical benefit from cetuximab was limited to those patients with *K-ras* wild-type tumors (21). This retrospective analysis elucidated the first predictive biomarker of anti-EGFR efficacy. Unfortunately, *K-ras* mutational status only provides physicians with a negative predictive biomarker as it only reveals the patients unlikely to receive any benefit from EGFR-directed therapy. Finally, results from the CAIRO-2 trial, evaluating XELOX/bevacizumab with or without cetuximab, and the PACCE trial, evaluating oxaliplatin or irinotecan-based chemotherapy with bevacizumab with or without panitumumab, have shown a negative clinical impact of adding dual anti-VEGF and anti-EGFR therapy. These studies highlight the challenges associated with combining biologic therapies as well as the need for specific patient selection to ensure treatment of the cohort most likely to benefit from therapy.

PROMISING TARGETS AND DRUGS IN DEVELOPMENT FOR CRC

Epidermal Growth Factor Receptor

Binding of EGFR leads to activation of cell signaling pathways and cell proliferation via various tyrosine kinases (22). Trials investigating the use of cetuximab and panitumumab with conventional chemotherapy have established a benefit in those patients with *K-ras* wild-type tumors (23). Though *K-ras* has helped clinicians determine which patients are unlikely to receive benefit from EGFR inhibition, other predictive biomarkers for EGFR monoclonal antibodies are currently under investigation, including alternative EGFR ligands, and mutations in *BRAF, PTEN,* and *PIK3CA* (24).

New drugs targeting EGFR are currently in development that improve antibody-dependent cellular toxicity (ADCC), increase degradation of EGFR, and target other HER membrane receptors. One example of improved ADCC comes from preclinical data involving lenalidomide. Though lenalidomide is used primarily in hematologic malignancies, in vitro data have shown that lenalidomide enhances the ability of IgG1-isotype antibodies to mediate ADCC of solid tumor cells, independent of *K-ras* mutation status when lenalidomide is combined with cetuximab (25,26). Sym004, a mixture of two anti-EGFR monoclonal antibodies directed against distinct nonoverlapping epitopes in EGFR extracellular domain III, has been shown to inhibit cancer cell growth and survival by blocking ligand-binding receptor activation and phosphorylation. However, unlike other EGFR antibodies, Sym004 has been shown to induce rapid and efficient removal of the receptor from the cancer cell surface by triggering EGFR internalization and degradation (27). Sym004 exhibited more pronounced growth inhibition in murine models, highlighting the possible efficacy of this strategy. Drugs targeting multiple EGFR receptors are currently in development, including MEHD7945A, a novel monoclonal antibody directed against EGFR/HER1 and HER3 (Table 19.1; 28).

Table 19.1 Current Drugs and Compounds in Development and Clinical Trials

Target	Drug/Compound	Phase
EGFR	Afatinib	II
	Nimotuzumab	II
	MEHD7945A	I
	RO5083945	I
	Sym004	I
VEGF	Aflibercept	III
	Brivanib	III
	Ramucirumab	III
	Regorafenib	III
	Pazopanib	Ib
IGF-1R	AMG479	II
	BMS-754807	II
	SCH-717454	II
	AXL1717	I
	Figitumumab	I
	OSI-906	I
	XL228	I
RAS/RAF	Vemurafenib	Ib/II
	GSK2118436	I
	Lonafarnib	I
	XL281	I
MEK	Selumetinib	II
	MSC1936369B	II
	E6201	I
	GSK1120212	I
	MEK162	I
	XL518	I
PI3K/AKT	Perifosine	III
	Everolimus	II
	PX-866	II
	BMK120	I
	BEZ235	I
	GDC-0941	I
	GSK2141795	I
	SF1126	I
	XL147	I
Wnt	Resveratrol	II
	AMG785	II
Notch	RO4929097	II
	MK0752	I
	PF03084014	I
	REGN421	I

Vascular Endothelial Growth Factor

VEGF-A interacts with both VEGFR-1 and VEGFR-2 to mediate angiogenesis. VEGFR-2 is the principal receptor that promotes the pro-angiogenic action of VEGF-A, and therefore has been the principal target of anti-angiogenic therapies. Angiogenesis and VEGF have been confirmed as viable targets for CRC for with a demonstrated improvement in response, progression-free survival (PFS), and OS when bevacizumab has been combined with conventional chemotherapy (20,29). Though the addition of bevacizumab has conferred a modest survival advantage, the relatively rapid development of drug resistance and progression of disease highlights the limitations of current angiogenic targeting.

An evolving hypothesis is that CRCs are able to evade VEGF pathway inhibitors through a number of distinct and interrelated mechanisms of evasive resistance including upregulation of alternative pro-angiogenic signals and protection of the tumor vasculature through the recruitment of pro-angiogenic inflammatory cells or by increasing protective pericyte coverage (30). In one phase II study of FOLFIRI in combination with bevacizumab, cytokine analyses demonstrated that alternate proangiogenic cytokines are modulated by therapy and are increased before disease progression. Prior to progression, levels of bFGF, PlGF, MMP-9, PDGF, and HGF were found to be significantly elevated.

Future antiangiogenic therapy will most likely attempt to target these evasive resistance mechanisms. Aflibercept is a fusion protein that functions as an inhibitor of VEGF-A, VEGF-B, and PlGF and achieved its primary endpoint of OS in the VELOUR phase III clinical trial for second-line treatment for metastatic CRC (31). This study suggests that targeting alternate VEGF ligands may be a successful strategy for overcoming bevacizumab resistance. Currently, there are numerous large molecule and small molecule VEGF inhibitors in development. Other drugs targeting alternate pro-angiogenic pathways are also in clinical trial testing including regorafinib (Ang-1,2), ramucirumab (VEGFR-2), brivanib (FGFR), ABT-869 (PDGFR), and AMG-102 (HGF/c-met; 32–36).

Insulin-Like Growth Factor

Insulin-like growth factor (IGF) signaling has been linked to increased cancer risk and more aggressive cancer behavior (37). In particular, IGF-1R is potentially promising in cancer treatment due to its effect on the RAS-RAF-MAPK and PI3K pathways. Studies in mouse models of colon cancer have shown that treatment with exogenous IGF-1 causes significantly increased rates of tumor development and metastasis (38). IGF-1R over expression has also been found in CRC and has been linked to tumor grade, poor survival, and decreased sensitivity to chemotherapy via downstream activation of cell survival signals (39–41).

Strategies to target the IGF pathway have mainly focused on the use of monoclonal antibodies to block IGF-1R (MK-0646) as well as intracellular tyrosine kinase inhibition (OSI-906; 42,43). Early trials have shown promising activity in CRC with a side effect profile consisting of fatigue, rash, hyperglycemia, and thrombocytopenia. One phase II study evaluated the monoclonal antibody IMC-A12 with and without cetuximab in patients with metastatic refractory CRC (44). Unfortunately, no antitumor activity was seen in the patients receiving IMC-A12 alone or in combination with cetuximab. Trials of other monoclonal antibodies directed against IGF-1R in combination with standard chemotherapy are currently ongoing in CRC.

RAS/RAF

Recurrent somatic mutations in *K-ras* and *BRAF* are found in colorectal carcinomas. *K-ras* mutations in codons 12 and 13 of exon 2 are present in 35%–40% of colorectal carcinomas and result in activation of the MAPK, PI3K, and other pathways (45). As stated previously, *K-ras* mutations predict a lack of benefit to current EGFR monoclonal antibodies. Unfortunately, inhibition of RAS has proven to be difficult. Farnesyl transferase inhibitors target the enzyme protein farnesyl transferase, which catalyzes the addition of a farnesyl isoprenoid moiety to the cysteine residue of RAS proteins, in hopes of inhibiting tumor growth. Unfortunately, a phase III trial of tipifarnib (R115777) showed no improvement in OS compared with best supportive care alone in refractory advanced CRC (46).

In the RAF family, mutations that constitutively activate this kinase occur predominantly in *BRAF*. Mutations in the BRAF V600E allele is present in approximately 10% of CRC and is mutually exclusive to *K-ras* mutations (47). Results from the CRYSTAL trial suggest that *BRAF* mutations are a poor prognostic marker and are not predictive for response to cetuximab (48). The discovery of oncogenic *BRAF* mutations has sparked vigorous efforts to pharmacologically block this kinase. This has been highlighted by the success in targeting *BRAF*-mutant melanoma with vemurafenib (49). Unfortunately, these results have not translated to CRC. A phase Ib/II trial of vemurafenib involving 21 patients with CRC showed very modest clinical activity with only 1 confirmed partial response (50). Further studies are ongoing with sorafenib in combination with chemotherapy.

MEK

RAF phosphorylates MEK, a kinase that activates ERK, and leads to cell proliferation (51). MEK activity can be increased via upstream mutations in the *K-ras* and *BRAF* pathways as discussed previously. Because of this, inhibition of MEK is a logical target for cancer therapeutics in patients with mutated *K-ras* or *BRAF*.

Unfortunately, early generation MEK inhibitors showed little clinical benefit in CRC in phase I and II trials (51,52). A second-generation MEK inhibitor, PD-0325901 showed preliminary clinical activity and an improved pharmacokinetic profile, but higher doses were associated with development of retinal vein occlusion (53). As a result, further development of this compound was discontinued. Selumetinib (AZD6244) has also been evaluated in the second- or third-line setting for metastatic CRC compared to capecitabine. AZD6244 showed similar efficacy to capecitabine in terms of the number of patients with a disease progression event with a tolerable side-effect profile (54). Further preclinical work has suggested that resistance to this compound may be mediated by upregulation of the Wnt pathway, suggesting a possible rational combination for AZD6244 (55). Preclinical work in breast cancer cell lines also demonstrate a negative feedback loop between MEK/MAPK and PI3K pathways facilitating survival during MEK blockade (56). Interruption of this feedback mechanism by targeting MEK and PI3K produced synergistic effects, suggesting a possible combination that may lead to better disease control.

PI3K

The PI3K pathway has a high frequency of alterations in cancer that has led to a surge in the development of PI3K inhibitors. PI3K can be activated by EGFR and RAS and activates AKT (57). Activated AKT modulates the function of numerous substrates related to the regulation of cell proliferation, including metabolism, cell survival, and angiogenesis. PTEN acts as a negative regulator of the PI3K-AKT pathway and inactivating mutations or a loss of PTEN expression leads to increased levels of PI3K products in cells (58). PTEN loss is present in 20%–40% of CRC and is associated with MSI (59). PIK3CA mutations can result in the upregulation of AKT in the absence of growth factors and are present in 15%–30% of CRC. Inhibition of the PI3K pathway has proven difficult because multiple signaling pathways converge and diverge at both PI3K and AKT. Mutations or amplifications of RTKs, PTEN, or RAS are likely to activate PI3K and other important pathways and to shut off negative feedback loops. Therefore rational combination strategies will be needed to overcome drug resistance.

Currently, multiple phase I/II trials are ongoing to explore the combination of everolimus (RAD001) in combination with standard treatment for metastatic CRC (NCT00849550, NCT01047293, NCT00597506, NCT00522665; 60). Perifosine is a synthetic alkylphospholipid that inhibits AKT signal transduction pathways, as well as MAPK and JNK. A small phase II trial of perifosine in combination with capecitabine was well-tolerated and showed an improvement in response rate, time to progression, and OS (61). The U.S. Food and Drug Administration has given this drug fast-track designation based on these results. A randomized phase III trial of perifosine and capecitabine versus capecitabine alone is currently ongoing (60).

Wnt

In CRC, Wnt pathway genetics continues to be dominated by mutation in the adenomatous polyposis coli (*APC*) gene. *APC* is one of the principal constituents of the β-catenin destruction complex. On Wnt stimulation, the β-catenin destruction complex dissociates, leading to the accumulation of nuclear β-catenin and transcription of Wnt pathway responsive genes. Germline mutations in *APC* cause familial adenomatous polyposis, and up to 90% of sporadic CRC show aberrant Wnt signaling activity, usually as the result of mutations in *APC* (62). The resulting chronic activation of the Wnt pathway drives the expansion of cells into benign adenomas, which then frequently progress to invasive colon carcinoma following additional genetic mutations. Given that nearly all colorectal tumors activate Wnt signaling, molecular targeting of this pathway is an attractive therapeutic option.

Despite heavy investment and interest in this critical pathway, drugs specifically designed to target Wnt have yet to show major clinical activity. However, a number of drugs are currently available for other diseases that may directly or indirectly target the Wnt pathway. NSAIDs have been proposed as a possible modulator of the Wnt pathway as reductions in prostaglandin levels by COX activity in the tumor or the surrounding stroma could account for the ability of NSAIDs to dampen the Wnt signaling pathway (63). NSAID treatment has been shown to reverse polyp growth in patients with FAP, and celecoxib has been shown to reduce the occurrence of colonic polyps after polypectomy (64–66). Trials involving COX-2 inhibitors in the advanced disease setting are currently ongoing. Antibody-based therapeutics directed against over expressed Wnt and Frizzled proteins are also currently in development. The monoclonal antibody AMG785 targeting sclerostin, a protein that inhibits LRP 5/6 receptors, is currently being evaluated in phase I/II trials in osteoporosis and has been generally well tolerated (67). Resveratrol, a stilbenoid found in grape skin and wine, is known to inhibit Wnt signaling, and a CRC prevention trial has found decreased levels of Wnt target genes as well as decreased CD133 expression (a colonic stem cell marker) in colonic epithelium with dietary supplementation of this agent (68). A phase II trial investigating the use of resveratrol in CRC in currently ongoing (60). Novel modulators of the Wnt signaling pathway are currently being investigated and are in preclinical development, including tankyrase inhibitors that have been shown to promote β-catenin degradation and stabilization of axin (69).

Notch

Notch is an evolutionarily conserved developmental pathway that is important in embryonic development and maintaining adult tissue homeostasis by influencing cell fate decisions (70). Dysregulation of the Notch pathway plays an integral role in the tumorigenesis of many human malignancies (71–74). Notch signaling plays an important role in the maintenance of normal intestinal epithelia and is essential for regulating the differentiation of colonic goblet cells and progenitor cells (75–77). The Notch ligand, Jagged1, messenger RNA was found to be expressed at a significantly higher level in the normal colonic mucosa and adenomas of patients with familial adenomatous polyposis, compared with normal intestinal mucosal tissues of healthy subjects (78). Another study involving a preclinical model of CRC showed that the Notch signaling pathway was significantly increased and activated in colon cancer-initiating cells (79). Treatment with a γ-secretase inhibitor induced apoptosis and the formation of terminally differentiated goblet cells. In a preclinical model of CRC, Notch-1 receptor was found to be upregulated at the time of cancer progression, and chemotherapy appeared to induce Notch-1 and Notch-1 intracellular domain (NICD) by an increase in the activity and expression of γ-secretase complex (80). Subsequent inhibition of Notch-1 signaling prevented the induction of NICD by chemotherapy and enhanced chemosensitivity was observed.

A phase I study of the selective γ-secretase inhibitor, RO4929097 has shown a favorable side-effect profile, and a phase II single agent trial for the third-line treatment of metastatic CRC (NCT01116687) and a phase I trial with cetuximab (NCT01198535) are ongoing (81). Other selective γ-secretase inhibitors currently being investigated include PF03084014 and MK0752. Extracellular inhibition of the Notch pathway via blockade of DLL-4 with REGN421 (a monoclonal antibody) is being investigated in a phase I study.

■ FUTURE DIRECTIONS AND STUDY DESIGNS IN ADJUVANT CRC

Since the MOSAIC trial was published in 2004, there have been no major recent advances for treatment in the adjuvant setting for resectable CRC (9). Trials evaluating the benefit of adding biologic therapy have failed to show a meaningful increase in disease-free survival (13,14). Controversy remains regarding the role of adjuvant chemotherapy in stage II patients. Prior studies failed to demonstrate a role for adjuvant chemotherapy for all stage II patients, and high-risk features commonly used to define a high-risk group most likely to benefit from treatment has also failed to improve survival (82,83).

Although few therapeutic changes appear to be on the horizon for the treatment of adjuvant colon cancer, studies are ongoing to determine the duration of treatment (3 months vs 6 months) as well as to evaluate the role of diagnostic imaging modalities to improve the overall approach to these patients (84). Another approach to adjuvant therapy for resected CRC involves the use of noncytotoxic therapy to evaluate the potential for preventing recurrence. Current trials with COX-2 inhibitors and statins are ongoing (60). Though the potential for benefit remains small, the risk of adverse effects helps these trials remain a low-risk, low-reward intervention in patients where investigators are attempting to avoid any harm following potentially curative surgery.

Because patients with resectable stage III CRC receive systemic therapy following surgical resection, it is often difficult to determine how effective standard adjuvant therapy is at treating micrometastases. Therefore, another potential model for a clinical trial in the adjuvant setting would be to treat potential patients in the neoadjuvant setting. This type of trial would have the potential to help guide adjuvant therapy following surgical resection. Patients would require imaging and endoscopy prior to enrollment, and those patients with T4 disease or node positive disease could be treated up front with systemic chemotherapy. At the time of surgery, a response marker (ie, imaging or pathology) could be used to determine how effective neoadjuvant therapy was. The patient could then go on to adjuvant therapy, based on the effectiveness of the neoadjuvant regimen.

■ FUTURE DIRECTIONS AND STUDY DESIGNS IN METASTATIC CRC

Despite significant advances in understanding the pathogenesis of CRC and an array of biologic agents currently in the pipeline, only two classes of biologic therapies are currently FDA approved for use in metastatic CRC. Challenges for the future include not only investigating the pathways critical to CRC growth and spread, but also the potential study designs that are implemented in order to treat the population most likely to derive a benefit from these novel therapies.

Clinical trial designs frequently do not mandate tumor tissue from all patients and attempt a post hoc analysis of biomarker status among those with available tissue from the original diagnostic biopsy. A novel trial design in metastatic non-small cell lung cancer (NSCLC) was highlighted by the Biomarker-Integrated Approaches of Targeted Therapy for Lung Cancer Elimination (BATTLE) trial (85). All NSCLC patients entering the trial underwent a core tumor biopsy for the purpose of obtaining biomarker status and were then randomized to 1 of 4 treatment arms. Biomarker analysis was performed with a large panel of mutation, gene copy number, and immunohistochemistry analyses performed on each sample. The results of these studies grouped patients into predefined biomarker signature groups, which could then be used to evaluate treatment-biomarker interactions. The initial cohort of patients was randomized equally into 4 different treatment arms and then was assessed by comparing the outcome of disease control rate with the biomarker status within each treatment arm. With this information, future randomization probabilities were adjusted using a Bayesian model. The pattern continually repeated so that the more patients with a particular signature did well on a particular therapy, the higher the probability of being assigned to that therapy for subsequent similar patients. Although it is currently unclear if a Bayesian trial design will more rapidly identify clinically significant biomarker-targeted therapy relationships compared with more common clinical trial designs, the BATTLE trial offered proof that a large clinical trial can include comprehensive pretreatment biopsies and genotyping for all participants.

An important consideration for future colorectal clinical trials is the population chosen to be studied. Patients with *BRAF* mutations are known to have poor overall prognosis with suboptimal response rates to standard therapies (47). This population is one that may benefit from a first-line clinical trial by either combining standard chemotherapy with a new agent, or possibly treating the patients in the first-line setting with a new agent alone. Another important consideration for future metastatic colorectal clinical trials is the timing of adding biologic therapy. In those patients that have unresectable disease, an OPTIMOX strategy of maintenance chemotherapy is usually employed if the patients have a response to standard chemotherapy. This "maintenance" period represents a possible window of opportunity to study biologic therapy, either in combination with 5-FU or as a single agent. In those patients with resectable disease, the time during which neoadjuvant chemotherapy is given also represents a window of opportunity to study biologic therapy. If tumor testing can be performed on a biopsy specimen prior to the initiation of therapy, a rational biologic agent can be chosen to hopefully improve response and disease stability. Following metastasectomy, results of biologic testing on the resected specimen may also be used to guide therapy following surgery in a clinical trial setting.

■ CONCLUSIONS

The treatment of metastatic CRC has seen significant advances over the last 30 years and has led to improvements in quality of life and OS. Though an expanded array of biologic agents is currently being investigated, only a few targeted agents are currently approved for use in metastatic CRC. Challenges for the future include not only developing novel compounds, but also determining which patients will derive the greatest benefits from these agents.

Biomarker development for each molecular target will need to continue in order to fully realize the potential of "personalized cancer therapy." Therefore, future trials will need to include the option of tissue or blood correlatives to elucidate the mechanisms of actions of these agents. Despite the complexity of each pathway and the heterogeneity of the patient population, our hope is that continued elucidation of colorectal biology and novel trial design will lead to improved treatment options for patients with metastatic CRC.

■ REFERENCES

1. Sauer R, Becker H, Hohenberger W, et al.; German Rectal Cancer Study Group. Preoperative versus postoperative chemoradiotherapy for rectal cancer. *N Engl J Med.* 2004;351(17):1731–1740.
2. Wolmark N, Fisher B, Rockette H, et al. Postoperative adjuvant chemotherapy or BCG for colon cancer: results from NSABP protocol C-01. *J Natl Cancer Inst.* 1988;80(1):30–36.
3. O'Connell MJ, Mailliard JA, Kahn MJ, et al. Controlled trial of fluorouracil and low-dose leucovorin given for 6 months as postoperative adjuvant therapy for colon cancer. *J Clin Oncol.* 1997;15(1):246–250.
4. Moertel CG, Fleming TR, Macdonald JS, et al. Levamisole and fluorouracil for adjuvant therapy of resected colon carcinoma. *N Engl J Med.* 1990;322(6):352–358.
5. Moertel C, Fleming T, Macdonald J, et al. Flurouracil plus levamisole as effective adjuvant therapy after resection of stage III colon carcinoma: a final report. *Ann Intern Med.* 1991;22:321–326.
6. Wolmark N, Rockette H, Fisher B, et al. The benefit of leucovorin-modulated fluorouracil as postoperative adjuvant therapy for primary colon cancer: results from National Surgical Adjuvant Breast and Bowel Project protocol C-03. *J Clin Oncol.* 1993;11(10):1879–1887.
7. Van Cutsem E, Hoff PM, Harper P, et al. Oral capecitabine vs intravenous 5-fluorouracil and leucovorin: integrated efficacy data and novel analyses from two large, randomised, phase III trials. *Br J Cancer.* 2004;90(6):1190–1197.
8. Scheithauer W, McKendrick J, Begbie S, et al.; X-ACT Study Group. Oral capecitabine as an alternative to i.v. 5-fluorouracil-based adjuvant therapy for colon cancer: safety results of a randomized, phase III trial. *Ann Oncol.* 2003;14(12):1735–1743.
9. André T, Boni C, Mounedji-Boudiaf L, et al.; Multicenter International Study of Oxaliplatin/5-Fluorouracil/Leucovorin in the Adjuvant Treatment of Colon Cancer (MOSAIC) Investigators. Oxaliplatin, fluorouracil, and leucovorin as adjuvant treatment for colon cancer. *N Engl J Med.* 2004;350(23):2343–2351.
10. Saltz LB, Niedzwiecki D, Hollis D, et al. Irinotecan fluorouracil plus leucovorin is not superior to fluorouracil plus leucovorin alone as adjuvant treatment for stage III colon cancer: results of CALGB 89803. *J Clin Oncol.* 2007;25(23):3456–3461.

11. Van Cutsem E, Labianca R, Bodoky G, et al. Randomized phase III trial comparing biweekly infusional fluorouracil/leucovorin alone or with irinotecan in the adjuvant treatment of stage III colon cancer: PETACC-3. *J Clin Oncol.* 2009;27(19):3117–3125.
12. Ychou M, Hohenberger W, Thezenas S, et al. A randomized phase III study comparing adjuvant 5-fluorouracil/folinic acid with FOLFIRI in patients following complete resection of liver metastases from colorectal cancer. *Ann Oncol.* 2009;20(12):1964–1970.
13. Allegra CJ, Yothers G, O'Connell MJ, et al. Phase III trial assessing bevacizumab in stages II and III carcinoma of the colon: results of NSABP protocol C-08. *J Clin Oncol.* 2011;29(1):11–16.
14. Goldberg R, Sargent D, Thibodeau S, et al. Adjuvant mFOLFOX6 plus or minus cetuximab (Cmab) in patients (pts) with K-ras mutant (m) resected stage III colon cancer (CC): NCCTG Intergroup Phase III Trial N0147. *J Clin Oncol.* 2010;28:abstr 3508.
15. Saltz LB, Cox JV, Blanke C, et al. Irinotecan plus fluorouracil and leucovorin for metastatic colorectal cancer. Irinotecan Study Group. *N Engl J Med.* 2000;343(13):905–914.
16. Goldberg RM, Sargent DJ, Morton RF, et al. A randomized controlled trial of fluorouracil plus leucovorin, irinotecan, and oxaliplatin combinations in patients with previously untreated metastatic colorectal cancer. *J Clin Oncol.* 2004;22(1):23–30.
17. Tournigand C, Cervantes A, Figer A, et al. OPTIMOX1: a randomized study of FOLFOX4 or FOLFOX7 with oxaliplatin in a stop-and-Go fashion in advanced colorectal cancer–a GERCOR study. *J Clin Oncol.* 2006;24(3):394–400.
18. Chibaudel B, Maindrault-Goebel F, Lledo G, et al. Can chemotherapy be discontinued in unresectable metastatic colorectal cancer? The GERCOR OPTIMOX2 Study. *J Clin Oncol.* 2009;27(34):5727–5733.
19. Folkman J. Tumor angiogenesis: a possible control point in tumor growth. *Ann Intern Med.* 1975;82(1):96–100.
20. Hurwitz H, Fehrenbacher L, Novotny W, et al. Bevacizumab plus irinotecan, fluorouracil, and leucovorin for metastatic colorectal cancer. *N Engl J Med.* 2004;350(23):2335–2342.
21. Van Cutsem E, Köhne CH, Láng I, et al. Cetuximab plus irinotecan, fluorouracil, and leucovorin as first-line treatment for metastatic colorectal cancer: updated analysis of overall survival according to tumor K-ras and BRAF mutation status. *J Clin Oncol.* 2011;29(15):2011–2019.
22. Carpenter G, Cohen S. Epidermal growth factor. *J Biol Chem.* 1990;265(14):7709–7712.
23. Petrelli F, Borgonovo K, Cabiddu M, Ghilardi M, Barni S. Cetuximab and panitumumab in K-ras wild-type colorectal cancer: a meta-analysis. *Int J Colorectal Dis.* 2011;26(7):823–833.
24. Barton S, Starling N, Swanton C. Predictive molecular markers of response to epidermal growth factor receptor(EGFR) family-targeted therapies. *Curr Cancer Drug Targets.* 2010;10(8):799–812.
25. Wu L, Adams M, Carter T, et al. lenalidomide enhances natural killer cell and monocyte-mediated antibody-dependent cellular cytotoxicity of rituximab-treated CD20+ tumor cells. *Clin Cancer Res.* 2008;14(14):4650–4657.
26. Wu L, Parton A, Lu L, Adams M, Schafer P, Bartlett JB. Lenalidomide enhances antibody-dependent cellular cytotoxicity of solid tumor cells *in vitro*: influence of host immune and tumor markers. *Cancer Immunol Immunother.* 2011;60(1):61–73.
27. Pedersen MW, Jacobsen HJ, Koefoed K, et al. Sym004: a novel synergistic anti-epidermal growth factor receptor antibody mixture with superior anticancer efficacy. *Cancer Res.* 2010;70(2):588–597.
28. Schaefer G. *Targeting EGFR and HER3 with a "two-in-one antibody"*, AACR 101st Annual Meeting. Washington, DC:2010.
29. Saltz LB, Clarke S, Díaz-Rubio E, et al. Bevacizumab in combination with oxaliplatin-based chemotherapy as first-line therapy in metastatic colorectal cancer: a randomized phase III study. *J Clin Oncol.* 2008;26(12):2013–2019.
30. Bergers G, Hanahan D. Modes of resistance to anti-angiogenic therapy. *Nat Rev Cancer.* 2008;8(8):592–603.
31. Cutsem EV, Tabernero J, Lakomy R, et al. Intravenous (IV) Aflibercept versus placebo in combination with irinotecan/5-FU (FOLFIRI) for second-line treatment of metastatic colorectal cancer (mCRC): results of a multinational phase III trial (EFC10262-VELOUR). *Ann Oncol.* 2011;22:v10–v18.
32. Wilhelm SM, Dumas J, Adnane L, et al. Regorafenib (BAY 73-4506): a new oral multikinase inhibitor of angiogenic, stromal and oncogenic receptor tyrosine kinases with potent preclinical antitumor activity. *Int J Cancer.* 2011;129(1):245–255.
33. Jonker DJ, Rosen LS, Sawyer MB, et al. A phase I study to determine the safety, pharmacokinetics and pharmacodynamics of a dual VEGFR and FGFR inhibitor, brivanib, in patients with advanced or metastatic solid tumors. *Ann Oncol.* 2011;22(6):1413–1419.
34. Wong CI, Koh TS, Soo R, et al. Phase I and biomarker study of ABT-869, a multiple receptor tyrosine kinase inhibitor, in patients with refractory solid malignancies. *J Clin Oncol.* 2009;27(28):4718–4726.
35. Rosen PJ, Sweeney CJ, Park DJ, et al. A phase Ib study of AMG 102 in combination with bevacizumab or motesanib in patients with advanced solid tumors. *Clin Cancer Res.* 2010;16(9):2677–2687.
36. Spratlin JL, Cohen RB, Eadens M, et al. Phase I pharmacologic and biologic study of ramucirumab (IMC-1121B), a fully human immunoglobulin G1 monoclonal antibody targeting the vascular endothelial growth factor receptor-2. *J Clin Oncol.* 2010;28(5):780–787.
37. Scagliotti GV, Novello S. The role of the insulin-like growth factor signaling pathway in non-small cell lung cancer and other solid tumors. *Cancer Treat Rev.* 2012;38(4):292–302.
38. Wu Y, Yakar S, Zhao L, Hennighausen L, LeRoith D. Circulating insulin-like growth factor-I levels regulate colon cancer growth and metastasis. *Cancer Res.* 2002;62(4):1030–1035.
39. Hakam A, Yeatman TJ, Lu L, et al. Expression of insulin-like growth factor-1 receptor in human colorectal cancer. *Hum Pathol.* 1999;30(10):1128–1133.
40. Pollak MN, Perdue JF, Margolese RG, Baer K, Richard M. Presence of somatomedin receptors on primary human breast and colon carcinomas. *Cancer Lett.* 1987;38(1–2):223–230.
41. Hopkins A, Crowe PJ, Yang JL. Effect of type 1 insulin-like growth factor receptor targeted therapy on chemotherapy in human cancer and the mechanisms involved. *J Cancer Res Clin Oncol.* 2010;136(5):639–650.
42. Higano C, Yu E, Whiting S, et al. A phase I, first in man study of weekly IMC-A12, a fully human insulin like growth factor-I receptor IgG1 monoclonal antibody, in patients with advanced solid tumors. *J Clin Oncol.* 2007;25:3505.
43. Lindsay C, Chan E, Evans T, et al. Phase I dose escalation study of continuous oral dosing of OSI-906, an insulin like growth factor-1 receptor (IGF-1R) tyrosine kinase inhibitor, in patients with advanced solid tumors. *J Clin Oncol.* 2009;27:2559.
44. Reidy DL, Vakiani E, Fakih MG, et al. Randomized, phase II study of the insulin-like growth factor-1 receptor inhibitor IMC-A12, with or without cetuximab, in patients with cetuximab- or panitumumab-refractory metastatic colorectal cancer. *J Clin Oncol.* 2010;28(27):4240–4246.
45. Bos JL, Fearon ER, Hamilton SR, et al. Prevalence of ras gene mutations in human colorectal cancers. *Nature.* 1987;327(6120):293–297.
46. Rao S, Cunningham D, de Gramont A, et al. Phase III double-blind placebo-controlled study of farnesyl transferase inhibitor R115777 in patients with refractory advanced colorectal cancer. *J Clin Oncol.* 2004;22(19):3950–3957.
47. Di Nicolantonio F, Martini M, Molinari F, et al. Wild-type BRAF is required for response to panitumumab or cetuximab in metastatic colorectal cancer. *J Clin Oncol.* 2008;26(35):5705–5712.
48. Cutsem EV, Lang I, Folprecht G, et al. Cetuximab plus folfiri: final data from the crystal study on the association of K-ras and braf biomarker status with treatment outcome. *J Clin Oncol.* 2010;28:3570.

49. Chapman PB, Hauschild A, Robert C, et al.; BRIM-3 Study Group. Improved survival with vemurafenib in melanoma with BRAF V600E mutation. *N Engl J Med.* 2011;364(26):2507–2516.
50. Kopetz S, Desai J, Chan E, et al. PLX4032 in metastatic colorectal cancer patients with mutant BRAF tumors. *J Clin Oncol.* 2010;28:3534.
51. Avruch J. MAP kinase pathways: the first twenty years. *Biochim Biophys Acta.* 2007;1773(8):1150–1160.
52. Rinehart J, Adjei AA, Lorusso PM, et al. Multicenter phase II study of the oral MEK inhibitor, CI-1040, in patients with advanced non-small-cell lung, breast, colon, and pancreatic cancer. *J Clin Oncol.* 2004;22(22):4456–4462.
53. LoRusso PM, Krishnamurthi SS, Rinehart JJ, et al. Phase I pharmacokinetic and pharmacodynamic study of the oral MAPK/ERK kinase inhibitor PD-0325901 in patients with advanced cancers. *Clin Cancer Res.* 2010;16(6):1924–1937.
54. Bennouna J, Lang I, Valladares-Ayerbes M, et al. A Phase II, open-label, randomised study to assess the efficacy and safety of the MEK1/2 inhibitor AZD6244 (ARRY-142886) versus capecitabine monotherapy in patients with colorectal cancer who have failed one or two prior chemotherapeutic regimens. *Invest New Drugs.* 2011;29(5):1021–1028.
55. Tentler JJ, Nallapareddy S, Tan AC, et al. Identification of predictive markers of response to the MEK1/2 inhibitor selumetinib (AZD6244) in K-ras-mutated colorectal cancer. *Mol Cancer Ther.* 2010;9(12):3351–3362.
56. Mirzoeva OK, Das D, Heiser LM, et al. Basal subtype and MAPK/ERK kinase (MEK)-phosphoinositide 3-kinase feedback signaling determine susceptibility of breast cancer cells to MEK inhibition. *Cancer Res.* 2009;69(2):565–572.
57. Osaki M, Oshimura M, Ito H. PI3K-Akt pathway: its functions and alterations in human cancer. *Apoptosis.* 2004;9(6):667–676.
58. Yuan TL, Cantley LC. PI3K pathway alterations in cancer: variations on a theme. *Oncogene.* 2008;27(41):5497–5510.
59. Lièvre A, Blons H, Laurent-Puig P. Oncogenic mutations as predictive factors in colorectal cancer. *Oncogene.* 2010; 29(21):3033–3043.
60. National Cancer Institute; University of Michigan. Resveratrol in treating patietns with colorectal cancer that can be removed by surgery. In: ClinicalTrials.gov [Internet]. Bethesda (MD): National Library of Medicine (US). 2000 - [cited 2013 Jul 1]. Available from http://clinicaltrials.gov/show/NCT00433576 NLM Identifier: NCT00433576.
61. Richards D, Nemunaitis J, Vukelja S, et al. Final results of a randomized phase II study of perifosine in combination with capecitabine (P-CAP) versus placebo plus capecitabine (CAP) in patients (pts) with second- or third-line metastatic colorectal cancer (mCRC). *J Clin Oncol.* 2010;28:3531.
62. Segditsas S, Tomlinson I. Colorectal cancer and genetic alterations in the Wnt pathway. *Oncogene.* 2006;25(57):7531–7537.
63. Barker N, Clevers H. Mining the Wnt pathway for cancer therapeutics. *Nat Rev Drug Discov.* 2006;5(12):997–1014.
64. Koehne CH, Dubois RN. COX-2 inhibition and colorectal cancer. *Semin Oncol.* 2004;31(2 Suppl 7):12–21.
65. Yang K, Fan K, Kurihara N, et al. Regional response leading to tumorigenesis after sulindac in small and large intestine of mice with Apc mutations. *Carcinogenesis.* 2003;24(3):605–611.
66. Arber N, Eagle CJ, Spicak J, et al.; PreSAP Trial Investigators. Celecoxib for the prevention of colorectal adenomatous polyps. *N Engl J Med.* 2006;355(9):885–895.
67. Padhi D, Jang G, Stouch B, Fang L, Posvar E. Single-dose, placebo-controlled, randomized study of AMG 785, a sclerostin monoclonal antibody. *J Bone Miner Res.* 2011;26(1):19–26.
68. Martinez M, Hope C, Planutis K, et al. Dietary grape-derived resveratrol for colon cancer prevention. *J Clin Oncol.* 2010;28:3622.
69. Huang SM, Mishina YM, Liu S, et al. Tankyrase inhibition stabilizes axin and antagonizes Wnt signalling. *Nature.* 2009; 461(7264):614–620.
70. Qiao L, Wong BCY. Role of Notch signaling in colorectal cancer. *Carcinogenesis.* 200930:1979–1986.
71. Fan X, Mikolaenko I, Elhassan I, et al. Notch1 and notch2 have opposite effects on embryonal brain tumor growth. *Cancer Res.* 2004;64(21):7787–7793.
72. Reedijk M, Odorcic S, Chang L, et al. High-level coexpression of JAG1 and NOTCH1 is observed in human breast cancer and is associated with poor overall survival. *Cancer Res.* 2005;65(18):8530–8537.
73. Santagata S, Demichelis F, Riva A, et al. JAGGED1 expression is associated with prostate cancer metastasis and recurrence. *Cancer Res.* 2004;64(19):6854–6857.
74. Konishi J, Kawaguchi KS, Vo H, et al. Gamma-secretase inhibitor prevents Notch3 activation and reduces proliferation in human lung cancers. *Cancer Res.* 2007;67(17):8051–8057.
75. Fre S, Huyghe M, Mourikis P, Robine S, Louvard D, Artavanis-Tsakonas S. Notch signals control the fate of immature progenitor cells in the intestine. *Nature.* 2005;435(7044): 964–968.
76. van de Wetering M, Sancho E, Verweij C, et al. The [beta]-catenin/tcf-4 complex imposes a crypt progenitor phenotype on colorectal cancer cells. *Cell.* 2002;111:241–250.
77. Riccio O, van Gijn ME, Bezdek AC, et al. Loss of intestinal crypt progenitor cells owing to inactivation of both Notch1 and Notch2 is accompanied by derepression of CDK inhibitors p27Kip1 and p57Kip2. *EMBO Rep.* 2008;9(4):377–383.
78. Rodilla V, Villanueva A, Obrador-Hevia A, et al. Jagged1 is the pathological link between Wnt and Notch pathways in colorectal cancer. *Proc Natl Acad Sci USA.* 2009;106(15):6315–6320.
79. Sikandar SS, Pate KT, Anderson S, et al. NOTCH signaling is required for formation and self-renewal of tumor-initiating cells and for repression of secretory cell differentiation in colon cancer. *Cancer Res.* 2010;70(4):1469–1478.
80. Meng RD, Shelton CC, Li YM, et al. gamma-Secretase inhibitors abrogate oxaliplatin-induced activation of the Notch-1 signaling pathway in colon cancer cells resulting in enhanced chemosensitivity. *Cancer Res.* 2009;69(2):573–582.
81. Tolcher A, Mikulski S, Messersmith W, et al. A phase I study of RO4929097, a novel gamma secretase inhibitor, in patients with advanced solid tumors. *J Clin Oncol.* 2010;28:2502.
82. Group QC. Adjuvant chemotherapy versus observation in patients with colorectal cancer: a randomised study. *Lancet.* 2007;370:2020–2029.
83. O'Connor ES, Greenblatt DY, LoConte NK, et al. Adjuvant chemotherapy for stage II colon cancer with poor prognostic features. *J Clin Oncol.* 2011;29(25):3381–3388.
84. NCI: FOLFOX-4. 3 months versus 6 months and bevacizumab as adjuvant therapy for patients with stage II/III colon cancer; 2010.
85. Kim ES, Herbst RS, Wistuba II, et al. The BATTLE trial: personalizing therapy for lung cancer. *Cancer Discov.* 2011; 1(1):44–53.

20 Future Directions in the Treatment of Colorectal Cancers: Designs for Biomarker-Driven Clinical Trials

QIAN SHI
SUMITHRA J. MANDREKAR
DANIEL J. SARGENT

■ INTRODUCTION

Colorectal cancer (CRC) remains the third most common cancer in the United States, with approximately 102,900 new cases diagnosed annually, and the second leading cause of cancer deaths (51,370 attributed deaths; 1). In recent decades, significant increases in our understanding of the molecular origins of CRC and characteristics of tumor aggressiveness have occurred, and have allowed the reclassification of CRC into molecular categories (2–5). With cancer treatment development focusing on molecular targeted therapies, it has become possible to define tools for more accurate diagnosis, prognosis assessment, selection of treatment for individual patients to achieve optimal clinical benefits, and the conduct of clinical trials in a cost-effective fashion by using surrogate endpoints (6–9).

The Biomarkers Definitions Working Group defined a biomarker to be "a characteristic that is objectively measured and evaluated as an indicator of normal biological processes, pathogenic processes, or pharmacologic responses to a therapeutic intervention" (10). Biomarkers include a large range of measures derived from tumor tissues, whole blood, plasma, serum, bone marrow, or urine. In this new era of targeted therapy in oncology, cellular, molecular, and genetic biomarkers have received great attention (9). From the perspective of clinical utility, biomarkers can be classified into three categories: prognostic biomarkers, predictive biomarkers, and surrogate endpoints. Prognostic and predictive biomarkers focus on individual patient risk-classification and treatment selection, whereas using a biomarker measure as a surrogate endpoint aids in the evaluation of the efficacy of a new treatment. It is critical to realize that the ultimate intended usage of a biomarker or a signature of multiple biomarkers defines its definition and the required validation methods (11–13). A prognostic biomarker predicts the natural history of the disease process in a given individual, and hence can aid the decision of whether a patient needs an intensive and possibly toxic treatment as opposed to no treatment or standard therapy. The clinical utility of a predictive biomarker can allow individualized therapy, since it can predict whether an individual patient will respond to a particular therapy or not. On the other hand, a surrogate endpoint is used to replace the primary clinical outcome in a clinical trial to inform the efficacy of a new treatment with greater cost effectiveness than traditional endpoints (such as overall survival) at the population level.

Prognostic and predictive biomarkers and surrogate endpoints share many properties, such as predictability over the disease course, comparativeness, and the requirement of validation (14). The challenges of validation become greater as considerations of a biomarker move from prognosis to prediction, and to being a potential surrogate endpoint. Strong predictive ability for an outcome regardless of treatment is sufficient for a prognostic biomarker, but not for a predictive biomarker. A prospectively designed single large randomized controlled trial (RCT) to test the interaction between the biomarker and treatment is sufficient for validating a predictive biomarker, but not for a surrogate endpoint, for which multiple randomized trials have to be gathered to test the association of treatment effects on the surrogate and primary outcomes. The focus of this chapter is on trial designs for validating prognostic biomarkers, predictive biomarkers, and surrogate endpoint, under the assumption that the biomarker can be assessed using a stable assay and that it has shown promising predictive ability in preliminary studies.

■ PROGNOSTIC BIOMARKERS

Historically a prognostic biomarker is defined as a single trait or signature of traits that predict the likely course of disease in the absence of treatment (15,16). In current oncology practices, it is rare that no effective treatment options exist; therefore, this definition has been expanded into the scenarios that involve systemic therapy (6,13). A validated prognostic biomarker can classify patients into subgroups where different treatment options are appropriate. For example, positive lymph-node (LN) involvement predicts a higher likelihood of recurrence or progression compared to negative LN involvement in many tumor types. Therefore, patients with negative LN involvement may not need aggressive (potentially toxic) treatment.

Although it is relatively straightforward to identify potential prognostic biomarkers by establishing strong correlation between the biomarker and a treatment-independent clinical endpoint based on small retrospective studies (17), it is recommended that the validation of a prognostic biomarker should be based on patients treated on clinical trials (11). Indeed, studies of prognostic factors many times are embedded in studies testing new therapies, ideally with a concurrent control arm (18). These trials usually include well-characterized patient cohorts treated with defined treatments with high-quality (ie, consistent) follow up on all patients for the primary endpoints. However, since the sample size is typically driven by the primary endpoints (ie, testing for an overall treatment effect), prespecifying a small number of prognostic biomarkers for validation can minimize the issues of multiple comparisons (18). A highly significant *p*-value and/or large effect sizes (odds ratio or hazard ratio) may not be sufficient in itself to validate a prognostic biomarker; measures of predictive accuracy and of explained variation are essential to reinforce the validity of a prognostic biomarker (9).

■ PREDICTIVE BIOMARKERS

A predictive biomarker is a marker that predicts the differential efficacy of a particular therapy, as assessed by a defined clinical endpoint, based on marker status (6,9,13). For molecularly targeted therapies, biomarkers related to the target or pathway are natural candidates for predictive biomarkers, eg, HER2/*neu* over expression in breast cancer for trastuzumab and mutations in KIT in GI stromal tumors for imatinib mesylate. In advanced CRC, *K-ras* mutation has been confirmed to predict a lack of benefit of anti-EGFR monoclonal antibodies panitumumab (19,20) and cetuximab (21–23) in multiple studies.

A validated predictive marker provides a powerful tool to guide the treatment decisions for individual patients. The presence of such a marker dictates a particular treatment that is most likely to provide benefit for a patient in terms of prolonged survival or delayed disease progression. On the other hand, the absence of such a marker in a patient can spare him/her from the toxicity of therapy known a priori to be ineffective, and avoid the time and cost of treatment for such patients, allowing them to seek better alternative treatment(s) (6,11,18,24,25).

Clinical Trial Designs for Validation of Predictive Biomarkers

There are two key aspects embedded in the goal of using a predictive marker to direct treatment decisions that must be accessed using appropriate methodology. First, accurate evaluation of the treatment effect is a critical component of validating a predictive marker, although it might be only restricted to a marker-defined subpopulation. Therefore, the same standards of evidence as needed to adopt a new therapeutic intervention are also required for predictive marker validation. Specifically, it is fundamentally essential to use an RCT in the validation of a predictive marker (7). When used in either the retrospective or prospective settings (see following sections), the RCT design minimizes the confounding effects of other prognostic factors by maintaining the comparability between patients treated in the comparison groups. Second, the ability to differentiate the subpopulations with respect to the treatment effect based on marker status is required in the validation process. The predictive value of a putative marker must be demonstrated by a significant difference in treatment effects on the outcomes of interest among different subpopulations. For example, the treatment prolongs patient survival significantly in marker-positive subgroup, but has harmful or no effect in marker-negative subgroup (optimally demonstrated through a significant statistical interaction test).

In general, clinical trial designs for validating a predictive biomarker can be grouped into retrospective and prospective settings. In prospective settings, validation designs can be further classified into (a) enrichment or targeted designs; (b) treatment-by-marker interaction designs. (c) marker-based strategy designs; and (d) adaptive designs. We will refer to the treatment-by-marker interaction and marker-based strategy designs as unselected designs in the following sections, since both biomarker-positive and biomarker-negative patients are included.

Retrospective Designs

When a prospective RCT may not be feasible due to ethical reasons or require unrealistically large sample size or long time to complete (13), retrospective validation using previously conducted prospective RCTs can provide the most important source of evidence, and bring forward effective treatments to marker defined subgroup of patients in a timely manner (9,13,26). One example is applying this "retrospective-prospective" approach to demonstrate the predictive value of *K-ras* gene status in advanced CRC. Several analyses based on the data from previously conducted RCTs in advanced CRC demonstrated that cetuximab (21–23) and panitumumab (19,20) are only effective in patients with *K-ras* wild type status.

However, there are several essential elements that are required to provide convincing evidence for a biomarker to be validated as a predictive marker based on retrospective data. First, in order to avoid selection bias, the samples on a large majority of patients should be available. Second, the analyses should be prospectively planned, specifically: (a) predefine the scoring system used for the biomarker measures to classify risk groups;

(b) state focused hypotheses; (c) define the statistical methods; and (d) clarify the interpretational guidelines, eg, level of statistical significance, magnitude of effect, and so on. In addition, if several series of independent RCTs are available, concordant results across trials will provide strong evidence for a robust predictive effect (9,13).

Enrichment or Targeted Designs

Enrichment or targeted designs have been proposed to evaluate a targeted therapy that is thought to have different activity in subgroups defined by a biomarker. In this design, only patients with biomarker-positive status (assuming this is on the group which the new agent will have efficacy impact) are enrolled and treated with the new agent. This is especially appealing when the proportion of truly benefiting patients is expected to be low (8). In such a situation, an enrichment design can improve the efficiency of testing a drug in a targeted subpopulation (larger effect size, hence smaller sample size) and possibly clearly and quickly define an effective treatment for a subset of patients (8,13).

This design was utilized to evaluate the efficacy of trastuzumab in HER2 positive patients with early stage of breast cancer. Simon and Maitournam demonstrated that the enrichment design has higher relative efficiency in terms of required sample size and number of patients to be screened compared to a traditional RCT design without incorporating biomarkers. The magnitude of the gained efficiency depends on the accuracy of the assay and the prevalence of the markers in the population (27,28). Other factors include the well-established reproducibility and accuracy of the assay, and the infeasibility of an unselected design based on previous knowledge (29).

Treatment-by-Marker Interaction Design

The treatment-by-marker interaction design uses the marker status as a stratification factor, and randomizes patients in the marker defined subgroups between experimental and control arms. The fundamental difference between this design and the common RCT is that only patients with a valid marker result are eligible and randomized. Therefore, the trial utilizing this design is truly a prospective marker validation trial that delivers the highest level of evidence (6,9,29,30). This approach was used in the Marker Validation of Erlotinib in Lung Cancer (MARVEL) trial, in which patients were tested for EFGR status and then randomized between erlotinib or pemetrexed as second-line treatment of non-small cell lung cancer (31).

The sample size planning for treatment-by-marker interaction design is based on the prespecified analysis plan. A separate evaluation of the treatment effect can be tested in the two marker-defined subgroups, or a preliminary test of interaction can be carried out first. Different sequential analysis plans can also be implemented. For example, when a preliminary test of interaction is not significant at a prespecified significance level, then the treatment arms can be compared in the overall population (ignoring the biomarker status). If the interaction is significant, then the experimental treatment can be compared to the control arm within the strata determined by the marker.

Marker-Based Strategy Design

In this design, patients are randomized to two arms—a biomarker directed arm and a biomarker independent arm. Patients in the biomarker directed arm receive the experimental therapy if their biomarker status is positive, or control treatment if their biomarker status is negative. Patients in the biomarker independent arm receive the control treatment (or are randomized between experimental and control treatment) regardless of their biomarker status (6,7, 18). This design fits the paradigm of evaluating treatment effectiveness, ie, the effect achieved when the treatment is used in broad clinical practice, since it naturally estimates the "averaged" treatment effect when a biomarker directed therapy will be the used in a certain population of patients compared to control treatments (32).

A limitation of this design is that, in the absence of a very large treatment effect, it results in a very large sample size due to the significant overlap between the treatment arms. That is, in this design there are patients in both the marker-directed and nonmarker-directed arms receiving the same therapy. As such, the hazard ratio for comparing the two arms is forced toward unity, and in general the marker by treatment interaction design is more efficient (29,33).

Adaptive Designs

A number of innovative adaptive designs have been proposed to validate putative predictive biomarkers. We briefly describe two—adaptive accrual based on interim analysis design (34) and the biomarker adaptive threshold design (35). The adaptive accrual design begins with accrual to both biomarker-positive and biomarker-negative subgroups. At the interim analysis time point, if the futility boundary is crossed for one of the subgroups, then the accrual to that group is terminated. Accrual to the other biomarker subgroup continues until the planned sample size is reached, plus the unaccrued patients from the other subgroup that was terminated due to the futility analysis (34).

The biomarker adaptive threshold design allows for the identification and validation of a cut point for a prespecified biomarker measured in an RCT. The advantages of this design are two-fold. This design preserves the ability to evaluate the overall treatment effect in the unselected population. Second, it allows for the prospective validation of a biomarker without a predefined cut off for risk group classification. This design involves testing the overall treatment effect and indentifying the optimal cut point for the biomarker (35). However, the fact that the data from the same trial are used for both defining and validating a marker cut-point challenges the external robustness of the findings. Freidlin et al (32) extended this design to combine the cut point development and validation in a complete cross-validation procedure, which considerably improved the performance of the original design.

Comparisons of Selected Validation Designs

A fundamental issue with the enrichment design is that it cannot assess whether the biomarker is truly predictive, since it does not provide any information regarding the lack or presence of the benefit of the experimental treatment among biomarker-negative patients. As in the HER2/*neu* example, the benefit of trastuzumab in patients with HER2/*neu* amplified tumors has been established by several large randomized trials (36). However, it has been suggested that trastuzumab is perhaps beneficial in patients beyond the specific HER2/*neu* status used in the adjuvant trails when the biomarker was retested in central laboratories (37,38). This suggests that an unselected design (treatment-by-marker interaction or marker-based strategy design) may be indicated even when the prior assumption is that the regimen will only work in marker-positive patients. In addition, in case of the therapy truly benefiting some subset of patients, if the biomarker targets the wrong subpopulation, then a promising regimen could mistakenly be abandoned (32).

The main spirit of the marker-based strategy design is to address the relevant question by comparing the new personalized treatment strategy arm that utilizes the biomarker status to direct the treatment to the standard approach arm without consideration of biomarker status. As previously mentioned, there are statistical issues that are problematic with this design (32). In this design, it is dictated that a portion of patients would receive the same treatment on both arms. This fact dilutes the between arm treatment difference as compared with enrichment design or treatment-by-biomarker interaction design, and thus the marker-based strategy design usually requires a much larger sample size than the interaction design (29,39). By contrast, the treatment-by-marker interaction design maximizes the advantage of randomization and allows one to address the relevant questions in both subpopulation level and overall population level. Furthermore, this design provides rigorous evidence to determine the best treatment in both the biomarker-positive and the biomarker-negative subgroups (32). However, there are also practical considerations factors that give the maker-based strategy design significant merit. For example, when there are a large number of regimens to be tested, or a treatment decision is to be based on a panel of biomarkers, the treatment-by-marker interaction design is not feasible but the strategy design could remain useful.

Surrogate Endpoints

Overall survival (OS) is historically the most standard phase III clinical trial primary endpoint in oncology, since it is sensitive to treatment effects and fully captures the goal of oncology studies—prolong patients' survival (40). However, using OS as an endpoint generally increases the duration and/or sample size of a clinical trial. For example, in early-stage cancer trials, in order to achieve sufficient statistical power, extended patient follow up or a large sample size due to the low-event rates is required. This clearly hinders the ability to rapidly develop effective therapies for life-threatening diseases. To overcome this problem, the use of a validated surrogate endpoint that can be measured earlier, more frequently, more conveniently, and/or at a lesser cost seems to be an attractive solution.

Over the past several decades, the need for a putative surrogate endpoint to be fully validated before its application in practice has been recognized by medical investigators, clinical trialists, statisticians, developers of therapeutic treatments, and regulators. A critical requirement of a valid surrogate endpoint is that the treatment effect observed on the surrogate endpoint should reliably and precisely predict the treatment effect on the primary clinical endpoint. This implies a stronger requirement than simply a significant correlation between the surrogate endpoint and the primary clinical endpoint.

Prentice (41) first established the foundation for validating a surrogate endpoint in a single trial setting. Since then, several statistical evaluation methods have been proposed for validating a putative surrogate endpoint (42–44). Recently, meta-analytic approaches have become widely accepted as the preferred method for evaluating and validating a putative surrogate endpoint. A hierarchical two-stage model, utilizing individual patients' data from multiple randomized clinical trials, allows both individual- and trial-level surrogacy estimations. In this approach, the trial-specific treatment effects on both the surrogate endpoint and the primary clinical endpoint, say OS, are estimated in the first stage of the model using a standard survival analysis approach. If multivariate survival models are used at this stage, then individual-level surrogacy can be estimated simultaneously. For trial-level surrogacy, there are common measures, such as the weighted least square (WLS) R^2 and Copula R^2. WLS R^2

is the coefficient of determination of the WLS regression between the treatment effects on OS and the surrogate endpoint across trials (45,46). The Copula R^2 is estimated based on the methods proposed by Burzykowski et al (47). Broadly speaking, values of $R^2 \geq 0.8$ (the lower bound of 95% CI ≥ 0.6) are considered indicative of a strong surrogacy, while values of R^2 between 0.6 and 0.8 are considered indicative of a modest surrogacy.

In oncology studies, there has been a long history of utilizing "surrogate" endpoints. For example, tumor shrinkage or delayed tumor growth, and improvement in levels of biomarkers, such as prostate-specific antigen (PSA) in prostate cancer, are known to be good prognostic factors for long-term clinical outcomes. Most of these measures, however, fail a formal surrogacy evaluation as correlation with clinical outcomes is insufficient to demonstrate prediction of treatment effects. Shi and Sargent summarized recent applications of evaluating surrogate endpoints in oncology studies including colorectal, prostate, and breast cancer (48). In adjuvant colorectal settings, Sargent et al successfully validated 3-year disease-free survival (DFS) as a surrogate endpoint for 5-year OS (6). In metastatic CRC, progression-free survival (PFS) has demonstrated promising surrogacy for OS in trials testing chemotherapies without biologic agents (49).

Using surrogate endpoints can deliver quicker answers to drug development questions, and thus are an attractive approach for clinical trials in oncology. However, before a biomarker can be used as a surrogate of the true clinical endpoint, formal validation from both the patient and trial level should be conducted. The evaluation and utilization of a surrogate endpoint involves compiling evidence from not only statistical estimations, but also from biological and/or pathological investigations and benefit-risk tradeoff examinations from regulatory perspectives.

■ DISCUSSION

In modern oncology, the rapidly increasing understanding of the biological mechanisms of disease development at the molecular level, enhanced laboratory assessment metrics, and new imaging techniques stimulate the desire for personalized patient disease management. Biomarkers can be integrated into this personalized disease management at different levels with different aspects: (a) avoiding toxic and aggressive therapy when a patient is classified with low risk of disease recurrence by a prognostic biomarker; (b) directing a patient to a particular (efficacious) regimen based on the results of a predictive biomarker; or (c) achieving rapid treatment effect evaluation of a new therapy by replacing the primary endpoint with a validated surrogate endpoint. In this chapter, we discussed the definition and clinical trial designs for validation of prognostic biomarkers, predictive biomarkers, and surrogate endpoints. It is worth noting that a combination of scientific, clinical, statistical, ethical, and practical considerations provide the guidance for the choice of the design for these biomarkers (6,9,13,48).

"Biomarkers in medicine" is a continuum with a wide range of biochemical markers, cellular markers, cytokine markers, genetic markers, physiological results, radiological measurements, physical signs, or pathological assessment (14). Moving from the lowest end forward on the continuum where many thousands of markers have shown some correlation with clinical outcomes, the "biomarker container" becomes vastly smaller when validated prognostic and predictive biomarkers are considered. It is further narrowed when it comes to the assessment of surrogate endpoints. This constriction of the "medical biomarker pool" is dedicated by the strength of the predictive relationship of the biomarker and the primary clinical outcome. Hence, the validation process presents greater challenges as the utility of the biomarker moves from the low to the high end of this "biomarkers in medicine" continuum. As the field of individualized oncology moves forward, the critical component required for the validation of prognostic and predictive biomarkers and surrogate endpoint requires a fit-for-purpose clinical validation design. Careful attention to this design principle will guide maximally efficient (and hopefully successful) future clinical trials.

■ REFERENCES

1. Jemal A, Siegel R, Xu J, Ward E. Cancer statistics, 2010. *CA Cancer J Clin.* 2010;60(5):277–300.
2. Kinzler KW, Vogelstein B, (eds). Colorectal tumors. In: Voelstein B, Kinzler K.W., eds. *The Genetic Basis of Human Cancer.* 2nd ed. McGraw-Hill: New York, NY; 2002;583–612.
3. Libutti SK, Saltz LB, Tepper JE. Colon Cancer. In: DeVita, VT, Jr, Lawrence, TS, Rosenberg, SA, eds. *Cancer: Principles and practice of Oncology.* Lippincott Williams & Wilkins: Philadelphia, PA: 2008;1232–1284.
4. Markowitz SD, Bertagnolli MM. Molecular origins of cancer: Molecular basis of colorectal cancer. *N Engl J Med.* 2009;361(25):2449–2460.
5. Gryfe R. Overview of colorectal cancer genetics. *Surg Oncol Clin N Am.* 2009;18(4):573–583.
6. Sargent DJ, Conley BA, Allegra C, Collette L. Clinical trial designs for predictive marker validation in cancer treatment trials. *J Clin Oncol.* 2005;23(9):2020–2027.
7. Mandrekar SJ, Grothey A, Goetz MP, Sargent DJ. Clinical trial designs for prospective validation of biomarkers. *Am J Pharmacogenomics.* 2005;5(5):317–325.
8. McShane LM, Hunsberger S, Adjei AA. Effective incorporation of biomarkers into phase II trials. *Clin Cancer Res.* 2009;15(6):1898–1905.
9. Buyse M, Sargent DJ, Grothey A, Matheson A, de Gramont A. Biomarkers and surrogate end points–the challenge of statistical validation. *Nat Rev Clin Oncol.* 2010;7(6):309–317.
10. Biomarkers and surrogate endpoints: preferred definitions and conceptual framework. *Clin Pharmacol Ther.* 2001;**69:**89–95.
11. Simon R. Validation of pharmacogenomic biomarker classifiers for treatment selection. *Cancer Biomark.* 2006;2(3–4):89–96.

12. Cummings J, Ward TH, Dive C. Fit-for-purpose biomarker method validation in anticancer drug development. *Drug Discov Today*. 2010;15(19–20):816–825.
13. Mandrekar SJ, Sargent DJ, eds. Clinical Validation of Biomarkers. In: *Biomarkers in Oncology*. 2010.
14. Lassere MN, Johnson KR, Boers M, et al. Definitions and validation criteria for biomarkers and surrogate endpoints: development and testing of a quantitative hierarchical levels of evidence schema. *J Rheumatol*. 2007;34(3):607–615.
15. Simon R, Altman DG. Statistical aspects of prognostic factor studies in oncology. *Br J Cancer*. 1994;69(6):979–985.
16. Hayes DF, Trock B, Harris AL. Assessing the clinical impact of prognostic factors: when is "statistically significant" clinically useful? *Breast Cancer Res Treat*. 1998;52(1–3):305–319.
17. Buyse M. Towards the validation of statistically reliable biomarkers. *Eur J Cancer*. 2007;41:89–95.
18. Sargent D, Allegra C. Issues in clinical trial design for tumor marker studies. *Semin Oncol*. 2002;29(3):222–230.
19. Amado RG, Wolf M, Peeters M, et al. Wild-type K-ras is required for panitumumab efficacy in patients with metastatic colorectal cancer. *J Clin Oncol*. 2008;26(10):1626–1634.
20. Freeman D, Juan T, Meropol NJ, et al. Association of K-ras gene mutations and clinical outcome in patients with metastatic colorectal cancer receiving panitumumab monotherapy. In: 14th European Cancer Conference, Barcelona, Spain, 2007
21. Karapetis CS, Khambata-Ford S, Jonker DJ, et al. K-ras mutations and benefit from cetuximab in advanced colorectal cancer. *N Engl J Med*. 2008;359(17):1757–1765.
22. Van Cutsem E, Lang I, D'haens G, et al. K-ras status and efficacy in the first-line treatment of patients with metastatic colorectal cancer (mCRC) treated with FOLFIRI with or without cetuximab: the CRYSTAL experience. *J Clin Oncol*. 2008;26.
23. Bokemeyer G, Bondarenko I, Hartmann JT, et al. K-ras status and efficacy of first-line treatment of patients with or without cetuximab: the OPUS experience. *J Clin Oncol*. 2008;26.
24. Simon R. Development and Validation of Biomarker Classifiers for Treatment Selection. *J Stat Plan Inference*. 2008;138(2):308–320.
25. Paik S. Clinical trial methods to discover and validate predictive markers for treatment response in cancer. *Biotechnol Annu Rev*. 2003;9:259–267.
26. Simon RM, Paik S, Hayes DF. Use of archived specimens in evaluation of prognostic and predictive biomarkers. *J Natl Cancer Inst*. 2009;101(21):1446–1452.
27. Simon R, Maitournam A. Evaluating the efficiency of targeted designs for randomized clinical trials. *Clin Cancer Res*. 2004;10(20):6759–6763.
28. Maitournam A, Simon R. On the efficiency of targeted clinical trials. *Stat Med*. 2005;24(3):329–339.
29. Mandrekar SJ, Sargent DJ. Clinical trial designs for predictive biomarker validation: one size does not fit all. *J Biopharm Stat*. 2009;19(3):530–542.
30. Mandrekar SJ, Sargent DJ. Clinical trial designs for predictive biomarker validation: theoretical considerations and practical challenges. *J Clin Oncol*. 2009;27(24):4027–4034.
31. Pemetrexed or Erlotinib as Second-Line Therapy in Treating Patients With Advanced Non-Small Cell Lung Cancer. In: http://www.clinicaltrials.gov/ct2/show/NCT00738881?term=NCT00738881&rank=1, 2009
32. Freidlin B, McShane LM, Korn EL. Randomized clinical trials with biomarkers: design issues. *J Natl Cancer Inst*. 2010;102(3):152–160.
33. Hoering A, Leblanc M, Crowley JJ. Randomized phase III clinical trial designs for targeted agents. *Clin Cancer Res*. 2008;14(14):4358–4367.
34. Wang SJ, O'Neill RT, Hung HM. Approaches to evaluation of treatment effect in randomized clinical trials with genomic subset. *Pharm Stat*. 2007;6(3):227–244.
35. Jiang W, Freidlin B, Simon R. Biomarker-adaptive threshold design: a procedure for evaluating treatment with possible biomarker-defined subset effect. *J Natl Cancer Inst*. 2007;99(13):1036–1043.
36. Romond EH, Perez EA, Bryant J, et al. Trastuzumab plus adjuvant chemotherapy for operable HER2-positive breast cancer. *N Engl J Med*. 2005;353(16):1673–1684.
37. Paik S, Kim C, Jeong J, et al. Benefit from adjuvant trastuzumab may not be confined to patient with IHC 3+ and/or FISH-positive tumors: central testing results from NSABP B-31. *J Clin Oncol*. 2007;25:511.
38. Perez EA, Romond EH, Suman VJ, et al. Updated results of the combined analysis of NCCTG N9831 and NSABP B-31 adjuvant chemotherapy with/without trastuzumab in patients with HER2-positive breast cancer. *J Clin Oncol*. 2007;25:512.
39. Young KY, Laird A, Zhou XH. The efficiency of clinical trial designs for predictive biomarker validation. *Clin Trials*. 2010;7(5):557–566.
40. Fleming TR, DeMets DL. Surrogate end points in clinical trials: are we being misled? *Ann Intern Med*. 1996;125(7):605–613.
41. Prentice RL. Surrogate endpoints in clinical trials: definition and operational criteria. *Stat Med*. 1989;8(4):431–440.
42. Burzykowski T, Molenberghs G, Buyse M. The Evaluation of Surrogate Endpoints (Statistics for Biology and Health). New York, NY: Springer; 2005.
43. Weir CJ, Walley RJ. Statistical evaluation of biomarkers as surrogate endpoints: a literature review. *Stat Med*. 2006;25(2):183–203.
44. Lassere MN. The Biomarker-Surrogacy Evaluation Schema: a review of the biomarker-surrogate literature and a proposal for a criterion-based, quantitative, multidimensional hierarchical levels of evidence schema for evaluating the status of biomarkers as surrogate endpoints. *Stat Methods Med Res*. 2008;17(3):303–340.
45. Sargent DJ, Wieand HS, Haller DG, et al. Disease-free survival versus overall survival as a primary end point for adjuvant colon cancer studies: individual patient data from 20,898 patients on 18 randomized trials. *J Clin Oncol*. 2005;23(34):8664–8670.
46. Sargent DJ, Patiyil S, Yothers G, et al.; ACCENT Group. End points for colon cancer adjuvant trials: observations and recommendations based on individual patient data from 20,898 patients enrolled onto 18 randomized trials from the ACCENT Group. *J Clin Oncol*. 2007;25(29):4569–4574.
47. Burzykowski T, Molenberghs G, Buyse M, Geys H, et al. Validation of surrogate end points in multiple randomized clinical trials with failure time end points. *Applied Statistics*. 2001;50:405–422.
48. Shi Q, Sargent DJ. Meta-analysis for the evaluation of surrogate endpoints in cancer clinical trials. *Int J Clin Oncol*. 2009;14(2):102–111.
49. Buyse M, Burzykowski T, Carroll K, et al. Progression-free survival is a surrogate for survival in advanced colorectal cancer. *J Clin Oncol*. 2007;25(33):5218–5224.

21 Colon Cancer Survivorship

JOHN KAUH
FADLO R. KHURI

■ INTRODUCTION

The evolution of colorectal cancer (CRC) care has steadily increased the cure rates for Stage II/III CRC as well as extending the survival of patients with metastatic CRC (1–9). This has resulted in ever-increasing numbers of patients living with CRC; current estimates place over 11 million patients with a diagnosis of CRC living in the United States (10). As the number of CRC survivors has grown, so has the importance of survivorship, which has rapidly become an integral component in the care of these patients. In recognition of the poorly understood needs of patients diagnosed with cancer, the National Cancer Institute (NCI) created the Office of Cancer Survivorship (OCS) in July 1996 to improve the quality of life (QOL) and survival of cancer survivors. Multiple cancer related organizations have created varying definitions of survivorship, but all share similar themes. The American Cancer Society (ACS) defines cancer survivorship as, "the state of being a cancer survivor, that is, having been diagnosed with cancer." The NCI describes survivorship as, "survivorship covers the physical, psychosocial, and economic issues of cancer, from diagnosis until the end of life. It focuses on the health and life of a person with cancer beyond the diagnosis and treatment phases. Survivorship includes issues related to the ability to get health care and follow-up treatment, late effects of treatment, second cancers, and QOL. Family members, friends, and caregivers are also part of the survivorship experience."

The 2006 survivorship report from the Institute of Medicine (IOM) recommends health care providers, patient advocates, and other stakeholders to work to raise the awareness of the needs of cancer survivors, and to establish cancer survivorship as a distinct phase of cancer care. Four critical components of comprehensive survivorship care identified in the IOM report included: prevention, surveillance, intervention, and coordination of care. Prevention focuses efforts to minimize risk of disease recurrence, new cancers, and late effects of cancer care. Surveillance focuses on detection of recurrence, new cancers, and assessment of late medical or psychosocial effects of cancer treatment. Intervention focuses on treatment of symptoms that may results from either the malignancy or the treatments themselves and covers issues ranging from medical concerns such as neuropathy to psychosocial issues such as depression or disability. Lastly, coordination of care focuses on integration of all members of the health care team (primary care providers, specialist, and social support staff).

A treatment summary/survivor care plan is recommended to facilitate care of cancer survivors and at a minimum include:

1. All diagnostic test results.
2. Tumor characteristics.
3. Dates of treatment.
4. Available psychosocial, nutritional, and other supportive services.
5. Full contact information of all treating physicians (primary care and specialists).
6. Identification of point of contact responsible for coordination of continued care.

The treatment summary is intended to be a comprehensive cancer care record covering diagnosis, staging, diagnostic imaging, treatments received, and toxicities at the conclusion of therapy. An expert panel convened by the American Society of Clinical Oncology (ASCO) has created a sample colon cancer treatment plan and summary, which is available online (11). Ultimately, the goal of a survivorship care plan is to improve communication among health care providers who in turn will facilitate coordination of follow up care. Additionally, the care plan may improve patients' understanding of their cancer diagnosis, treatment, and ongoing surveillance; resulting in increased compliance and patient satisfaction. Ongoing research to assess and improve care plans will need to be completed.

COMPLICATIONS OF ACUTE CRC TREATMENT

CRC survivorship is multifaceted and for many patients completing acute therapy, treatment-related toxicities are a major concern. Chemotherapy can lead to both short-term and long-term toxicities. Short-term toxicities are well characterized with CRC chemotherapeutics, but with the exception of fluorouracil (5-FU), experience with all other agents is limited to less than 15 years.

Chemotherapy Issues Facing Survivors

5-Fluorouracil

5-FU has been in clinical use since 1958. The long-term effects of 5-FU appear to be minimal as no long-term complications have been reported despite its extensive clinical history. Regarding fertility and reproductive performance, 5-FU has not been adequately studied in animals to permit full evaluation; however, studies on male rats indicate transient infertility as a result of effects on sperm (12). Given this information, male patients should be counseled appropriately.

Oxaliplatin

Oxaliplatin is a platinum-based drug approved for use in combination with 5-FU in the treatment of metastatic CRC and the adjuvant treatment of Stage III colon cancer in patients who have undergone complete resection of the primary tumor (13). Although most side effects of oxaliplatin are temporary and limited to the acute treatment period, neuropathy can become a debilitating toxicity that may emerge after the completion of acute therapy (14–17). Oxaliplatin is associated with two types of neuropathy, acute, and chronic. The acute sensory neuropathy usually occurs within hours to 2 days of dosing and resolves within 14 days. The symptoms may be precipitated/exacerbated by exposure to cold temperatures. The sensory neuropathy can be particularly distressing as patients can develop jaw spasm, dysarthria, and pharyngolaryngeal dysesthesia without actual laryngospasm or bronchospasm characterized by subjective sensations of dysphagia or dyspnea.

The chronic form of sensory neuropathy is characterized by paresthesias, dysesthesias, hypoesthesias, and proprioception deficits that can interfere with activities of daily living and can develop without prior acute neuropathy, albeit the majority of patients (80%) who develop grade 3 neuropathy progress from prior grade 1 or 2 states. These symptoms improve in most patients upon discontinuation of oxaliplatin; however, some patients will have to suffer with lifelong debilitating sequelae. In the adjuvant colon cancer trial (MOSAIC), the incidence of peripheral sensory neuropathy was reported with a frequency of 92% (all grades) and 13% (grade 3). At 28 days after the last treatment, 60% of all patients had any grade (grade 1 = 40%, grade 2 = 16%, grade 3 = 5%) peripheral sensory neuropathy decreasing to 39% at 6 months follow up (grade 1 = 31%, grade 2 = 7%, grade 3 = 1%) and 21% at 18 months of follow up (grade 1 = 17%, grade 2 = 3%, grade 3 = 1%; 18; Table 21.1).

Data regarding oxaliplatin effects on fertility are sparse but male dog studies revealed testicular degeneration and atrophy when administered the equivalent of one-sixth of the recommended human dose suggesting a decrease in male fertility. The oxaliplatin prescribing information recommends counseling on sperm storage before starting treatment as irreversible infertility is a potential risk.

Irinotecan

Irinotecan, a derivative of camptothecin interferes with topoisomerase I and is approved for the treatment of metastatic CRC (19). The most common and notorious toxicity associated irinotecan is diarrhea, which comes in two forms: early and late. Early diarrhea is due to the cholinergic effects while late diarrhea generally occurring more than 24 hours after drug administration and can be prolonged, leading to life threatening dehydration and electrolyte imbalances, is due to GI mucosal toxicity. Irinotecan is myelosuppressive and in the setting of concurrent severe diarrhea has been noted to cause patient deaths, thus irinotecan-associated diarrhea requires aggressive treatment.

Long-term carcinogenicity studies with irinotecan have not been conducted, but neither irinotecan nor SN-38 (active metabolite of irinotecan) were found to be mutagenic in the in vitro Ames assay. No significant adverse effects on fertility and general reproductive performance were observed after intravenous administration of irinotecan in doses of up to 6 mg/kg/day to rats and rabbits. Although irinotecan is only approved for treatment of metastatic CRC, there are long-term survivors previously treated with irinotecan prior to curative metastectomy. In the future, increased rates of second malignancies may be noted given the long-term sequelae associated with other topoisomerase inhibitors such as etoposide.

Table 21.1 NCI Common Toxicity Criteria—Version 1, Utilized in MOSAIC Trial Sensory Neuropathy

Grade	Definition
0	No change or none
1	Mild paresthesias, loss of deep tendon reflexes
2	Mild or moderate objective sensory loss, moderate paresthesias
3	Severe objective sensory loss or paresthesias that interfere with function
4	Not applicable

Bevacizumab

Bevacizumab is a humanized monoclonal antibody that binds vascular endothelial growth factor (VEGF) and prevents the interaction of VEGF to its receptors (Flt-1 and KDR; 20). Bevacizumab is indicated for the treatment of metastatic CRC in combination with 5-FU-based chemotherapy. Although bevacizumab is only approved for the treatment of metastatic CRC, there are patients with resectable metastatic disease who receive bevacizumab in the perioperative setting who may have to deal with the long-term sequelae of complications related to its antiangiogenic effects. In a small phase II study, Willett et al administered bevacizumab and chemoradiation preoperatively for resectable rectal cancer and reported a low adverse event rate, but did note the following: one anastomotic leak, one fistula, one myocardial infarction (MI), and one deep venous thrombosis (DVT), all occurring greater than 90 days after surgery/bevacizumab (21). Given our relatively, short experience with this agent, new long-term toxicities such as wound healing complications or increased cardiovascular disease rates, may emerge for long-term survivors.

In addition to vascular complication, bevacizumab is associated with renal and central nervous system (CNS) toxicities. Bevacizumab-associated proteinuria ranges from 0.7%–7.4% across multiple clinical trials and fortunately, nephrotic syndrome occurred in only a small proportion of patients (less than 1%) receiving bevacizumab in clinical trials, albeit in some instances with fatal outcome. Reversible posterior leukoencephalopathy syndrome (RPLS) is a neurological disorder that can present with headache, seizure, lethargy, confusion, blindness, and other visual and neurologic disturbances; it was first described in 1996 and has been reported with an incidence of less than 0.1% in clinical studies (22). The onset of symptoms occurred from 16 hours to 1 year after initiation of bevacizumab. The symptoms tend to resolve after a period of time, although visual changes can persist (23,24).

Long-term effects on fertility are poorly studied; however, reproduction studies in rabbits treated with approximately 1 to 12 times the recommended human dose of bevacizumab resulted in teratogenicity.

Cetuximab and Panitumumab

Cetuximab is a chimeric monoclonal antibody directed against the extracellular domain of the epidermal growth factor receptor (EGFR) and is approved for the treatment of both head and neck (H&N) cancer and advanced CRC (25). Panitumumab is a fully human monoclonal antibody directed against EGFR approved for use in advanced CRC (26). Cetuximab and panitumumab gained approval in the United States in 2004 and 2006, respectively. Both agents have similar toxicity profiles and since both agents are relatively new, long-term toxicity data are limited. The most significant toxicity associated with this class of agent is acneiform rash, which can be disfiguring and functionally debilitating in up to 15% of patients. The dermatologic toxicities can be particularly emotionally distressing to patients already facing stressors associated with systemic chemotherapies and is a toxicity that requires particular attention to detail. Fortunately, the dermatologic toxicity is temporary and usually resolves at the conclusion of therapy with EGFR inhibitors.

This class of agent is only approved for use in advanced CRC; therefore, long-term toxicity it not relatable to general CRC survivors. However, a small proportion of resectable metastatic CRC patients will be long-term survivors following EGFR inhibitor therapy. Undoubtedly, if long-term toxicities exist for EGFR inhibitors, they will come to light in the future in long-term CRC survivors as well as in the H&N survivors.

The data regarding EGFR inhibitor effects on reproduction are very limited and there are no adequate and well-controlled studies of cetuximab or panitumumab regarding fertility to make recommendations to survivors.

Long-Term Sequelae of CRC Treatment

Psychosocial Issues

There is a relative dearth of psychosocial studies of CRC survivors. The incidence of depression is reported to be higher in CRC survivors (14%) vs the general patient population (10%), but do compare favorably to the prevalence of depression in survivors of other malignances: H&N—18% at 3 years, Hodgkin's disease—27%, and breast cancer—25% at 3 years (27–31). Overall, CRC survivors appear to cope well with psychosocial stressors. Ramsey et al reported a cohort survey study of 272 patients with CRC who have survived at least 5 years from diagnosis. The subjects were recruited from the cancer surveillance system (CSS), a registry of cancer cases for residents of western Washington State, and answered survey questions about QOL and colon cancer specific issues (3,27,32). Most survivors reported a high QOL life irrespective of stage at diagnosis and time from diagnosis. Noncancer related comorbid conditions and low socioeconomic status appeared to be more of an influence in overall QOL. Trentham-Dietz et al completed a cohort survey study of Wisconsin women diagnosed with colon cancer from 1990 to 1991 (33). Of the original 726 women, 443 women were alive in 1999, and 307 patients responded to the survey. With a mean follow up of 9 years, the authors concluded that female long-term survivors of CRC appear to report health-related QOL comparable with that of age-matched women in the general population. These data suggest that over the long term, noncancer factors such as age, weight, and comorbid conditions play important roles in determining the long-term well-being of survivors than factors related to initial colon cancer diagnosis. The same cohort of Wisconsin women were also interrogated regarding social support and it was found that patients with larger social networks and frequent social interactions appear to correlate with improved mental health (34). In summary, these data suggest CRC survivors adjust well to treatment-related sequelae, especially those survivors with strong social support networks. In most cases, long-term complications from cancer treatment are less important than noncancer related issues in determining overall QOL for CRC survivors.

Rectal Cancer Related Quality of Life

As the prognosis of rectal cancer patients has improved over time, functional outcome has become increasingly more important. Although the rectum is simply a continuation of the colon, due to its anatomic location (pelvic and retroperitoneal), additional issues in the care of rectal cancer patients must be addressed (1). Most low rectal cancer survivors will successfully learn to cope with permanent colostomies, but the assistance of entero-stomal health care providers can greatly ease the transition from precolostomy life to the postsurgical period. Baumel et al reported on a cohort of 1082 patients who underwent placement of a colostomy or ileostomy; 55% reported change in sexual activity and 63% reported a change in working life highlighting the need for enterostomal care support for this patient population (35). Additionally, a Chinese rectal cancer study reported significantly higher rates of "embarrassment" with bowel movements in stoma patients versus nonstoma patients ($P = .00001$; 36).

After survivors navigate through the adjustment period, most patients appear to accept their stoma without long-term emotional distress. Peng et al reported 92% of nonstoma patients had a body image score of 100 (out of a possible 100), while 80.8% of stoma patients had a score of 100 and the majority of patients (94%) were found to be satisfied with their stoma appliance as reported by Baumel (35,36). Overall, rectal cancer survivors appear to have similar high QOL scores as seen in the general CRC survivor population (37,38). Rauch et al reported survey results from 121 European patients who were in complete remission 2 or more years after the diagnosis and treatment of rectal cancer (39). When compared to an age-matched population without a diagnosis of rectal cancer, study subjects reported less pain than the control group. Surprisingly, patients with stomas were found to have better social functions in terms of less anxiety and higher self-esteem than the general population.

Potential stoma related issues are not limited to the patient but can also affect the emotional well-being of spouses. Cakmak reported an increase in time spent at home by spouses and a significant decline in sexual activity following placement of a permanent colostomy (40). These data suggest that not only should the social and sexual aspects of life following a colostomy be counseled with the patient but also include the spouse.

Damage to pelvic autonomic nerves as a result of surgical trauma or radiation, leading to fibrosis and neurovascular dysfunction, can result in both urinary and sexual dysfunction (41). Common urinary dysfunction symptoms include: overflow incontinence, stress incontinence, or urinary retention. Effective treatments for urinary dysfunction are lacking; multiple treatments exist, but there is a dearth of prospective trial data. Pelvic floor muscle training is most commonly tried as first-line therapy, but it is of limited use in patients with nerve damage. Sacral nerve stimulation can be utilized if pelvic floor muscle training proves unsuccessful; however, the technology is unproven and can be difficult to implement.

Sexual dysfunction following rectal cancer treatment is a multifaceted problem (42). Poor self-image, fatigue, loss of independence, depression, and changes in personal relationships may all contribute to sexual dysfunction. In the Dutch total mesorectal excision (TME) trial, sexual dysfunction was reported by 62% of women (dyspareunia—59%, vaginal dryness—57%) and 76% of men (erectile dysfunction [ED]—80%, ejaculatory problems—72%; 43). In addition to surgical trauma, ED can be attributed to multiple etiologies. Radiotherapy has been shown to induce hypogonadism resulting in low testosterone levels and arteriosclerosis leading to vascular insufficiency as causes of ED (44,45). ED can best be treated with phosphodiesterase-5 inhibitors, which have a response rate upwards of 87% in this patient population (46). The treatment of female sexual dysfunction is more problematic as little clinical data exist, and even the pathophysiology remains obscure. Radiation can lead to fibrosis and adhesions resulting in shortening of the vaginal canal and pelvic RT can lead to early ovarian failure resulting in vaginal dryness and dyspareunia (47–49). Mechanical intervention with lubrication for vaginal dryness and vaginal dilators to prevent vaginal stenosis can be attempted, while a trial of topical estrogens for symptoms of dyspareunia is a reasonable initial treatment option.

Issues Pertinent to Survivor Family Members

Most CRC occur in a sporadic fashion and inherited genetic syndromes account for less than 10% of individuals with CRC (50). However, upward of 25% of CRC cases can be considered familial but with no known identifiable inherited syndrome. It has been recommended that testing should be limited to patients whose family history suggests an inherited syndrome or exhibits specific features of inherited cancer syndrome such as colon cancer before the age of 50. If a genetic mutation is identified in the cancer patient, additional first-degree relatives can then be tested. However, if the results of particular tests are negative, additional genetic screening for family members is not recommended as the likelihood of finding a mutation is low. As a standard, all genetic testing should only be performed in the setting of a consultation with a trained medical geneticist to review potential limitations of test results and the psychological, medical, and legal implications for test results.

Financial Considerations

A diagnosis of malignancy not only leads to psychological stress but also to financial stresses. The explosion of new therapeutics for the treatment of CRC has been equaled by the explosion of the costs of new agents. For example, the drug costs alone for a 6-month course of adjuvant FOLFOX is estimated to be over $72,000 and a patient with traditional Medicare Part B would be expected to pay over $3600 out of pocket and in 2003, the elderly spent an estimated 22% of their income on average for health care (51). The medical community has had a proud tradition of offering the most effective treatments regardless of cost; however, given the exponentially escalating costs associated with delivering state-of-the-art care, health care providers must become much more cognizant of the financial demands placed on cancer survivors.

Many patients require temporary or long-term financial assistance to not only cover direct health care cost but also to supplement income lost to time away from work during treatment. Private disability insurance provides some support but only 30%–40% of patients have access to short- and long-term disability plans (52). For those patients without access to private disability insurance, the federal government offers assistance programs to those who qualify. The Supplemental Security Income (SSI) program provides minimal income for aged, blind, or disabled individuals. Disability as defined by SSI is someone who has a medically determined physical or mental impairment that is expected to last at least 12 continuous months or result in death and for those over the age of 18, the impairment must prevent him or her from doing any substantial gainful activity. SSI should not be considered an income replacement but truly an income supplemental program, as in 2011 the highest federal SSI payment was $674 per month for a person and $1011 per month for a couple. The Social Security Disability Insurance (SSDI) is an insurance program that provides payments to persons with disabilities based on their history of social security earnings. Unlike the SSI program that requires no prior work history, SSDI requires documented prior participation in the labor force. To be eligible, an individual must be unable to work at all, in any job for at least 12 months, or be in the terminal stages of illness. Income is determined by prior contributions to the Social Security program.

In addition to state and federal programs, volunteer cancer organizations also provide critical information and supportive services to survivors:

- The ACS offers volunteer service such as the Road to Recovery program, which provides transportation to and from treatment for people who have cancer who do not have a ride or are unable to drive themselves. The ACS also offers the "Hope Lodge" at various locations providing lodging to patients during active cancer treatment.
- CancerCare is a nonprofit volunteer agency that provides supportive services to qualified cancer patients including transportation, home care, child care, and medical supplies.
- Fertile Hope is a national Livestrong initiative dedicated to providing information and support for cancer patients and survivors facing reproductive issues as a result of cancer treatments.

Although some cancer survivors are physically unable to work, data suggest most cancer survivors resume working after completing acute cancer therapy. A 2002 study reported 67% of survivors of lung cancer, CRC, breast, or prostate cancer were employed 5 to 7 years after initial diagnosis. Survivors who stopped working did so because of: retirement (54%), poor health/disability (24%), quit (4%), or business closed (9%; 53). For those survivors that wished to work but could not find jobs, Rothstein et al reported data suggesting survivors with occupations requiring manual labor suffer a significantly higher likelihood of difficulty in obtaining employment (54).

Once survivors navigate the financial difficulties of acute cancer treatment, they will be faced with potential discrimination in finding jobs and insurance policies. Although the health reform acts of 2010 prevent denial of coverage based upon prior medical history the law does not limit insurance premiums, thus health insurance premiums could become untenable for self-employed persons or persons working for small businesses that do not have a large pool of participants to dilute the risk. Four federal laws, the Americans with Disabilities Act, the Family and Medical Leave Act (FMLA), the Employee Retirement and Income Security Act (ERISA), and the Federal Rehabilitation Act, provide cancer survivors with some protection against employment discrimination, but does not fully protect survivors from future discrimination (52). Many states also have similar state laws preventing discrimination as well. In the future, state and federal agencies will need to work together to create policies to assist cancer survivors to ensure their access to employment and health care.

■ SCREENING

Upward of 40% of individuals treated for CRC will have their disease recur or develop second primary cancers. Routine surveillance has been recommended to identify patients at an earlier disease state that may render their recurrent disease potentially resectable as well as locating new primary tumors (55). In a surveillance study by Green et al, the medical records of 3278 patients treated on Intergroup 0089 (a phase III study of 5-FU, leucovorin, and levamisole in high-risk Stage II and III colon cancer) were examined (56). Occurrence of endoscopic or radiologic discovery of colon cancer was the primary end point. Forty-two cases of second primary invasive colon cancer were found, which translated into an incidence of 1.5% at 5 years. This rate was compared with the rates of first colon cancer in two reference groups; the general population (SEER data) and patients who had a history of adenomatous polyps. Standardized incidence ratios were 1.6 and 6.8, respectively, suggesting the incidence of second primary CRC remains high supporting the concept of intensive surveillance strategies.

There have been multiple prospective randomized trials of surveillance following curative treatment of CRC with various surveillance strategies. The results have been mixed with most studies reporting no survival benefit. Makela reported a Scandinavian prospective trial of conventional vs intensive follow up after radical surgery for CRC (57). One hundred six patients were randomized to one of two follow up schedules; with a minimum of 5 years of follow up, the intensive group discovered recurrences earlier (10 months vs 15 months); however, the 5-year survivals were similar for both groups (54% conventional vs 59% intensive). The authors concluded that earlier detection of recurrence did not lead to improved resectability or OS. Ohlsson reported a randomized Swedish trial of intense vs conventional follow up in 107 patients (58). Five-year survival was 67% in the conventional group and 75% in the intensive follow-up group ($p \geq 0.05$). Kjeldsen reported a Danish study of 597 patients randomized to virtually no follow up or frequent follow up visits (59). Both groups had a 26% recurrence rate but the patients in the intensive follow up group were diagnosed with recurrence on average 9 months earlier. However, no improvement in overall survival was noted between the two groups. Schoemaker reported an Australian study of 325 patients with 5-year follow up and reported no difference in survival between two groups (60). Only one symptomatic curable metachronous colon tumor was detected and computed tomography (CT) did not increase detection of curable liver metastases. The authors concluded that yearly colonoscopy, liver CT, and chest x-ray will not improve survival from CRC when added to symptoms and simple screening review. Lastly, Rodriguez-Moranta reported a trial from Spain in which 259 patients were randomized to "simple" vs "intensive" surveillance. Although the overall study population did not have a survival benefit (HR, 0.87; 95% CI, 0.49 to 1.54; $P = .62$), a subset of Stage II patient did appear to have improved outcome with the intensive screening (HR, 0.34; 95% CI, 0.12 to 0.98, $P = .03$; 61).

In contrast to the aforementioned trials, Pietra reported an Italian study of 207 patients randomized to conventional vs intensive follow up; local recurrences were detected in 20% of the conventional group and 25% of the intensive surveillance group (62). Curative metastectomy was feasible in 2 patients (10%) in the conventional group and 17 patients (65%) in the intensive group. The 5-year survival was 58.3% for the conventional group and 73% for the intensive group ($P < .02$), supporting the use of an intensive follow up regimen. Secco et al also reported data supporting intensive surveillance; utilizing a risk-adapted approach to intensive surveillance for high-risk individuals improved OS and had similar costs to low-intensity surveillance (63). High-risk disease characteristics included: adenocarcinoma of low rectum status post low anterior resection, T3 lesion of the left colon, carcinoembryonic antigen (CEA) ≥ 7.5 ng/mL, Dukes C, poorly differentiated grade (G3), mucinous adenocarcinoma, or signet ring cells. Patients with an absence of high-risk features were considered low risk.

Utilizing data from randomized trials, there have been three meta-analyses often cited in the medical literature (Table 21.2). All three meta-analyses results were in favor of intensive screening with 5-year mortality relative risks from 0.80 to 0.81 in the Figeredo and Renehan studies, respectively, and an odds ratio of 0.67 in the Jeffery study (64–66). Based upon these results, several professional cancer associations have recommended intensive screening (Table 21.3). Although surveillance recommendations vary slightly among organizations (Table 21.4), all guidelines recommend the most intensive monitoring (H&P, CEA, colonoscopy, and CT scans) within the first 3 years of surgery as 80% of relapses occur during this time period (67). The utility of CEA (glycoprotein involved in cell adhesion) was demonstrated by Chau et al. In a cohort of 530 patients, 154 developed recurrent disease after curative surgery followed by adjuvant 5-FU. Forty-five patients (29%) had an elevated CEA at time of recurrence and 49 (32%) had CT imaging demonstrating recurrence (68). Of the 33 patients who underwent attempted curative surgery, 13 (27%) were in the CT group and 8 (18%) were in the CEA group. These data support the role of CEA in CRC surveillance following curative treatment.

Despite the previously completed randomized trials and meta-analyses, controversies regarding the true benefit of intensive screening schedules remain. As of 2011 there are two large prospective randomized surveillance trials that have fully accrued but not yet reported. The UK Follow-Up After Colorectal Surgery (FACS) trial is a 1200 patient study designed to assess the effect on the number

Table 21.2 Meta-Analyses in Favor of Intensive Surveillance

	No. of Patients		5 Year Mortality (%)			
	Control	Intensive Surveillance	Control	Intensive Surveillance	Effect on 5-Year Mortality	95% CI
Renehan	676	666	37%	30%	Relative risk = 0.81	0.70 to 0.94
Figueredo	821	858	37%	30%	Relative risk = 0.80	0.70 to 0.91
Jeffery	676	666	37%	30%	Odds ratio = 0.67	0.53 to 0.84

Table 21.3 Surveillance Guidelines

	ASCO (74)	NCCN (55)	AGA/ACS/USPTF (75)	ESMO (76)
History and physical	Every 3 to 6 mo × 3 yr then annually	Every 3 to 6 mo × 2 yr then every 6 mo for 3 yr		Every 3 to 6 mo × 3 yr then Every 6 to 12 mo × 2 yr
Fecal occult blood test	Not recommended	No recommendation		Symptom directed
Complete blood count	Not recommended	No recommendation		Symptom directed
Liver function test	Not recommended	No recommendation		Symptom directed
CEA	If patient is a candidate for curative surgery, check every 3 mo for at least 3 yr	If patient is a candidate for curative surgery then check every 3 mo × 2 yr then every 6 mo × 3 yr		Every 3 to 6 mo × 3 yr then Every 6 to 12 mo × 2 yr
Chest x-ray	Not recommended	No recommendation		Symptom directed
Flexible sigmoidoscopy	For patients who have not received pelvic radiation direct imaging of the rectum at periodic interval suggested For patients who have received pelvic radiation direct visualization of rectum other than colonoscopy not recommended	No recommendation		Rectosigmoidoscopy every 6 mo × 2 yr for patients with cancer of distal sigmoidal cancer
Colonoscopy	Every 3 to 5 yr to detect new cancers and polyps	1 yr after primary therapy Repeat 1 yr if abnormal Repeat every 3 yr if normal	1 yr after initial surgery 3 yr after initial surgery every 5 yr	1 yr after primary therapy then every 3 to 5 yr
CT of chest/abdomen	If patient candidate for curative surgery then check yearly × 3 yr	No recommendation		Every 6 to 12 mo × 3 yr for high risk patients
US of abdomen	No recommendation	No recommendation		Substitute for CT if needed
MRI of abdomen	No recommendation	No recommendation		Symptom directed

Table 21.4 Randomized Surveillance Studies

	Arm	Follow-Up Interval	Screening Tests		5-Year OS	*P* Value
Makela	Control *n* = 54	q3 mo × 2 yr q yr × 3 yr	• H&P • CBC • FOBT • Sigmoidoscopy (rectal/ sigmoid only)	• CEA • CXR	54%	.5
	Intensive Group *n* = 52	q3 mo × 2 yr q yr × 3 yr	• H&P • CBC • Liver US—every 6 mo • CT A/P—yearly • Colonoscopy 3 mo postop then q yr	• FOBT • CEA • CXR	59%	
Ohlsson	Control *n* = 54	q3 mo × 2 yr q yr × 3 yr	• FOBT		67%	>.05
	Intensive Group *n* = 53	q3 mo × 2 yr q6 mo × 2 yr q yr × 1 yr	• H&P • Proctosigmoidoscopy • CEA, AP, GGT • Colonoscopy—q yr • CT—every 6 mo × 2 yr	• FOBT • CXR	75%	
Pietra	Control *n* = 103	q6 mo × 1 yr q yr	• H&P • CXR—yearly • Colonoscopy—yearly	• US • CEA	58%	<.02
	Intensive Group *n* = 104	q3 mo × 2 yr q6 mo × 3 yr q yr	• H&P • Colonoscopy— yearly • CT—yearly	• US • CEA • CXR—q yr	73%	
Kjeldsen	Control *n* = 290	5 yr postop 10 yr postop 15 yr postop	• H&P • DRE • FOBT • Colonoscopy	• CXR • CBC • ESR • LFT	70%	.48
	Intensive Group *n* = 307	q6 mo × 3 yr q12 mo × 2 yr 10 yr postop 15 yr postop	• H&P • Digital rectal exam • FOBT • Colonoscopy	• CXR • CBC • ESR • LFT	68%	
Shoemaker	Control *n* = 158	q3 mo × 2yr q6 mo × 5 yr	• H&P • CBC • LFT	• CEA • FOBT	65%	.07
	Intensive Group *n* = 167	q3 mo × 2yr q6 mo × 5 yr	• H&P • CXR—yearly • CT—yearly • Colonoscopy—yearly	• CBC • LFT • CEA • FOBT	74%	
Secca	Control High Risk *n* = 84		• H&P • Laboratory studies		32%	<.05
	Risk Adaptive High Risk *n* = 108		• H&P • Laboratory studies • CEA every 3 mo × 2 yr, then every 4 mo × 1 yr, then every 6 mo × 2 yr • Abd/pel US every 6 mo × 3 yr then yearly × 2 yr • CXR yearly • Sigmoidoscopy yearly (rectal cancer only)		50%	
	Control Low Risk *n* = 61		• H&P • Laboratory studies		60%	<.01
	Risk Adaptive		• H&P		80%	

(Continued)

Table 21.4 *(Continued)*

	Arm	Follow-Up Interval	Screening Tests		5-Year OS	*P* Value
	Low Risk *n* = 84		• Laboratory studies • CEA every 6 mo × 2 yr, then yearly × 3 yr • Abd/pel US every 6 mo × 2 yr, then yearly • CXR yearly • Sigmoidoscopy yearly × 2 yr then every 2 yr (rectal cancer only)			
Rodriguez-Moranta	Control *n* = 132	q3 mo × 2 yr then q6 mo × 3 yr	• H&P • CEA • Colonoscopy—1 yr and 3 yr postop	• CBC • LFT	Stage II/III patients	
	Intensive Group *n* = 127	q3 mo × 2 yr then q6 mo × 3 yr	• H&P • CEA • CXR—q yr • Colonoscopy—yearly • CT A/P or Abd US—every 6 mo × 2 yr then yearly	• CBC • LFT		
Wang	Control *n* = 161	q3 mo × 1 yr then q6 mo × 2 yr then q12 mo × 2 yr	• H&P • CT or US • Colonoscopy—6, 30, 60 months postop only	• CEA • CXR	73%	>.05
	Intensive Group *n* = 165	q3 mo × 1 yr then q6 mo × 2 yr then q12 mo × 2 yr	• H&P • CT or US • Colonoscopy—every visit	• CEA • CXR	77%	

of surgically treatable recurrences diagnosed during routine follow up in primary care with three more intensive methods of follow up. The GILDA (Gruppo Italiano di Lavoro per la Diagnosi Anticipata) trial has also completed accrual (1500 patients) and results are awaited. These two large trials should be able to definitively determine the role of intensive surveillance following curative surgery for CRC.

PREVENTIVE HEALTH MAINTENANCE

Once patients complete acute cancer treatments, they must then transition into the survivorship plan, which is multifaceted and requires multidisciplinary care involving Medical Oncology, Physiatry, Primary Care, Surgery, Gastroenterology, and others. Health maintenance activities must be resumed to minimize risk of preventable disease such as proceeding with vaccinations against influenza and pneumococcal infection, dental care, and age/sex-appropriate screening for cardiovascular disease and second primary malignancies such as breast, cervical, and prostate.

Survivors should be encouraged to resume normal physical activity and in some cases increase their level of exercise beyond their baseline levels prior to cancer diagnosis. In addition to lowering rates of obesity, diabetes, and cardiovascular disease, physical activity levels correlate with CRC disease recurrence as well the development of additional primary cancers. Diets rich in red meat, processed grains, low in vegetables, and unprocessed grains have been associated with increased levels of circulating insulin-like growth factor, which is implicated in the promotion of colon cancer (69).

Data from the Health Professionals Follow-up Study (HPFS) of 668 men with a history of Stage I to III CRC revealed a significant protective effect of exercise and CRC-specific mortality and overall mortality (70). Compared to men who participate in little physical activity (less than or equal to 3 Metabolic Equivalent of Task [MET] hours per week), men who engaged in more than 27 MET hours per week had a hazard ratio for CRC-specific mortality of 0.47 (95% CI, 0.24–0.92). The benefit was seen regardless of age, disease stage, body mass index (BMI), diagnosis year, tumor location, and prediagnosis physical activity. In a prospective observation study of 832 patients with Stage III colon cancer enrolled on CALGB 89803 (phase III trial of irinotecan plus 5-FU/leucovorin [IFL] vs 5-FU/leucovorin alone [FL] in Stage III colon cancer) increasing levels of physical activity correlated with reduced risk of recurrent disease (71).

These data suggest exercise is a preventive treatment that should be stressed to all CRC survivors.

Related to physical activity levels, high BMI is associated with poor CRC outcomes. A retrospective study in a cohort of 4288 patient with Dukes B and C colon treated on National Surgical Adjuvant Breast and Bowel Project (NSABP) trials following surgery revealed risk of recurrence, second primary cancer, and mortality were all higher for obese patients. In patients with BMI > 35 kg/m^2, risk of recurrence or development of second primary cancers were significantly higher (HR, 1.38; 95% CI, 1.10–1.736) as was overall mortality (HR, 1.28; CI 95%, 1.04–1.57) and CRC specific mortality (HR, 1.36; 95% CI, 1.06–1.73; 72).

In addition to exercise, survivors should also be counseled against diets rich in red meat and processed grains. In a prospective observational study of 1009 patients who were enrolled in CALGB 89803, subjects were surveyed for their dietary habits (73). Diets were divided into two major patterns, the "prudent" diet (high intake of fruits, vegetables, poultry, and fish) and the "Western" diet (high intake of meat, fat, refined grains, and dessert). The patients were then categorized into quintiles based upon consumption levels of the Western diet. With a median follow-up of 5.3 years, high intake of Western dietary pattern was associated with a significantly worse disease-free survival compared with patients in the lowest quintile of Western dietary pattern. The highest quintile had a hazard ratio for disease-free survival of 3.25 (95% CI, 2.04–5.19; *P* <.001) and overall survival 2.32 (95% CI, 1.36–3.96).

CONCLUSION

Successes in the treatment of CRC have resulted in increasing numbers of CRC survivors. With implementation of the OCS by the NIH, research to develop and evaluate programs improving survivorship care has been evolving. Ultimately, the end goal will be to provide a seamless transition from active cancer treatment to surveillance for CRC survivors while providing supportive services to offer a holistic approach to CRC survivors.

REFERENCES

1. Sauer R, Becker H, Hohenberger W, et al.; German Rectal Cancer Study Group. Preoperative versus postoperative chemoradiotherapy for rectal cancer. *N Engl J Med.* 2004;351(17):1731–1740.
2. Twelves C, Wong A, Nowacki MP, et al. Capecitabine as adjuvant treatment for stage III colon cancer. *N Engl J Med.* 2005;352(26):2696–2704.
3. Allegra CJ, Yothers G, O'Connell MJ, et al. Phase III trial assessing bevacizumab in stages II and III carcinoma of the colon: results of NSABP protocol C-08. *J Clin Oncol.* 2011;29(1):11–16.
4. Saltz LB, Cox JV, Blanke C, et al. Irinotecan plus fluorouracil and leucovorin for metastatic colorectal cancer. Irinotecan Study Group. *N Engl J Med.* 2000;343(13):905–914.
5. de Gramont A, Buyse M, Abrahantes JC, et al. Reintroduction of oxaliplatin is associated with improved survival in advanced colorectal cancer. *J Clin Oncol.* 2007;25(22):3224–3229.
6. de Gramont A, Figer A, Seymour M, et al. Leucovorin and fluorouracil with or without oxaliplatin as first-line treatment in advanced colorectal cancer. *J Clin Oncol.* 2000;18(16):2938–2947.
7. Tournigand C, André T, Achille E, et al. FOLFIRI followed by FOLFOX6 or the reverse sequence in advanced colorectal cancer: a randomized GERCOR study. *J Clin Oncol.* 2004;22(2):229–237.
8. Tournigand C, Cervantes A, Figer A, et al. OPTIMOX1: a randomized study of FOLFOX4 or FOLFOX7 with oxaliplatin in a stop-and-Go fashion in advanced colorectal cancer–a GERCOR study. *J Clin Oncol.* 2006;24(3):394–400.
9. Goldberg RM, Sargent DJ, Morton RF, et al. A randomized controlled trial of fluorouracil plus leucovorin, irinotecan, and oxaliplatin combinations in patients with previously untreated metastatic colorectal cancer. *J Clin Oncol.* 2004;22(1):23–30.
10. Rowland JH, Bellizzi KM. Cancer survivors and survivorship research: a reflection on today's successes and tomorrow's challenges. *Hematol Oncol Clin North Am.* 2008;22(2):181–200, v.
11. ASCO Chemotherpay Treatment Plan and Summary. American Society of Clinical Oncology. Accessed at http://www.asco.org/ASCOv2/Practice+%26+Guidelines/Quality+Care/Quality+Measurement+%26+Improvement/Chemotherapy+Treatment+Plan+and+Summary.
12. Fluorouracil Prescribing Information.
13. Oxaliplatin Prescribing Information, Inc.
14. Choi J, Kong K, Mozaffar T, Holcombe RF. Delayed oxaliplatin-associated neurotoxicity following adjuvant chemotherapy for stage III colon cancer. *Anticancer Drugs.* 2006;17(1):103–105.
15. Kuebler JP, Wieand HS, O'Connell MJ, et al. Oxaliplatin combined with weekly bolus fluorouracil and leucovorin as surgical adjuvant chemotherapy for stage II and III colon cancer: results from NSABP C-07. *J Clin Oncol.* 2007;25(16):2198–2204.
16. Land SR, Kopec JA, Cecchini RS, et al. Neurotoxicity from oxaliplatin combined with weekly bolus fluorouracil and leucovorin as surgical adjuvant chemotherapy for stage II and III colon cancer: NSABP C-07. *J Clin Oncol.* 2007;25(16):2205–2211.
17. Ramanathan RK, Rothenberg ML, de Gramont A, et al. Incidence and evolution of oxaliplatin-induced peripheral sensory neuropathy in diabetic patients with colorectal cancer: a pooled analysis of three phase III studies. *Ann Oncol.* 2010;21(4):754–758.
18. André T, Boni C, Mounedji-Boudiaf L, et al.; Multicenter International Study of Oxaliplatin/5-Fluorouracil/Leucovorin in the Adjuvant Treatment of Colon Cancer (MOSAIC) Investigators. Oxaliplatin, fluorouracil, and leucovorin as adjuvant treatment for colon cancer. *N Engl J Med.* 2004;350(23):2343–2351.
19. Irinotecan Prescribing Information.
20. Bevacizumab Prescribing Information.
21. Willett CG, Duda DG, Ancukiewicz M, et al. A safety and survival analysis of neoadjuvant bevacizumab with standard chemoradiation in a phase I/II study compared with standard chemoradiation in locally advanced rectal cancer. *Oncologist.* 2010;15(8):845–851.
22. Hinchey J, Chaves C, Appignani B, et al. A reversible posterior leukoencephalopathy syndrome. *N Engl J Med.* 1996;334(8):494–500.
23. Garg RK. Posterior leukoencephalopathy syndrome. *Postgrad Med J.* 2001;77(903):24–28.
24. Pula JH, Eggenberger E. Posterior reversible encephalopathy syndrome. *Curr Opin Ophthalmol.* 2008;19(6):479–484.
25. Cetuximab Prescribing Information.
26. Panitumumab Prescribing Information.

27. Ramsey SD, Berry K, Moinpour C, Giedzinska A, Andersen MR. Quality of life in long term survivors of colorectal cancer. *Am J Gastroenterol.* 2002;97(5):1228–1234.
28. Day R, Ganz PA, Costantino JP, Cronin WM, Wickerham DL, Fisher B. Health-related quality of life and tamoxifen in breast cancer prevention: a report from the National Surgical Adjuvant Breast and Bowel Project P-1 Study. *J Clin Oncol.* 1999;17(9):2659–2669.
29. List MA, Stracks J. Evaluation of quality of life in patients definitively treated for squamous carcinoma of the head and neck. *Curr Opin Oncol.* 2000;12(3):215–220.
30. Loge JH, Abrahamsen AF, Ekeberg O, Hannisdal E, Kaasa S. Psychological distress after cancer cure: a survey of 459 Hodgkin's disease survivors. *Br J Cancer.* 1997;76(6):791–796.
31. Burgess C, Cornelius V, Love S, Graham J, Richards M, Ramirez A. Depression and anxiety in women with early breast cancer: five year observational cohort study. *BMJ.* 2005;330 (7493):702.
32. Ramsey SD, Andersen MR, Etzioni R, et al. Quality of life in survivors of colorectal carcinoma. *Cancer.* 2000;88(6):1294–1303.
33. Trentham-Dietz A, Remington PL, Moinpour CM, Hampton JM, Sapp AL, Newcomb PA. Health-related quality of life in female long-term colorectal cancer survivors. *Oncologist.* 2003;8(4):342–349.
34. Sapp AL, Trentham-Dietz A, Newcomb PA, Hampton JM, Moinpour CM, Remington PL. Social networks and quality of life among female long-term colorectal cancer survivors. *Cancer.* 2003;98(8):1749–1758.
35. Baumel H, Fabre JM, Manderscheid JC, Domergue J, Visset J. [Medicosocial consequences of permanent digestive stomas. A national multicenter retrospective study]. *Presse Med.* 1994;23(40):1849–1853.
36. Peng J, Shi D, Goodman KA, et al. Early results of quality of life for curatively treated rectal cancers in Chinese patients with EORTC QLQ-CR29. *Radiat Oncol.* 2011;6:93.
37. Gelber RD, Goldhirsch A, Cole BF, Wieand HS, Schroeder G, Krook JE. A quality-adjusted time without symptoms or toxicity (Q-TWiST) analysis of adjuvant radiation therapy and chemotherapy for resectable rectal cancer. *J Natl Cancer Inst.* 1996;88(15):1039–1045.
38. Barnett GC, De Meerleer G, Gulliford SL, Sydes MR, Elliott RM, Dearnaley DP. The Impact of Clinical Factors on the Development of Late Radiation Toxicity: Results from the Medical Research Council RT01 Trial (ISRCTN47772397). *Clin Oncol (R Coll Radiol).* 2011.
39. Rauch P, Miny J, Conroy T, Neyton L, Guillemin F. Quality of life among disease-free survivors of rectal cancer. *J Clin Oncol.* 2004;22(2):354–360.
40. Cakmak A, Aylaz G, Kuzu MA. Permanent stoma not only affects patients' quality of life but also that of their spouses. *World J Surg.* 2010;34(12):2872–2876.
41. Lange MM, van de Velde CJ. Urinary and sexual dysfunction after rectal cancer treatment. *Nat Rev Urol.* 2011;8(1):51–57.
42. Ho VP, Lee Y, Stein SL, Temple LK. Sexual function after treatment for rectal cancer: a review. *Dis Colon Rectum.* 2011;54(1):113–125.
43. Kapiteijn E, Marijnen CA, Nagtegaal ID, et al.; Dutch Colorectal Cancer Group. Preoperative radiotherapy combined with total mesorectal excision for resectable rectal cancer. *N Engl J Med.* 2001;345(9):638–646.
44. Bruheim K, Guren MG, Dahl AA, et al. Sexual function in males after radiotherapy for rectal cancer. *Int J Radiat Oncol Biol Phys.* 2010;76(4):1012–1017.
45. Zelefsky MJ, Eid JF. Elucidating the etiology of erectile dysfunction after definitive therapy for prostatic cancer. *Int J Radiat Oncol Biol Phys.* 1998;40(1):129–133.
46. Nishizawa Y, Ito M, Saito N, Suzuki T, Sugito M, Tanaka T. Male sexual dysfunction after rectal cancer surgery. *Int J Colorectal Dis.* 2011.
47. Bachmann GA, Leiblum SR. The impact of hormones on menopausal sexuality: a literature review. *Menopause.* 2004;11(1):120–130.
48. Grigsby PW, Russell A, Bruner D, et al. Late injury of cancer therapy on the female reproductive tract. *Int J Radiat Oncol Biol Phys.* 1995;31(5):1281–1299.
49. Ogilvy-Stuart AL, Shalet SM. Effect of radiation on the human reproductive system. *Environ Health Perspect.* 1993;101(Suppl 2):109–116.
50. Calvert PM, Frucht H. The genetics of colorectal cancer. *Ann Intern Med.* 2002;137(7):603–612.
51. Schrag D. The price tag on progress–chemotherapy for colorectal cancer. *N Engl J Med.* 2004;351(4):317–319.
52. Hewitt ME, Ganz PA, Institute of Medicine (U.S.), American Society of Clinical Oncology (U.S.). From cancer patient to cancer survivor: lost in transition: an American Society of Clinical Oncology and Institute of Medicine Symposium. Washington, DC: National Academies Press; 2006.
53. Bradley CJ, Bednarek HL. Employment patterns of long-term cancer survivors. *Psychooncology.* 2002;11(3):188–198.
54. Rothstein MA, Kennedy K, Ritchie KJ, Pyle K. Are cancer patients subject to employment discrimination? *Oncology (Williston Park, NY).* 1995;9(12):1303–6; discussion 1311.
55. Engstrom PF, Arnoletti JP, Benson AB 3rd, et al.; National Comprehensive Cancer Network. NCCN Clinical Practice Guidelines in Oncology: colon cancer. *J Natl Compr Canc Netw.* 2009;7(8):778–831.
56. Green RJ, Metlay JP, Propert K, et al. Surveillance for second primary colorectal cancer after adjuvant chemotherapy: an analysis of Intergroup 0089. *Ann Intern Med.* 2002;136(4):261–269.
57. Mäkelä JT, Laitinen SO, Kairaluoma MI. Five-year follow-up after radical surgery for colorectal cancer. Results of a prospective randomized trial. *Arch Surg.* 1995;130(10):1062–1067.
58. Ohlsson B, Breland U, Ekberg H, Graffner H, Tranberg KG. Follow-up after curative surgery for colorectal carcinoma. Randomized comparison with no follow-up. *Dis Colon Rectum.* 1995;38(6):619–626.
59. Kjeldsen BJ, Kronborg O, Fenger C, Jørgensen OD. A prospective randomized study of follow-up after radical surgery for colorectal cancer. *Br J Surg.* 1997;84(5):666–669.
60. Schoemaker D, Black R, Giles L, Toouli J. Yearly colonoscopy, liver CT, and chest radiography do not influence 5-year survival of colorectal cancer patients. *Gastroenterology.* 1998;114(1):7–14.
61. Rodríguez-Moranta F, Saló J, Arcusa A, et al. Postoperative surveillance in patients with colorectal cancer who have undergone curative resection: a prospective, multicenter, randomized, controlled trial. *J Clin Oncol.* 2006;24(3):386–393.
62. Pietra N, Sarli L, Costi R, Ouchemi C, Grattarola M, Peracchia A. Role of follow-up in management of local recurrences of colorectal cancer: a prospective, randomized study. *Dis Colon Rectum.* 1998;41(9):1127–1133.
63. Secco GB, Fardelli R, Gianquinto D, et al. Efficacy and cost of risk-adapted follow-up in patients after colorectal cancer surgery: a prospective, randomized and controlled trial. *Eur J Surg Oncol.* 2002;28(4):418–423.
64. Figueredo A, Rumble RB, Maroun J, et al.; Gastrointestinal Cancer Disease Site Group of Cancer Care Ontario's Program in Evidence-based Care. Follow-up of patients with curatively resected colorectal cancer: a practice guideline. *BMC Cancer.* 2003;3:26.
65. Jeffery GM, Hickey BE, Hider P. Follow-up strategies for patients treated for non-metastatic colorectal cancer. *Cochrane Database Syst Rev.* 2002:CD002200.
66. Renehan AG, Egger M, Saunders MP, O'Dwyer ST. Impact on survival of intensive follow up after curative resection for colorectal cancer: systematic review and meta-analysis of randomised trials. *BMJ.* 2002;324(7341):813.
67. Sargent D, Sobrero A, Grothey A, et al. Evidence for cure by adjuvant therapy in colon cancer: observations based on individual

patient data from 20,898 patients on 18 randomized trials. *J Clin Oncol.* 2009;27(6):872–877.

68. Chau I, Allen MJ, Cunningham D, et al. The value of routine serum carcino-embryonic antigen measurement and computed tomography in the surveillance of patients after adjuvant chemotherapy for colorectal cancer. *J Clin Oncol.* 2004;22(8):1420–1429.
69. Meyerhardt JA, Ma J, Courneya KS. Energetics in colorectal and prostate cancer. *J Clin Oncol.* 2010;28(26):4066–4073.
70. Meyerhardt JA, Giovannucci EL, Ogino S, et al. Physical activity and male colorectal cancer survival. *Arch Intern Med.* 2009;169(22):2102–2108.
71. Meyerhardt JA, Heseltine D, Niedzwiecki D, et al. Impact of physical activity on cancer recurrence and survival in patients with stage III colon cancer: findings from CALGB 89803. *J Clin Oncol.* 2006;24(22):3535–3541.
72. Dignam JJ, Polite BN, Yothers G, et al. Body mass index and outcomes in patients who receive adjuvant chemotherapy for colon cancer. *J Natl Cancer Inst.* 2006;98(22):1647–1654.
73. Meyerhardt JA, Niedzwiecki D, Hollis D, et al. Association of dietary patterns with cancer recurrence and survival in patients with stage III colon cancer. *JAMA.* 2007;298(7):754–764.
74. Desch CE, Benson AB 3rd, Somerfield MR, et al.; American Society of Clinical Oncology. Colorectal cancer surveillance: 2005 update of an American Society of Clinical Oncology practice guideline. *J Clin Oncol.* 2005;23(33):8512–8519.
75. Rex DK, Kahi CJ, Levin B, et al.; American Cancer Society; US Multi-Society Task Force on Colorectal Cancer. Guidelines for colonoscopy surveillance after cancer resection: a consensus update by the American Cancer Society and the US Multi-Society Task Force on Colorectal Cancer. *Gastroenterology.* 2006;130(6):1865–1871.
76. Labianca R, Nordlinger B, Beretta GD, Brouquet A, Cervantes A; ESMO Guidelines Working Group. Primary colon cancer: ESMO Clinical Practice Guidelines for diagnosis, adjuvant treatment and follow-up. *Ann Oncol.* 2010;21(Suppl 5): v70–v77.

22 Patient Advocacy: What Does That Mean, and Why Should I Care?

NANCY ROACH

Patient advocates (PAs) and patient advocacy organizations (PAOs) have become an integral part of the health care and research landscape. While there is significant literature available that examines their evolution and impact over the years (1), this chapter focuses on opportunities in patient advocacy, using real-life examples.

> Advocacy means taking action to bring about the change you are seeking. When I first started advocating for my own health care, I felt productive, knowing I was getting the best in health care. When I started advocating on the Hill (Congress) or in my hometown, I left offices knowing I was making a difference and showing what I was passionate about. I felt empowered and I was not just doing it for myself, but others who no longer could voice their opinion or those yet to be diagnosed. (*Pamela Seijo, colorectal cancer survivor and advocate*)

A PA is defined as an individual impacted by a disease, either directly or indirectly, who seeks to help others. PAs frequently are self-identified, and their paths as advocates are frequently very different. There are PAs who:

- Regularly provide educational information to chemotherapy patients.
- Provide one-on-one support to other patients; eg, volunteering as a patient navigator.
- Support or direct efforts to raise money to support research or PAOs.
- Speak locally and nationally about issues such as screening and research funding.
- Lobby elected officials.
- Serve on a variety of scientific or medical advisory boards that make decisions which directly impact patients, such as the FDA Oncology Drug Advisory Committee or the National Cancer Institute (NCI) advisory boards.

■ ADVOCATING FOR ONESELF

There is no formal path to becoming a PA. Patients and their loved ones may be shocked and devastated by a diagnosis of cancer (2). They are suddenly immersed in a new world that involves facing their own mortality, learning new terminology, and making life-changing decisions. The first job of a patient and/or loved ones is taking the time to cope with a new reality (vs. their) their new reality—in essence, being their own advocate. In this situation, patients may need help with understanding their diagnosis and treatment options. In an ongoing series of focus groups with patients conducted by Fight Colorectal Cancer, patients strongly indicated that they like getting medical information from their health care team and from credible online resources. About half of the patients received written information about treatment and side effects from their health care team, while all patients surveyed would have liked getting this type of information. Many patients indicated that they would have appreciated additional information about complementary treatments, and a written treatment plan.

> My doctor asked me what I understood about my diagnosis. He used that as a jump-off point to help me know what I needed to learn to take my next step. (*Anon, from online conversation*)

Patients and loved ones are faced with a bewildering amount of information as they begin to learn about their diagnosis and treatment. There are many online resources that provide information that can support patient–physician interactions:

- National PAOs generally have well-vetted resources available on their websites or in print, and will send copies to physicians' offices. Many have call lines that provide an additional venue for education.
- The American Cancer Society has identified treatment and survivorship plans which can be completed and personalized by physicians (www.cancer.org/treatment/survivorshipduringandaftertreatment/survivorshipcareplans/index). The list includes the

American Society of Clinical Oncology's colorectal cancer-specific plans.

- The Agency for Healthcare Research and Quality has created a "question builder" which helps patients identify and prioritize questions for their doctor visits (www.ahrq.gov/questions/qb/).
- The National Cancer Institute (NCI) provides information about complementary and alternative therapies (www.cancer.gov/cancertopics/cam).
- The National Center for Complementary and Alternative Medicine has tips for evaluating web-based resources (http://nccam.nih.gov/health/webresources).

Patients may find it helpful if their clinician provides them with a list of credible online resources and hints on how to spot cancer-related quackery.

> Patients are often overwhelmed by information, and may have a hard time identifying the key questions for their doctor appointments. For example, before surgery, a patient may have questions about chemotherapy and may not realize that they might want to learn more about the surgical plans. We help them prioritize their questions to make sure their appointments are productive. (*Kim Ryan, Fight Colorectal Cancer Director of Patient Services*)

Patients also want to connect with other patients to share personal experiences and questions about treatment and side effects. Many national PAOs have ways to connect patients with patients:

- Local support groups or "virtual" support groups.
- Local fundraising efforts.
- Conferences focused on survivorship and care.
- Conferences focused on advocacy.

In addition, the growing impact of social media such as Facebook and Twitter has given patients countless ways to find information, support, and other patients. These forums allow patients to learn from each other.

Advocating for Others: Becoming a Patient Advocate

As time passes, patients and loved ones may decide to become advocates on behalf of others. This is the first step in becoming a PA.

> When I was fighting my own battle against Stage III colorectal cancer (CRC), I vowed that if I was lucky enough to beat the odds and survive, I would help those people I met in the waiting rooms or walking the hospital halls, and do something to honor the memory of the people I'd met along the way who did not make it. Now I raise money to fund research through a national CRC patient advocacy organization. We want bright young researchers focusing their careers on CRC, and this is how I can make that happen. (*Andrea Kramer, Stage III survivor*)

A PAO is defined as a nonprofit organization that seeks to support individual patients, patient outcomes, or societal outcomes. A PAO may do this through:

- Patient education, such as informational booklets, website content, and answer lines.
- Patient services and support such as counseling, support groups, and clinical trials matching.
- Public awareness campaigns to increase public knowledge of disease issues.
- Legislative and regulatory efforts to improve patient outcomes through increased research funding, better coverage, and access to care.
- Direct funding of research and engagement with the research process.

There are numerous PAOs active in CRC, from local groups that fundraise for a local institution to national groups that lobby Congress. Since the landscape of online resources evolves daily, a comprehensive list is not possible. Reputable national organizations that provide support and opportunities for patients are given in table 22.1.

Table 22.1 National Patient Advocacy Organizations

Organization Name	Website	Unique Features
American Cancer Society	Cancer.org	Highly detailed patient information; strong local presence; multiple structured opportunities to volunteer (eg, patient navigator program)
Cancer Support Community	CancerSupport Community.org	Focus on support and survivorship; local and virtual support groups
Colon Cancer Alliance	CCAlliance.org	Focus on support; annual conference on care and survivorship; buddy program for volunteers; local runs
Fight Colorectal Cancer	FightColorectal Cancer.org	Focus on advocacy and policy; annual congressional training and lobby day; research advocacy training; direct funding of research
National Comprehensive Cancer Network	NCCN.org	Detailed patient booklet for colon cancer; detailed physician guidelines for colon and rectal cancer
Patient Advocate Foundation Colorectal Care Line	Colorectal careline.org	Focus on reimbursement and access to care, including appeals assistance

Engaging with PAOs allows patients to make an impact on a disease that changed their lives, and to help others. This type of engagement is seen as a cornerstone of survivorship (3). Physicians may want to understand the difference among various organizations so that they can guide patients who ask how they can make a difference. For example, if a patient wants to work for public policy that improves access to care or screening, they could be directed to a PAO that focuses on policy. If a patient wants to help other patients, they could be directed to a PAO that offers support programs, or to a local hospital support group. Patients should be urged to ask questions of the PAO, especially with regards to fundraising, to ensure that the PAO is legitimate. Guidestar (guidestar.org) provides a comprehensive list of nonprofits and identifies key questions to ask.

In addition, many PAOs, especially smaller ones, can benefit from engagement with both community oncologists and academic center researchers. Physicians can:

- Review material for correctness.
- Suggest topics for booklets and webinars.
- Engage in advocacy opportunities with elected officials (a doctor and patient can tell the story about the need for research funding or access to care very compellingly).
- Help PAOs develop a network of informed, engaged patients and caregivers.

Physicians interested in getting involved can contact organizations directly.

PERSONAL STATEMENT ABOUT ADVOCACY

> I am motivated to be an advocate because I have seen it work. And because I know this disease is preventable. This disease can be beaten. It will take multidisciplinary approach and doctors will not be the sole community from which victory arises. Advocacy is very much part of the big picture ... Together, we are making a change. (*Josh Wimberly, colorectal cancer survivor and advocate*)

Research Advocacy

Over time, patients and loved ones have become part of the research process. The publicly funded NCI National Clinical Trial Network engages PAs in multiple ways such as:

- Cooperative group committees and data safety monitoring committees.
- Institutional review boards.
- NCI scientific steering committees and task forces.
- NCI advisory committees.

One advocacy organization defines research advocacy as follows:

> Research advocates represent patients at tables where research decisions are made. We may review basic science grants for the Department of Defense, or participate in meetings where clinical trials are designed. We are there to comment and ask questions from the patient perspective. If a phase 3 trial is positive, will the results change how patients are treated? If a basic research proposal pans out, could the results help patients down the line? (*Fight Colorectal Cancer Research Advocacy Training and Support*)

Research advocates are asked to present the collective patient experience, which is created when a person has knowledge of multiple disease experiences and conveys this collective perspective rather than his or her own exclusive experience. Their impact can be profound:

> You ask the questions the clinicians do not ask, you remind them that their patients are people like themselves and not charts. You work with them to design better trials and increase accrual. You make the clinical trials enterprise a much better place for the patients. (*Personal correspondence to N. Roach*)

Patients who are interested in becoming involved in the research process can contact NCI's Office of Advocacy Relations (nciadvocacy@mail.nih.gov; 301–594-3194) for additional information and referral to specific organizations.

ENGAGING WITH PATIENT ADVOCACY ORGANIZATIONS

Advocacy: Changing Lives, Changing the World

> Advocacy is about helping patients, and with our collective voices, changing the world. We want to change the world that allows CRC to go undiagnosed until it is advanced, when treatment is difficult—and more expensive. We want to change the world where people can't afford care without going into bankruptcy. We want to change the world where vital research that could save lives and dollars goes unfunded year after year. We work toward these changes by connecting with real power players in Washington, D.C. We testify before Congress. We stand with (or up to) politicians when important decisions are being debated. We make sure that patient voices are in the rooms where committees meet, rules are made and budgets are written, which affect people's daily lives. (*Fight Colorectal Cancer 2012 Annual Report*)

REFERENCES

1. Earp JL, French EA, Gilkey MB. (2007). Patient Advocacy for Healthcare Quality: Strategies for Achieving Patient Centered Care, Jones and Barlett Publishers (note: this book references much of the research that's been done about the impact of advocates and advocacy organizations).
2. Hegel MT, Moore CP, Collins ED, et al. Distress, psychiatric syndromes, and impairment of function in women with newly diagnosed breast cancer. *Cancer.* 2006;107(12):2924–2931.
3. Clark EJ, Stovall EL. Advocacy: the cornerstone of cancer survivorship. *Cancer Pract.* 1996;4(5):239–244.

Index